Cardiac Hypertrophy and Failure

Cardiac Hypertrophy and Failure

Editor: Jace Xavier

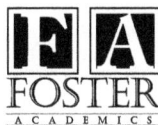

FA FOSTER
A C A D E M I C S

www.fosteracademics.com

www.fosteracademics.com

FA
FOSTER
ACADEMICS

Cataloging-in-Publication Data

Cardiac hypertrophy and failure / edited by Jace Xavier.
p. cm.
Includes bibliographical references and index.
ISBN 978-1-63242-885-1
1. Heart--Hypertrophy. 2. Heart failure. 3. Heart--Diseases. 4. Heart--Size. I. Xavier, Jace.
RC685.H9 C37 2020
616.12--dc23

Foster Academics,
118-35 Queens Blvd., Suite 400,
Forest Hills, NY 11375, USA

ISBN 978-1-63242-885-1 (Hardback)

Contents

Preface

The heart must respond to myriad physiological and pathophysiological stimuli to maintain sufficient cardiac output over a complete lifespan. To meet such demands on a daily basis, the heart relies on the myocardial reserve, whereby it can alter cardiac output in response to any sudden increase in demand. However, sustained and progressive demands on the heart can lead to cardiac hypertrophy. Hypertension, post-myocardial infarction remodeling and valvular abnormalities are common disease states that result in prolonged hemodynamic demand. If there is no relief from the pathogenic stimulus, it ultimately leads to impaired ventricular relaxation, filling and eventual cardiac failure. Hypertrophy can result from both adaptive (eccentric) and maladaptive (concentric) conditions. Concentric hypertrophy can result from various stressors such as congenital heart defects, hypertension, valvular defects and primary defects of the myocardium. This kind of hypertrophy can result in a dilated ventricle, which is incapable of effectively pumping blood. This can lead to heart failure. Eccentric hypertrophy often arises as a response to exercise or pregnancy. It is largely considered to be a healthy response to high cardiac demand, but comes with associated risks. Some of the diverse topics covered in this book address the varied clinical aspects of cardiac hypertrophy and failure. It consists of contributions made by international experts. It aims to equip students and experts with the advanced topics and upcoming concepts in this area.

The information contained in this book is the result of intensive hard work done by researchers in this field. All due efforts have been made to make this book serve as a complete guiding source for students and researchers. The topics in this book have been comprehensively explained to help readers understand the growing trends in the field.

I would like to thank the entire group of writers who made sincere efforts in this book and my family who supported me in my efforts of working on this book. I take this opportunity to thank all those who have been a guiding force throughout my life.

Editor

PARP-Inhibitor Treatment Prevents Hypertension Induced Cardiac Remodeling by Favorable Modulation of Heat Shock Proteins, Akt-1/GSK-3β and Several PKC Isoforms

Laszlo Deres[1,2], Eva Bartha[1], Anita Palfi[1], Krisztian Eros[1,2], Adam Riba[1,2], Janos Lantos[3], Tamas Kalai[4], Kalman Hideg[4], Balazs Sumegi[2,5,6], Ferenc Gallyas[5,6], Kalman Toth[1], Robert Halmosi[1,2]*

1 First Department of Medicine, Division of Cardiology, University of Pécs, Pécs, Hungary, **2** Szentagothai Janos Research Center, University of Pécs, Medical School, Pécs, Hungary, **3** Department of Surgical Research and Techniques, University of Pécs, Pécs, Hungary, **4** Department of Organic and Medicinal Chemistry, University of Pécs, Pécs, Hungary, **5** Department of Biochemistry and Medical Chemistry, Medical School, University of Pécs, Pécs, Hungary, **6** MTA-PTE Nuclear-Mitochondrial Interactions Research Group, Pécs, Hungary

Abstract

Spontaneously hypertensive rat (SHR) is a suitable model for studies of the complications of hypertension. It is known that activation of poly(ADP-ribose) polymerase enzyme (PARP) plays an important role in the development of postinfarction as well as long-term hypertension induced heart failure. In this study, we examined whether PARP-inhibitor (L-2286) treatment could prevent the development of hypertensive cardiopathy in SHRs. 6-week-old SHR animals were treated with L-2286 (SHR-L group) or placebo (SHR-C group) for 24 weeks. Wistar-Kyoto rats were used as aged-matched, normotensive controls (WKY group). Echocardiography was performed, brain-derived natriuretic peptide (BNP) activity and blood pressure were determined at the end of the study. We detected the extent of fibrotic areas. The amount of heat-shock proteins (Hsps) and the phosphorylation state of Akt-1^{Ser473}, glycogen synthase kinase (GSK)-3β^{Ser9}, forkhead transcription factor (FKHR)^{Ser256}, mitogen activated protein kinases (MAPKs), and protein kinase C (PKC) isoenzymes were monitored. The elevated blood pressure in SHRs was not influenced by PARP-inhibitor treatment. Systolic left ventricular function and BNP activity did not differ among the three groups. L-2286 treatment decreased the marked left ventricular (LV) hypertrophy which was developed in SHRs. Interstitial collagen deposition was also decreased by L-2286 treatment. The phosphorylation of extracellular signal-regulated kinase (ERK)1/2$^{Thr183-Tyr185}$, Akt-1^{Ser473}, GSK-3β^{Ser9}, FKHR^{Ser256}, and PKC ε^{Ser729} and the level of Hsp90 were increased, while the activity of PKC α/βII$^{Thr638/641}$, ζ/λ$^{410/403}$ were mitigated by L-2286 administration. We could detect signs of LV hypertrophy without congestive heart failure in SHR groups. This alteration was prevented by PARP inhibition. Our results suggest that PARP-inhibitor treatment has protective effect already in the early stage of hypertensive myocardial remodeling.

Editor: Rajesh Gopalrao Katare, University of Otago, New Zealand

Funding: The work was supported by Hungarian National Research Foundations (OTKA F-46594, OTKA K-73738, OTKA K-81123, OTKA NN-109841). This research was realized in the frames of SROP 4.2.1.B-10/2/KONV-2010-0002, 4.2.4. A/2-11-1-2012-0001. The funders had no role in study design, data collection and analysis, decision to publish, or preparation of the manuscript.

* Email: dr.halmosi.robert@gmail.com

Introduction

Left ventricular hypertrophy (LVH) represents the heart's response to increased biomechanical stress such as arterial hypertension or valvular heart disease. Cardiac hypertrophy has traditionally been considered a compensatory mechanism required to normalize wall tension and to maintain cardiac output. However, recent clinical studies as well as several animal models have shown that cardiac hypertrophy is rather a maladaptive process, ultimately leading to heart failure (HF) and sudden cardiac death independent of the underlying cause of hypertrophy [1].

Both physiologic and pathologic stimulation-induced cellular adaptations of the heart are typically initiated by stress-responsive signaling pathways, which serve as central transducers of cardiac hypertrophic growth and/or ventricular dilation. These signaling pathways include extracellular signal-regulated protein kinases (ERK), p38 mitogen-activated protein kinases (p38-MAPK), c-Jun NH$_2$-terminal kinases (JNK) and several protein kinase C (PKC) isoforms [2]. These pathways and the Akt-1/glycogen synthase kinase-3β (GSK-3β) signaling cascade have all been demonstrated to alter their activation state in response to hypertrophic stimuli, and may therefore contribute to myocardial remodeling [3].

The poly(ADP-ribose) polymerase (PARP) enzyme becomes activated in response to DNA single-strand breaks that can be excessive as a response to free radicals and oxidative cell damage. PARP is an energy-consuming enzyme that transfers ADP-ribose to nuclear proteins. As a result of this process, the intracellular

NAD$^+$ and ATP levels decrease remarkably resulting in cell dysfunction and cell death via the necrotic route. Therefore, PARP-activation contributes to the pathogenesis of various cardiovascular diseases including endothelial dysfunction, ischemia-reperfusion injury and myocardial infarction, as well as HF. Several studies reported that endothelial dysfunction associated with hypertension also depends on PARP activity and can be prevented by its pharmacological inhibition [4,5].

It has been shown previously that our experimental agent, an isoquinoline derivative PARP-inhibitor, L-2286 (Fig. 1) had a beneficial effect against oxidative cell damage, against ischemia-reperfusion injury and the development of postinfarction or long-term high blood pressure-induced heart failure. Although the molecule have a slight scavenger characteristic, its forementioned effects were mediated mainly by influencing the Akt-1/GSK-3β, MAPK and PKC signal transduction factors [3,6,7].

Hypertension in spontaneously hypertensive rat (SHR) is similar to that of human in numerous ways such as the occurence of long-term, stable LVH followed by a transition to HF [8,9,10]. It makes SHR a useful tool for studying the development of LVH [9] and HF, well separated from each other in time. Therefore, our present study aimed to clarify whether pharmacological PARP-inhibition has protective effect in an SHR model against the development of the early stage of hypertensive cardiac remodeling.

Materials and Methods

Ethics Statement

The investigation conforms to the Guide for the Care and Use of Laboratory Animals published by the U.S. National Insitutes of Health (NIH Publication No. 85-23, revised 1996), and was approved by the Animal Research Review Committee of the University of Pecs, Medical School.

Experimental protocol

Six weeks old male WKY-strain Wistar Kyoto and spontaneously hypertensive rats (Charles River Laboratories, Budapest, Hungary) were used. Animals were kept under standard conditions throughout the experiment; 12 h light-dark cycle, water and rat chow provided ad libitum. SHRs were randomly divided into two groups; SHR-L and SHR-C. SHR-L group was treated with L-2286 (2-[(2-piperidin-1-ylethyl)thio]quinazolin-4(3H)-one), a wa-ter-soluble PARP-inhibitor (5 mg/b.w. in kg/day, n = 12), while SHR-C group received only placebo (n = 11, SHR-C) p. os for 24 weeks [11,12]. WKY rats were used as age-matched controls (n = 10). Dosage of L-2286 administered in drinking water was based on preliminary data about the volume of daily consumption [3,6]. At the beginning and at the end of the 24-week-long period, echocardiographic measurements were performed. Invasive blood pressure measurements were carried out on 3 rats of each group at the end of the study. These rats were anesthetized with ketamine hydrochloride (Richter Gedeon Ltd., Budapest, Hungary) intra-peritoneally and a polyethylene catheter (Portex, London, UK) was inserted into their left femoral artery. Systolic, diastolic and

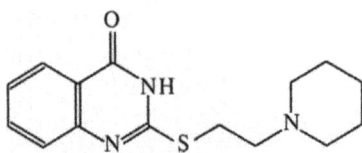

Figure 1. Chemical structure of L-2286 (2-[(2-Piperidine-1-ylethyl)thio]quinazolin-4(3H)-one).

mean arterial blood pressure was determined by CardioMed System CM-2005 (Medi-Stim AS, Oslo, Norway). Animals were euthanized with an overdose of ketamine hydrochloride intraper-itoneally and heparinized with sodium heparin (100 IU/rat i.p., Biochemie GmbH, Kundl, Austria). After the sacrifice, blood was collected to determine the concentration of plasma brain-derived natriuretic peptide (BNP), and hearts were removed, the atria and great vessels were trimmed from the ventricles and weight of the ventricles was measured, which was then normalized to body mass (index of cardiac hypertrophy). The lung wet weight-to-dry weight ratio (an index of pulmonary congestion) was also measured in 7–9 experimental animals [3]. Hearts were freeze-clamped and were stored at −70°C or fixed in 10% formalin. In order to detect the extent of fibrotic areas, histologic samples were stained with Masson's trichrome. The phosphorylation state of Akt-1/GSK-3β, MAPK and PKC signaling molecules were monitored by Western blotting.

Determination of plasma B-type natriuretic peptide

Blood samples were collected into Lavender Vacutainer tubes containing EDTA and aprotinin (0.6 IU/ml of blood), and were centrifuged at 1600 g for 15 minutes at 4°C to separate the plasma. Supernatants were collected and kept at −70°C. BNP-45 were determined by enzyme immunoassay method as the manufacturer proposed (BNP-45, Rat EIA Kit, Phoenix Pharma-ceuticals Inc., CA, USA).

Histology

Ventricles fixed in formalin were embedded in paraffin, and 5 μm thick sections were cut from base to apex. Sections were stained with Masson's trichrome staining to detect the interstitial fibrosis, and quantified by the NIH ImageJ image processing program as described previously [3].

Western blot analysis

Fifty milligrams of heart samples were homogenized in ice-cold 50 mM Tris buffer, pH 8.0 containing protease inhibitor cocktail 1:100, and 50 mM sodium vanadate (Sigma-Aldrich Co., Budapest, Hungary), and were harvested in 2x concentrated sodium dodecyl sulphate (SDS)-polyacrylamide gel electrophoresis sample buffer. Proteins were separated on 10% or 12% SDS-polyacrylamide gel and transferred to nitrocellulose membranes. After blocking (2 h with 3% nonfat milk in Tris-buffered saline), membranes were probed overnight at 4°C with primary antibodies recognizing the following antigenes: phospho-specific Akt-1/protein kinase B-α Ser^{473} (1:1000), Actin (1:10000), phospho-specific glycogen synthase kinase (GSK)-3β Ser^9 (1:1000), phospho-specific extracellular signal-regulated kinase (ERK 1/2) Thr^{202}-Tyr^{204} (1:1000), phospho-specific p38 mitogen-activated protein kinase (p38-MAPK) Thr^{180}-Gly-Tyr^{182} (1:1000), phospho-specific c-Jun N-terminal kinase (JNK) Thr^{183}-Tyr^{185} (1:1000), phospho-specific protein kinase C (PKC) (pan) βII Ser^{660} (1:1000), phospho-specific protein kinase C α/βII (PKC α/βII) Thr$^{638/641}$ (1:1000), phospho-specific protein kinase C δ (PKC δ) Thr^{505} (1:1000), phospho-specific protein kinase C ζ/λ (PKC ζ/λ) Thr$^{410/403}$ (1:1000), phospho-specific protein kinase C ε (PKC ε) Ser^{729} (1:1000), anti-poly(ADP-ribose) (anti-PAR, 1:5000), phos-pho-Foxo1A (forkhead transcription factor, FKHR Ser^{256}, 1:1000), Heat shock protein 72 (Hsp72, 1:20000), Heat shock protein 90 (Hsp90, 1:1000). Antibodies were purchased from Cell Signaling Technology (Beverly, MA, USA) except from actin, which was bought from Sigma-Aldrich Co, (Budapest, Hungary), phospho-specific PKC ε, which was purchased from Upstate (London, UK), anti-PAR, which was purchased from Alexis

Table 1. Effect of L-2286 treatment on gravimetric parameters and on plasma BNP in SHR.

	WKY	SHR-C	SHR-L
SAP^{30w}, (mmHg)	129±7	192±9^b	186±5^b
DAP^{30w}, (mmHg)	89±5	127±8^b	125±4^b
MAP^{30w}, (mmHg)	103±7	149±5^b	146±7^b
BW^{6w} (g)	71.01±1.89	72.02±2.36	69.9±3.21
BW (g)	393±14.01	323.8±11.27^a	321.86±6.8^{a,c}
WV (g)	1.16±0.17	1.45±0.18^b	1.24±0.24^{b,c}
WV/BW (mg/g)	2.95±0.17	4.48±0.12^b	3.85±0.15^{b,c}
Lung wet weight/dry weight	4.84±0.92	4.79±0.84	4.77±0.99
p-BNP (ng/ml)	2.19±0.011	2.33±0.034	2.31±0.031

WKY: normotensive age-matched control rats, n = 7, SHR-C: SHR age-matched control rats, n = 8, SHR-L: SHR treated with L-2286 for 24 weeks, n = 9. SAP, DAP, MAP^{30w}: systolic, diastolic and mean arterial blood pressure at 30-week-old age (n = 3 from each group). BW^{6w}: body weight of 6-week-old rats, BW: body weight, WV: weights of ventricles, BNP: plasma b-type natriuretic peptide. Values are means±S.E.M.
^{a}<0.01 (vs. WKY group),
^{b}<0.05 (vs. WKY group),
^{c}<0.05 (vs. SHR-C).

Biotechnology (London, UK), Hsp90, which was bought from Santa Cruz Biotechnology (Wembley, UK), Hsp72, which was purchased from StressGene Biomol GmbH (Hamburg, Germany). Membranes were washed six times for 5 min in Tris-buffered saline, pH 7.5 containing 0.2% Tween before addition of goat anti-rabbit horseradish peroxidase-conjugated secondary antibody (1:3000 dilution, Bio-Rad, Budapest, Hungary). The antibody-antigen complexes were visualized by means of enhanced

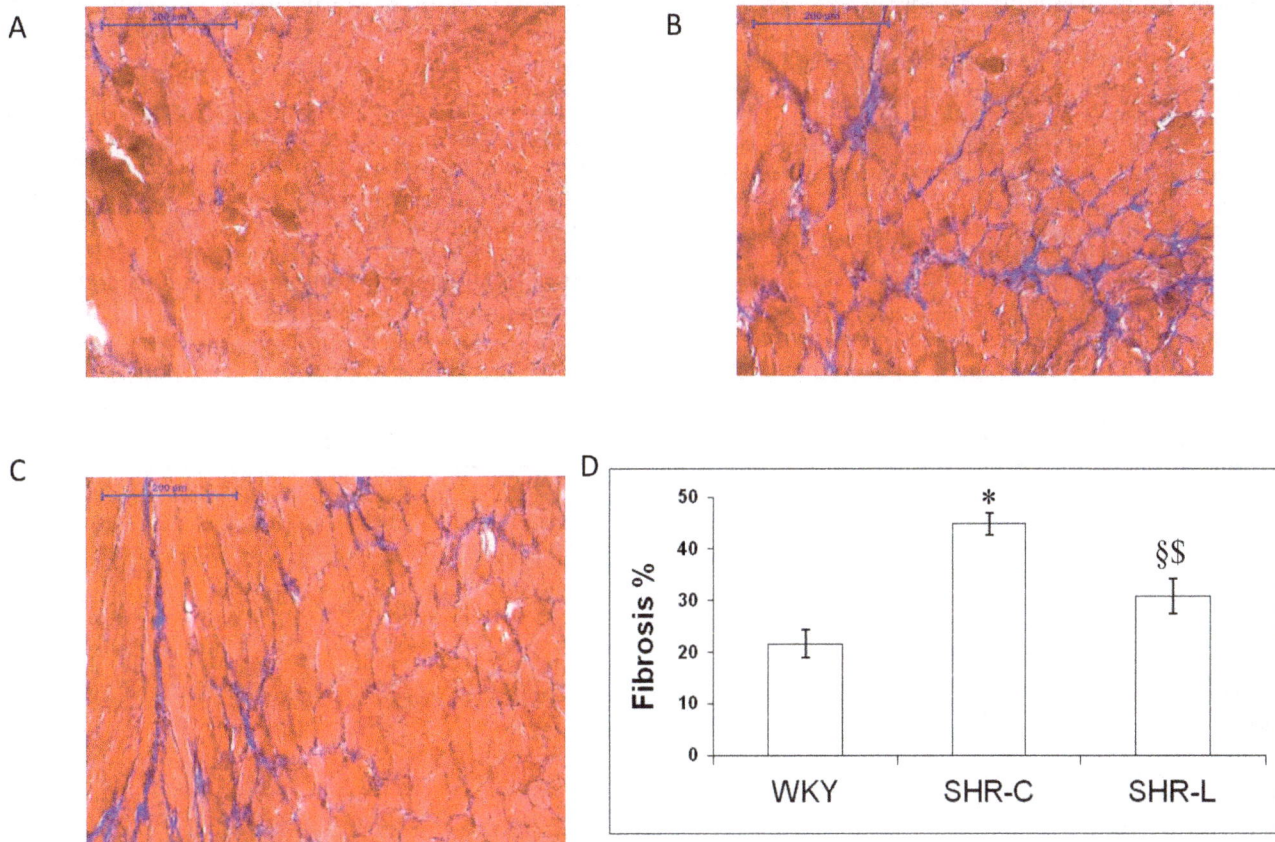

Figure 2. L-2286 treatment decreased the deposition of interstitial collagen. Sections stained with Masson's trichrome (n = 5). Scale bars mean 200 µm. Magnifications 10-fold. WKY (A): normotensive age-matched control rats. SHR-C (B): 30 week-old spontaneously hypertensive rats, SHR-L (C): 30 week-old spontaneously hypertensive rats treated with L-2286 for 24 week. D: Denzitometric evaluation of the sections is shown. *p< 0.01 vs. WKY, §p<0.05 vs. WKY, $p<0.05 vs. SHR-C.

Table 2. L-2286 treatment moderately influenced the echocardiographic parameters in 6 weeks old SHRs.

	WKY	SHR-C	SHR-L
EF (%)[6w]	67.26±0.525	68.4±1.77	68.23±1.81
FS[6w]	38.63±4.47	38.03±5.52	39.35±4.15
LVEDV[6w] (ml)	147.27±13.88	149.56±16.78	149.11±14.43
LVESV[6w] (ml)	46.63±4.47	48.03±5.52	47.35±5.45
Septum[6w] (mm)	1.2±0.07	1.18±0.05	1.17±0.12
PW[6w] (mm)	1.19±0.07	1.16±0.067	1.14±0.04
LV mass[6w] (uncorrected)	344.14±35.49	351.66±36.23	354.77±33.23

WKY: normotensive age-matched control rats, n = 7, SHR-C: SHR age-matched control rats, n = 8, SHR-L: n = 9, SHR treated with L-2286 for 24 weeks. EF[6w]: ejection fraction, FS[6w]: fractional shortening, LVEDV[6w]: left ventricular (LV) end-diastolic volume, LVESV[6w]: LV end-systolic volume, Septum[6w]: thickness of septum, PW[6w]: thickness of posterior wall, LV mass[6w]: weights of LVs.

chemiluminescence. After scanning, results were quantified by NIH ImageJ program. Pixel densities of bands were normalized to that of the loading controls.

Noninvasive evaluation of cardiac functions and dimensions

At the start of the experiment, all animals were examined by echocardiography to exclude rats with any heart abnormalities. Transthoracic two-dimensional echocardiography was performed under inhalation anesthesia at the beginning of the experiment and on the day of sacrifice. Rats were lightly anesthetized with a mixture of 1.5% isoflurane (Forane, Abbott Laboratories, Hungary) and 98.5% oxygen. The chest of animals was shaved, acoustic coupling gel was applied and warming pad was used to maintain normothermia. Rats were imaged in the left lateral decubitus position. Cardiac dimensions and functions were measured from short- and long-axis views at the mid-papillary level by a VEVO 770 high-resolution ultrasound imaging system (VisualSonics, Toronto, Canada) equipped with a 25 MHz transducer. LV fractional shortening (FS), ejection fraction (EF), LV end-diastolic volume (LVEDV), LV end-systolic volume (LVESV), and the thickness of septum and posterior wall were determined. FS (%) was calculated by $100x((LVID_d-LVID_s)/LVID_d)$ (LVID: LV inside dimension; d: diastolic; s: systolic), EF

(%) was calculated by $100x((LVEDV-LVESV)/LVEDV)$, relative wall thickness (RWT) was calculated by (PW thickness + interventricular septal thickness)/$LVID_d$.

Statistical analysis

All data are expressed as mean±SEM. First of all the homogeneity of the groups was tested by F-test (Levene's test). There were no significant differences among the groups. Comparisons among groups were made using one-way ANOVA (SPSS for Windows 11.0). For post hoc comparison Bonferroni test was chosen. Values of p<0.05 were considered statistically significant.

Results

Effect of L-2286 on normotensive WKY rats was also examined, but the investigated parameters did not differ significantly from the non-treated WKY animals. Therefore, data of L-2286 treated WKY rats were not shown to avoid unnecessary redundancies.

Effect of PARP inhibition on gravimetric parameters of spontaneously hypertensive rats

Body weights did not differ significantly among the three groups (WKY: 71.01±0.11 g, SHR-C: 72.03±2.36 g, SHR-L:

Table 3. L-2286 treatment moderately influenced the echocardiographic parameters in 30 weeks old SHRs.

	WKY	SHR-C	SHR-L
EF (%)[30w]	69.1±2.4	68.72±2.1	69.01±3.2
FS[30w]	39.8±1.9	39.04±1.85	40.57±2.66
LVEDV[30w] (ml)	279.18±18.18	335.87±10.36[a]	326.94±9.18[a]
LVESV[30w] (ml)	85.77±8.56	96.85±10.36[a]	99.81±11.85[a]
Septum[30w] (mm)	1.43±0.04	1.93±0.04[a]	1.79±0.05[a,b]
PW[30w] (mm)	1.54±0.08	2.15±0.12[a]	1.87±0.03[a,b]
RWT[30w]	0.38±0.05	0.504±0.02[a]	0.445±0.012[a,b]
LV mass[30w] (uncorrected)	1002.81±59.5	1370.35±79.87[a]	1121.13±53.23[a,b]
LV mass[30]/BW[30] (mg/g)	2.73±0.7	4.23±0.8[a]	3.70±0.3[a,b]

WKY: normotensive age-matched control rats, n = 7, SHR-C: SHR age-matched control rats, n = 8, SHR-L: n = 9, SHR treated with L-2286 for 24 weeks. EF[30w]: ejection fraction, F[30w]: fractional shortening, LVEDV[30w]: left ventricular (LV) end-diastolic volume, LVESV[30w]: LV end-systolic volume, Septum[30w]: thickness of septum, PW[30w]: thickness of posterior wall, RWT[30w]: relative wall thickness, LV mass[30w]: weights of LVs. Values are mean±S.E.M.
[a]p<0.05 (vs. WKY group),
[b]p<0.05 (vs. SHR-C group).

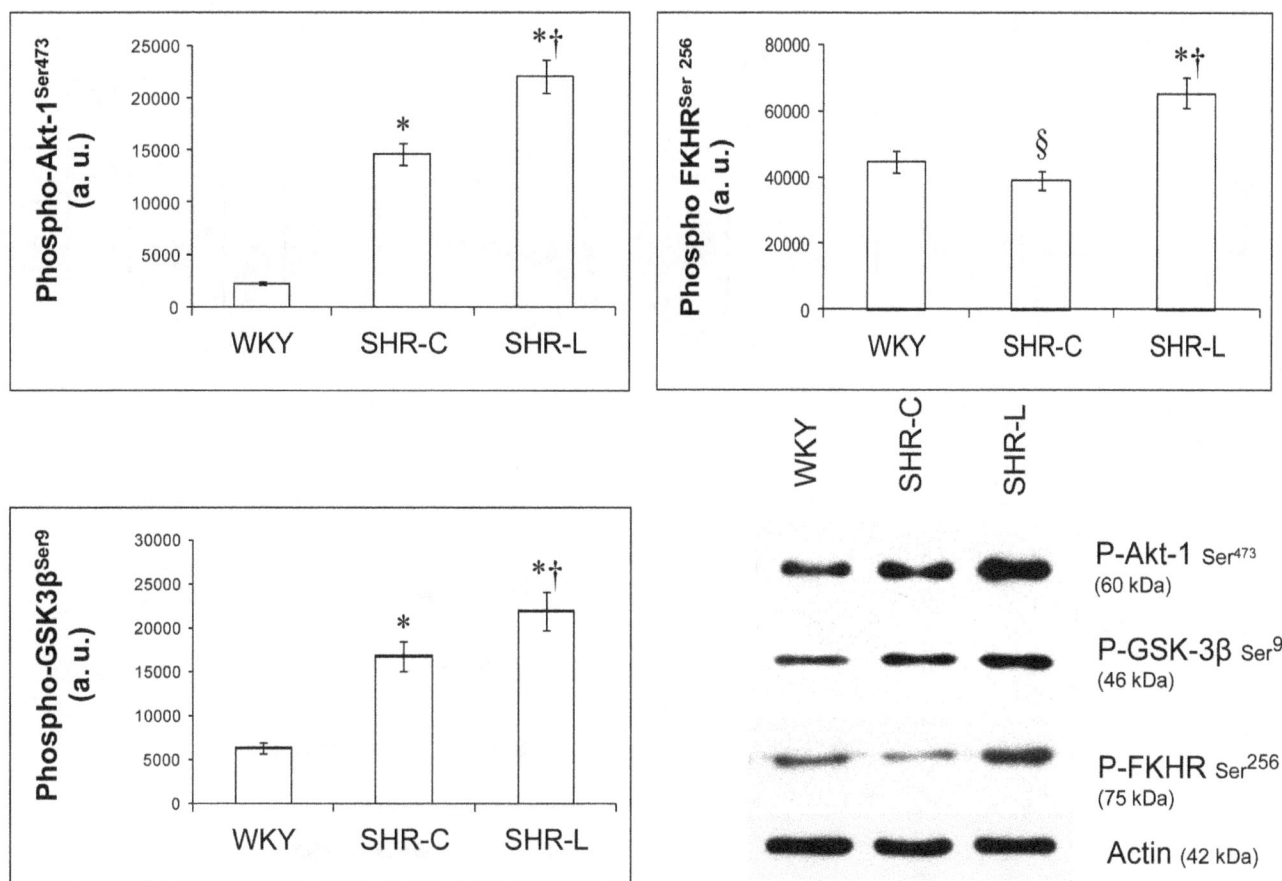

Figure 3. Effect of L-2286 treatment on Akt-1^{Ser473}/GSK-3β^{Ser9}, FKHR^{Ser256} pathway. Representative Western blot analysis of Akt-1^{Ser473}, GSK-3β^{Ser9}, FKHR^{Ser256} phosphorylation and densitometric evaluation is shown (n = 4). Actin was used as loading control. Values are means±S.E.M. WKY: normotensive age-matched control rats. SHR-C: 30 week-old spontaneously hypertensive rats, SHR-L: 30 week-old spontaneously hypertensive rats treated with L-2286 for 24 weeks. *p<0.01 vs. WKY, †p<0.01 vs. SHR-C, §p<0.05 vs. WKY.

69.92±3.21 g, 6-week-old rats) at the beginning of our study. However, at the end of the 24-week-long treatment period, body weights of WKY group were significantly higher than those of SHR-C and SHR-L groups (WKY: 392.7±14.01 g, SHR-C: 323.8±11.27 g, SHR-L: 321.9±6.84 g, p<0.01 WKY vs. SHR groups, 30-week-old rats). The degree of myocardial hypertrophy was determined by ventricular weight to body weight ratio (WV/BW, mg/g). This parameter was significantly increased in SHR groups compared to the WKY group (WV/BW: WKY: 2.95±0.17, SHR-C: 4.48±0.12, SHR-L: 3.85±0.15, p<0.05 WKY vs. SHR groups). Similar results were obtained in case of weights of ventricles (WV, WKY: 1.16±0.17 g, SHR-C: 1.45±0.18 g, SHR-L: 1.24±0.24 g, p<0.05 WKY vs. SHR groups). The WV and WV/BW ratios were significantly decreased by L-2286 treatment (p<0.05 SHR-L vs. SHR-C). The lung wet weight-to-dry weight ratio was not elevated significantly in SHR-C and SHR-L compared to WKY groups (Table 1). All these results indicate the presence of cardiac hypertrophy without congestive heart failure in the SHR-C group that was ameliorated in the SHR-L group.

L-2286 treatment did not influence the levels of plasma BNP and blood pressure

Slightly elevated plasma BNP levels were found both in SHR-C and SHR-L groups (not significant vs. WKY group). Although plasma BNP level was a little higher in SHR-C group than in SHR-L group, this difference was also not statistically significant (Table 1). In both SHR groups, blood pressure was significantly elevated compared to the WKY group (p<0.05). L-2286 treatment did not decrease significantly the elevated blood pressure (Table 1).

L-2286 decreased the interstitial collagen deposition in the myocardium

Histological analysis revealed slight interstitial collagen deposition in the WKY group. Chronic high blood pressure caused significantly higher collagen deposition in SHR-C rats that was significantly diminished (p<0.05) in the SHR-L group (Fig. 2).

PARP inhibition decreased the left ventricular hypertrophy in spontaneously hypertensive rats

At the beginning of the study the echocardiographic parameters of the three groups did not differ significantly from each other (Table 2). At the age of 30 weeks there was no significant difference in LV systolic functions (EF and FS) between the WKY and SHR groups. Heart rate did not differ significantly during the anesthesia among the groups. LVESV and LVEDV were increased significantly in SHRs (p<0.05 WKY vs. SHR-C and SHR-L), and these unfavorable alterations were not reduced by L-2286 treatment. The thickness of the septum, and the posterior

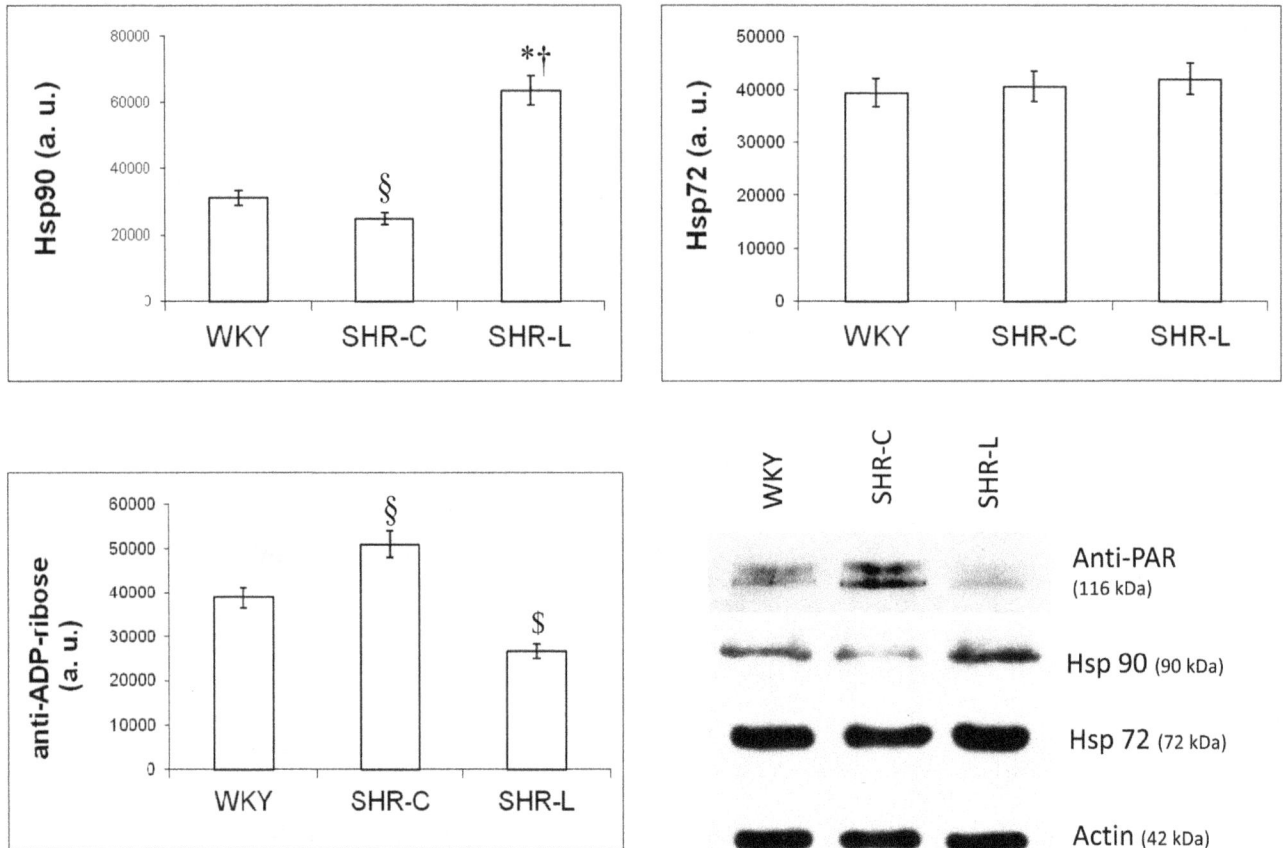

Figure 4. Effect of L-2286 treatment on the level of Hsp72, 90 and poly(ADP-ribos)ylation. Representative Western-blot analysis of Hsp72, 90, anti-PAR and densitometric evaluations are shown (n = 4). Actin was used as loading control. Values are means ± S.E.M. WKY: normotensive age-matched control rats. SHR-C: 30 week-old spontaneously hypertensive rats, SHR-L: 30 week-old spontaneously hypertensive rats treated with L-2286 for 24 weeks. $^{*}p<0.01$ vs. WKY, $^{†}p<0.01$ v.s SHR-C, $^{§}p<0.05$ vs. WKY, $^{\$}p<0.05$ vs. SHR-C.

wall and the relative wall thickness were also increased in SHR groups (indicating the presence of ventricular hypertrophy) comparing to the WKY group ($p<0.05$), and these parameters could be significantly reduced by the administration of L-2286 ($p<0.05$ SHR-C vs. SHR-L group) (Table 3).

Effect of L-2286 treatment on poly-ADP-ribosylation as well as on the phosphorylation state of Akt-1^{Ser473}/GSK-3β^{Ser9} and FKHR^{Ser256}

Akt-1^{Ser473} was moderately phosphorylated in WKY group. In SHR-C group, the phosphorylation of Akt-1^{Ser473} was more pronounced ($p<0.01$ vs. WKY). Moreover, in SHR-L rats the L-2286 treatment caused further elevation in Akt-1^{Ser473} phosphorylation ($p<0.01$ vs. WKY and SHR-C groups) (Fig. 3). The same result was obtained in the case of GSK-3β^{Ser9} phosphorylation (Fig. 3).

Another target protein of Akt-1^{Ser473} (besides GSK3β^{Ser9}) is FKHR^{Ser256}. Consistently with the result of Akt-1^{Ser473} phosphorylation, the strongest phosphorylation (therefore inhibition) could be observed in SHR-L group ($p<0.01$ vs. SHR-C and WKY). The lowest phosphorylation and therefore the highest activity of FKHR was seen in SHR-C group ($p<0.05$ vs. WKY, Fig. 3). To detect the effectivity of L-2286, the ADP-ribosylation of the

samples were analysed by Western-blot. The lowest degree of ADP-ribosylation was present in SHR-L group, and the most pronounced ADP-ribosylation was seen in SHR-C group ($p<0.05$ vs. WKY) (Fig. 4).

Effect of L-2286 on the amount of Hsp72 and 90

There was no significant difference among the three groups in the level of Hsp72. On the other hand, the level of Hsp90 was elevated in SHR-L group compared to WKY and SHR-C groups ($p<0.01$ SHR-L vs. WKY or SHR-C groups), and the lowest amount of this protein was present in WKY samples (Fig. 4).

Effect of L-2286 administration on MAPKs

Phosphorylation of p38-MAPK$^{Thr180-Gly-Tyr182}$, ERK 1/2$^{Thr183-Tyr185}$ and JNK was the lowest in the WKY group compared to SHR-C and SHR-L groups (p38-MAPK$^{Thr180-Gly-Tyr182}$: $p<0.01$ vs. SHR groups, ERK 1/2: $p<0.05$ vs. SHR groups, JNK: $p<0.05$ vs. SHR groups). In the case of p38-MAPK$^{Thr180-Gly-Tyr182}$, ERK 1/2$^{Thr183-Tyr185}$ and JNK, their phosphorylation was elevated in both SHR-C and SHR-L groups, but there were no significant differences between the two SHR groups (Fig. 5, JNK: data not shown).

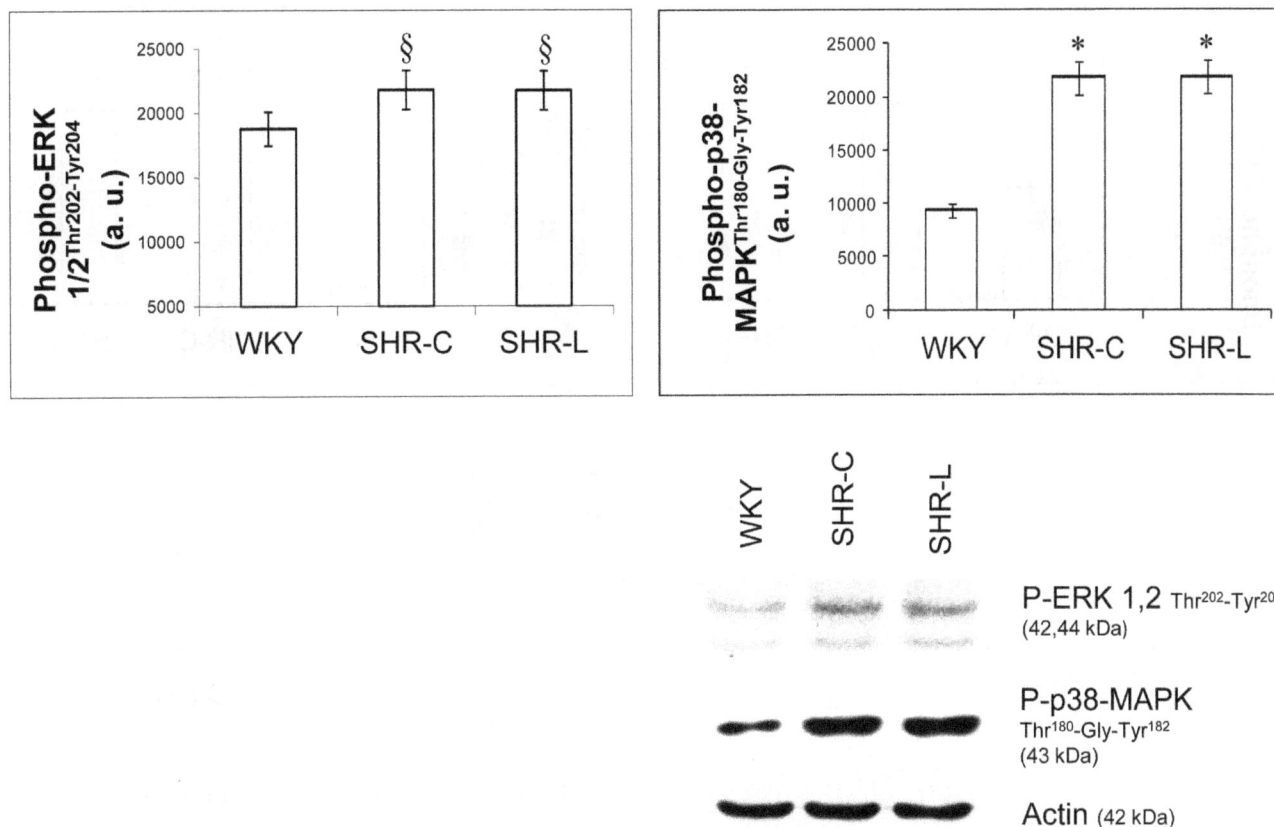

Figure 5. Effect of L-2286 on the phosphorylation state of MAPK pathway. Representative Western blot analysis of ERK 1/2[Thr183-Tyr185], and p38-MAPK[Thr180-Gly-Tyr182] phosphorylation and densitometric evaluation is shown (n = 4). Actin was used as loading control. Values are means±S.E.M. WKY: normotensive age-matched control rats, SHR-C: 30 week-old spontaneously hypertensive rats, SHR-L: 30 week-old spontaneously hypertensive rats treated with L-2286 for 24 weeks. [§]$p < 0.05$ vs. WKY [*]$p < 0.01$ vs. WKY.

Influence of L-2286 treatment on the phosphorylation state of several PKC isoforms

The overall (pan) phosphorylation of PKC (pan βII^{Ser660}) was low in the WKY group and became significantly higher in SHR-C and SHR-L groups ($p < 0.01$ WKY vs. SHR groups). Administration of L-2286 could not affect the phosphorylation state of PKC pan βII Ser^{660} in SHR-L group compared to the SHR-C group (Fig. 6).

The lowest phosphorylation could be observed in the WKY group in case of PKC $\alpha/\beta II^{Thr638/641}$, δ^{Thr505}, $\zeta/\lambda^{Thr410/403}$ and ε^{Ser729} ($p < 0.01$ vs. SHR groups). As PKC ζ antibody, we used a combined antibody (i.e. PKC ζ/λ Thr$^{410/403}$), which did not discriminate between PKC ζ and λ; PKC λ being structurally highly homologous to PKC ζ in the COOH-terminal end of the molecule [12]. L-2286 treatment decreased significantly the phosphorylation of PKC $\alpha/\beta II^{Thr638/641}$ and ζ, while it could increase the phosphorylation of ε^{Ser729} (PKC $\alpha/\beta II^{Thr638/641}$, ζ, ε^{Ser729}: $p < 0.01$, SHR-L vs. SHR-C) (Fig. 6,7). In the case of PKC δ^{Thr505} there was no significant difference between the SHR groups (Fig. 7).

Discussion

The major findings of this study are that chronic inhibition of nuclear PARP enzyme reduces excessive ADP-ribosylation of nuclear proteins, beneficially influences the intracellular signaling pathways and thus prevents the development of cardiac hypertrophy, which is an early consequence of hypertension. We used the SHR model that is a relevant animal model of essential hypertension in humans [13]. Our study began at a very early age (6-week-old) of SHRs, because at this age the blood pressure of animals is still normal and the hearts show no signs of remodeling. However, by the end of the study (30 weeks), marked signs of hypertensive cardiopathy develop in SHRs.

Previously, we have proved that PARP-inhibition could inhibit the transition of hypertensive cardiopathy to end-stage heart failure [6], but there is no data about the role of PAPR-inhibitors against the development of early consequences of hypertension.

Hypertension is a major risk factor for cardiovascular mortality and morbidity, and it is associated with left ventricular hypertrophy and diastolic dysfunction and later with systolic dysfunction and it can lead to heart failure. There is a strong correlation between left ventricular mass and the development of cardiovascular pathogies [14]. The development of long-term hypertension-induced myocardial remodeling can be explained by different mechanism in the literature, but generally, oxidative stress and abnormal signaling are considered as molecular basis of the disease. Peroxynitrite and other reactive species induce oxidative DNA damage and consequent activation of the nuclear enzyme PARP. In related animal models of the disease, pharmacological inhibition of PARP provides significant therapeutic benefits [15].

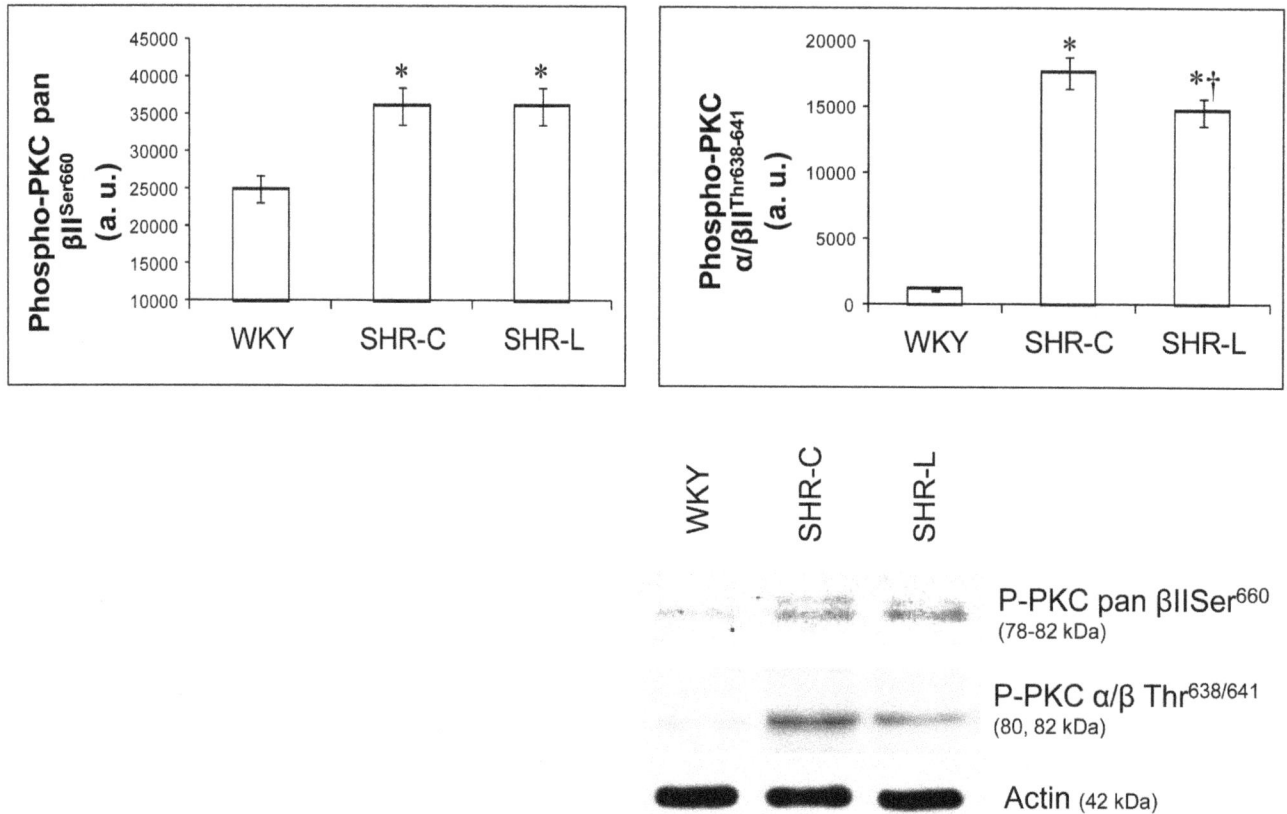

Figure 6. Effect of L-2286 administration on the activity of PKC isoenzymes. Representative Western blot analysis of PKC pan βII^{Ser660} and PKC α/βII$^{Thr638/641}$ phosphorylation and densitometric evaluations are shown (n = 4). Values are means±S.E.M. WKY: normotensive age-matched control rats. SHR-C: 30 week-old spontaneously hypertensive rats, SHR-L: 30 week-old spontaneously hypertensive rats treated with L-2286 for 24 weeks. *p<0.01 vs. WKY, †p<0.01 vs. SHR-C.

PARP inhibition and gravimetric parameters in SHR

Significant LV hypertrophy develops by the age of 3 months in SHR animals but it is more often studied closer to 6 months of age [16]. In our SHR rats myocardial hypertrophy developed, as increased WV/BW ratio could be observed. We could not observe any obvious signs of HF, because BNP activity and the index of pulmonary congestion was not elevated compared to the WKY group.

PARP inhibition and interstitial collagen deposition in SHR

Chronic hypertension leads to excessive collagen deposition (fibrosis) as part of the process of cardiovascular remodeling. In our previous studies, when SHR or postinfarcted animals exhibited overt heart failure, L-2286 also prevented interstitial fibrosis and adverse structural remodeling [3,6]. In the present study, our results suggest that PARP inhibitor treatment can exert marked antifibrotic effect already in this early stage of hypertensive heart disease.

PARP inhibition and echocardiographic parameters

In our experiment the systolic LV function was not decreased in SHR rats during the 24-week-long treatment. It is in accordance with several other studies [8,9,10] involving different experimental models of pressure overload-induced hypertrophy. During the development of hypertension, alterations in LV geometry may also occur as an adaptation to increased pressure overload. In

hypertensive patients, LV geometry can be classified into four patterns on the basis of LV mass index and RWT and these patterns have been shown to be closely related to LV function and to patients' prognosis [17,18,19]. In this study, increased RWT and increased WV/BW were found, which indicates concentric LV hypertrophy [9]. L-2286 treatment decreased significantly the signs of left ventricular hypertrophy (wall thickness and RWT) even though the elevated blood pressure of SHR rats was not influenced by PARP inhibition.

L-2286 treatment and the activity of Akt-1^{Ser473}/ GSK3β^{Ser9} and FKHR^{Ser256} pathway

Previous works demonstrated that PARP inhibitors can induce the phosphorylation and activation of Akt-1 in reperfused myocardium, thus raising the possibility that the protective effect of PARP inhibition can be mediated through the activation of the prosurvival phosphatidylinositol-3-kinase (PI3-kinase)/Akt-1 pathway [20]. Akt-1 is a key molecule in the signaling cascade of physiological hypertrophy [21]. Recent results demonstrate an important role of Akt/m-TOR signaling in cardiac angiogenesis, whose disruption contributes to the transition from hypertrophy to HF [1]. In our experiment, the phosphorylation of Akt-1^{Ser473} was far the lowest in WKY group and the highest in SHR-L group. Phosphorylation and therefore the inhibition of GSK-3β^{Ser9} and Foxo1 (FKHR) (downstream targets of Akt-1) [22,23] were also determined. This showed the same pattern as the phosphorylation of Akt-1. The similar results were obtained in our studies using

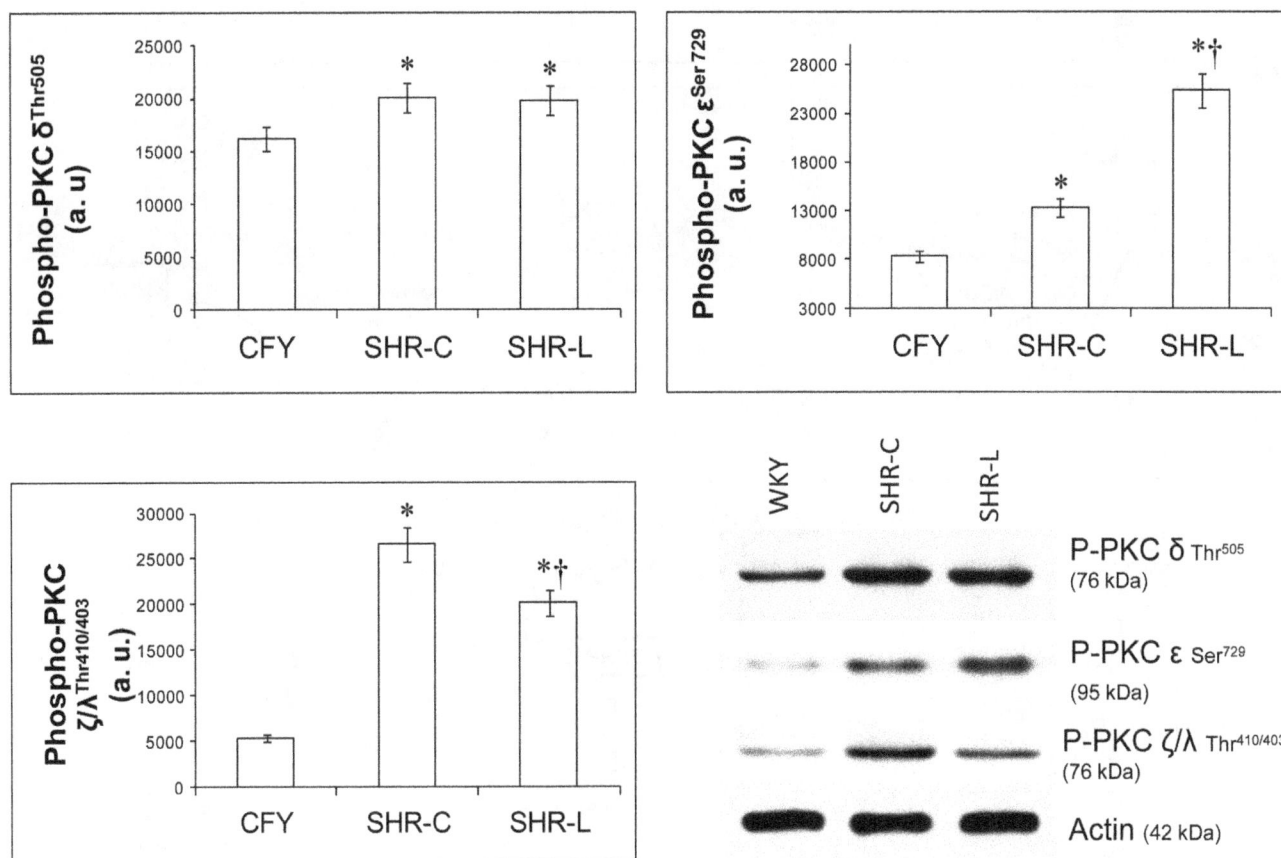

Figure 7. Effect of L-2286 administration of PKC isoenzymes. Representative Western blot analysis of PKC δ^{Thr505}, ε^{Ser729} and $\zeta/\lambda^{Thr410/403}$ phosphorylation and densitometric evaluation is shown (n = 4). Actin was used as loading control. Values are means±S.E.M. WKY: normotensive age-matched control rats. SHR-C: 30 week-old spontaneously hypertensive rats, SHR-L: 30 week-old spontaneously hypertensive rats treated with L-2286 for 24 weeks. *p<0.01 vs. WKY, †p<0.01 vs. SHR-C.

PARP inhibitors [20,24] or by suppressing PARP-1 activation by siRNA technique [25]. These results may indicate that SHR-C animals tried to compensate for the adverse effects of chronic hypertension, but failed to do so. On the other hand, L-2286 treatment further elevated Akt activation that could, at least partially, account for the beneficial changes in the cardial remodeling of the SHR-L animals.

L-2286 administration and levels of Hsp 72 and 90

Cellular stress leads to the expression of Hsp's [26]. They are known to protect the myocardium from the damaging effects of ischemia and reperfusion [27]. According to the results of Jiang et al [27] and Shinohara et al [28] the Hsp's can preserve the mitochondrial respiratory function and structure which are damaged in case of cell death. The flux of pro-apoptotic proteins can be induced by various stimuli, one of them is the decreased level of ATP. This can be induced by overactivation of PARP-1, which consumes too much ATP in certain pathologic conditions [29]. In case of Hsp90 in our study, the level of it was increased by long-term L-2286 treatment. Besides the activation of Akt-1^{Ser473}, this can contribute to the cell survival in L-2286 treated rats. The level of Hsp72 was not influenced significantly by L-2286 administration in our investigation.

L-2286 administration and MAPKs in young SHR

Previous works demonstrated that PARP inhibitors have a moderate effect on MAPKs in acute phase of myocardial infarction and in postinfarction heart failure [3,20]. MAPKs are ubiquitously expressed and their activation is observed in different heart diseases, including hypertrophic cardiomyopathy, dilated cardiomyopathy, and ischemic/reperfusion injury in human and animal models [30]. In our study, the phosphorylation of p38-MAPK$^{Thr180-Gly-Tyr182}$, JNK and ERK 1/2$^{Thr183-Tyr185}$ was elevated both in SHR-C and SHR-L groups. Our results are consistent with the results of Kacimi et Gerdes [31] using spontaneously hypertensive heart failure (SHHF) rats. L-2286 treatment did not influence the phosphorylation of p38-MAPK and JNK. The role of JNK and p38-MAPK-signaling in cardiac hypertrophy is not fully clarified [1]. However, both p38-MAPK and JNK transduction cascades have been implicated in the regulation of hypertrophic response as well as cardiomyopathy and HF [32]. JNK activity was not altered by L-2286 treatment in SHR animals, similarly to Hsp72 level. This result is in accordance with previous data [28] demonstrating that Hsp72 downregulates JNK by accelerating its dephosphorylation.

The elevated blood pressure may induced ERK activation [33]. Accordingly, activation of ERK1/2 was the lowest in WKY group, and was higher in SHR-C. Phosphorylation of ERK1/2 was not

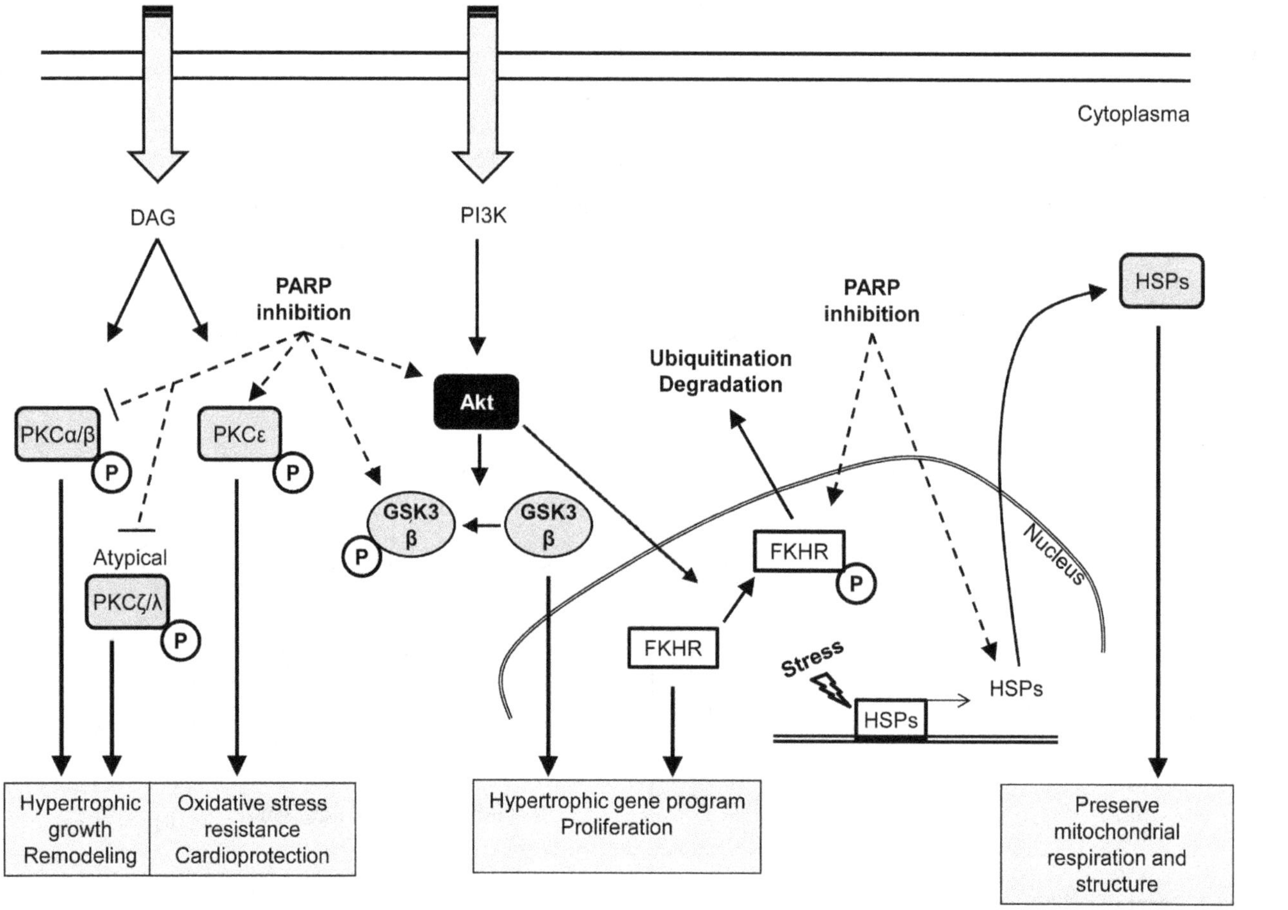

Figure 8. Summary of pathway alterations due to L-2286 treatment.

elevated by L-2286 administration in this study. The in vivo role of ERK in cardiac hypertrophy has been demonstrated in several genetically engineered animal models. Cardiac-specific expression of constitutively activated MEK1 promotes cardiac hypertrophy without compromised function or long-term animal survival, suggesting that activation of ERK activity promotes a compensated form of hypertrophy [30]. All these results suggest that MAPK activation did not participate significantly in mediating the adverse cardiac effects of chronic hypertension in our model.

PARP inhibition and PKC pathways in young SHR

PARP inhibitors were found to affect PKC isoenzymes [3,17]. The levels of all PKC isoforms increased in SHR groups compared to the WKY group in our study. Our results are in agreement with Koide et al. [34] using Dahl Salt-Sensitive rats in cardiac hypertrophy stage. Recent studies suggested that PKC is critically involved in the development of cardiac remodeling and HF. The data also suggest that individual PKC isoforms have different effects on cell signaling pathways, variously leading to changes in cardiac contractility, hypertrophic response and tolerance to myocardial ischaemia in the heart [34].

Activation of PKC pan βII^{Ser660} and δ^{Thr505} were not altered by L-2286 treatment, while activation of $\alpha/\beta II^{Thr638/641}$ and ζ/λ $^{Thr410/403}$ were attenuated and activation of ϵ^{Ser729} was augmented by L-2286. These alterations can mediate – at least partly – the favourable cardiovascular effects of L-2286, similarly as it was found in previous works [3,20].

PKC α is the most extensively expressed among the myocardial PKC isoforms, and it is a key regulator of cardiomyocyte hypertrophic growth [35,36]. PKC α was sufficient to stimulate cell hypertrophy [37]. Transgenic mice overexpressing PKC $\beta2$ exhibited cardiac hypertrophy and decreased LV performance; this depressed cardiac function improved after the administration of a PKC β-selective inhibitor [38]. Previous reports suggest that PKC α and β and PKC ζ/λ are involved in the development of cardiac hypertrophy and HF. Additionally, PKC ϵ plays a role in physiological hypertrophic responses [34,39], has cardioprotective effect [40] and by interacting with Akt-1 and affecting Bcl-2 promote vascular cytoprotection [41]. Accordingly, in our study, both the activity of Akt-1^{Ser473} and PKCϵ^{Ser729} were elevated by L-2286 administration.

Conclusions

In our study, we examined the effect of a PARP inhibitor (L-2286) in SHR at the stage of LV hypertrophy. L-2286 exerted a beneficial effect on the progression of myocardial hypertrophy (thickness of PW and septum, RWT) and myocardial fibrosis. In the background of these changes, we did not observe any blood pressure lowering effect of PARP-inhibition. According to our results, PARP-inhibition can exert this antihypertrophic effect due to the activation of several prosurvival (especially Akt-1/GSK-3β, FKHR, PKCϵ and Hsp90) and the inhibition of prohypertrophic (PKC- $\alpha/\beta II$, - ζ/λ) protein kinases (Fig.8).

Acknowledgments

We are grateful for Bertalan Horvath and Laszlo Giran for their excellent technical support.

References

1. Luedde M, Katus HA, Frey N (2006) Novel molecular targets in the treatment of cardiac hypertrophy. Recent Pat Cardiovasc Drug Discov 1: 1–20.
2. Baines CP, Molkentin JD (2005) STRESS signaling pathways that modulate cardiac myocyte apoptosis. J Mol Cell Cardiol 38: 47–62.
3. Palfi A, Toth A, Hanto K, Deres P, Szabados E, et al. (2006) PARP inhibition prevents postinfarction myocardial remodeling and heart failure via the protein kinase C/glycogen synthase kinase-3β pathway. J Mol Cell Cardiol 41: 149–159.
4. Szabó Cs, Pacher P, Zsengellér Zs, Vaslin A, Komjáti K, et al. (2004) Angiotensi II-mediated endothelial dysfunction: role of poly(ADP-ribose) polymerase activation. Mol Med 10: 28–35.
5. Pacher P, Mabley JG, Soriano FG, Liaudet L, Szabó C (2002) Activation of poly(ADP-ribose) polymerase contributes to the endothelial dysfunction associated with hypertension and aging. Int J Mol Med 9: 659–664.
6. Bartha E, Solti I, Kereskai L, Lantos J, Plozer E, et al. (2009) PARP inhibition delays transition of hypertensive cardiopathy to heart failure in spontaneously hypertensive rats. Cardiovasc Res 83: 501–510.
7. Racz B, Hanto K, Tapodi A, Solti I, Kalman N, et al. (2010) Regulation of MKP-1 expression and MAPK activation by PARP-1 in oxidative stress: a new mechanism for the cytoplasmic effect of PARP-1 activation. Free Radic Biol Med 49: 1978–1988.
8. Ito N, Ohishi M, Yamamoto K, Tatara Y, Shiota A, et al. (2007) Renin-Angiotensin inhibition reverses advanced cardiac remodeling in aging spontaneously hypertensive rats. Am J Hypertens 20: 792–799.
9. Kokubo M, Uemura A, Matsubara T, Murohara T (2005) Noninvasive evaluation of the time course of change in cardiac function in spontaneously hypertensive rats by echocardiography. Hypertens Res 28: 601–609.
10. Meurrens K, Ruf S, Ross G, Schleef R, van Holt K, et al. (2007) Smoking accelerates the progression of hypertension-induced myocardial hypertrophy to heart failure in spontaneously hypertensive rats. Cardiovasc Res 76: 311–322.
11. Kulcsar Gy, Kalai T, Osz E, Sar CP, Jeko J, et al. (2006) Synthesis and study of new 4-quinazolinone inhibitors of the DNA repair enzyme poly(ADP-ribose) polymerase (PARP). Arkivoc IV:121–131.
12. Hideg K, Kálai T, Sümegi B (2003) Quinazoline derivates and their use for preparation of pharmaceutical compositions having PARP-Enzyme inhibitory effect. WO2004/096779, Hung Pat PO301173.
13. Pfeffer JM, Pfeffer MA, Mirsky I, Braunwald E (1982) Regression of left ventricular hypertrophy and prevention of left ventricular dysfunction by captopril in the spontaneously hypertensive rat. Proc Natl Acad Sci U S A. 79(10):3310–4.
14. Lip GY, Felmeden DC, Li-Saw-Hee FL, Beevers DG (2000) Hypertensive heart disease. A complex syndrome or a hypertensive 'cardiomyopathy'? Eur Heart J; 21: 1653–1665.
15. Pacher P, Szabo C (2008) Role of the peroxynitrite-poly(ADP-ribose) polymerase pathway in human disease. Am J Pathol 173: 2–13.
16. McCrossan ZA, Billeter R, White E (2004) Transmural changes in size, contractile and electrical properties of SHR left ventricular myocytes during compensated hypertrophy. Cardiovasc Res 63: 283–292.
17. Cooper RS, Simmons BE, Castaner A, Santhanam V, Ghali J, et al. (1990) Left ventricular hypertrophy is associated with worse survival independent of ventricular function and number of coronary arteries severely narrowed. Am J Cardiol. 65(7):441–445.
18. Levy D, Garrison RJ, Savage DD, Kannel WB, Castelli WP (1990) Prognostic implications of echocardiographically determined left ventricular mass in the Framingham Heart Study. N Engl J Med. 322: 1561–1566.
19. Koren MJ, Devereux RB, Casale PN, Savage DD, Laregh JH (1991) Relation of left ventricular mass and geometry to morbidity and mortality in uncomplicated essential hypertension. Ann Intern Med. 114: 345–352.
20. Pálfi A, Tóth A, Kulcsár G, Hantó K, Deres P, et al. (2005) The role of Akt and MAP kinase systems in the protective effect of PARP inhibition in Langendorff perfused and in isoproterenol-damaged rat hearts. J Pharmacol Exp Ther 315: 273–282.
21. Taniike M, Yamaguchi O, Tsujimoto I, Hikoso S, Takeda T, et al. (2008) Apoptosis signal-regulating kinase 1/p38 signaling pathway negatively regulates physiological hypertrophy. Circulation 117: 545–552.
22. Li HH, Willis MS, Lockyer P, Miller N, McDonough H, et al. (2007) Atrogin-1 inhibits Akt-dependent cardiac hypertrophy in mice via ubiquitin-dependent coactivation of Forkhead proteins. J Clin Invest 117: 3211–3223.
23. Ni YG, Berenji K, Wang N, Oh M, Sachan N, et al. (2006) Foxo transcription factors blunt cardiac hypertrophy by inhibiting calcineurin signaling. Circulation 114: 1159–1168.
24. Kovacs K, Toth A, Deres P, Kalai T, Hideg K, et al. (2006) Critical role of PI3-kinase/Akt activation in the PARP inhibitor induced heart function recovery during ischemia-reperfusion. Biochem Pharmacol 71: 441–452.
25. Tapodi A, Debreceni B, Hanto K, Bognar Z, Wittmann I, et al. (2005) Pivotal role of Akt activation in mitochondrial protection and cell survival by poly(ADP-ribose)polymerase-1 inhibition in oxidative stress. J Biol Chem 280: 35767–3575.
26. Sóti Cs, Nagy E, Giricz Z, Vígh L, Csermely P, et al. (2005) Heat shock proteins as emerging therapeutic targets. Br J Pharmacol 146: 769–780.
27. Jiang B, Xiao W, Shi Y, Liu M, Xiao X (2005) Heat shock pretreatment inhibited the release of Smac/DIABLO from mitochondria and apoptosis induced by hydrogen peroxide in cardiomyocytes and C_2C_{12} myogenic cells. Cell Stress Chaperones 10: 252–262.
28. Shinohara T, Takahashi N, Kohno H, Yamanaka K, Ooie T, et al. (2007) Mitochondria are targets for geranylgeranylacetone-induced cardioprotection against ischemia-reperfusion in rat heart. Am J Physiol Heart Circ Physiol 293:H1892–H1899.
29. Pacher P, Szabó C (2007) Role of poly(ADP-ribose) polymerase 1 (PARP-1) in cardiovascular diseases: The therapeutic potential of PARP inhibitors. Cardiovasc Drug Rev 25: 235–260.
30. Wang Y (2007) Mitogen-Activated Protein Kinases in heart development and diseases. Circulation 116: 1413–1423.
31. Kacimi R, Gerdes AM (2003) Alterations in G protein and MAP Kinase signaling pathways during cardiac remodeling in hypertension and heart failure. Hypertension 41: 968–977.
32. Liang Q, Molkentin JD (2003) Redefining the roles of p38 and JNK signaling in cardiac hypertrophy: dichotomy between cultured myocytes and animal models. J Mol Cell Cardiol 35: 1385–1394.
33. Bogoyevitch MA (2000) Signalling via stress-activated mitogen-activated protein kinases in the cardiovascular system. Cardiovas Res 45: 826–842.
34. Koide Y, Tamura K, Suzuki A, Kitamura K, Yokoyama K, et al. (2003) Differential induction of protein kinase C isoforms at the cardiac hypertrophy stage and congestive heart failure stage in Dahl salt-sensitive rats. Hypertens Res 26: 421–426.
35. Dorn GW II, Force T (2005) Protein kinase cascades in the regulation of cardiac hypertrophy. J Clin Invest 115: 527–537.
36. García-Hoz C, Sánchez-Fernández G, García-Escudero R, Fernández-Velasco M, Palacios-García J, et al. (2012) Protein Kinase C (PKC)ζ-mediated Gαq Stimulation of ERK5 Protein Pathway in Cardiomyocytes and Cardiac Fibroblasts JBiolChem. 287: 7792–7802.
37. Braz JC, Bueno OF, De Windt LJ, Molkentin JD (2002) PKC alpha regulates the hypertrophic growth of cardiomyocytes through extracellular signal-regulated kinase1/2 (ERK1/2) J. Cell Biol. 156: 905–919.
38. Takeishi Y, Chu G, Kirkpatrick DM, Li Z, Wakasaki H, et al. (1998) In vivo phosphorylation of cardiac troponin I by protein kinase Cbeta2 decreases cardiomyocyte calcium responsiveness and contractility in transgenic mouse hearts. J Clin Invest. 102: 72–78.
39. Inagaki K, Iwanaga Y, Sarai N, Onozawa Y, Takenaka H, et al. (2002) Tissue angiotensin II during progression or ventricular hypertrophy to heart failure in hypertensive rats; differential effects on PKC epsilon and PKC beta. J Mol Cell Cardiol. 34: 1377–1385.
40. Dorn GW II, Souroujon MC, Liron T, Chen CH, Gray MO, et al. (1999) Sustained in vivo cardiac protection by a rationally designed peptide that causes epsilon protein kinase C translocation. Proc Natl Acad Sci USA 96: 12798–12803.
41. Steinberg R, Harari OA, Lidington EA, Boyle JJ, Nohadani M, et al. (2007) A protein kinase Cepsilon-anti-apoptotic kinase signalling complex protects human vascular endothelial cells against apoptosis through induction of Bcl-2. J Biol Chem 282: 32288–32297.

Author Contributions

Conceived and designed the experiments: LD EB AP TK KH BS FG KT RH. Performed the experiments: LD EB KE AR. Analyzed the data: LD KE GF SB KT RH. Contributed reagents/materials/analysis tools: JL TK KH. Wrote the paper: LD EB RH.

The Effects of 17-Methoxyl-7-Hydroxy-Benzene-Furanchalcone on the Pressure Overload-Induced Progression of Cardiac Hypertrophy to Cardiac Failure

Jianchun Huang[1,♥], XiaoJun Tang[2,♥], Xingmei Liang[1], Qingwei Wen[1], Shijun Zhang[1], Feifei Xuan[1], Jie Jian[1], Xing Lin[1], Renbin Huang[1]*

1 Pharmaceutical College, Guangxi Medical University, Nanning, Guangxi, China, 2 Department of Laboratory Medicine, Guangxi Medical College, Nanning, Guangxi, China

Abstract

We investigated the effects of 17-methoxyl-7-hydroxy-benzene-furanchalcone (MHBFC), which was isolated from the roots of *Millettia pulchra* (Benth.) Kurz var. *Laxior* (Dunn) Z.Wei (Papilionaceae) (MKL), on the progression of cardiac hypertrophy to failure in a rat model of abdominal aortic banding (AAB)-induced pressure overloading. Endothelial dysfunction is central to pressure overload-induced cardiac hypertrophy and failure. It would be useful to clarify whether MHBFC could prevent this dysfunction. The effects of pressure overload were assessed in male Sprague–Dawley rats 6 weeks after AAB using the progression of cardiac hypertrophy to heart failure as the endpoint. The AAB-treated rats exhibited a greater progression to heart failure and had significantly elevated blood pressure, systolic and diastolic cardiac dysfunction, and evidence of left ventricular hypertrophy (LVH). LVH was characterized by increases in the ratios of heart and left ventricular weights to body weight, increased myocyte cross-sectional areas, myocardial and perivascular fibrosis, and elevated cardiac hydroxyproline. These symptoms could be prevented by treatment with MHBFC at daily oral doses of 6 and 12 mg/kg for 6 weeks. The progression to cardiac failure, which was demonstrated by increases in relative lung and right ventricular weights, cardiac function disorders and overexpression of atrial natriuretic peptide (ANP) mRNA, could also be prevented. Furthermore, MHBFC partialy rescued the downregulated nitric oxide signaling system, whereas inhibited the upregulated endothelin signaling system, normalizing the balance between these two systems. MHBFC protected the endothelium and prevented the pressure overload-induced progression of cardiac hypertrophy to cardiac failure.

Editor: Luis Eduardo M. Quintas, Universidade Federal do Rio de Janeiro, Brazil

Funding: This work was supported by the Guangxi Scientific Research and Technology Development Research Projects (No. 0630002-2A); the Guangxi Natural Science Foundation (No. 2013GXNSFAA019175); the Fund of Guangxi Key Laboratory of Functional Phytochemicals Research and Utilization (No. FPRU2013-3); and the Outstanding Doctoral Dissertation Breeding Program in the Guangxi Zhuang Autonomous Region (No. YCBZ2012013). The funders had no role in study design, data collection and analysis, decision to publish, or preparation of the manuscript.

Competing Interests: The authors expect to develop a novel drug for the treatment of hypertensive heart disease with high quality and low toxicity.

* E-mail: huangrenbin518@163.com

♥ These authors contributed equally to this work.

Introduction

Hypertension is a continuum that starts with a rise in blood pressure, evolves to left ventricular hypertrophy (LVH), proteinuria or endothelial dysfunction, and, insofar as it is not adequately treated or controlled, finally leads to the development of complications, the most relevant of which are stroke and heart failure [1]. Hypertensive disease is the most frequent background of LVH, and it is generally felt that anti-hypertensive treatment should not only lower blood pressure but also cause the regression of LVH [2]. Various noxious sequelae of cardiovascular diseases and conditions, such as coronary heart disease, stroke, congestive heart failure, and sudden death, are known to be aggravated by LVH [3]. Endothelial dysfunction is known to play important roles in the pathogenesis and progressiveness of hypertensive heart disease [4,5]. The pathophysiological mechanisms of endothelial dysfunction that are related to a decrease in the bioavailability of NO as well as to augmented ET-1 synthesis, release, or activity [6]. Thus, a subsequent decrease in NO bioavailability is fundamental to the LVH process. In hypertension, reduction of BP *per se* does not seem to restore endothelial function. Angiotensin receptor blockers and angiotensin-converting enzyme inhibitors have been shown to be especially beneficial [7–9]. There is current evidence demonstrating that the best drugs that achieve these goals are renin-angiotensin system blockers (ACEI or angiotensin-receptor blocking agents) and calcium channel blockers, as evidenced by three large trials, LIFE ASCOT and ACCOMPLIISH, with more than 40000 patients [1]. In animal models of hypertension, oxidative excess leads to endothelial dysfunction as evidenced by improvement of the impaired endothelium-dependent relaxation after use of antioxidants [10]. Oxidative excess in hypertensive patients leads to diminished NO [11] and correlates with the degree of impairment of endothelium-dependent vasodilation and with cardiovascular events [12]. Recently, increased attention has been focused on traditional Chinese herbal treatments because of their unique decrease in oxidative stress efficacy and little adverse reactions.

Table 1. Oligonucleotide primers used for reverse transcription-polymerase chain reaction.

Target gene	Accession no.	Primers (5′–3′)	Cycle program T (°C)	Length(bp)
ANP	NM-012612	F: GGC TCC TTC TCC ATC ACC AA	52	268
		R: TCT GAG ACG GGT TGA CTT CC		
ET-1	NM-012548	F: TGG CTT TCC AAG GAG CTC	58	394
		R: GCT TGG CAG AAA TTC CAG		
ECE	NM-053596	F: TGA GCA CCC TGA AAT GGA	56	488
		R: CTG CTG CTT GAA TGC CTC		
β-Actin	NM_031144.3	F: AGG CAT CCT GAC CCT GAA GTA C	60	389
		R: TCT TCA TGA GGT AGT CTG TCA G		
β-Actin	NM_031144.3	F: AAC CCT AAG GCC AAC CGT GAA AAG	60	240
		R: TCA TGA GGT GGT AGT CTG TCA GGT		

Millettia pulchra (Benth.) Kurz var. *Laxior* (Dunn) Z.Wei (Papilionaceae) (MKL) is a traditional Chinese medicinal herb that is extensively distributed in the Guangxi Province of China. Our previous studies have demonstrated that extracts of MKL roots have antihypertensive, antioxidative, anti-inflammatory effects [13–16]. Additionally, the drugs of these previous studies were the total extracts of MKL roots, and MHBFC is a flavonoid monomer that was originally isolated from a 60% ethanol extract from MKL roots [17]. Previous studies have demonstrated that MHBFC could scavenge hydroxyl radicals and oxyradicals [18], enhance the cardiocyte survival rate in hypoxia/reoxygenation injury [19], and protect the heart against myocardial ischemia *in vitro* and *in vivo* [20]. Based on the above information, we hypothesized that MHBFC might be effective in the treatment of hypertensive heart disease. Here, for the first time, we investigated its effects on cardiovascular remodeling that is induced by a pressure overload as well as the potential mechanisms that are involved.

The abdominal aortic stenosis model using rats is a pressure-overload model that is similar to the progression of hypertensive heart disease. In this condition, LVH with myocyte hypertrophy and interstitial fibrosis develops in response to a sustained elevation of LV systolic pressure in the presence of systemic hypertension 6 weeks after abdominal aortic banding (AAB) [21,22]. Here, we investigated the effects of MHBFC on cardiac hypertrophy and cardiac failure that was induced by pressure overloading using AAB in rats, exploring the potential mechanisms that were involved in endothelial protection. From our data, we suggest that MHBFC might be effective in the treatment of hypertensive heart disease via the molecular pathways that are involved in endothelial protection.

Materials and Methods

2.1: Chemicals

MHBFC (purity >95%) was isolated from MKL by the Department of Pharmacology, Guangxi Medical University

Table 2. Effect of MHBFC on heart rate (HR) and systolic blood pressure (SBP) in different groups during the course of the experiments ($\overline{X} \pm S$, n = 6).

Group	0 week	2 week	4 week	6 week
Heart rate (b.p.m.)				
Sham	359±37	361±38	358±21	360±23
Model	361±33	380±25	388±23[#]	389±21[#]
MHBFC 6 mg/kg	365±32	372±20	372±20	371±26
MHBFC 12 mg/kg	356±29	373±26	369±29	365±29
Lisenopril 15 mg/kg	364±36	373±41	368±39	365±41
Systolic blood pressure (tail-cuff) (mmHg)				
Sham	105.53±8.44	104.87±8.21	106.09±6.97	105.87±7.92
Model	103.80±4.73	116.40±5.13[#]	118.31±4.08[##]	121.64±4.50[##]
MHBFC 6 mg/kg	104.19±4.93	113.18±4.17	111.20±3.94*	110.02±3.62**
MHBFC 12 mg/kg	104.55±5.74	110.55±6.97	107.97±7.32*	107.08±8.31**
Lisenopril 15 mg/kg	104.30±6.38	108.72±4.38*	106.20±3.67**	105.09±4.00**

[#]P<0.05,
[##]P<0.01 vs Sham group;
*P<0.05,
**P<0.01 vs Model group.

Table 3. Effects of MHBFC on carotid ASBP, ADBP, AMBP and body weight in pressure-overload rats ($\overline{X} \pm S$, n = 6).

Group	ASBP (kPa)	ADBP (kPa)	AMBP (kPa)	body weight (g)
Sham	16.38±1.06	12.62±1.44	13.53±1.56	303.75±8.87
Model	24.58±2.44##	16.75±1.90##	19.20±1.72##	296.18±6.79
MHBFC 6 mg/kg	22.23±1.06	14.40±1.46*	16.57±1.05**	297.81±6.57
MHBFC 12 mg/kg	19.43±2.57 **§	13.53±1.52**	15.85±1.27**	296.20±7.93
Lisenopril 15 mg/kg	19.78±2.37 **	13.30±1.85**	15.35±2.37**	300.54±10.42

ASBP: aorta systolic blood pressure; ADBP: aorta diastolic blood pressure; AMBP: aortamean blood pressure.
##$P < 0.01$ vs Sham group;
*$P < 0.05$,
**$P < 0.01$ vs Model group;
§$P < 0.05$ vs MHBFC 6 mg/kg.

(Guangxi, China), characterized by UV, IR, ESI-MS, NMR, and X-ray monocrystal diffraction [17,20]. NG-nitro-L-arginine methyl ester (L-NAME) was purchased from Shanghai Yuanye Bio-Technology Co., Ltd. All other chemicals and materials were obtained from local commercial sources.

2.2: Abdominal Aortic Banding Model and Protocol

Male Sprague–Dawley rats with a body weight of 130–160 g were obtained from the Guangxi Medical Laboratory Animal Center. Rats were housed under standard conditions (temperature at 20–25°C, relative humidity at 50–60%). The animal experiments were approved by the Animal Ethics Committee of the Guangxi Medical University and performed in accordance with their guidelines. After surgery, the rats were divided randomly into 7 groups (n = 6): sham-operated group, animals underwent a similar procedure without banding the aorta; model group, pressure-overloaded rats induced by AAB above the renal arteries and treated with distilled water; AAB rats treated with MHBFC 6 or 12 mg kg^{-1}day^{-1}; AAB rats treated with lisinopril, an angiotensin-converting enzyme I (ACEI), 15 mg kg^{-1}day^{-1} (the effects of lisinopril on the LVH that was induced by pressure overload has been well documented. In this study, lisinopril was used as a positive control drug to demonstrate the reliability of AAB rats under our experimental conditions); AAB rats treated with L-NAME 50 mg kg^{-1}day^{-1}; and AAB rats treated with MHBFC 12 mg kg^{-1}day^{-1} plus L-NAME 50 mg kg^{-1}day^{-1}. No significant difference was found among all of the experimental rats in age and body weight before surgery, using a pressure-overload model as described previously with minor modifications [22].

Briefly, the rats were anaesthetized with a 10% chloral hydrate (3 ml kg^{-1}, intraperitoneal injection). Under sterile conditions, the abdominal aorta above the kidneys was exposed through a midline abdominal incision and constricted at the suprarenal level by a 4-0 silk suture tied around both the aorta and a blunted 22 gauge needle, which was then pulled out. A similar procedure was performed for Sham, without the ligature. The drugs were dissolved in distilled water and administered orally via a gastric tube. MHBFC or vehicle was orally administered once a day in 2 mL kg^{-1} for 6 weeks after surgery. At the last day of 0, 2, 4 and 6 weeks, the relevant transducer was connected to a MS 4000 biological signal quantitative analytical system (Longfeida Technology Co., Ltd.), conscious systolic blood pressure (SBP) and heart rates (HRs) were monitored by the tail-cuff method as we described previously [20], and the researchers blinded to the identity of the rats during the recordings. No significant difference was found among all of the experimental groups in body weight, SBP and HRs at 0 week.

2.3: Hemodynamics and Cardiac Remodeling Index

On day 42, all animals were anesthetized with 10% chloral hydrate (3 ml kg^{-1}, intraperitoneal injection), the right carotid arteries were cannulated with a polyethylene catheter that was connected to a Statham transducer, and the mean carotid pressures were measured.

Then, the polyethylene cannula was inserted along the right coronary artery into the left ventricle, and electrodes were plugged in the limbs for electrocardiography. The relevant transducer was connected to an MS 4000 organism signal quantitative analytical

Table 4. Effects of MHBFC on left ventricular function in pressure-overload rats ($\overline{X} \pm S$, n = 6).

Group	HR(beats/min)	LVEDP(kPa)	LVSP(kPa)	+dp/dt$_{max}$(kPa/s)	−dp/dtmax(kPa/s)
Sham	382.3±32.0	4.02±1.24	15.90±1.99	432.00±44.96	404.62±38.46
Model	411.7±33.2	1.18±0.97##	19.72±1.75##	533.95±35.82##	482.58±29.57##
MHBFC 6 mg/kg	379.0±33.4	2.07±0.97	17.45±1.56*	492.22±27.13*	451.12±30.68
MHBFC 12 mg/kg	362.8±40.9*	3.28±1.14**	16.25±1.04**	466.47±47.04*	421.20±28.83**
Lisenopril 15 mg/kg	366.7±32.1*	3.05±1.03**	15.85±1.94**	464.85±38.06**	419.80±19.97**

HR: heart rate; LVSP: left ventricular systolic pressure; LVEDP: left ventricular end-diastolic pressure; +dp/dtmax: maximal rate of left ventricular systolic pressure; −dp/dtmax: maximal rate of left ventricular diastolic pressure.
##$P < 0.01$ vs Sham group;
*$P < 0.05$,
**$P < 0.01$ vs Model group.

Table 5. Effect of MHBFC on aorta remodeling in pressure-overload rats. ($\overline{X}\pm S$, n=6).

Group	TAA/×10³ μm²	LA/×10³ μm²	CSA/×10³ μm²	CSA/TAA/%	AD/μm	Lumen/μm	Media/μm	Media/Lumen/%
Sham	4135.26±388.12	2794.80±253.49	1340.47±275.61	32.26±4.42	2293.01±109.16	1885.26±85.23	203.88±37.95	10.84±2.12
Model	6115.76±668.19##	3713.86±456.52##	2401.90±240.50##	39.34±1.72##	2787.69±153.14##	2171.62±134.66##	308.04±17.51##	14.21±0.92##
MHBFC 6 mg/kg	5191.13±656.23*	3312.68±469.27	1878.44±206.92**	36.29±1.85*	2567.12±165.47*	2049.72±149.55	258.70±14.90**	12.66±0.93*
MHBFC 12 mg/kg	4418.90±815.12**	2962.43±559.09*	1456.47±259.56**$	32.99±0.81**$$	2364.39±215.87**	1935.63±180.40*	214.38±18.80**$$	11.08±0.37**$$
Lisenopril 15 mg/kg	4496.72±448.41**	3061.18±323.87*	1435.55±145.42**	31.96±1.46**	2390.94±118.50**	1972.41±104.92*	209.26±12.77**	10.62±0.64**

TAA: Area of total aorta; LA: Area of lumen; CSA: cross-sectional area; AD: aorta diameter.
##$p<0.01$ vs Sham group;
*$p<0.05$,
**$p<0.01$ vs Model group;
$$p<0.05$,
$$$p<0.01$ vs MHBFC 6 mg/kg.

system (Longfeida Technology Co., Ltd.), and the hemodynamic parameters (including HR, SP, DP, AP, LVSP, LVEDP, +dp/dtmax, and −dp/dtmax) were recorded.

Thereafter, blood samples were collected and animals were killed by exsanguination. The thoracic cavity was opened to expose the still-beating heart. The hearts and lungs were rapidly removed, rinsed in ice-cold 0.9% NaCl solution, blotted, and weighed. The heart-weight index (HW/BW) was calculated by dividing heart weight by body weight, and then the left ventricles (including interventricular septum) and right ventricular free walls were collected separately and weighed. The left ventricular-weight index (LVW/BW), right ventricular-weight index (RVW/BW), and lung index (LW/BW) were then calculated.

2.4: Histological Analysis

The hearts were immersion-fixed in neutral 10% buffered formalin, and paraffin sections (5 mm) were cut. The myocyte cross-sectional area and myocardial fibrosis were quantitatively analyzed with the Image J2× software. For the measurement of the cross-sectional area, 50 cells (per animal, in hematoxylin and eosin stain, ×400) from the left ventricular lateral-mid free wall (including epicardial and endocardial portions) were randomly selected and analyzed. Myocardial fibrosis in the tissue sections was quantitatively analyzed by morphometry in two ways (in Masson's trichrome stained sections, ×100): (i) The perivascular fibrosis of arteries was evaluated in short-axis images of intramuscular arteries and arterioles (at least 10 per animal). The area occupied by the artery (A) and the area of fibrosis surrounding the artery (B) were traced and calculated. The perivascular fibrosis index was defined as B/A. (ii) The collagen in myocardial interstitial spaces, excluding perivascular areas, was visualized, and the whole areas of the sections were scanned. The total interstitial fibrosis index was defined as the sum of the total area of collagen in the entire visual field, divided by the sum of total connective tissue area, plus the myocardial area in the entire visual field. All of the images were digitalized and transformed into binary images, and the areas occupied by collagen were calculated by an automatic area-quantification program in the Image J2× software.

After treatment for 6 weeks, the animals were killed, the sections at the same spot along the aorta were obtained and the structural changes of aorta were investigated using a light microscope. The total aortic area (TAA), lumen area (LA), cross-sectional area (CSA), aorta diameter (AD), luminal radius (L), and media thickness (M) of aorta were recorded under a light microscope, and the ratio of M/L was calculated.

2.5: Nitric Oxide, Endothelin-1, and Hydroxyproline Measurement

Within 30 s after collection, heparinized blood was centrifuged for 10 min at 3000 rpm, and all samples were stored at −80°C until assayed. Because of its instability in physiological solutions, most of the NO is rapidly converted to nitrite (NO_2^-) and further to nitrate (NO_3^-). Plasma levels of NO_2^-/NO_3^- were measured using a NO detection kit according to the manufacturer's instructions. Briefly, nitrate was converted to nitrite using aspergillus nitrite reductase, and the total nitrite was measured with the Griess reagent. The absorbance was determined at 540 nm with a spectrophotometer. ET-1 was measured using a rat Endothelin 1 Elisa kit (CUSABIO BIOTECH Co., Ltd.) according to the manufacturer's instructions. The contents of hydroxyproline in cardiac muscle were measured using a commercial kit (Nanjing Jiancheng Bioengineering Institute, Nanjing, China) according to the manufacturer's instructions.

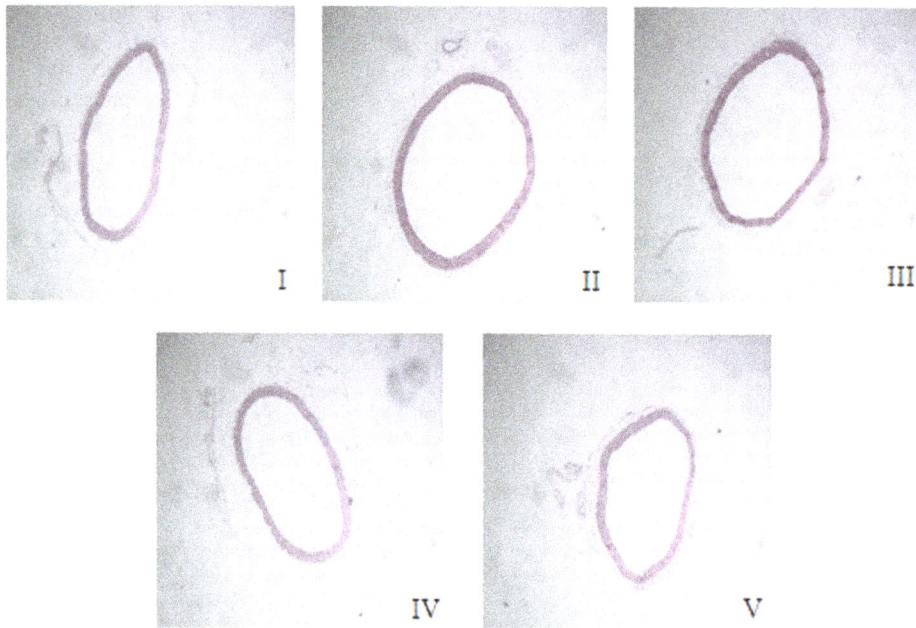

Figure 1. Representative figure of aorta remodeling in different groups. I: Sham group; II: Model group; III: MHBFC 6 mg kg^{-1} group; IV: MHBFC 12 mg kg^{-1} group; V: Lisinopril 15 mg kg^{-1} group. The hypertensive vascular remodelling was observed by increases in the area of the total aorta, aorta lumen and aorta cross-sectional, which could be prevented by treatment with MHBFC at all doses for 6 weeks.

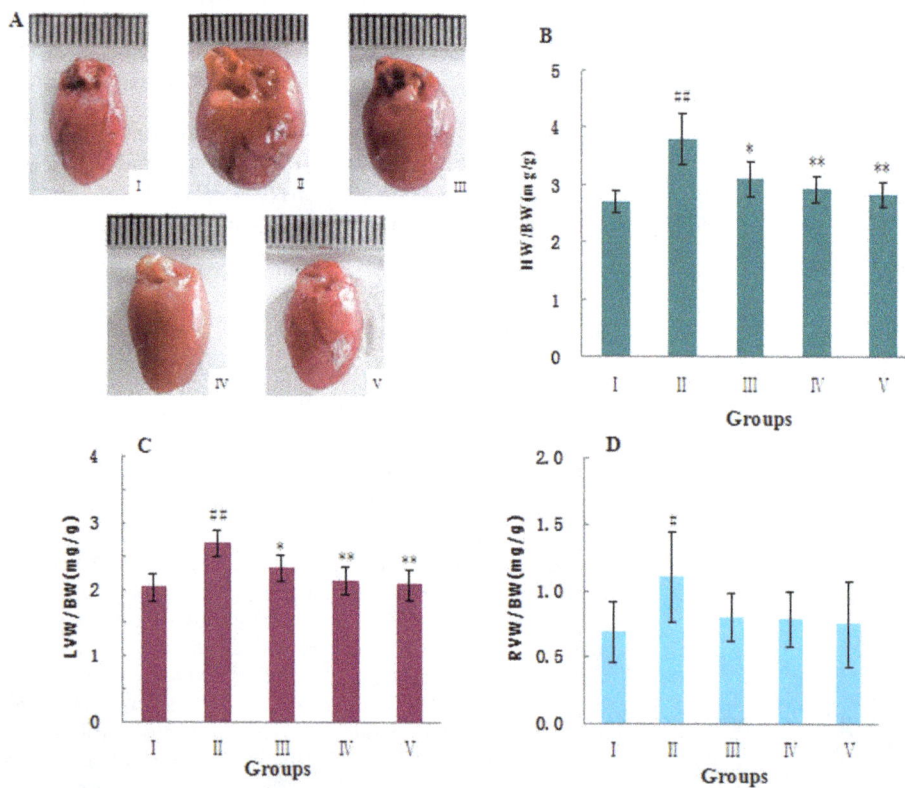

Figure 2. Effects of MHBFC on HW, HW/BW, LVW/BW, and RVW/BW in pressure-overload rats. (A) Representative figure of heart macroscopic image; (B–D) statistic results. I: Sham group; II: Model group; III: MHBFC 6 mg kg^{-1} group; IV: MHBFC 12 mg kg^{-1} group; V: Lisinopril 15 mg kg^{-1} group. Cardiac hypertrophy was characterized by increases in the HW/BW, LVW/BW, and RVW/BW ratios, which could be reversed by MHBFC at all doses for 6 weeks. The data are expressed as the mean±SD, n = 6. [#]P<0.05, [##]P<0.01 vs. Sham group; *P<0.05, **P<0.01 vs. Model group.

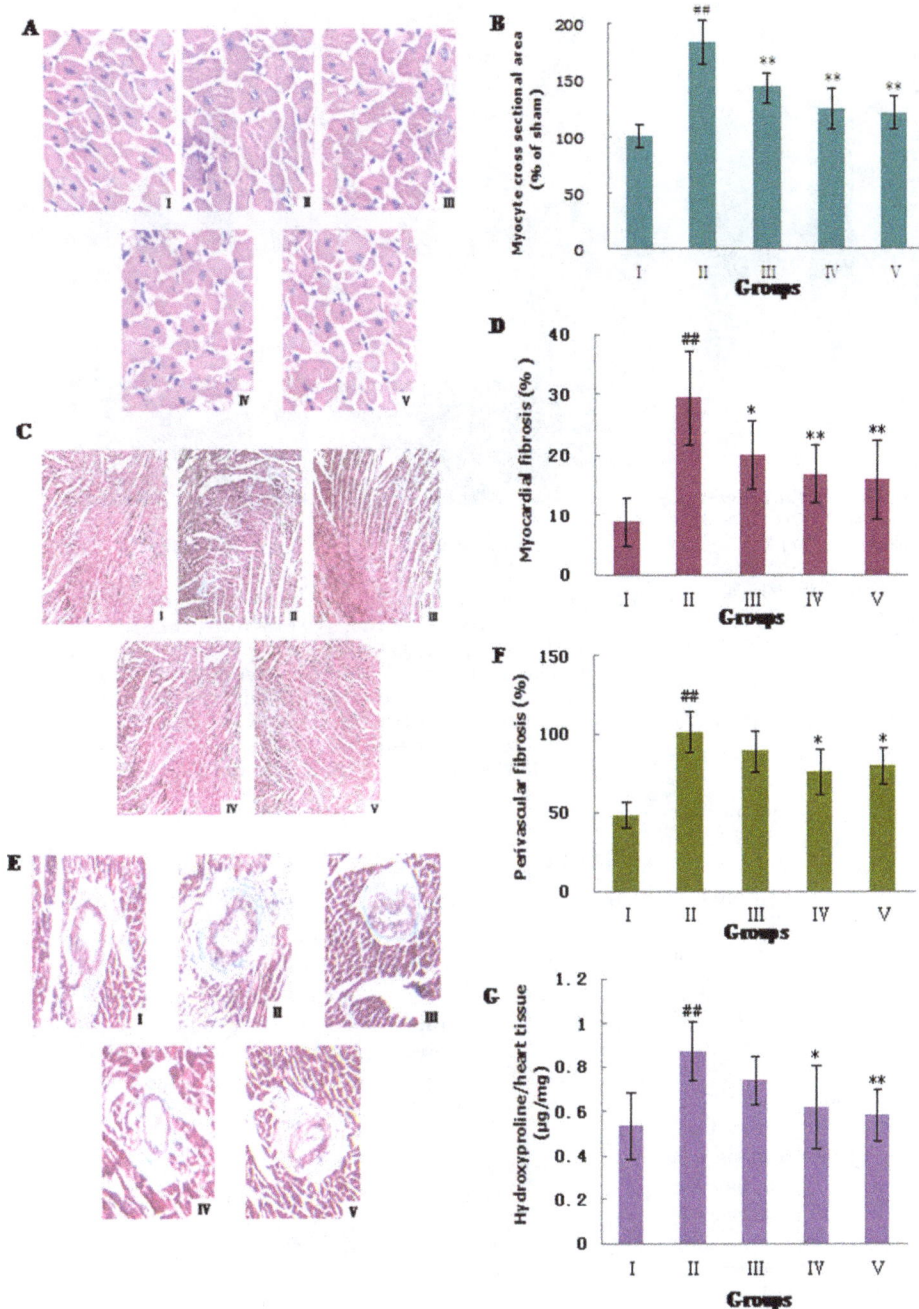

Figure 3. Effects of MHBFC on myocyte cross-sectional area, myocardial fibrosis, perivascular fibrosis, and hydroxyproline content in cardiac tissue of pressure-overload rats. (A) Representative figure of myocyte cross-section (HE stain, ×400); (B) statistic results of myocyte cross-section area; (C) representative figure of myocardial fibrosis (Masson's stain, ×100); (D) statistic results of myocardial fibrosis; (E) representative figure of perivascular fibrosis (Masson's stain, ×100); (F) statistic results of perivascular fibrosis; (G) hydroxyproline content in cardiac tissue. I: Sham group; II: Model group; III: MHBFC 6 mg kg^{-1} group; IV: MHBFC 12 mg kg^{-1} group; V: Lisinopril 15 mg kg^{-1} group. The myocyte cross-sectional area, levels of myocardial and perivascular fibrosis, and the hydroxyproline content all increased significantly when compared with the sham-operated rats. MHBFC at dose of 12 mg/kg for 6 weeks could reverse all these pathological changes in LVH parameters, and MHBFC at dose of 6 mg/kg for 6 weeks could reduced the myocyte cross-sectional area and level of myocardial fibrosis. The data are expressed as the mean±SD, n = 6. #P<0.05, ##P<0.01 vs. Sham group; *P<0.05, **P<0.01 vs. Model group.

2.6: Immunohistochemistry of Endothelial Nitric Oxide Synthase, Endothelin Receptor A, and Endothelin Receptor B Expression

Immunohistochemical staining was performed using an Ultra-Sensitive TM S-P kit according to the manufacturer's instructions.

Briefly, the sections were deparaffinized and microwave-treated for 10 min twice in 10 mM sodium citrate (pH 6.0). Endogenous peroxidase was blocked by incubating the sections in endogenous peroxidase blocking solution for 10 min at room temperature. Rabbit polyclonal antibodies against endothelial NO synthase (eNOS), endothelin receptor A (ET$_A$), and endothelin receptor B

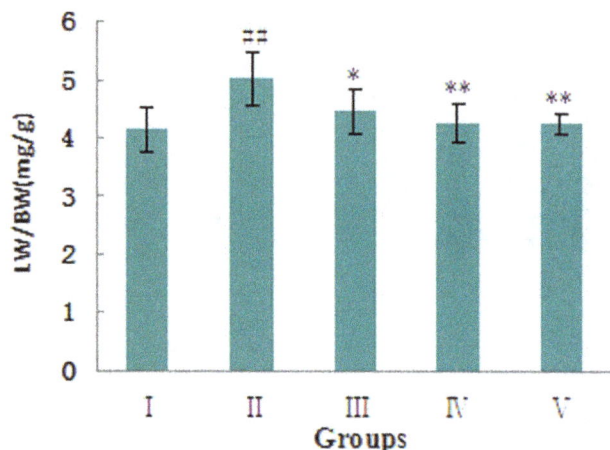

Figure 4. Effects of MHBFC on lung index (LW/BW) in pressure-overload rats. I: Sham group; II: Model group; III: MHBFC 6 mg kg^{-1} group; IV: MHBFC 12 mg kg^{-1} group; V: Lisinopril 15 mg kg^{-1} group. The LW/BW ratio increased when compared with sham-operated rats, which could be completely reversed by treatment with MHBFC at all doses for 6 weeks. The data are expressed as the mean±SD, n=6. [#]P<0.05, [##]P<0.01 vs. Sham group; [*]P<0.05, [**]P<0.01 vs. Model group.

(ET$_B$) proteins were used as primary antibodies in a 1:100 dilution at 4°C for 18 h. After washing three times with phosphate-buffered saline (PBS), sections were incubated with biotin-conjugated anti-rabbit secondary antibody for 10 min. The sections were then washed three times with PBS, treated with streptavidin-peroxidase for 10 min, and then washed again with PBS three times. Lastly, the specimens were incubated in diaminobenzidine for 5 min, followed by hematoxylin counter-staining. Images from all sections were acquired using a digital camera system. Confocal images were then transferred to a personal computer using the image analysis software package Image J2×.

2.7: Reverse Transcription-polymerase Chain Reaction

Total RNA was extracted from the LV tissue of rats using TRIzol reagent according to the manufacturer's instructions. The total RNA was then converted to cDNA using reverse transcriptase with random hexamer priming. PCR was performed by standard methods, as described in a previous report [22], using synthetic gene-specific primers for ANP, ET-1, endothelin-converting enzyme (ECE), and β-Actin (Table 1). The parallel amplification of rat β-Actin was performed for reference, and the intensity of each band was quantified using densitometry. The intensity of each gene band was expressed relative to the corresponding densities of the β-Actin bands from the same RNA samples.

2.8: Statistical Analysis

The results were presented as the means ± SD, and a statistical analysis was performed with the Sigma Stat (version 13.0) statistical program (SPSS Inc., Chicago, IL, USA). Differences between groups were tested for statistical significance using a one-way analysis of variance (ANOVA) performed with S-N-K post-test. Differences were considered statistically significant at P-values that were less than 0.05.

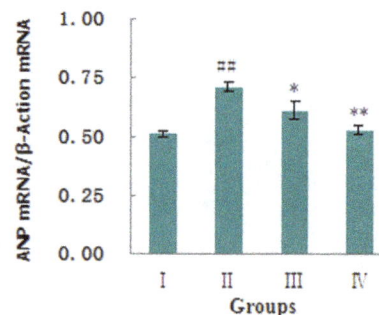

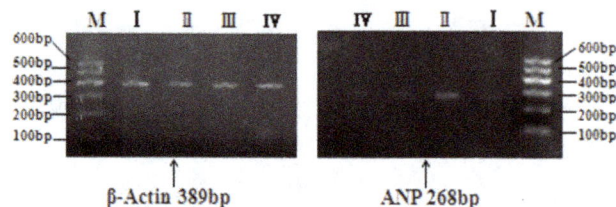

Figure 5. Effects of MHBFC on atrial natriuretic peptide (ANP) mRNA expression in LV tissue of pressure-overload rats. I: Sham group; II: Model group; III: MHBFC 6 mg kg^{-1} group; IV: MHBFC 12 mg kg^{-1} group. ANP is the molecular marker of heart failure. The ANP mRNAs were overexpressed compared with sham-operated rats, which could be completely reversed by treatment with MHBFC at all doses for 6 weeks. The data are expressed as the mean±SD, n=3. [#]P<0.05, [##]P<0.01 vs. Sham group; [*]P<0.05, [**]P<0.01 vs. Model group.

Results

3.1: Hemodynamic Effects of MHBFC

After applying AAB above the renal arteries, the HR and SBP didn't show significant difference between the groups at 0 week but increased significantly at 2, 4 and 6 weeks compared with sham-operated rats. MHBFC, at the daily oral doses of 6 and 12 mg kg^{-1} for 6 weeks, prevented increases in HR and SBP (Table 2). The carotid arterial pressure and cardiac functions were measured 6 weeks after AAB. As shown in Table 3, compared with those measurements in sham-operated rats, right carotid aorta systolic blood pressure (ASBP), diastolic blood pressure (ADBP) and aorta mean blood pressure (AMBP) were significantly elevated in AAB-treated rats. These features were prevented by treatment with MHBFC at all doses for 6 weeks. The measurements of the in vivo function of LV for all groups are shown in Table 4. Systolic cardiac parameters, including LVSP, +dp/dt_{max} and diastolic cardiac parameter −dp/dt_{max}, were all significantly elevated in AAB-treated rats. In contrast, LVEDP decreased significantly. These changes could also be prevented by treatment with MHBFC.

3.2: MHBFC Reverses the Aortic Remodeling that was Induced by a Pressure Overload

The hypertensive vascular remodeling of the upper thoracic aorta that was exposed to a pressure overload by narrowing the abdominal aorta was observed 6 weeks after AAB. The values of the area of the TAA, LA, CSA, AR, Lumen, Media and M/L ratio of the aorta in AAB-treated rats increased significantly compared with sham-operated rats. These changes could be prevented by treatment with MHBFC at all doses for 6 weeks (Table 5, Figure 1).

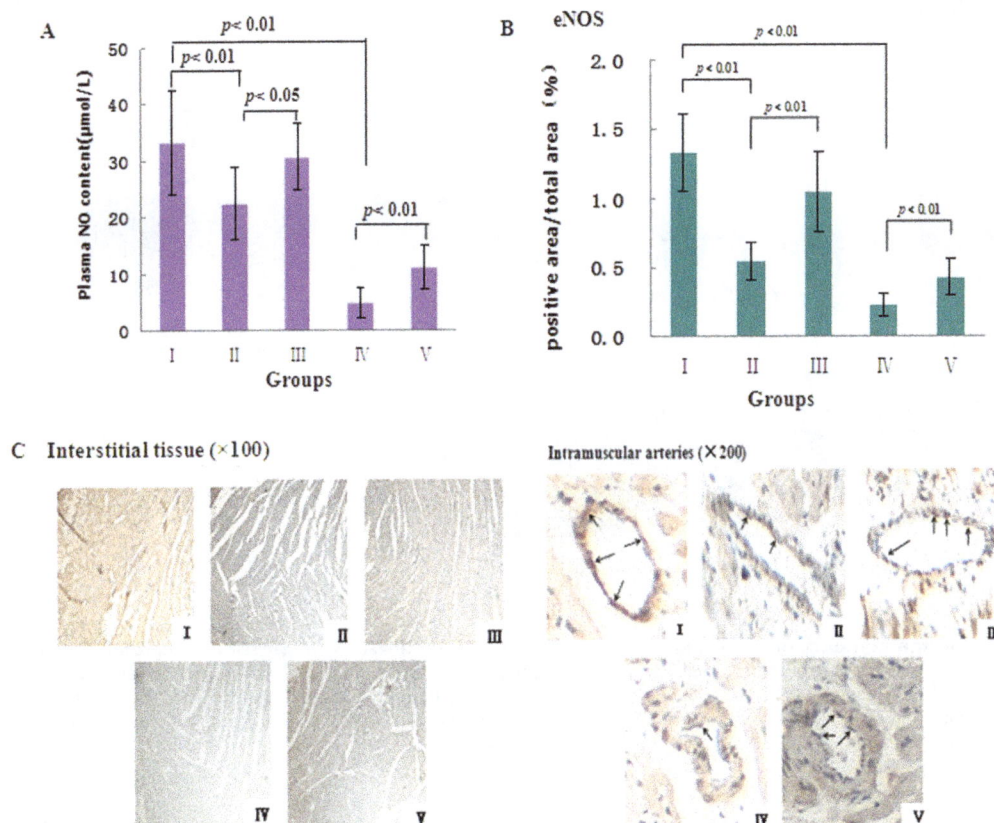

Figure 6. Effects of MHBFC on plasma nitric oxide content (A), endothelial nitric oxide synthase (eNOS) protein (B and C) expression in cardiac tissue of pressure-overload rats. I: Sham group; II:Model group; III: MHBFC 12 mg/kg group; IV: L-NAME 50 mg/kg; V: MHBFC 12 mg/kg +L-NAME 50 mg/kg; M, marker. (C) eNOS protein expression tested with immunohistology stain in interstitial tissue of myocardium and intramuscular arteries in hearts. Compared with the sham-operated rats, the plasma nitric oxide levels and the eNOS protein expression levels in the AAB-treated rat hearts decreased significantly, and this decrease could be prevented by treatment with MHBFC at 12 mg kg^{-1}. L-NAME at 50 mg kg^{-1} could abolish these facilitatory effects of MHBFC. The data are expressed as the mean±SD, n = 3–6. #P<0.05, ##P<0.01 vs. Sham group; *P<0.05, **P<0.01 vs. Model group.

3.3: MHBFC Improves the Left Ventricular Hypertrophy Induced by a Pressure Overload

Results for all groups at 6 weeks after AAB are shown in Figure 2. LVH was characterized by increases in the HW/BW and LVW/BW ratios, whereas the BW showed no significant difference between groups (Table 3). The histology of the hearts from the AAB-treated rats showed that the myocyte cross-sectional area as well as the levels of myocardial and perivascular fibrosis all increased significantly compared with the sham-operated rats (Figure 3A–F). The hydroxyproline content reflected the collagen level in cardiac tissue, and the degree of myocardial fibrosis increased by 64.78% in AAB-treated rats when compared with sham-operated controls (Figure 3G). MHBFC at dose of 12 mg/kg for 6 weeks could reverse all these pathological changes in LVH parameters, and MHBFC at dose of 6 mg/kg for 6 weeks could reduce the myocyte cross-sectional area and level of myocardial fibrosis.

3.4: MHBFC Prevents the Progression of Hypertrophy to Cardiac Failure

The initiation and transition from LVH to heart failure in AAB-treated rats is characterized by right ventricular hypertrophy, pulmonary congestion and overexpression of ANP, which is a molecular marker for heart failure. [23] The RVW/BW

(Figure 2D) and LW/BW (Figure 4) ratios were increased, and the ANP mRNAs (Figures 5) were overexpressed when compared with sham-operated rats. These changes could be completely reversed by treatment with MHBFC at all doses for 6 weeks.

3.5: Endothelial Mechanisms

A battery of tests was performed to investigate the endothelial mechanisms by which MHBFC reverses cardiac remodeling in the AAB-treated rats.

3.5.1: Nitric oxide pathway. The plasma NO levels of AAB-treated rats decreased significantly 6 weeks after AAB (P<0.01), and this decrease could be prevented by treatment with MHBFC (Figure 6A). L-NAME (50 mg kg^{-1}), which is an inhibitor of NOS, could abolish these facilitatory effects of MHBFC (Figure 6A). Compared with the sham-operated rats, the eNOS protein expression levels in the AAB-treated rat hearts decreased significantly (P<0.01). MHBFC at 12 mg/kg significantly increased the eNOS protein expression levels (P<0.01 vs. model), which could also be abolished by treatment with L-NAME (Figure 6B–C). Thus, the enhanced NO signaling system, which was induced by MHBFC treatment, might be responsible for reversing the cardiac remodeling that was induced by a pressure overload.

3.5.2: Endothelin pathway. The plasma concentrations and the gene expression levels of ET-1 and ECE increased significantly

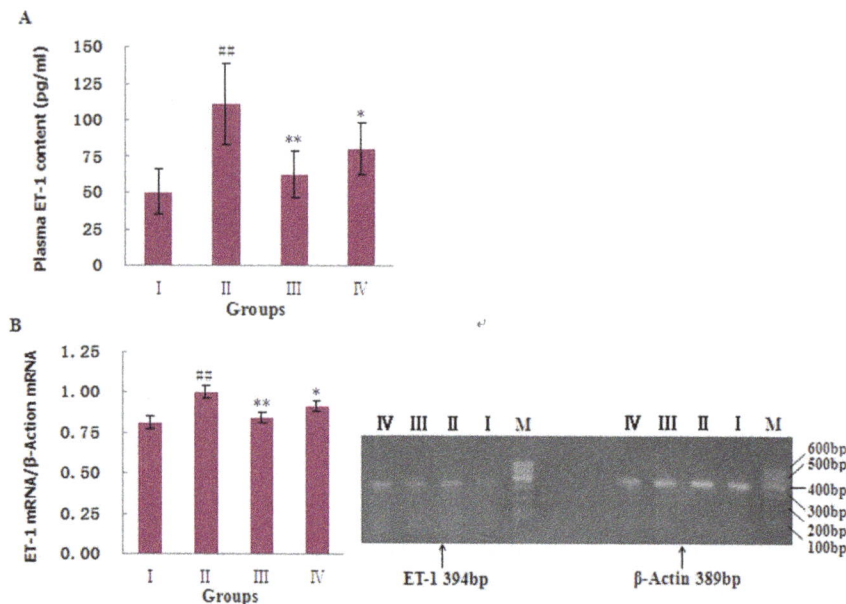

Figure 7. Effects of MHBFC on plasma contents of endothelin-1(ET-1) (A), and ET-1 mRNA (B) expression in cardiac tissue of pressure-overload rats. I: Sham group; II: Model group; III: MHBFC 12 mg kg^{-1} group; IV: MHBFC 6 mg kg^{-1} group; M, marker. The plasma contents and gene expression levels of ET-1 increased significantly 6 weeks after abdominal aortic banding. Treatment with MHBFC for 6 weeks at all doses significantly decreased the plasma contents and overexpression of ET-1 in cardiac tissue to nearly normal levels. The data are expressed as the mean±SD, n = 3–6. $^{\#}P<0.05$, $^{\#\#}P<0.01$ vs. Sham group; $^{*}P<0.05$, $^{**}P<0.01$ vs. Model group.

6 weeks after AAB (P<0.01; Figures 7 and 8A). The cardiac tissue protein levels of ET$_A$ and ET$_B$, as measured by immunohisto-chemistry, also increased significantly in the AAB-treated rats (P< 0.01; Figure 8B–C). Thus, pressure overloading in the AAB-treated rats caused increased synthesis and release of ET-1, as well as increased expression levels of endothelin receptors. Treatment with MHBFC for 6 weeks significantly decreased the elevated plasma levels of ET-1, the overexpression of ET-1 and ECE genes, and the increased production of ET$_A$ and ET$_B$ proteins in cardiac tissue to nearly normal levels (Figures 8). Thus, MHBFC appeared to counteract the cardiac remodeling, which was induced by a pressure overload, by inhibiting the endothelin signaling system.

Discussion

Most hypertensive animals that are used in various models of hypertension develop cardiac hypertrophy leading to heart failure, which has been characterized extensively, parallel with the rise in blood pressure. Examples of such models are various types of hypertensive rats (in particular, the spontaneously hypertensive rat) and rats, guinea pigs or ferrets that are subjected to aortic or pulmonary artery banding [24]. In this model, the abdominal aorta is banded above the renal arteries in rats to induce cardiovascular remodeling and hypertension [25]. Early hypertension arises from the activation of the renin–angiotensin system (RAS), and compensatory LVH develops, which eventually leads to heart failure. In the present experiment, decompensatory cardiac remodeling was characterized by pulmonary congestion and right ventricular hypertrophy (RVH) 6 weeks after AAB [21,22]. This AAB rat model was characterized by LVH, LV functional disorders, pulmonary congestion, and RVH, along with hypertension.

MHBFC is a new compound that we have isolated and identified from a 60% ethanol extract of the MKL root. Our previous studies have demonstrated that extracts of MKL roots

have antihypertensive, antioxidative, anti-inflammatory effects [13–16]. However, the possible clinical use of MHBFC for the treatment of hypertensive heart disease has not been studied. Using an aortic stenosis model, this study is the first to evaluate the improvement by MHBFC on cardiovascular remodeling induced by pressure overloading. The results suggest that MHBFC can prevent hypertension, cardiovascular remodeling, and the progression of cardiac hypertrophy to heart failure, which is induced by pressure overloading. Thus, MHBFC might be a suitable therapy for patients with hypertensive heart disease.

LVH has been recognized as an important cardiovascular risk factor. Hypertensive disease is the most frequent background of LVH, and it is generally felt that anti-hypertensive treatment should not only lower blood pressure but also cause the regression of LVH [2,26]. That MHBFC improved LVH in our study indicates that MHBFC is beneficial against hypertensive cardiovascular events; this result is promising because an antihypertensive drug that can decrease BP effectively does not necessarily mean that it can reverse LVH. LVH is the one of the major causes of heart failure [27,28], and because ANP plays an important role in the regulation of cardiovascular homeostasis that maintains blood pressure, ANP has emerged as a potentially important clinical biomarker of LVH [29,30]. In the present study, the finding of pulmonary congestion, RVH, and the overexpression of ANP mRNAs indicated that cardiac functions were decompensatory in this rat model and that LVH progressed gradually to heart failure. MHBFC could effectively prevent this progression; therefore, MHBFC might be beneficial against hypertensive heart disease and congestive heart failure.

Hypertension evokes detrimental changes in the arterial vessel wall that facilitate stiffening and thus lead to a further rise in mean blood pressure, eventually causing heart failure [31]. Here, we observed hypertensive vascular remodeling of the upper thoracic aorta that was exposed to a pressure overload and systemic hypertension that was induced by narrowing the abdominal aorta;

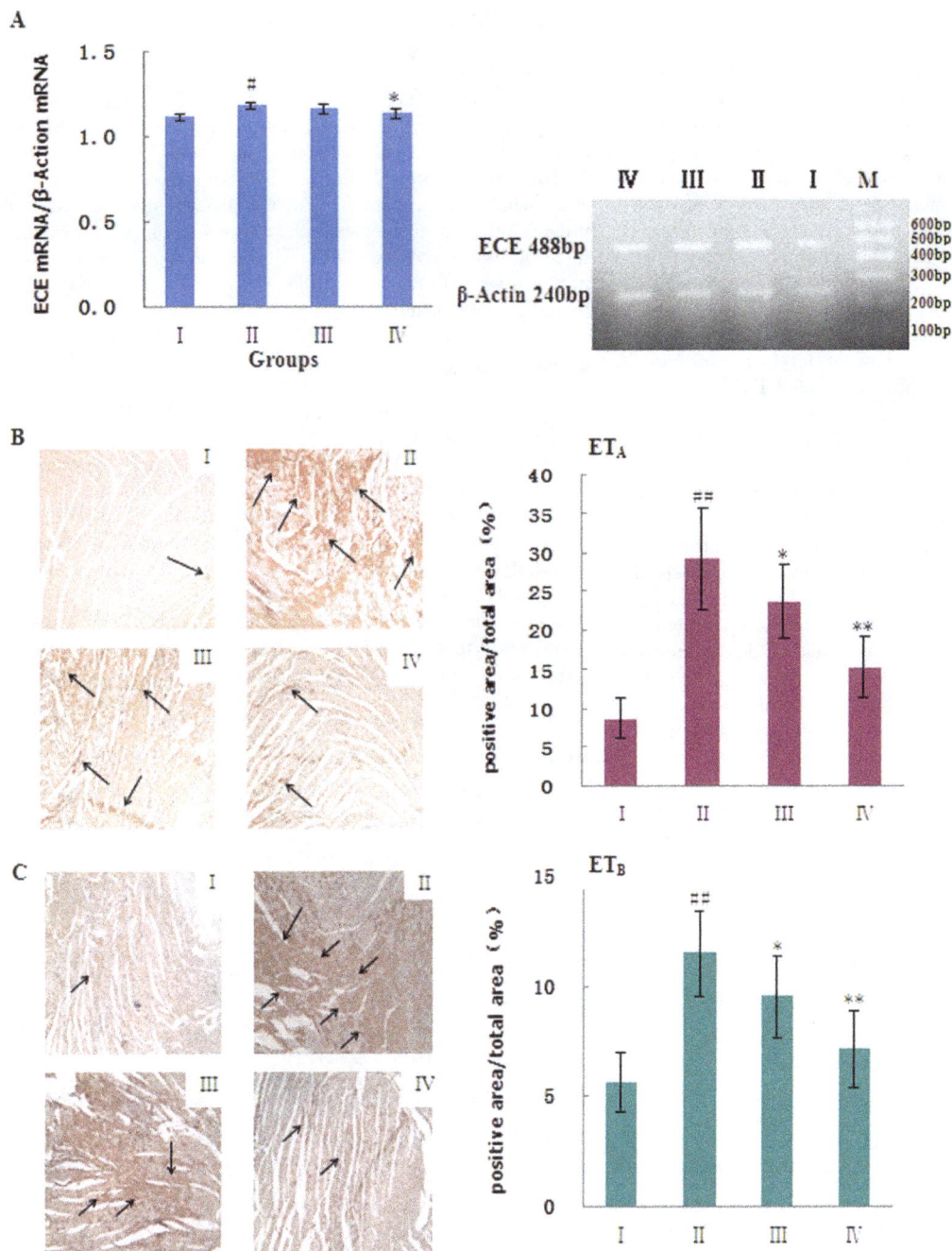

Figure 8. Effects of MHBFC on endothelin-converting enzyme (ECE) mRNA (A), endothelin receptor A (ET$_A$) (B, immunohistology stain, ×100), and endothelin receptor B (ET$_B$) (C, immunohistology stain, ×100) expression in cardiac tissue of pressure-overload rats. I: Sham group; II: Model group; III: MHBFC 6 mg kg^{-1} group; IV: MHBFC 12 mg kg^{-1} group; M, marker. The gene expression levels of ECE and the cardiac tissue protein levels of ET$_A$ and ET$_B$ measured by immunohistochemistry increased significantly 6 weeks after abdominal aortic banding. Treatment with MHBFC for 6 weeks significantly decreased the overexpression of ECE genes and the increased production of ET$_A$ and ET$_B$ proteins in cardiac tissue to nearly normal levels. The data are expressed as the mean±SD, n = 3–6. $^{#}P<0.05$, $^{##}P<0.01$ vs. Sham group; $^{*}P<0.05$, $^{**}P<0.01$ vs. Model group.

these symptoms could be reversed by treatment with MHBFC. These results suggest that MHBFC can reverse both cardiac remodeling and vascular modeling.

The dysfunction of the endothelium has been implicated in the pathophysiology of different forms of cardiovascular disease, including hypertension, coronary artery disease, chronic heart failure, peripheral artery disease etc. The pathophysiological mechanisms of endothelial dysfunction were related to a decrease in the bioavailability of NO as well as from augmented ET-1 synthesis, release, or activity [6]. Because the dysregulation of the NO and endothelin systems is important in the pathogenesis of cardiac remodeling, restoring the balance between NO and ET-1 may be an attractive therapeutic strategy for cardiac remodeling. The pathogenesis of many cardiovascular diseases is associated with reduced nitric oxide (NO) bioavailability and/or increased endothelial NO synthase (eNOS)-dependent superoxide formation. In the cardiovascular system, the signaling molecule NO, which is produced by the enzyme eNOS, has a crucial role in maintaining normal vascular function, which is mediated by its vasodilating capacity and through a variety of antiatherogenic effects [32,33]. There is evidence demonstrating that pharmacological interventions that are designed to increase eNOS-derived NO constitute a promising therapeutic approach for the amelioration of postinfarction ventricular remodeling and heart failure [34].

Endothelin (ET-1, in particular) is regarded as an autocrine/paracrine factor in the development of cardiac hypertrophy both in vivo and in vitro [35]. The actions of ET-1 are mediated through the activation of the G-protein-coupled ET_A and ET_B receptors, which are found in a variety of cells in the cardiovascular system. Based on the biological effects that are induced by ET-1, including profound vasoconstriction, proinflammatory actions, mitogenic, proliferative, and fibrotic effects, ET-1 is implicated as an important factor in the development of cardiac hypertrophy and heart failure [36,37]. ET-1 and the ET_A and ET_B receptors have been implicated in the pathogenesis of hypertension and in cardiac remodeling. For this reason, endothelin receptor antagonists, which are now becoming available, are being investigated as potential anti-proliferative agents [35].

In the present study, we found that MHBFC could improve the function of the NO signaling system through increasing the gene and protein expression of eNOS, resulting in augmented serum NO contents. This drug also modulated the endothelin signaling system by suppressing the synthesis and release of endothelin into the blood, which diminishes the expression of ET_A and ET_B in cardiac tissue, as well by as inhibiting the responses to endothelin.

Thus, MHBFC could restore the balance between the NO and endothelin signaling systems in situations of endothelial dysfunction, resulting in endothelial protection. Furthermore, our previous studies have showed that MHBFC has potential therapeutic efficacy on the in vitro cardiocyte apoptosis model and in vivo myocardial ischemia rat model [20], Therefore, MHBFC might directly affect on the cardiomyocyte through its endothelial pathway and prevent the pressure overload-induced progression of cardiac hypertrophy to cardiac failure, but whether these effects are secondary to its effects on the vascular system have not been very clear now, and the possible mechanisms remain to be further investigated.

Conclusions

In conclusion, the present study has shown that MHBFC offers cardiac antihypertrophic properties and helps maintain hemodynamic homeostasis. MHBFC counteracted cardiac hypertrophy and prevented the progression of cardiac hypertrophy to cardiac failure that was induced by a pressure overload. The molecular mechanism was related to its regulation of endothelial function, including the augmentation of NO release and inhibition of the ET-1 system. The further mechanisms that MHBFC interferes with the pressure overload-induced progression of cardiac hypertrophy to cardiac failure will be investigate in our further research, for example the eNOS knock-out mouse model will be used to clarify if the effects of MHBFC are eNOS dependent.

Author Contributions

Conceived and designed the experiments: JH RH. Performed the experiments: JH XT XL QW SZ FX JJ. Analyzed the data: JH XT XL. Contributed reagents/materials/analysis tools: XT JJ XL RH. Wrote the paper: JH.

References

1. Mc Murray A (2008) Combined Therapy with Angiotensin-Converting Enzyme Inhibitors and Calcium Channel Blockers is the Treatment of Choice to Reduce Cardiovascular Risk in Patients with Hypertension. Revista argentina de cardiologia 76(4): 295–299.
2. Van Zwieten P (2000) The influence of antihypertensive drug treatment on the prevention and regression of left ventricular hypertrophy. Cardiovascular research 45: 82–91.
3. Frohlich ED (2001) Local Hemodynamic Changes in Hypertension Insights for Therapeutic Preservation of Target Organs. Hypertension 38: 1388–1394.
4. Scherrer-Crosbie M, Ullrich R, Bloch KD, Nakajima H, Nasseri B, et al. (2001) Endothelial nitric oxide synthase limits left ventricular remodeling after myocardial infarction in mice. Circulation 104: 1286–1291.
5. Kobayashi N, Mori Y, Nakano S, Tsubokou Y, Shirataki H, et al. (2001) Celiprolol stimulates endothelial nitric oxide synthase expression and improves myocardial remodeling in deoxycorticosterone acetate-salt hypertensive rats. J Hypertens 19: 795–801.
6. Endemann DH, Schiffrin EL (2004) Endothelial dysfunction. Journal of the American Society of Nephrology 15: 1983–1992.
7. Schiffrin EL, Park JB, Intengan HD, Touyz RM (2000) Correction of arterial structure and endothelial dysfunction in human essential hypertension by the angiotensin receptor antagonist losartan. Circulation 101: 1653–1659.
8. Schiffrin EL, Park JB, Pu Q (2002) Effect of crossing over hypertensive patients from a beta-blocker to an angiotensin receptor antagonist on resistance artery structure and on endothelial function. J Hypertens 20: 71–78.
9. Schiffrin EL (1996) Correction of remodeling and function of small arteries in human hypertension by cilazapril, an angiotensin I-converting enzyme inhibitor. Journal of cardiovascular pharmacology 27: 13–18.
10. Chen X, Touyz RM, Park JB, Schiffrin EL (2001) Antioxidant effects of vitamins C and E are associated with altered activation of vascular NADPH oxidase and superoxide dismutase in stroke-prone SHR. Hypertension 38: 606–611.
11. Taddei S, Virdis A, Ghiadoni L, Magagna A, Salvetti A (1998) Vitamin C improves endothelium-dependent vasodilation by restoring nitric oxide activity in essential hypertension. Circulation 97: 2222–2229.
12. Heitzer T, Schlinzig T, Krohn K, Meinertz T, Münzel T (2001) Endothelial dysfunction, oxidative stress, and risk of cardiovascular events in patients with coronary artery disease. Circulation 104: 2673–2678.
13. Huang RB, Jiao Y, Jiang WZ (2003) Effect of Yulangsan extract on the cardiac hemodynamics and the coronary flow in rats. Chinese Journal of Hospital Pharmacy 6: 726–727.
14. Huang RB, Lv JH, Zhang XD (2010) Effects of yulangsan flavonoids on myocardial ischemia reperfusion injury in isolated rat hearts. West China Journal of Pharmaceutical Sciences 25(3): 287–289.
15. Huang YH, Chen J, Huang RB, Lin X, Wang NP (2008) Anti-inflammatory effect of Yulangsan extracts and the mechanisms. Chinese Journal of New Drugs 20: 1764–1767.
16. Jiao Y, Duan XQ, Huang RB (2004) Scavenging and inhibiting effect of Yulangsan extract on superoxide anion free radical and hydroxy free radical. Journal of Guangxi Medical University 1: 22–23.
17. Jian J, Huang JC, Jao Y, Tan HD, Huang RB (2011) Isolation and preparation of chalcone compounds from tuber of Millettia pulchra var. laxior by pre-HPLC. Chinese Traditional Herbal Drugs 42(7): 1313–1316.
18. Jian J, Li YW, Jiang WZ, Huang RB (2009) The effect of two chalcone monomers from Yulangsan on scavenging free radicals. Chinese Journal of Gerontology 29(18): 73–74.
19. Jian J, Liu X, Huang RB, Jiang WZ (2009) Protection and its mechanism of two flavone morphons from Yulangsan on hypoxia-reoxygenation induced injury in myocardial cells. Chinese Pharmacological Bulletin 7: 942–945.
20. Jian J, Qing FZ, Zhang SJ, Huang JC, Huang RB (2012) The effect of 17-methoxyl-7-hydroxy-benzene-furanchalcone isolated from Millettia Pulchra on myocardial ischemia in vitro and in vivo. Planta Medica 78 (12): 1324–1331.
21. Dhalla NS, Golfman L, Liu X, Sasaki H, Elimban V, et al. (1999) Subcellular Remodeling and Heart Dysfunction in Cardiac Hypertrophy due to Pressure Overloada. Annals of the New York Academy of Sciences 874: 100–110.
22. Gao S, Long CL, Wang RH, Wang H (2009) K_{ATP} activation prevents progression of cardiac hypertrophy to failure induced by pressure overload via protecting endothelial function. Cardiovascular research 83: 444–456.
23. Grantham JA, Burnett Jr JC (1997) BNP: increasing importance in the pathophysiology and diagnosis of congestive heart failure. Circulation 96: 388.
24. Friberg P, Nordlander M (1990) Influence of left ventricular and coronary vascular hypertrophy on cardiac performance. J Hypertens 8: 879–889.
25. Owens GK, Reidy MA (1985) Hyperplastic growth response of vascular smooth muscle cells following induction of acute hypertension in rats by aortic coarctation. Circulation research 57: 695–705.

26. Savage D, Garrison R, Kannel W, Levy D, Anderson S, et al. (1987) The spectrum of left ventricular hypertrophy in a general population sample: the Framingham Study. Circulation 75: I26.

27. Berk BC, Fujiwara K, Lehoux S (2007) ECM remodeling in hypertensive heart disease. Journal of Clinical Investigation 117: 568–575.

28. Benjamin EJ, Levy D (1999) Why is left ventricular hypertrophy so predictive of morbidity and mortality? The American journal of the medical sciences 317: 168–175.

29. Stephenson T, Pipkin FB (1990) Atrial natriuretic factor: the heart as an endocrine organ. Archives of disease in childhood 65: 1293.

30. Woodard GE, Rosado JA (2008) Natriuretic peptides in vascular physiology and pathology. International review of cell and molecular biology 268: 59–93.

31. Pfisterer L, Feldner A, Hecker M, Korff T (2012) Hypertension impairs myocardin function: a novel mechanism facilitating arterial remodelling. Cardiovascular research 96: 120–129.

32. Zhang Y, Janssens SP, Wingler K, Schmidt HH, Moens AL (2011) Modulating endothelial nitric oxide synthase: a new cardiovascular therapeutic strategy. American Journal of Physiology-Heart and Circulatory Physiology 301: H634–H646.

33. Janssens S, Pokreisz P, Schoonjans L, Pellens M, Vermeersch P, et al. (2004) Cardiomyocyte-specific overexpression of nitric oxide synthase 3 improves left ventricular performance and reduces compensatory hypertrophy after myocardial infarction. Circulation research 94: 1256–1262.

34. Fraccarollo D, Widder JD, Galuppo P, Thum T, Tsikas D, et al. (2008) Improvement in left ventricular remodeling by the endothelial nitric oxide synthase enhancer AVE9488 after experimental myocardial infarction. Circulation 118: 818–827.

35. Fraccarollo D, Hu K, Galuppo P, Gaudron P, Ertl G (1997) Chronic Endothelin Receptor Blockade Attenuates Progressive Ventricular Dilation and Improves Cardiac Function in Rats With Myocardial Infarction Possible Involvement of Myocardial Endothelin System in Ventricular Remodeling. Circulation 96: 3963–3973.

36. Böhm F, Pernow J (2007) The importance of endothelin-1 for vascular dysfunction in cardiovascular disease. Cardiovascular research 76: 8–18.

37. Clozel M, Salloukh H (2005) Role of endothelin in fibrosis and anti-fibrotic potential of bosentan. Annals of medicine 37: 2–12.

Angiotensin II Reduces Cardiac AdipoR1 Expression through AT1 Receptor/ROS/ERK1/2/c-Myc Pathway

Li Li[1⌖], Zhi-Guo Zhang[1⌖], Hong Lei[1], Cheng Wang[1], Li-Peng Wu[2], Jin-Yu Wang[1], Feng-Ying Fu[3], Wei-Guo Zhu[2], Li-Ling Wu[1]*

1 Department of Physiology and Pathophysiology, Peking University Health Science Center, and Key Laboratory of Molecular Cardiovascular Sciences, Ministry of Education, Beijing, China, 2 Department of Biochemistry and Molecular Biology, Peking University Health Science Center, Beijing, China, 3 Key Laboratory of Cardiovascular Molecular Biology and Regulatory Peptides, Ministry of Health, Beijing, China

Abstract

Adiponectin, an abundant adipose tissue-derived protein, exerts protective effect against cardiovascular disease. Adiponectin receptors (AdipoR1 and AdipoR2) mediate the beneficial effects of adiponectin on the cardiovascular system. However, the alteration of AdipoRs in cardiac remodeling is not fully elucidated. Here, we investigated the effect of angiotensin II (AngII) on cardiac AdipoRs expression and explored the possible molecular mechanism. AngII infusion into rats induced cardiac hypertrophy, reduced AdipoR1 but not AdipoR2 expression, and attenuated the phosphorylations of adenosine monophosphate-activated protein kinase and acetyl coenzyme A carboxylase, and those effects were all reversed by losartan, an AngII type 1 (AT1) receptor blocker. AngII reduced expression of AdipoR1 mRNA and protein in cultured neonatal rat cardiomyocytes, which was abolished by losartan, but not by PD123319, an AT2 receptor antagonist. The antioxidants including reactive oxygen species (ROS) scavenger NAC, NADPH oxidase inhibitor apocynin, Nox2 inhibitor peptide gp91 ds-tat, and mitochondrial electron transport chain complex I inhibitor rotenone attenuated AngII-induced production of ROS and phosphorylation of extracellular signal-regulated kinase (ERK) 1/2. AngII-reduced AdipoR1 expression was reversed by pretreatment with NAC, apocynin, gp91 ds-tat, rotenone, and an ERK1/2 inhibitor PD98059. Chromatin immunoprecipitation assay demonstrated that AngII provoked the recruitment of c-Myc onto the promoter region of AdipoR1, which was attenuated by PD98059. Moreover, AngII-induced DNA binding activity of c-Myc was inhibited by losartan, NAC, apocynin, gp91 ds-tat, rotenone, and PD98059. c-Myc small interfering RNA abolished the inhibitory effect of AngII on AdipoR1 expression. Our results suggest that AngII inhibits cardiac AdipoR1 expression in vivo and in vitro and AT1 receptor/ROS/ERK1/2/c-Myc pathway is required for the downregulation of AdipoR1 induced by AngII.

Editor: Qingbo Xu, King's College London, University of London, United Kingdom

Funding: This work was supported by grants from the National Nature Science Foundation of China (Nos. 30871014 and 30973316) and the National Basic Research Program of China (973 Program 2007CB512004). The funders had no role in study design, data collection and analysis, decision to publish, or preparation of the manuscript.

Competing Interests: The authors have declared that no competing interests exist.

* E-mail: pathophy@bjmu.edu.cn

⌖ These authors contributed equally to this work.

Introduction

Adiponectin is an abundant adipose tissue-derived protein with important metabolic modulation and energy homeostasis effects [1]. Adiponectin participates in the regulation of cardiovascular function and its circulating level may be a predictor of cardiovascular outcomes [2]. For instance, high plasma adiponectin levels are associated with a reduced risk of myocardial infarction in men, whereas low plasma adiponectin levels are found in patients with coronary artery disease [3]. Plasma adiponectin concentration is significantly lower in hypertensive patients than that in normotensive men, which indicates that hypoadiponectinemia is an independent risk factor for hypertension [4]. There is growing evidence to demonstrate a negative correlation between circulating adiponectin and cardiac hypertrophy [5,6]. Pressure overload in adiponectin-deficient mice results in enhanced concentric cardiac hypertrophy and adenovirus-mediated supplementation of adiponectin protects against the development of cardiac hypertrophy [7]. Therefore, adiponectin is an important endogenous adipokine protecting against cardiovascular disease.

Two types of adiponectin receptors (AdipoRs), AdipoR1 and AdipoR2, mediate most effects of adiponectin via activating adenosine monophosphate-activated protein kinase (AMPK) [8]. Downregulation of AdipoRs may play a role in metabolic syndrome and cardiovascular disease. Decreased expressions of AdipoR1 and AdipoR2 are found in skeletal muscle and adipose tissue of ob-/ob- mice [9] and in aortic tissues of rats fed with high-fat diet [10]. Expression of AdipoR1 is significantly decreased in infarcted mice heart [11]. AdipoRs also contribute to the inhibitory effect of adiponectin on endothelin-1- induced hypertrophy in cultured cardiomyocytes [12]. However, expression of AdipoRs in the process of cardiac remodeling has not been fully evaluated.

Angiotensin II (AngII), the major component of renin-angiotensin system (RAS), exerts vasoconstrictive, growth-promoting, and remodeling effects on the cardiovascular system [13]. Lower plasma adiponectin concentrations in patients with essential hypertension are elevated when administrated with AngII type 1 receptor (AT1) blocker or angiotensin converting enzyme inhibitor (ACEI) [14]. AngII infusion into rats decreases plasma concentration of adiponectin and adiponectin mRNA expression in adipose tissue [15]. These observations elicit that AngII is involved in the regulation of adiponectin synthesis and secretion. However, whether AngII interferes with cardiac adiponectin signaling cascade by regulating the expression of AdipoRs and its underlying mechanism is unknown.

The present study was designed to investigate the effect of AngII on AdipoRs expression in rats exposed to continuous infusion of AngII and in cultured neonatal rat cardiomyocytes. We also explored the possible molecular mechanism by which AngII regulates AdipoRs expression.

Materials and Methods

Materials

AngII, PD123319, CGP42112A, N-acetyl cysteine (NAC), apocynin, retenone, allopurinol, PD98059, SB202190, and SP600125 were purchased from Sigma-Aldrich Co. (St. Louis, MO, USA). Losartan was from Merck & Co. (Whitehouse Station, NJ, USA). gp91 ds-tat and scrambled gp91 ds-tat were from Anaspec (San Jose, CA, USA). Antibodies for AdipoR1, AdipoR2, phospho- and total extracellular signal-regulated kinase 1/2 (ERK1/2), nuclear factor (NF)-κB, and actin were from Santa Cruz Biotechnology (Santa Cruz, CA, USA). Antibodies for phospho- and total AMPK, and phospho- and total acetyl coenzyme A carboxylase (ACC) were from Cell Signaling Technology (Beverly, MA, USA). Anti-c-Myc antibody was from Upstate (Billerica, MA, USA). Anti-signal transducer and activator of transcription (STAT) 5 antibody was from Abcam (Cambridge, UK).

In vivo rat model of continuous AngII infusion

All experimental procedures were approved by the Ethics Committee of Animal Research, Peking University Health Science Center, and the investigation conformed to the guidelines of the National Institutes of Health for the care and use of laboratory animals. Male Sprague-Dawley (SD) rats weighing 250 to 280 g were randomly divided into control, AngII, and losartan groups. An osmotic mini-pump (model 2004, Durect Corp., Cupertino, CA, USA) was subcutaneously embedded in rats under anesthesia with sodium pentobarbital (50 mg/kg, IP). AngII (400 ng/kg/min) or normal saline was infused constantly for 28 days. In the losartan group, rats also received losartan (10 mg/kg/day orally) during AngII infusion. At day 28, rats were anesthetized by sodium pentobarbital (50 mg/kg, IP). The right carotid artery was cannulated with polyethylene tubing connected to a Model TCB-500 transducer control unit (Millar Instruments, Houston, TX, USA). Hemodynamic parameters were recorded on a PowerLab data-acquisition system (ADInstruments, Sydney, Australia). Blood was collected and plasma was separated by centrifugation. Hearts, blood vessels, skeletal muscle, and adipose tissue were then excised for further investigation.

Enzyme-linked immunosorbent assay (ELISA)

Plasma total adiponectin was determined with a rat adiponectin ELISA kit (Phoenix Pharmaceuticals Inc., Belmont, CA, USA).

Culture of neonatal rat ventricular myocytes

Primary neonatal rat ventricular myocytes (NRVMs) was cultured as described previously [16]. Briefly, ventricles of 1–3 day-old SD rats were minced and digested in phosphate-buffered saline (PBS) containing 0.1% trypsin (Invitrogen Co., Carlsbad, CA, USA) and 0.05% type I collagenase (Invitrogen) at 37°C. Cells were pelleted and suspended in Dulbecco's modified Eagle's medium (DMEM) containing 10% fetal bovine serum (FBS, Invitrogen). A single preplating step was used to allow fibroblasts to attach to culture plates. Non-adherent cardiomyocytes were cultured for 3 to 4 days and placed in serum-free medium for 24 h before experiments. The identity of NRVMs was confirmed by morphological examination and by staining with anti-sarcomeric α-actin antibody; most (>95%) of the cells were identified as NRVMs.

Quantitative real-time RT-PCR (qRT-PCR)

Total RNA of myocardial tissues or NRVMs was isolated by use of Trizol reagent (Invitrogen) and cDNA was generated from total RNA by use of the RevertAid First Strand cDNA Synthesis Kit (Fermentas, Burlington, ON, Canada). qRT-PCR was performed using following primer sets: AdipoR1 (forward, 5'-GGTTCTTCCTCATGGCTGTGA-3', reverse, 5'-AGGTGAA-GATACCCCACAGGT-3'), AdipoR2 (forward, 5'-GGCCTCCTCTTGGGATCTACT-3', reverse, 5'-GTTGGCGCATGGTACTCATAC-3') and β-actin (forward, 5'-ATGTTTGTGATGGGCGTGAACC-3', reverse, 5'-CCCAGCATCGAAGGTAGAGGA-3'). Amplifications were performed in 35 cycles using an opticon continuous fluorescence detection system (MJ Research Inc., Waltham, MA, USA) with SYBR green fluorescence (Molecular Probes, Eugene, OR, USA). Each cycle consisted of a 45 s at 94°C, a 45 s at 56°C, and a 60 s at 72°C. All data were quantified by use of the comparative CT method, normalized to β-actin.

Western blot analysis

Myocardial tissues or NRVMs were lysed in a buffer containing 50 mM Tris-HCl, pH 7.2, 0.1% sodium deoxycholate, 1% Triton X-100, 5 mM EDTA, 5 mM EGTA, 150 mM NaCl, 40 mM NaF, 2.175 mM sodium orthovanadate, 0.1% SDS, 0.1% aprotinin, and 1 mM phenylmethylsulfonyl fluoride. The lysates were centrifuged at 10 000×g for 10 min (4°C) and the supernatant was collected. Equal amounts of protein (50 μg), assayed using the Lowry's method [17], underwent SDS-PAGE and were transferred to polyvinylidene difluoride membranes. Membranes were incubated with primary antibodies and then probed with horseradish peroxidase-conjugated secondary antibodies. Blots were visualized using an enhanced chemiluminescence kit (Amersham Biosciences Inc., Piscataway, NJ, USA). The densities of bands were quantified using Quantity One software (Bio-Rad, Hercules, CA, USA).

Immunohistochemical staining

NRVMs were fixed in 4% paraformaldehyde and permeabilized in 0.2% Triton X-100 in PBS. NRVMs were stained with anti-AdipoR1 or AdipoR2 antibody overnight at 4°C, then fluorescence-labeled secondary antibody for 2 h at 37°C. Nuclei were stained with 4, 6-diamidino-2-phenylindole (DAPI, Sigma-Aldrich). Fluorescence images were captured on the Olympus confocal microscope (Olympus Corp., Tokyo, Japan). AdipoRs-positive areas were quantified by use of Image J software (National Institute of Health, Bethesda, MD, USA). Fluorescence density of AdipoRs was expressed as the positive area corrected for the number of nuclei.

Ventricles were fixed in 10% phosphate-buffered formalin and embedded in paraffin. Deparaffined sections (5 μm thickness) were incubated with primary antibody against AdipoR1 or AdipoR2 overnight at 4°C, then horseradish peroxidase (HRP)-conjugated secondary antibody. Immunoreactions were visualized with 3-3′ diaminobenzidine tetrahydrochloride. The nuclei were counterstained with hematoxylin. Negative controls involved omission of primary antibodies. Microscopy images were analyzed by use of Leica QWin image analysis software (Leica, Wetzlar, Germany). Staining density was expressed as positive area corrected for the numbers of nuclei.

Analysis of reactive oxygen species (ROS)

Intracellular ROS level was determined by using the cell-permeable, redox-sensitive fluorophore, 2′,7′-dichlorofluorescin diacetate (DCF-DA) (Molecular Probes, Eugene, OR, USA). NRVMs were incubated with 20 μM DCF-DA for 30 min and DCF fluorescence was visualized using the Olympus confocal microscope and analyzed with Image J software. All experiments were done with minimal exposure to light, and fluorescence was normalized to cell count.

Chromatin immunoprecipitation (ChIP) assay

ChIP assay was performed as described by Wu et al [18]. Briefly, NRVMs were cross-linked with 1% formaldehyde, and collected into the lysis buffer (1% SDS, 10 mM EDTA, 50 mM Tris-HCl, pH 8.1, 1× protease inhibitor cocktail). After sonication, the lysates underwent immunoclearing and were immunoprecipitated with anti-c-Myc, anti-STAT5, or anti-NF-κB antibody, and equivalent concentration of normal rabbit IgG (Santa Cruz) served as negative control. After incubation with protein A Sepharose and salmon sperm DNA and a sequential washing, precipitates were heated at 65°C for 6 h to reverse the formaldehyde cross-linking. DNA fragments were purified with TIANquick Midi Purification Kit (Tiangen Biotech Co., Ltd., Beijing, China). PCR analysis was performed using the following primer sets: c-Myc site 1 (forward, 5′-TGTAGCTGTCTTCA-GACACACCA-3′, reverse, 5′-TGTCTTTATTTGGGCTGGA-GAG-3′), c-Myc site 2 (forward, 5′-ATGAGAGA-GAAGGGCTGGAGA-3′, reverse, 5′-TCGCTGTCTTCAGACACACCA-3′), c-Myc site 3 (forward, 5′-AGATGGCTCAGCGGTTAAGAG-3′, reverse, 5′-TGTAGCTGTCTTCAGATACACCAGA-3′), STAT5 site 1 (forward, 5′-AGCCAAGCCTGTAACTCAGCA-3′, reverse, 5′-CAGGACCTCTGGAGGAGCAGT-3′), STAT5 site 2 (forward, 5′-TGAGAGAGAGAGAGAGCCAGGA-3′, reverse, 5′-TCAGGCTCTGCCAACTACTGAC-3′), and NF-κB (forward, 5′-AGCCAGCCAGGCCGTAAGTGT-3′, reverse, 5′-CCGGAAATGTTTACGGTGGAC-3′).

Electrophoretic mobility shift assay (EMSA)

Nuclear protein fractions were separated as described [19]. Detection of DNA-protein interactions involved the nonisotopic method of the LightShift™ chemiluminescent EMSA kit (Pierce Biotechnology, Rockford, IL, USA). Briefly, nuclear extract protein was incubated with biotin-labeled DNA probes containing the consensus sequence 5′- AGAGATTCAACCACATGGTG-CAGCTAG-3′ (sense). After reaction, DNA-protein complexes underwent 6% native PAGE and were transferred to a nitrocellulose membrane, then cross-linked to the membrane at 120 mJ/cm^2 and detected by use of horseradish peroxidase-conjugated streptavidin according to the manufacturer's instructions.

Small interfering RNA (siRNA)

NRVMs were seeded at a density of 3×10^5 cells per well of six-well plates. After 48–72 h culture, cells were transfected with siRNA of interest by use of Lipofectamine 2000 (Invitrogen). The potent siRNA for rat c-Myc was designed by use of the siRNA Target Finder (Ambion Inc., Austin, TX, USA), based on the Rattus norvegicus mRNA sequences deposited at the NIH-PubMed database, and were submitted to BLAST analysis to assure specificity. The potent rat c-Myc siRNA 5′-GAAGAA-CAAGAUGAUGAGGTT-3′ (sense) and a nonspecific control siRNA were synthesized by GeneChem Co. (Shanghai, China).

Hematoxylin and eosin staining

Deparaffined heart sections (5 μm thickness) were stained with hematoxylin and eosin for routine histological examination. Images were captured from six hearts in each group and cardiac myocyte cross-sectional surface area was evaluated by use of Leica QWin image analysis software. One hundred myocytes per heart were counted, and the average area was determined.

Statistical analysis

Data are expressed as mean ± SE. Data were compared by one-way ANOVA for multiple groups, followed by Bonferroni's tests by use of GraphPad Prism 5.0 (GraphPad Software, San Diego, CA, USA). $P < 0.05$ was considered statistically significant.

Results

1. AngII infusion induces cardiac hypertrophy, reduces plasma adiponectin levels, inhibits cardiac AdipoR1 expression, and decreases phosphorylation of AMPK and ACC in vivo

1.1 Effect of AngII on cardiac hypertrophy and ERK1/2 phosphorylation. Hemodynamic parameters on day 28 were shown in Table S1. Systolic blood pressure (SBP), diastolic blood pressure (DBP), dP/dt max, dP/dt min and left ventricular end-diastolic pressure (LVEDP) were increased in AngII-treated rats compared with those in controls (P<0.01), but were all suppressed by losartan, a specific AngII type 1 (AT1) receptor blocker. The cross-sectional surface area of cardiac myocytes (Figure S1A) and the ratio of heart weight to body weight (HW/BW, Figure S1B) were significantly increased (P<0.01) in AngII group. These results indicated that AngII infusion for 28 days resulted in cardiac hypertrophy. In addition, AngII infusion enhanced the phosphorylation of ERK1/2, a critical mediator in controlling the hypertrophic response (Figure S1C). Losartan attenuated AngII-induced cardiac hypertrophy and ERK1/2 phosphorylation (Figure S1A–C).

1.2 Effect of AngII on plasma adiponectin levels, myocardial AdipoRs expression, and phosphorylations of AMPK and ACC. Plasma adiponectin levels in AngII-infused rats were significantly lower than that in controls, and losartan treatment prevented the AngII-induced decrease in circulating adiponectin levels (Figure 1A). Expression of AdipoR1 mRNA and protein in the AngII-induced hypertrophic heart was significantly decreased, which was reversed by losartan (Figure 1B and C). Immunostaining results showed that AdipoR1 was distributed widely in ventricular myocytes in control group. AngII infusion reduced the positive staining density of myocardial AdipoR1, which was reversed by losartan (Figure 1D). The negative control image was shown in Figure S2. Phosphorylations of AMPK-α at Thr-172 (Figure 1E) and ACC at Ser-79 (Figure 1F), a direct downstream target of AMPK, were attenuated in the hypertrophic hearts, and those effects were reversed by losartan administration. However, there was no significant difference of myocardial AdipoR2 mRNA and protein expression among the control, AngII, and losartan groups (Figure S3).

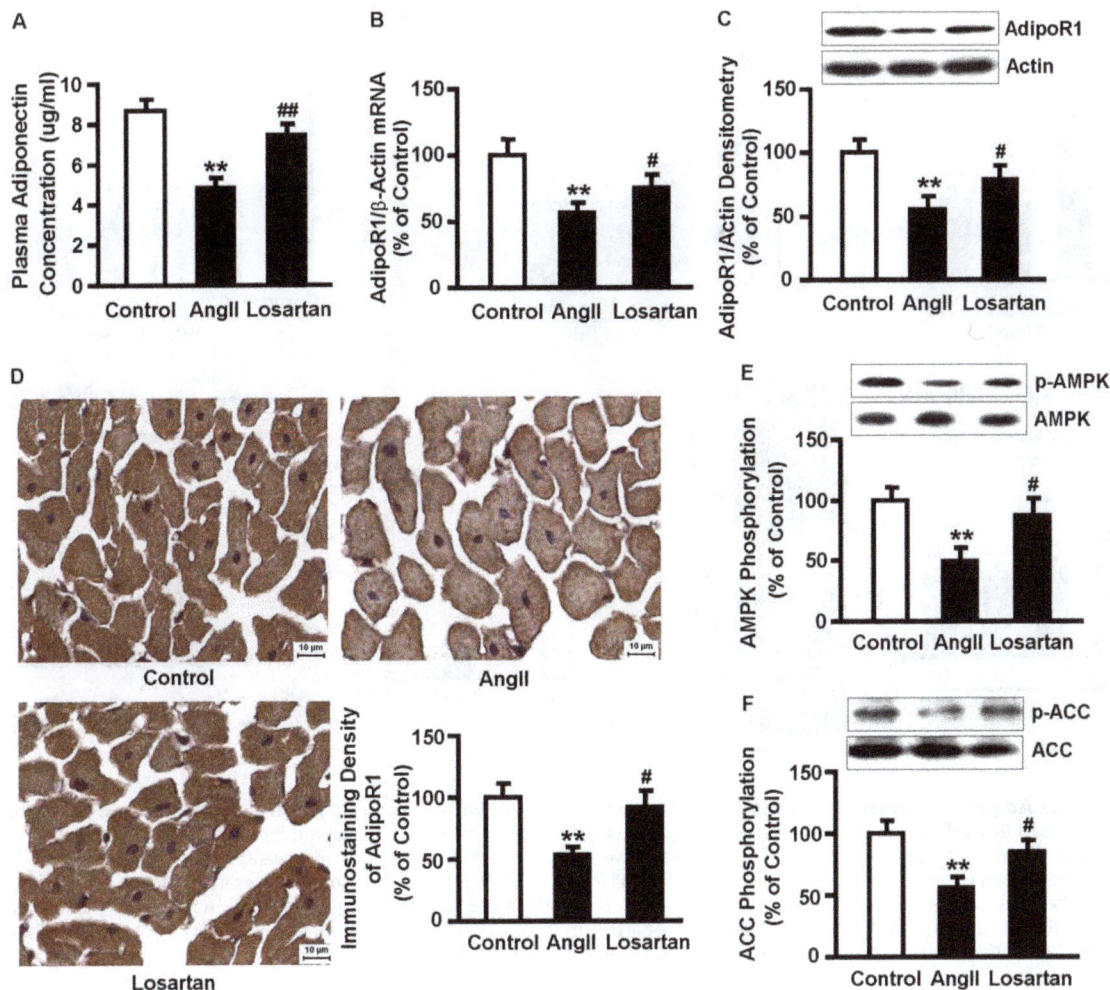

Figure 1. AngII infusion reduces plasma adiponectin levels, inhibits cardiac AdipoR1 expression, and decreases phosphorylation of AMPK and ACC. (A) Plasma adiponectin levels in the control, AngII, and losartan groups were detected by ELISA. (B) Levels of AdipoR1 mRNA were analyzed by qRT-PCR, and β-actin was used as an internal control. (C) Myocardial extracts were immunoblotted with antibody specific for AdipoR1. Blots were reprobed with actin to confirm equal loading. (D) Representative immunostaining images and averaged bar graphs of AdipoR1 density. AdipoR1 is shown in brown and cell nuclei in blue. Scale bar represents 10 μm (6 fields in each sample were scanned and averaged). (E) Myocardial extracts were immunoblotted with antibody specific for p-AMPKα at Thr-172. Blots were reprobed with antibody for AMPK to confirm equal loading. (F) Myocardial extracts were immunoblotted with antibody specific for p-ACC at Ser-79. Blots were reprobed with antibody for ACC to confirm equal loading. Data represent mean ± SE. n = 6 in each group. **$P < 0.01$ vs. control. #$P < 0.05$, ##$P < 0.01$ vs. AngII.

1.3 Effect of AngII on AdipoRs expression in skeletal muscle, adipose tissue, and blood vessels. There was no significant difference of AdipoRs protein expression in skeletal muscle and adipose tissue among the control, AngII, and losartan groups (Figure S4A–D). AdipoR1 protein expression in blood vessels was increased by 45.2% in AngII group when compared with that in control group, which was attenuated by losartan treatment ($P < 0.05$, Figure S4E). Expression of AdipoR2 protein in blood vessels did not change in AngII-infused rats (Figure S4F).

2. AngII decreases AdipoR1 expression in NRVMs

To determine the effect of AngII on AdipoRs expression in vitro, NRVMs were incubated with 0.1 μmol/L AngII for the indicated times. Expression of AdipoR1 mRNA and protein was significantly decreased after exposure to AngII for 36 and 48 h ($P < 0.01$, Figure 2A and B). Incubation with 0.1, 1, and 10 μmol/L AngII for 48 h decreased the level of AdipoR1 mRNA by 45.6% ($P < 0.01$), 50.9% ($P < 0.01$), and 56.9% ($P < 0.01$), respectively (Figure 2C). AngII-reduced AdipoR1 protein expression was parallel with a decrease in its mRNA level ($P < 0.01$, Figure 2D). Immunofluorescence staining showed that AdipoR1 was widespread in the cytoplasm and membrane in unstimulated control cells. The fluorescence densities were attenuated significantly after AngII incubation for 48 h ($P < 0.01$, Figure 2E) AMPK phosphorylation was enhanced upon incubation with 1 μg/ml globular adiponectin for 10 min, and this effect was dramatically attenu-

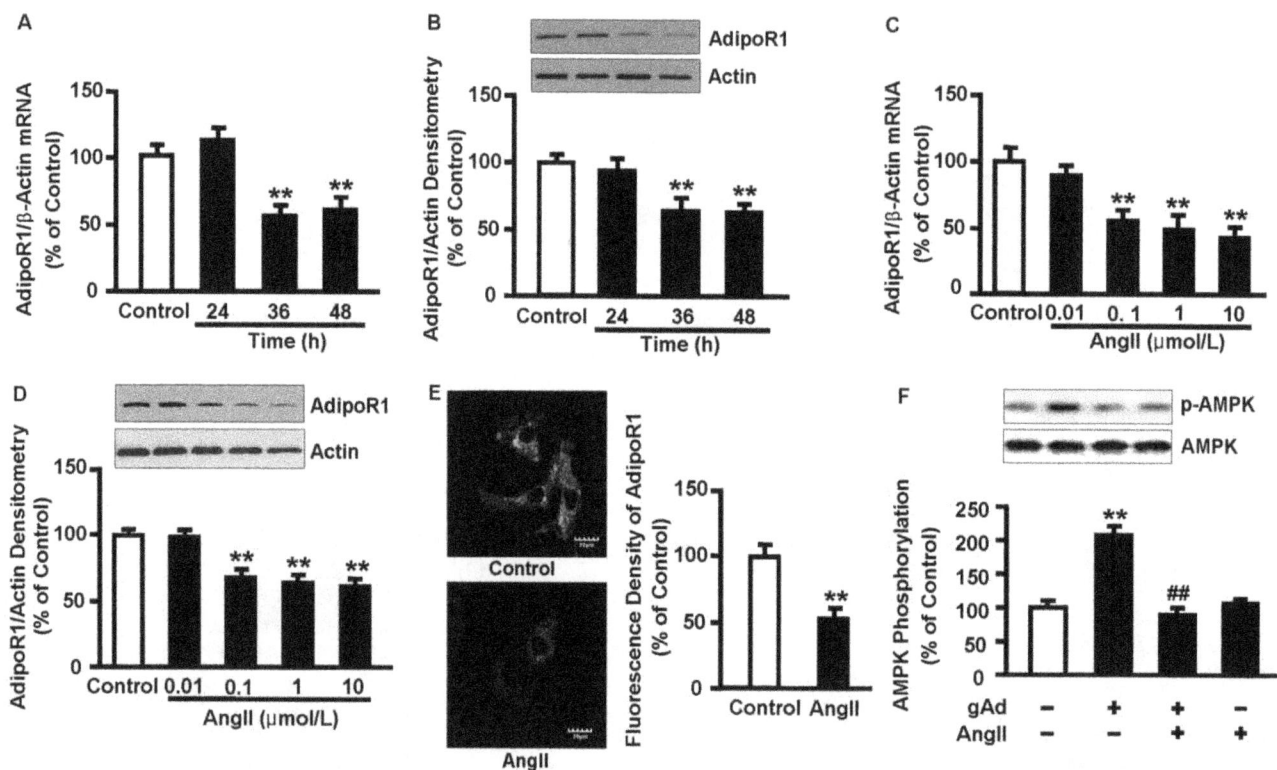

Figure 2. AngII decreases AdipoR1 expression in NRVMs. NRVMs were incubated with 0.1 μmol/L AngII for the indicated times, or treated with AngII at the indicated concentrations for 48 h. (A, C) Levels of AdipoR1 mRNA were analyzed by qRT-PCR. (B, D) Expression of AdipoR1 protein was determined by Western blot analysis. (E) Representative immunofluorescence images and averaged bar graphs of AdipoR1 density in unstimulated control NRVMs and cells treated with 0.1 μmol/L AngII for 48 h. Green fluorescence signals represent AdipoR1 protein. Scale bar represents 20 μm (6 fields in each sample were scanned and averaged). (F) NRVMs were pretreated with 0.1 μmol/L AngII for 48 h and then stimulated with 1 μg/ml globular adiponectin for 10 min. AMPK phosphorylation in cell lysates was determined by Western blot analysis. Data represent mean ± SE of three independent experiments. **$P<0.01$ vs. control. ##$P<0.01$ vs. AngII.

ated in AngII-pretreated NRVMs (Figure 2F). Expression of AdipoR2 had no change upon incubation with AngII (Figure S5).

3. The AngII-induced decrease in AdipoR1 expression is AT1 receptor-dependent

To determine the receptor subtypes mediating the inhibitory effect of AngII on AdipoR1 expression, NRVMs were pretreated with 10 μmol/L losartan or 1 μmol/L PD123319, an AT2 receptor antagonist, for 1 h and then stimulated with 0.1 μmol/L AngII for 48 h. Expression of AdipoR1 mRNA and protein was downregulated by AngII, which was reversed significantly when pretreated with losartan. However, the suppressive effect of AngII on AdipoR1 expression was not affected by PD123319. Furthermore, CGP42112A, a specific AT2 receptor agonist, did not change the expression of AdipoR1 (Figure 3A and B). Losartan and PD123319 alone had no effect on AdipoR1 expression (data not shown).

4. The AngII-induced decrease in AdipoR1 expression involves ERK1/2 activation and ROS production

4.1 Effect of mitogen-activated protein kinase inhibitors on AngII-reduced AdipoR1 expression. To explore the role of mitogen-activated protein kinase (MAPK) in AngII-reduced AdipoR1 expression, we employed SB202190 (5 μmol/L), a selective p38MAPK inhibitor, PD98059 (10 μmol/L), an ERK1/2 upstream kinase inhibitor, and SP600125 (10 μmol/L), a c-Jun-N-terminal kinase (JNK) inhibitor to preincubate NRVMs

for 1 h, and then stimulated with 0.1 μmol/L AngII for 48 h. PD98059 reversed AngII-reduced AdipoR1 expression. SB202190 and SP600125 did not affect AngII-induced AdipoR1 downregulation (Figure 4A and B). Each of the inhibitors alone had no effect on AdipoR1 expression (Figure S6A).

4.2 Effect of the pharmacological inhibition of ROS on AngII-induced ERK1/2 phosphorylation and AdipoR1 downregulation. We explored whether ROS was involved in the activation of ERK1/2 and downregulation of AdipoR1 in response to AngII. Fluorescence density of DCF was significantly increased after AngII treatment for 30 min. AngII-increased ROS production was eliminated by the ROS scavenger NAC (10 mmol/L), the NADPH oxidase inhibitor apocynin (100 μmol/L), and the inhibitor of the mitochondrial electron transport chain complex I rotenone (10 μmol/L), but not by the inhibitor of xanthine oxidase allopurinol (100 μmol/L) (Figure 4C). AngII-mediated ERK1/2 phosphorylation was also attenuated by the antioxidants including NAC, apocynin, and rotenone, but not allopurinol (Figure 4D). Similarly, the inhibitory effect of AngII on AdipoR1 expression was reversed by NAC, apocynin, and rotenone, but not by allopurinol (Figure 4E). Each of the inhibitors alone had no effect on ERK1/2 phosphorylation and AdipoR1 expression (Figure S6B and C).

4.3 Effect of Nox2 inhibitor on AngII-induced ERK1/2 phosphorylation and AdipoR1 downregulation. The catalytic subunit gp91phox (Nox2), a major isoform of NADPH oxidase expressed in cardiomyocytes, is critical for cardiac

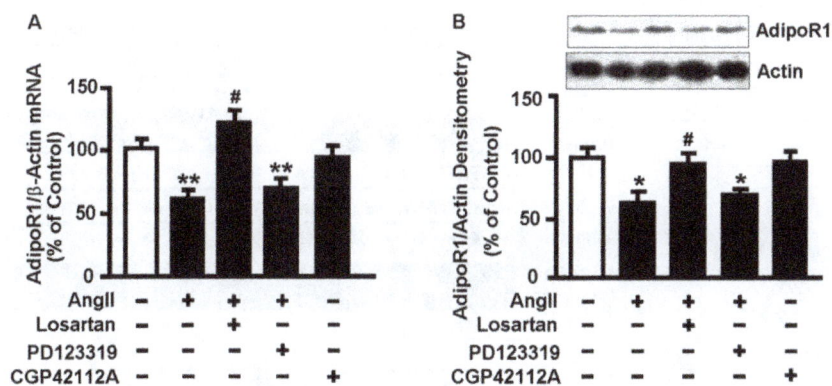

Figure 3. The AngII-induced decrease in AdipoR1 expression is AT1 receptor-dependent. NRVMs were pretreated with losartan (10 μmol/L) or PD123319 (1 μmol/L) for 1 h and then stimulated with 0.1 μmol/L AngII for 48 h, or incubated with CGP42112A (1 μmol/L) for 48 h. (A) Levels of AdipoR1 mRNA were analyzed by qRT-PCR, and β-actin was used as an internal control. (B) Western blot was performed to detect levels of AdipoR1 and actin protein expression. Data represent mean ± SE of three independent experiments. *$P<0.05$, **$P<0.01$ vs. control. #$P<0.05$ vs. AngII.

hypertrophy in response to chronic AngII infusion [20]. We then employed gp91 ds-tat, a Nox2 inhibitor peptide, to examine the role of Nox2 in this process. Pretreatment with gp91 ds-tat attenuated AngII-induced ROS production (Figure S7) and was associated with an 81.2% reduction in ERK1/2 phosphorylation induced by AngII ($P<0.01$, Figure 4F). AngII-reduced AdipoR1

expression was reversed markedly by gp91 ds-tat ($P<0.05$, Figure 4G).

5. AngII promotes binding of c-Myc to the AdipoR1 promoter region and it requires ERK1/2 involvement

To further reveal the transcription mechanism of AngII-mediated AdipoR1 expression, we screened the DNA sequence

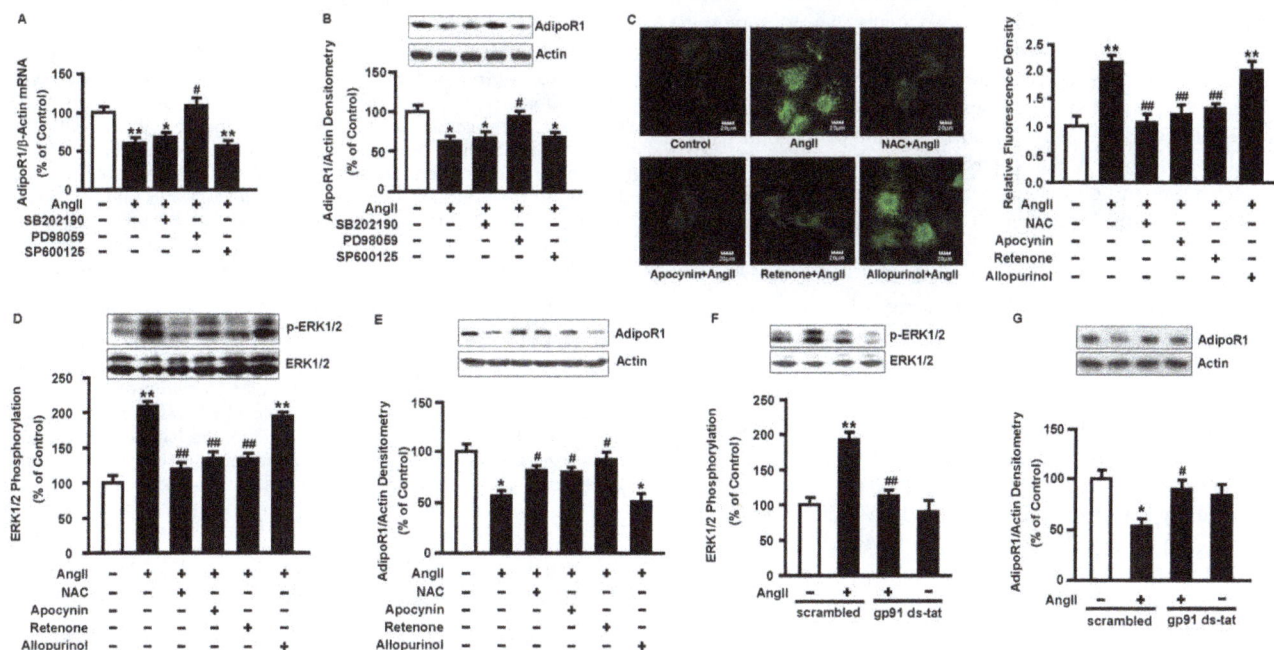

Figure 4. The AngII-induced decrease in AdipoR1 expression involves ERK1/2 activation and ROS production. (A, B) NRVMs were pretreated with SB202190 (5 μmol/L), PD98059 (10 μmol/L), or SP600125 (10 μmol/L) for 1 h, then stimulated with 0.1 μmol/L AngII for 48 h. Expression of AdipoR1 mRNA and protein was analyzed by qRT-PCR and Western blot respectively. (C) Representative fluorescence images and histogram of relative fluorescence density of ROS. NRVMs were pretreated with NAC (10 mmol/L), apocynin (100 μmol/L), rotenone (10 μmol/L), or allopurinol (100 μmol/L) for 1 h, followed by DCF-DA incubation for 30 min, and then stimulated with 0.1 μmol/L AngII for 30 min. DCF fluorescence was visualized using confocal microscopy. The green color represents ROS and the fluorescence density was normalized to cell count. Scale bar represents 20 μm (6 fields in each sample were scanned and averaged). (D, E) NRVMs were pretreated with NAC (10 mmol/L), apocynin (100 μmol/L), rotenone (10 μmol/L), or allopurinol (100 μmol/L) for 1 h and then stimulated with 0.1 μmol/L AngII for 30 min (D) or 48 h (E). Western blot was performed to detect levels of p-ERK1/2 (D) or AdipoR1 (E). Blots were reprobed with antibody for ERK1/2 (D) or actin (E) to confirm equal loading. (F, G) NRVMs were pretreated with 10 μmol/L gp91 ds-tat or scrambled gp91 ds-tat for 1 h and then stimulated with 0.1 μmol/L AngII for 30 min (F) or 48 h (G). Western blot was performed to detect levels of p-ERK1/2 (F) or AdipoR1 (G). Data represent mean ± SE of three independent experiments. *$P<0.05$, **$P<0.01$ vs. control. #$P<0.05$, ##$P<0.01$ vs. AngII.

Table 1. Putative binding sites of c-Myc, STAT5, and NF-κB in the promoter region of AdipoR1.

	Sequence	Chromosomal Location
c-Myc site 1	CaaccaCATGgtg	−1051 to −1039
c-Myc site 2	CaaccaCATGgtg	−2036 to −2024
c-Myc site 3	CaaccaCATGgtg	−2515 to −2503
STAT5 site 1	atccTTCTgcgaactgcac	−2636 to −2618
STAT5 site 2	aaaaTTCTtcgaatggtac	−2830 to −2812
NF-κB site	gcGGGActggccc	−225 to −213

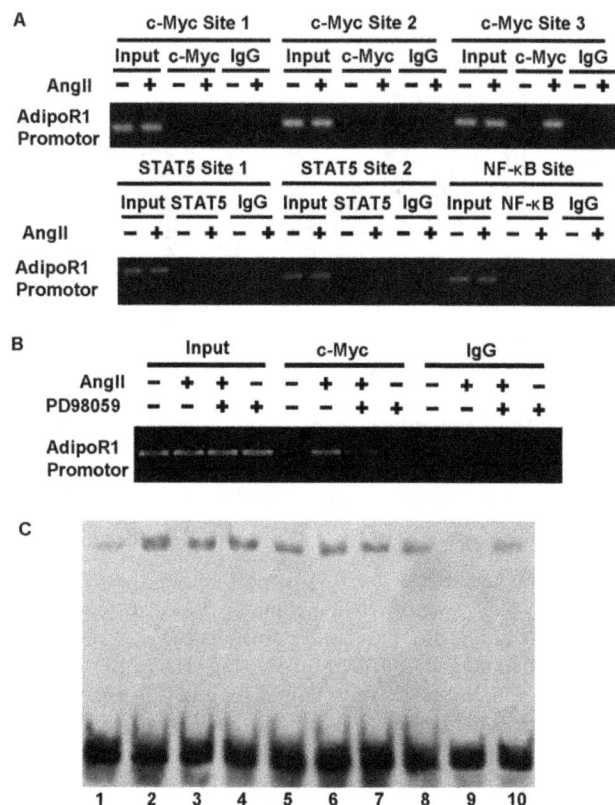

of rat AdipoR1 promoter region by use of Genomatix from the UCSC Genome Browser Database (http://www.genome.ucsc.edu) and identified six putative binding sites located between −3000 and −200 on AdipoR1 promoter sequence for three cardiovascular-related transcription factors, including three for c-Myc, two for STAT5, and one for NF-κB (Table 1). ChIP assay showed that AngII provoked the recruitment of c-Myc to its putative binding site 3 between −2515 and −2503 located on the AdipoR1 promoter region. AngII did not affect the binding of c-Myc to sites 1 and 2, and had no influence on the binding of STAT5 and NF-κB to their corresponding putative binding sites (Figure 5A). PD98059 preincubation partially, but significantly, inhibited the binding of c-Myc to AdipoR1 promoter region induced by AngII (Figure 5B). EMSA results showed that AngII treatment for 48 h increased the DNA binding activity of c-Myc (lane 2). Enhanced c-Myc binding activity was significantly attenuated by losartan, NAC, apocynin, rotenone, gp91 ds-tat, and PD98059 (lane 3–8). Unlabeled wild-type oligonucleotide completely competed the control band off (lane 9), whereas unlabeled mutant oligonucleotide failed to compete (lane 10), demonstrating the specificity of the DNA-protein complex (Figure 5C).

6. AngII decreases AdipoR1 expression in a c-Myc-dependent manner

To further examine the effect of c-Myc on AngII-reduced AdipoR1 expression, NRVMs were transfected with control or c-Myc siRNA (100 nmol/L) for 48 h and serum-deprived for 24 h, then incubated with 0.1 μmol/L AngII for 48 h. c-Myc siRNA greatly reduced c-Myc protein level ($P<0.01$, Figure 6A) and abolished the suppressive effect of AngII on AdipoR1 expression ($P<0.01$, Figure 6B). Transfection with c-Myc siRNA alone had no effect on protein expression of AdipoR1.

Discussion

In the present study, we demonstrated that AngII reduced AdipoR1 but not AdipoR2 expression both in hearts of AngII-infused rats and in cultured neonatal rat cardiomyocytes. We also found that AT1 receptor, ROS derived from NADPH oxidase and mitochondria, and ERK1/2 were critical for AngII-reduced AdipoR1 expression. The recruitment of c-Myc to AdipoR1 promoter region was required for the transcription modulation of AngII on AdipoR1 expression. Moreover, the AT1 receptor/ROS/ERK1/2 pathway was involved in AngII-induced DNA binding activity of c-Myc. These results suggest that the downregulation of cardiac AdipoR1 by AngII may play an important role in the progression of cardiac remodeling. This

Figure 5. AngII promotes binding of c-Myc to the AdipoR1 promoter region and it requires ERK1/2 involvement. (A) NRVMs were stimulated with 0.1 μmol/L AngII for 48 h. Sheared chromatin prepared from cardiomyocytes was immunoprecipitated with the indicated antibodies (control IgG, anti-c-Myc, anti-STAT5 or anti-NF-κB antibodies). The immunoprecipitated DNA was used as a template for PCR using the indicated primer sets. (B) NRVMs were pretreated with 10 μmol/L PD98059 for 1 h, then stimulated with 0.1 μmol/L AngII for 48 h. Chromatin fragments were immunoprecipitated with anti-c-Myc antibody or normal rabbit IgG. Immunoprecipitated chromatin was quantified with RT-PCR. (C) NRVMs were pretreated with losartan (10 μmol/L, lane 3), NAC (10 mmol/L, lane 4), apocynin (100 μmol/L, lane 5), rotenone (10 μmol/L, lane 6), gp91 ds-tat (10 μmol/L, lane 7) or PD98059 (10 μmol/L, lane 8) for 1 h, and then stimulated with 0.1 μmol/L AngII for 48 h. DNA binding activity of c-Myc was determined by EMSA with nuclear extracts of NRVMs and DNA probes. Lane 1, control; lane 2, AngII; lane 3–8, inhibitors; lane 9, with 100-fold molar excess of unlabeled oligonucleotide; lane 10, with 100-fold molar excess of unlabeled mutant oligonucleotide.

research focused on the mechanism involved in AngII-reduced AdipoR1 expression in cardiomyocytes will hopefully lead to novel strategies for clinical cardioprotection.

Adiponectin is an endogenous protective protein that acts as a modulator in energy metabolism and cardiovascular function [1,2]. Adiponectin and AdipoRs play important roles in alleviating pathological cardiac hypertrophy. Low levels of adiponectin are associated with a further progression of left ventricular hypertrophy in patients presenting with hypertension, left ventricular diastolic dysfunction and hypertrophy [21,22]. Adiponectin-deficient mice have enhanced concentric cardiac hypertrophy and increased mortality in response to AngII infusion and aortic constriction, which is attenuated by adiponectin supplementation [7]. As the critical components in the adiponectin signaling cascade, AdipoRs are proved to mediate the protective action of adiponectin against insulin resistance, type 2 diabetes, and

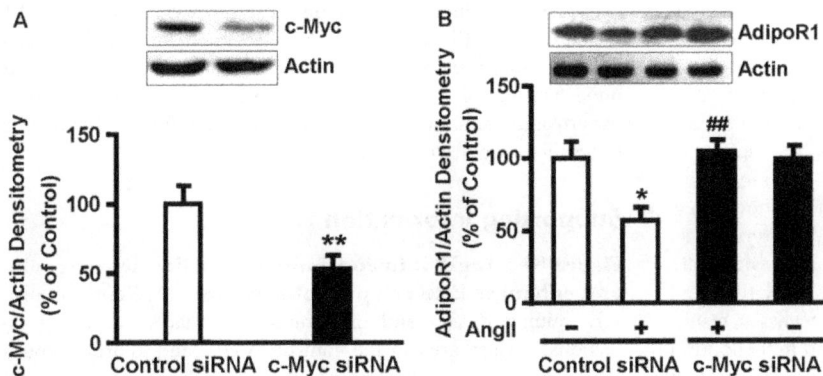

Figure 6. AngII decreases AdipoR1 expression in a c-Myc-dependent manner. (A) NRVMs were transfected with c-Myc or control siRNA (100 nmol/L) for 48 h. Western blot was performed to detect levels of c-Myc and actin. (B) NRVMs were transfected with c-Myc or control siRNA (100 nmol/L) for 48 h and serum-deprived for 24 h, followed by incubation with 0.1 μmol/L AngII for 48 h. The level of AdipoR1 protein was analyzed by Western blot analysis with actin as an internal control. Data represent mean ± SE of three independent experiments. *$P<0.05$, **$P<0.01$ vs. control. ##$P<0.01$ vs. AngII.

cardiomyocytes hypertrophy [12,23]. A series of studies have indicate that AdipoR1 expression is downregulated in various organs under pathological conditions, such as in the pancreas and liver of *ob-/ob-* and *db-/db-* mice [24], in the adipose tissue of obese diabetic KKAy mice and patients with obesity [25,26], in the soleus muscle of obese Zucker rats [27], and in hyperglycemia- and hyperinsulinemia- stimulated L6 myoblasts [28]. In type 2 diabetic rats induced by high-fat and high-sugar diets, cardiac hypertrophy and decreased heart function are associated with decreased myocardial AdipoR1 expression and AMPK phosphorylation [29]. Expression of AdipoR1 is also reduced in infarcted mice heart and tumor necrosis factor-α-treated cardiomyocytes [11]. Here, we provided evidence that AdipoR1 expression was decreased in hearts, increased in blood vessels, and did not change in skeletal muscle and adipose tissue in AngII-infused rats. Several studies have also shown the diverse action of hormones or drugs on AdipoRs expression in different tissues. Rosiglitazone treatment for 8 weeks improves the histological lesions in liver of nonalcoholic steatohepatitis rats, increases mRNA and protein expressions of AdipoR1 and AdipoR2 in liver and visceral fat, with down-regulation of the two receptors in muscle [30]. Leptin decreases AdipoR2 expression in rat liver and stomach, but increases its expression in adipose tissue [31]. The downregulation of AdipoR1 by AngII in cultured neonatal cardiomyocytes revealed the direct inhibitory effect of AngII on AdipoR1 expression. AdipoR2 expression did not change in our *in vivo* rat model and in cultured cardiomyocytes. Decreased AMPK phosphorylation indicated that the function of AdipoR1 was suppressed in hearts of AngII-infused rats and in AngII-treated cardiomyocytes. Previous studies have demonstrated that transfection of siRNA specific for AdipoR1 or AdipoR2 reverses the stimulatory effect of adiponectin on AMPK activation and the suppressive effect of adiponectin on endothelin-1-induced cellular hypertrophy in cardiomyocytes [12]. Considered together, our results suggest that the reduced AdipoR1 expression by AngII may contribute to the attenuated adiponectin signaling, thereby reducing the protective effect of adiponectin and resulting in abnormal metabolic change and cardiac hypertrophy.

AngII binds to and activates AT1 and AT2 receptors, which seem to induce phenotypically opposite responses [32]. It would be of interest to determine the exact subtype involved in the AngII-reduced AdipoR1 expression. The decreased expression of AdipoR1 by AngII was abolished by losartan, but not affected

by PD123319. Furthermore, activation of AT2 receptor with CGP42112A had no influence on AdipoR1 expression. These results indicate that the inhibitory effect of AngII on AdipoR1 expression is mediated thoroughly by AT1 receptor. The prevention effect of losartan on the AngII-reduced AdipoR1 expression will provide further understanding of the pathogenesis of cardiac hypertrophy and provide novel insights into this anti-remodeling therapy.

AngII regulates cell behavior through several mechanisms downstream of AT1 receptor, including stimulation of MAPK cascades. ERK1/2, p38MAPK, and JNK are three major members of the MAPK family, but the exact signal molecule responsible for AdipoR1 expression in this process is still poorly understood. We found that the suppressive effect of AngII on AdipoR1 expression was prevented by PD98059, but not by SB202190 and SP600125, which indicates that ERK1/2 is critical for AngII-reduced AdipoR1 expression in cardiomyocytes.

Increased ROS production mediates the hypertrophic response in cardiomyocytes to stretch or to neurohormonal stimuli such as AngII [33]. Suppression of ROS formation inhibits AngII-induced cardiomyocyte hypertrophy [34]. There are four enzymatic systems including NADPH oxidase, xanthine oxidase, uncoupled NO synthase, and the mitochondrial electron transport chain that produce ROS predominantly in mammalian cells [35–37]. We showed here that AngII-stimulated ROS production in cardiomyocytes resulted mainly from NADPH oxidase and mitochondrial electron transport enzyme. The crucial role of NADPH oxidase and mitochondrial oxidative stress in AngII-induced cardiac hypertrophy has been implicated in a series of studies [33]. Recent evidence also indicates a linking between these two sources for ROS production. In cardiomyocytes and vascular smooth muscle cells, AngII enhances the production of ROS through the activation of NADPH oxidase, which in turn triggers mitochondrial ATP dependent K^+ channel opening and mitochondrial ROS production [38,39]. ROS has been proposed to result in ERK1/2 activation and modulate the subsequent development of cardiac hypertrophy in response to different stimuli such as pressure overload, serotonin, AngII, and isoproterenol [40]. We then explored the ROS-mediated signal transduction involved in AngII-reduced AdipoR1 expression. We found that NAC, apocynin, and rotenone blocked the increase of ERK1/2 phosphorylation and the decrease of AdipoR1 expression by AngII, but inhibition of xanthine oxidase with allopurinol did not affect AngII-induced ERK1/2 activation and AdipoR1 downregulation. Nox2 NADPH oxidase is normally quiescent in cardiomyocytes and is activated through binding the cytosolic regulatory components to generate superoxide anion by stimuli such as G protein-coupled receptor agonists, growth factors, and cytokines [41]. Nox2 plays an important role in the hypertrophic response to AngII and myocardial infarction [20,42,43]. Nox2 knock-out mice subjected to AngII infusion or myocardial infarction show a less extent of cardiac hypertrophy than the matched wild-type mice. The current study demonstrated that Nox2 inhibition with gp91 ds-tat attenuated AngII-induced ERK1/2 phosphorylation and reversed AngII-reduced AdipoR1 expression. These results confirm that NADPH oxidase, especially Nox2, and mitochondria are major sources for ROS production in response to AngII in cardiomyocytes and are critical for the subsequent ERK1/2 activation, thereby being required for AngII-reduced AdipoR1 expression.

Although AdipoRs expression is mediated by various physiological and pathological factors, the precise mechanism involved in AdipoRs transcription regulation has not been fully evaluated. Recently, an insulin-responsive repressor element, termed nuclear inhibitory protein, has been identified in the AdipoR1 promoter region of C2C12 cells [44]. Our previous study has demonstrated that insulin decreases cardiac AdipoR1 expression via the PI3K/Akt pathway and that FoxO1 plays an important role in insulin-mediated AdipoR1 transcription by binding directly to the AdipoR1 promoter [45]. In the present study, we identified the putative binding sites located on AdipoR1 promoter region for c-Myc, STAT5 and NF-κB which are activated by AngII [46,47]. ChIP analysis provided the evidence that AngII provoked the binding of c-Myc, but not STAT5 or NF-κB, to the AdipoR1 promoter region in cardiomyocytes. The suppressive effect of AngII on AdipoR1 expression was abolished by c-Myc siRNA, suggesting that c-Myc acts negatively on AdipoR1 transcription. There is a growing body of evidence to implicate the crucial role of c-Myc in provoking cardiac hypertrophy *in vivo* and in cultured cardiomyocytes [48,49]. Inactivation of c-Myc in the adult myocardium attenuates hypertrophic growth and decreases the expression of glycolytic and mitochondrial biogenesis genes in response to hemodynamic load, which implies that c-Myc is an important regulator of energy metabolism in the heart in response to hypertrophic stimulus [50]. Our data give the information that c-Myc plays an important role in the transcription regulation of AdipoR1 by AngII and provide an alternative mechanism about c-Myc activation in regulating hypertrophic response. A series of studies have indicated that ERK1/2 responds to different stimuli and mediates the expression and activation of c-Myc in a plethora of cell types; examples are AngII-induced c-Myc expression in astrocytes [51], and serum- or thrombin-induced c-Myc phosphorylation in vascular smooth muscle cells [52]. We demonstrated here that AT1 receptor, ROS generation, and ERK1/2 activation were required for AngII-induced DNA binding activity of c-Myc.

Conclusions

In summary, we demonstrate that AngII reduces the expression of AdipoR1 but not AdipoR2 in hearts of AngII-infused rat model and in cultured neonatal cardiomyocytes. AngII decreases AdipoR1 expression through its AT1 receptor. ROS generated from NADPH oxidase, especially Nox2, and mitochondria and the sequential activation of ERK1/2 are involved in AngII-reduced AdipoR1 expression. Moreover, c-Myc plays an important role in AngII-mediated AdipoR1 transcription regulation in cardiomyo-

cytes through binding to AdipoR1 promoter directly. The AT1 receptor/ROS/ERK1/2 pathway is required for AngII-induced DNA binding activity of c-Myc. These findings may improve our understanding of the molecular mechanisms involved in cardiac hypertrophy and provide new insights into future therapeutic targets for cardiac remodeling.

Supporting Information

Figure S1   AngII infusion induces cardiac hypertrophy and enhances ERK1/2 phosphorylation. (A) Representative HE staining images and histogram of cardiac myocytes cross-sectional surface area in the control, AngII, and losartan groups (100 myocytes in each section were scanned and averaged). (B) Averaged bar graphs of HW/BW in the control, AngII, and losartan groups. (C) Myocardial extracts were immunoblotted with antibody specific for p-ERK1/2. Membranes were stripped and re-probed to normalize the blotted samples with anti-ERK1/2 antibody. Relative densities of p-ERK1/2 were quantified by scanning densitometry and normalized to percentage of control. Data represent mean ± SE. n = 6 in each group. **P<0.01 vs. control. ##P<0.01 vs. AngII.

Figure S2   The negative control image of AdipoR1 immunostaining. Deparaffined heart sections (5 μm thickness) were incubated with PBS overnight at 4°C, then horseradish peroxidase (HRP)-conjugated secondary antibody. Immunoreactions were visualized with 3-3′ diaminobenzidine tetrahydrochloride. The nuclei were counterstained with hematoxylin. Cell nuclei is shown in blue. Scale bar represents 10 μm.

Figure S3   AdipoR2 expression in the control, AngII, and losartan groups. (A) Levels of AdipoR2 mRNA were analyzed by qRT-PCR, and β-actin was used as an internal control. (B) Expression of AdipoR2 protein was determined by Western blot analysis. (C) Representative immunostaining images and averaged bar graphs of AdipoR2 density. AdipoR2 is shown in brown and cell nuclei in blue. Scale bar represents 10 μm (6 fields in each sample were scanned and averaged). Data represent mean ± SE. n = 6 in each group.

Figure S4   Effect of AngII on AdipoRs expression in skeletal muscle, adipose tissue, and blood vessels. Protein lysates from skeletal muscle (A, B), adipose tissue (C, D), and blood vessels (E, F) were immunoblotted with antibody specific for AdipoR1 (A, C, E) or AdipoR2 (B, D, F). Blots were reprobed with actin to confirm equal loading. Data represent mean ± SE. n = 6 in each group. *P<0.05 vs. control. #P<0.05 vs. AngII.

Figure S5   Effect of AngII on AdipoR2 expression in NRVMs. (A, B) NRVMs were incubated with 0.1 μmol/L AngII for the indicated times, or treated with AngII at the indicated concentrations for 48 h. Levels of AdipoR2 mRNA were analyzed by qRT-PCR. (C) Representative immunofluorescence images and averaged bar graphs of AdipoR2 density in unstimulated control NRVMs and cells treated with 0.1 μmol/L AngII for 48 h. Green fluorescence signals represent AdipoR2 protein. Scale bar represents 20 μm (6 fields in each sample were scanned and averaged). Data represent mean ± SE of three independent experiments.

Figure S6 Effect of pharmacological inhibitors of MAPK, ROS scavengers, and the specific inhibitors of ROS-producing enzymes on ERK1/2 phosphorylation or AdipoR1 expression. (A) NRVMs were treated with SB202190 (5 μmol/L), PD98059 (10 μmol/L), or SP600125 (10 μmol/L) for 1 h. Western blot was performed to detect levels of AdipoR1 and actin. (B, C) NRVMs were treated with NAC (10 mmol/L), apocynin (100 μmol/L), rotenone (10 μmol/L), or allopurinol (100 μmol/L) for 1 h. Western blot was performed to detect levels of p-ERK1/2 (B) and AdipoR1 (C). Data represent mean ± SE of three independent experiments.

Figure S7 Representative fluorescence images and histogram of relative fluorescence density of ROS. NRVMs were pretreated with 10 μmol/L gp91 ds-tat or scrambled gp91 ds-tat for 1 h, followed by DCF-DA incubation for 30 min, and then stimulated with 0.1 μmol/L AngII for 30 min. DCF fluorescence was visualized using confocal microscopy. The green color represents ROS and the fluorescence density was normalized to cell count. Scale bar represents 20 μm

(6 fields in each sample were scanned and averaged). Data represent mean ± SE of three independent experiments. **$P<0.01$ vs. control. ##$P<0.01$ vs. AngII.

Table S1 Hemodynamic parameters with control, angiotensin II, and losartan treatment. AngII, angiotensin II; SBP, systolic blood pressure; DBP, diastolic blood pressure; dP/dt max, peak rate of left ventricular pressure increase; dP/dt min, peak rate of left ventricular pressure decrease; LVEDP, left ventricular end-diastolic pressure. Data are mean ± SE. **$P<0.01$ vs. control. ##$P<0.01$ vs. AngII.

Author Contributions

Conceived and designed the experiments: LLW LL ZGZ. Performed the experiments: LL ZGZ HL CW FYF JYW. Analyzed the data: LL ZGZ. Contributed reagents/materials/analysis tools: LPW WGZ. Wrote the paper: LL LLW ZGZ.

References

1. Matsuzawa Y, Funahashi T, Kihara S, Shimomura I (2004) Adiponectin and metabolic syndrome. Arterioscler Thromb Vasc Biol 24:29–33.
2. Hopkins TA, Ouchi N, Shibata R, Walsh K (2007) Adiponectin actions in the cardiovascular system. Cardiovasc Res 74:11–18.
3. Tobias P, Cynthia JG, Gokhan SH, Nader R, Frank BH, et al. (2004) Plasma adiponectin levels and risk of myocardial infarction in men. JAMA 291:1730–1737.
4. Iwashima Y, Katsuya T, Ishikawa K, Ouchi N, Ohishi M, et al. (2004) Hypoadiponectinemia is an independent risk factor for hypertension. Hypertension 43:1318–1323.
5. Kozakova M, Muscelli E, Flyvbjerg A, Frystyk J, Morizzo C, et al. (2008) Adiponectin and left ventricular structure and function in healthy adults. J Clin Endocrinol Metab 93:2811–2818.
6. Mitsuhashi H, Yatsuya H, Tamakoshi K, Matsushita K, Otsuka R, et al. (2007) Adiponectin level and left ventricular hypertrophy in Japanese men. Hypertension 49:1448–1454.
7. Shibata R, Ouchi N, Ito M, Kihara S, Shiojima I, et al. (2004) Adiponectin-mediated modulation of hypertrophic signals in the heart. Nat Med 10:1384–1389.
8. Yamauchi T, Kamon J, Ito Y, Tsuchida A, Yokomizo T, et al. (2003) Cloning of adiponectin receptors that mediate antidiabetic metabolic effects. Nat Med 423:762–769.
9. Tsuchida A, Yamauchi T, Ito Y, Hada Y, Maki T, et al. (2004) Insulin/Foxo1 pathway regulates expression levels of adiponectin receptors and adiponectin sensitivity. J Biol Chem 279:30817–30822.
10. Li R, Xu M, Wang X, Wang Y, Lau WB, et al. (2010) Reduced vascular responsiveness to adiponectin in hyperlipidemic rats-mechanisms and significance. J Mol Cell Cardiol 49:508–515.
11. Saito Y, Fujioka D, Kawabata K, Kobayashi T, Yano T, et al. (2007) Statin reverses reduction of adiponectin receptor expression in infarcted heart and in TNF-α-treated cardiomyocytes in association with improved glucose uptake. Am J Physiol Heart Circ Physiol 293:H3490–3497.
12. Fujioka D, Kawabata K, Saito Y, Kobayashi T, Nakamura T, et al. (2006) Role of adiponectin receptors in endothelin-induced cellular hypertrophy in cultured cardiomyocytes and their expression in infarcted heart. Am J Physiol Heart Circ Physiol 290: H2409–2416.
13. Unger T (2002) The role of the renin-angiotensin system in the development of cardiovascular disease. Am J Cardiol 89:3A–9A.
14. Furuhashi M, Ura N, Higashiura K, Murakami H, Tanaka M, et al. (2003) Blockade of the renin-angiotensin system increases adiponectin concentrations in patients with essential hypertension. Hypertension 42:76–81.
15. Ran J, Hirano T, Fukui T, Saito K, Kageyama H, et al. (2006) Angiotensin II infusion decreases plasma adiponectin level via its type 1 receptor in rats: an implication for hypertension-related insulin resistance. Metabolism 55:478–488.
16. Li L, Wu L, Wang C, Liu L, Zhao Y (2007) Adiponectin modulates carnitine palmitoyltransferase-1 through AMPK signaling cascade in rat cardiomyocytes. Regul Pept 139:72–79.
17. Lowry OH, Rosebrough NJ, Farr AL, Randall RJ (1951) Protein measurement with the folin phenol reagent. J Biol Chem 93:265–275.
18. Wu LP, Wang X, Li L, Zhao Y, Lu S, et al. (2008) Histone deacetylase inhibitor depsipeptide activates silenced genes through decreasing both CpG and H3K9 methylation on the promoter. Mol Cell Biol 28:3219–3235.
19. Zhao Y, Liu J, Li L, Liu L, Wu L (2005) Role of Ras/PKCζ/MEK/ERK1/2 signaling pathway in angiotensin II-induced vascular smooth muscle cell proliferation. Regul Pept 128:43–50.
20. Bendall JK, Cave AC, Heymes C, Gall N, Shah AM (2002) Pivotal role of a gp91phox-containing NADPH oxidase in angiotensin II-induced cardiac hypertrophy in mice. Circulation 105:293–296.
21. Hong SJ, Park CG, Seo HS, Oh DJ, Ro YM (2004) Associations among plasma adiponectin, hypertension, left ventricular diastolic function and left ventricular mass index. Blood Press 13:236–242.
22. Pääkkö T, Ukkola O, Ikäheimo M, Kesäniemi YA (2010) Plasma adiponectin levels are associated with left ventricular hypertrophy in a random sample of middle-aged subjects. Ann Med 42:131–137.
23. Yamauchi T, Nio Y, Maki T, Kobayashi M, Takazawa T, et al. (2007) Targeted disruption of AdipoR1 and AdipoR2 causes abrogation of adiponectin binding and metabolic actions. Nat Med 13:332–339.
24. Wade TE, Mathur A, Lu D, Swartz-Basile DA, Pitt HA, et al. (2009) Adiponectin receptor-1 expression is decreased in the pancreas of obese mice. J Surg Res 154:78–84.
25. Fu L, Isobe K, Zeng Q, Suzukawa K, Takekoshi K, et al. (2008) The effects of β₃-adrenoceptor agonist CL-316,243 on adiponectin, adiponectin receptors and tumor necrosis factor-α expressions in adipose tissues of obese diabetic KKAy mice. Eur J Pharmacol 584:202–206.
26. Rasmussen MS, Lihn AS, Pedersen SB, Bruun JM, Rasmussen M, et al. (2006) Adiponectin receptors in human adipose tissue: effects of obesity, weight loss, and fat depots. Obesity 14:28–35.
27. Chang SP, Chen YH, Chang WC, Liu IM, Cheng JT (2006) Increase of adiponectin receptor gene expression by physical exercise in soleus muscle of obese Zucker rats. Eur J Appl Physiol 97:189–195.
28. Fang X, Palanivel R, Zhou X, Liu Y, Xu A, et al. (2005) Hyperglycemia- and hyperinsulinemia-induced alteration of adiponectin receptor expression and adiponectin effects in L6 myoblasts. J Mol Endocrinol 35:465–476.
29. Guo Z, Zheng C, Qin Z, Wei P (2010) Effect of telmisartan on the expression of cardiac adiponectin and its receptor 1 in type 2 diabetic rats. J Pharm Pharmacol 63:87–94.
30. Liu S, Wu HJ, Zhang ZQ, Chen Q, Liu B, et al. (2011) The ameliorating effect of rosiglitazone on experimental nonalcoholic steatohepatitis is associated with regulating adiponectin receptor expression in rats. Eur J Pharmacol 650:384–389.
31. González CR, Caminos JE, Gallego R, Tovar S, Vázquez MJ, et al. (2010) Adiponectin receptor 2 is regulated by nutritional status, leptin and pregnancy in a tissue-specific manner. Physiol Behav 99:91–99.
32. AbdAlla S, Lother H, Abdel-tawab AM, Quitterer U (2001) The angiotensin II AT2 receptor is an AT1 receptor antagonist. J Biol Chem 276:39721–39726.
33. Seddon M, Looi YH, Shah AM (2007) Oxidative stress and redox signalling in cardiac hypertrophy and heart failure. Heart 93:903–907.
34. Laskowski A, Woodman OL, Cao AH, Drummond GR, Marshall T, et al. (2006) Antioxidant actions contribute to the antihypertrophic effects of atrial natriuretic peptide in neonatal rat cardiomyocytes. Cardiovasc Res 72:112–123.
35. Brandes RP, Weissmann N, Schröder K (2010) NADPH oxidases in cardiovascular disease. Free Radic Biol Med 49:687–706.
36. Park J, Lee J, Choi C (2011) Mitochondrial network determines intracellular ROS dynamics and sensitivity to oxidative stress through switching inter-mitochondrial messengers. PLoS One 6:e23211.

37. Afanas'ev I (2011) ROS and RNS signaling in heart disorders: could antioxidant treatment be successful? Oxid Med Cell Longev 2011:293769.

38. De Giusti VC, Garciarena CD, Aiello EA (2009) Role of reactive oxygen species (ROS) in angiotensin II-induced stimulation of the cardiac Na^+/HCO_3^- cotransport. J Mol Cell Cardiol 47:716–722.

39. Dikalov S (2011) Cross talk between mitochondria and NADPH oxidases. Free Radic Biol Med 51:1289–1301.

40. Santos CX, Anilkumar N, Zhang M, Brewer AC, Shah AM (2011) Redox signaling in cardiac myocytes. Free Radic Biol Med 50:777–793.

41. Bedard K, Krause KH (2007) The NOX family of ROS-generating NADPH oxidases: physiology and pathophysiology. Physiol Rev 87:245–313.

42. Zhang M, Perino A, Ghigo A, Hirsch E, Shah AM (2012) NADPH oxidases in heart failure: poachers or gamekeepers? Antioxid Redox Signal [Epub ahead of print]

43. Looi YH, Grieve DJ, Siva A, Walker SJ, Anilkumar N, et al. (2008) Involvement of Nox2 NADPH oxidase in adverse cardiac remodeling after myocardial infarction. Hypertension 51:319–325.

44. Sun X, He J, Mao C, Han R, Wang Z, et al. (2008) Negative regulation of adiponectin receptor 1 promoter by insulin via a repressive nuclear inhibitory protein element. FEBS Lett 582:3401–3407.

45. Cui XB, Wang C, Li L, Fan D, Zhou Y, et al. (2012) Insulin decreases myocardial adiponectin receptor 1 expression via PI3K/Akt and FoxO1

46. Touyz RM, Berry C (2002) Recent advances in angiotensin II signaling. Braz J Med Biol Res 35:1001–1015.

47. McWhinney CD, Dostal D, Baker K (1998) Angiotensin II activates Stat5 through Jak2 kinase in cardiac myocytes. J Mol Cell Cardiol 30:751–761.

48. Xiao G, Mao S, Baumgarten G, Serrano J, Jordan MC, et al. (2001) Inducible activation of c-Myc in adult myocardium *in vivo* provokes cardiac myocyte hypertrophy and reactivation of DNA synthesis. Circ Res 89:1122–1129.

49. Zhong W, Mao S, Tobis S, Angelis E, Jordan MC, et al. (2006) Hypertrophic growth in cardiac myocytes is mediated by Myc through a Cyclin D2-dependent pathway. EMBO J 25:3869–3879.

50. Ahuja P, Zhao P, Angelis E, Ruan H, Korge P, et al. (2010) Myc controls transcriptional regulation of cardiac metabolism and mitochondrial biogenesis in response to pathological stress in mice. J Clin Invest 120:1494–1505.

51. Delaney J, Chiarello R, Villar D, Kandalam U, Castejon AM, et al. (2008) Regulation of c-fos, c-jun and c-myc gene expression by angiotensin II in primary cultured rat astrocytes: role of ERK1/2 MAP kinases. Neurochem Res 33:545–550.

52. Schauwienold D, Plum C, Helbing T, Voigt P, Bobbert T, et al. (2003) ERK1/2- dependent contractile protein expression in vascular smooth muscle cells. Hypertension 41:546–552.

pathway. Cardiovasc Res 93:69–78.

3,3′-Diindolylmethane Protects against Cardiac Hypertrophy via 5′-Adenosine Monophosphate-Activated Protein Kinase-α2

Jing Zong[1,2◗], **Wei Deng**[1,2◗], **Heng Zhou**[1,2], **Zhou-yan Bian**[1,2], **Jia Dai**[1,2], **Yuan Yuan**[1,2], **Jie-yu Zhang**[1,2], **Rui Zhang**[1,2], **Yan Zhang**[1,2], **Qing-qing Wu**[1,2], **Hai-peng Guo**[3], **Hong-liang Li**[1,2], **Qi-zhu Tang**[1,2]*

1 Department of Cardiology, Renmin Hospital of Wuhan University, Wuhan, China, **2** Cardiovascular Research Institute of Wuhan University, Wuhan, China, **3** The Key Laboratory of Cardiovascular Remodeling and Function Research, Chinese Ministry of Education and Chinese Ministry of Health, Qilu Hospital of Shandong University, Jinan, China

Abstract

Purpose: 3,3′-Diindolylmethane (DIM) is a natural component of cruciferous plants. It has strong antioxidant and anti-angiogenic effects and promotes the apoptosis of a variety of tumor cells. However, little is known about the critical role of DIM on cardiac hypertrophy. In the present study, we investigated the effects of DIM on cardiac hypertrophy.

Methods: Multiple molecular techniques such as Western blot analysis, real-time PCR to determine RNA expression levels of hypertrophic, fibrotic and oxidative stress markers, and histological analysis including H&E for histopathology, PSR for collagen deposition, WGA for myocyte cross-sectional area, and immunohistochemical staining for protein expression were used.

Results: In pre-treatment and reverse experiments, C57/BL6 mouse chow containing 0.05% DIM (dose 100 mg/kg/d DIM) was administered one week prior to surgery or one week after surgery, respectively, and continued for 8 weeks after surgery. In both experiments, DIM reduced to cardiac hypertrophy and fibrosis induced by aortic banding through the activation of 5′-adenosine monophosphate-activated protein kinase-α2 (AMPKα2) and inhibition of mammalian target of the rapamycin (mTOR) signaling pathway. Furthermore, DIM protected against cardiac oxidative stress by regulating expression of estrogen-related receptor-alpha (ERRα) and NRF2 etc. The cardioprotective effects of DIM were ablated in mice lacking functional AMPKα2.

Conclusion: DIM significantly improves left ventricular function via the activation of AMPKα2 in a murine model of cardiac hypertrophy.

Editor: Xiongwen Chen, Temple University, United States of America

Funding: This work was supported by the National Nature Science Foundation of China [30901628, 30972954, 81000036 and 81000095]; and the Fundamental Research Funds for the Central Universities of China [20103020201000193]. The funders had no role in study design, data collection and analysis, decision to publish, or preparation of the manuscript.

Competing Interests: The authors have declared that no competing interests exist.

* E-mail: qztang@whu.edu.cn

◗ These authors contributed equally to this work.

Introduction

Cardiac hypertrophy is a chronic compensatory condition, in which the heart has suffered from long-term overload. Cardiac hypertrophy can be divided into physiological hypertrophy and pathological hypertrophy [1]. Physiological hypertrophy is a reversible condition that is mainly found in the development of healthy people and pregnant or exercising person. Pathological hypertrophy is mainly characterized by the accumulation of various stimulatory signals (such as heart damage, neurohormonal factors, and aortic stenosis) and is a compensatory response. Initially, in response to a variety of stimuli, myocardial cells increase in size to improve myocardial contractile function and increase myocardial contractility. When the stimulatory factors are sustained, the compensatory mechanism becomes a decompensatory mechanism that eventually leads to heart failure [2,3]. However, the mechanisms participate in the process of cardiac hypertrophy have not been clearly demonstrated. Up to now, there is no effective method to prevent and treat cardiac hypertrophy. Therapies for cardiac hypertrophy still focus on regulating hemodynamics. Thus, pharmacological interventions targeting the molecular changes involved in cardiac hypertrophy may provide promising approaches for protecting against cardiac hypertrophy and progression to heart failure.

DIM is the major in vivo product derived from the acid-catalyzed condensation of I3C which is a *Brassica* food plant extract material. Studies have found that DIM has a variety of anti-cancer effects, in pancreatic [4], prostate [5] and breast cancer [6]. Moreover, recent studies have shown that DIM has an anti-angiogenic effect. I3C and DIM play anti-angiogenic roles through partly inhibiting of extracellular signal receptor-regulated kinase1/2 (ERK1/2) activity. Compared with I3C, DIM has a stronger role in anti-angiogenesis by inhibiting Akt activity [7]. In addition to participation in the anti-cancer and anti-angiogenic effects, DIM has anti-inflammatory effects. Pervious research has found that in murine macrophages DIM inhibits LPS-induced proinflammatory cytokine release. DIM inhibits the inflammatory response by attenuate the nuclear factor-κB (NF-κB) activity and activator protein 1 (AP-1) signaling pathway [8]. However, the effects of DIM on cardiac hypertrophy and the related signaling mechanisms are not yet clear. Therefore, we aimed to determine whether DIM attenuates cardiac hypertrophy induced by pressure-overload.

In the present study, we show that DIM protects against cardiac hypertrophy by promoting AMPKα phosphorylation. AMPK is a serine/threonine protein kinase that plays an important role in the cardiovascular system [9]. Previous studies have shown that AMPK activation can protect the heart from ischemic injury [10], cell death induced by reactive oxygen species [11] and pressure overload-induced cardiac hypertrophy [12]. In hypertrophic hearts subjected to chronic pressure overload, the activity of both AMPKα1 and AMPKα2 is increased [13]. AMPKα2 was proved to protect against pressure overload-induced ventricular hypertrophy and dysfunction [12]. Increasing number of studies suggest that DIM has various properties, including eliminating free radicals, activating apoptotic signaling pathways, antioxidant and anti-angiogenic effects, and promoting the apoptosis of a variety of tumor cells [4,7,14,15]. DIM can affect mitogen-activated protein kinases (MAPKs), phosphoinositide 3-kinase (PI3K)/Akt and the NF-κB signaling pathway to play anti-cancer, anti-angiogenic and anti-inflammatory roles. The molecular mechanisms of DIM inhibition of the hypertrophic response remain unknown. The purpose of this study were, therefore, to determine whether DIM can attenuate cardiac hypertrophy and fibrosis induced by pressure overload in mice, as well as to identify the molecular mechanisms that may be responsible for its putative effects. In addition, to determine whether the cardioprotective effects of DIM ameliorated in mice lacking functional AMPKα2.

Materials and Methods

Materials

Antibodies against total and phosphorylated AMPKα, mTOR, S6, phosphorylated p70 ribosomal protein S6 kinase (p70S6K), phosphorylated translation initiation factor binding protein (4E-BP1) and GAPDH were purchased from Cell Signaling Technology. Antibodies against total p70S6K, total and phosphorylated eukaryotic initiation factor 4E (eIF4E), total translation initiation factor binding protein (4E-BP1) and NRF2 were purchased from Bioworld Technology. Antibodies against Estrogen Related Receptor alpha (ERRα) was purchased from Abcam Inc. The bicinchoninic acid protein assay kit was purchased from Pierce. DIM (>98% purity as determined by HPLC analysis) was purchased from Shanghai Medical Technology Development Co., Ltd. Harmony.

Animal and Animal Models

All animal procedures were performed in accordance with the Guide for the Care and Use of Laboratory Animals published by the US National Institutes of Health (NIH Publication No. 85-23, revised 1996) and approved by the Animal Care and Use Committee of Renmin Hospital of Wuhan University. Adult male C57/BL6 mice and AMPKα2 knockout mice (C57/BL6 back-ground) (8–10 weeks old) were used in the current study. The diet was based on commonly used diets in rodent intervention studies. Aortic banding (AB) was performed as described previously [16,17]. Surgery and subsequent analyses were performed in a blinded fashion for all groups. Mice (15–20 per group) received normal feed or feed containing 0.05% DIM (dose: 100 mg/kg/day DIM). After 1 week we subjected the mice to either chronic pressure overload generated by AB or sham surgery as the control group. Mice were randomly assigned into four groups as DIM+sham, DIM+AB, Vehicle+sham, and Vehicle+AB. In a reverse experiment, normal feed containing 0.05% DIM was administered to mice for 7 weeks beginning 1 week after aortic banding surgery to 8 weeks after surgery. Mice were randomly assigned into four groups: DIM(R)+sham, DIM(R)+AB, Vehicle+sham, and Vehicle+AB. AMPKα2 knockout (KO) mice were randomly assigned to four groups: KO+sham, KO+AB, KO+-DIM+sham, and KO+DIM+AB. Mouse chow feed containing 0.05% DIM was initiated one week prior to surgery and continued for 4 weeks after surgery. After the mice were killed, the hearts were dissected and weighed to compare heart weight/body weight (HW/BW, mg/g) and heart weight/tibia length (HW/TL, mg/mm) ratios in DIM-treated and vehicle-treated mice.

Echocardiography and Hemodynamics

Echocardiography was performed by Mylab30CV (ESAOTE S.P.A) with a 10 MHz linear array ultrasound transducer. The LV was assessed in both parasternal long-axis and short-axis views at a frame rate of 50 Hz. End-systole and end-diastole were defined as the phase in which the smallest or largest area of LV was obtained, respectively. Left ventricular end-diastolic diameter (LVEDD) and left ventricular end-systolic diameter (LVESD) were measured from the LV M-mode tracing with a sweep speed of 50 mm/s at the mid-papillary muscle level.

For hemodynamic measurements, mice were anesthetized with 1.5% isoflurane, microtip catheter transducer (SPR-839, Millar Instruments, Houston, TX, USA) was inserted into the right carotid artery and advanced into the left ventricle. The pressure signals and heart rate were recorded continuously with a Millar Pressure-Volume System (MPVS-400, Millar Instruments, Houston, TX, USA), and the data were processed by PVAN data analysis software.

Histological Analysis

Hearts were excised, washed with saline solution, and placed in 10% formalin. Hearts were cut transversely close to the apex to visualize the left and right ventricles. Several sections of heart (4–5 μm thick) were prepared and stained with H&E for histopathology or PSR for collagen deposition and visualized by light microscopy. For myocyte cross-sectional area, sections were stained for membranes with FITC-conjugated WGA (Invitrogen) and for nuclei with DAPI. A single myocyte was measured with a digital quantitative image digital analysis system (Image Pro-Plus, version 6.0). The outline of 100 myocytes was traced in each group.

Immunohistochemistry

The procedures were described previously [18]. Heart sections were heated using the pressure cooker method for antigen retrieval. For immunohistochemistry (IHC), the sections were blocked with 3% H_2O_2, incubated with anti-NRF2 (Bioworld, rabbit) overnight at 4°C, then incubated with an anti-rabbit EnVisionTM+/HRP reagent, and stained using a DAB detection kit.

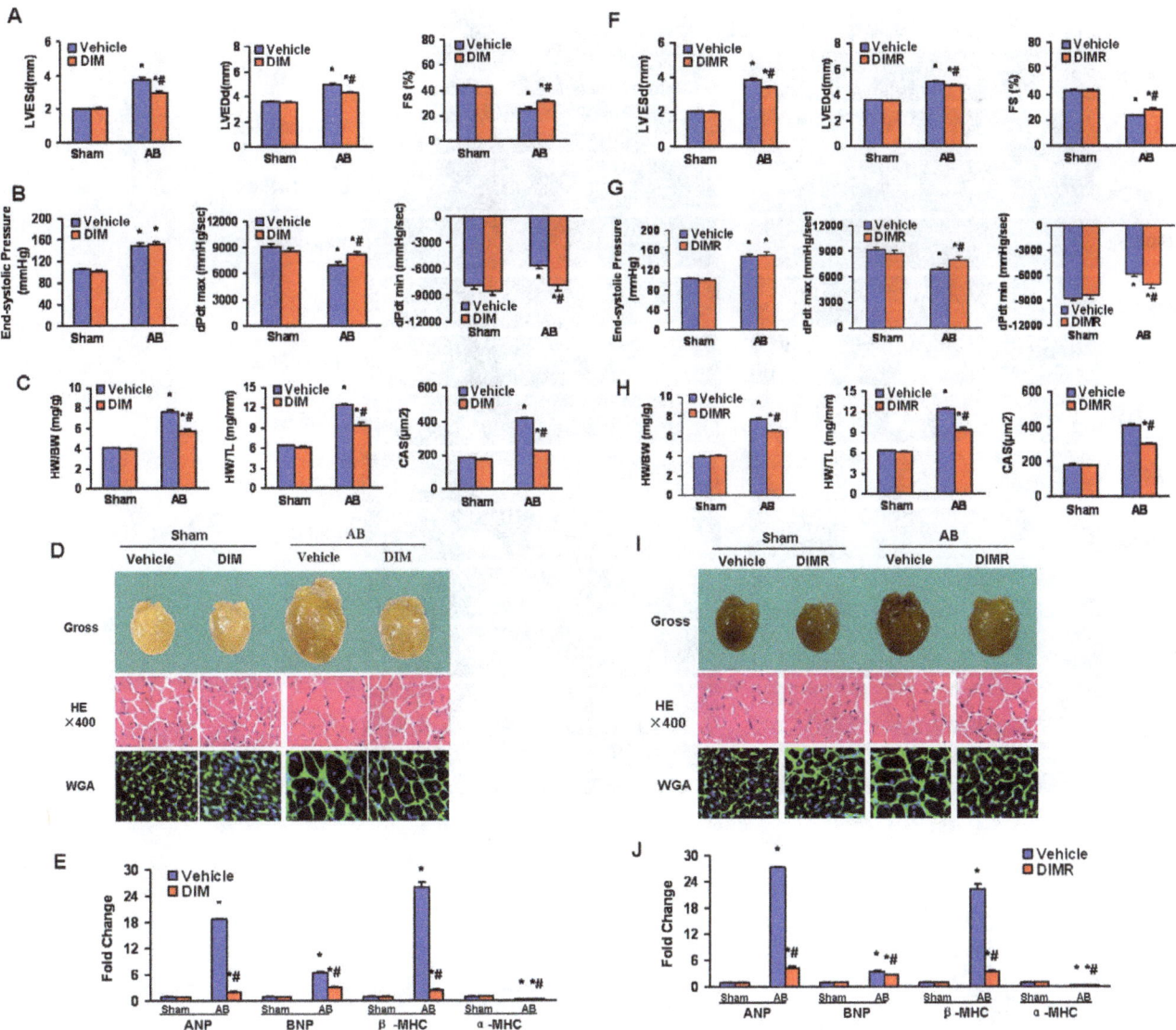

Figure 1. DIM attenuated cardiac hypertrophy induced by pressure overload. (A and B) A, Echocardiography results and B, pressure volume results from four groups of mice at 8 weeks after AB or sham surgery. (C) Statistical results of HW/BW ratio, HW/TL ratio (n = 12) and myocyte cross-sectional areas (n = 100 cells per section) at 8 weeks after AB or sham surgery. (D) Histology: representative gross hearts (top), H&E staining (middle), and WGA–FITC staining (bottom) at 8 weeks after AB or sham surgery. (E) Real-time PCR analysis of hypertrophic markers including ANP, BNP, α-MHC and β-MHC from hearts of mice in the indicated groups (n = 6). (F and G) F, Echocardiography and G, pressure volume results from four groups of mice at 8 weeks after AB or sham surgery in reverse experiments. (H) Statistical results of HW/BW ratio, HW/TL ratio (n = 9) and myocyte cross-sectional areas (n = 100 cells per section) at 8 weeks after AB or sham surgery in reverse experiments. (I) Histology: representative gross hearts (top), H&E staining (middle), and WGA–FITC staining (bottom) at 8 weeks after AB or sham surgery in reverse experiments. (J) Real-time PCR analysis of hypertrophic markers including ANP, BNP, α-MHC and β-MHC, from hearts of mice in the indicated groups in reverse experiment (n = 6). Values are expressed as the mean±SEM. *P<0.05 compared with the corresponding sham group. #P<0.05 vs Vehicle+AB group.

Quantitative Real-time RT-PCR and Western Blotting

Real-time PCR was used to detect those RNA expression levels of hypertrophic and fibrotic markers. Total RNA was extracted from frozen, pulverized mouse cardiac tissue using TRIzol (Roche), and cDNA was synthesized using oligo (dT) primers with the Advantage RT-for-PCR kit (Roche). We performed PCR with LightCycler 480 SYBR Green 1 Master Mix (Roche) and normalized results against glyceraldehyde-3-phosphate dehydrogenase (GAPDH) gene expression. For Western blotting, cardiac tissues were lysed in RIPA lysis buffer. Fifty micrograms of cell lysate was used for SDS/PAGE, and proteins were subsequently transferred to an polyvinylidene difluoride membranes (Millipore).

Specific protein expression levels were normalized to the GAPDH protein level for total cell lysate and cytosolic proteins on the same polyvinylidene difluoride membrane. The quantification of Western blots bands was performed with the Odyssey infrared imaging system (Li-Cor Biosciences). The secondary antibodies anti-rabbit IRdye 800 and anti-mouse IRdye 800 (Li-Cor Biosciences) were used at 1:10000 in Odyssey blocking buffer for 1 hour. The blots were scanned with the infrared Li-Cor scanner, allowing for the simultaneous detection of two targets (antiphospho and anti-total protein) in the same experiment.

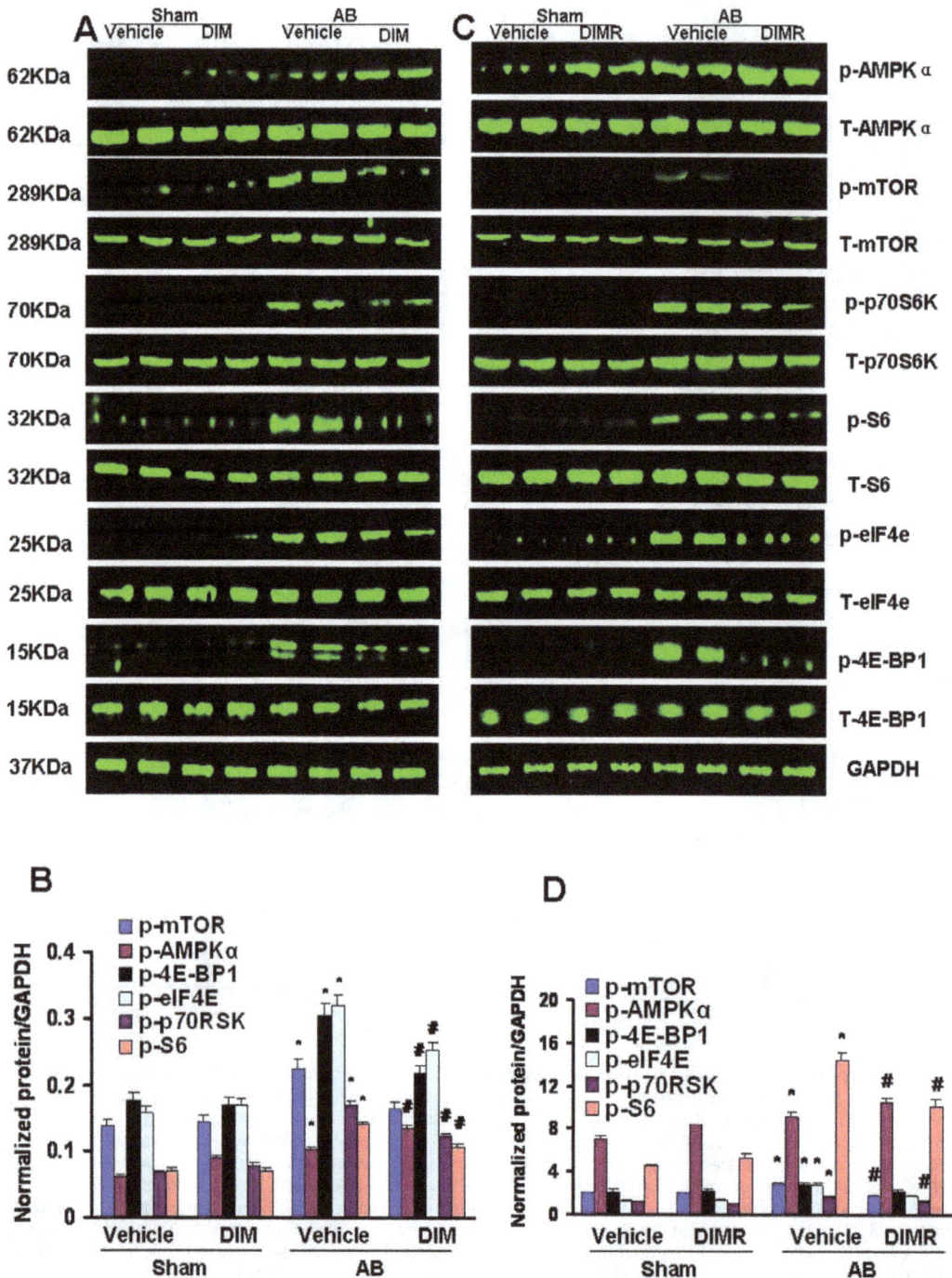

Figure 2. The effect of DIM on AMPKα and mTOR/p-70S6K signaling. (A and B) The protein levels of phosphorylated and total AMPKα, mTOR, p70S6K, S6, eIF4e and 4E-BP1 in mice from indicated groups. A, Representative Western blots. B, Quantitative results (n = 6). (C and D) The protein levels of phosphorylated and total AMPKα, mTOR, p70S6K, S6, eIF4e and 4E-BP1 in mice from indicated groups in reverse experiments (n = 6). C, Representative Western blots. D, Quantitative results. Values are expressed as the mean±SEM. *$P<0.05$ compared with the corresponding sham group. #$P<0.05$ vs Vehicle+AB group.

Statistical Analysis

Data are expressed as the means ± SEM. Differences among groups were tested by two-way ANOVA followed by a *post hoc* Tukey test. Comparisons between two groups were performed by unpaired Student's *t*-test. $P<0.05$ was considered to be significantly different.

Results

DIM Attenuated Cardiac Hypertrophy Induced by Pressure Overload in WT Mice

Both DIM-treated and vehicle-treated mice were submitted to AB or a sham surgery for 8 weeks to determine whether DIM antagonized and reversed the hypertrophic response to pressure

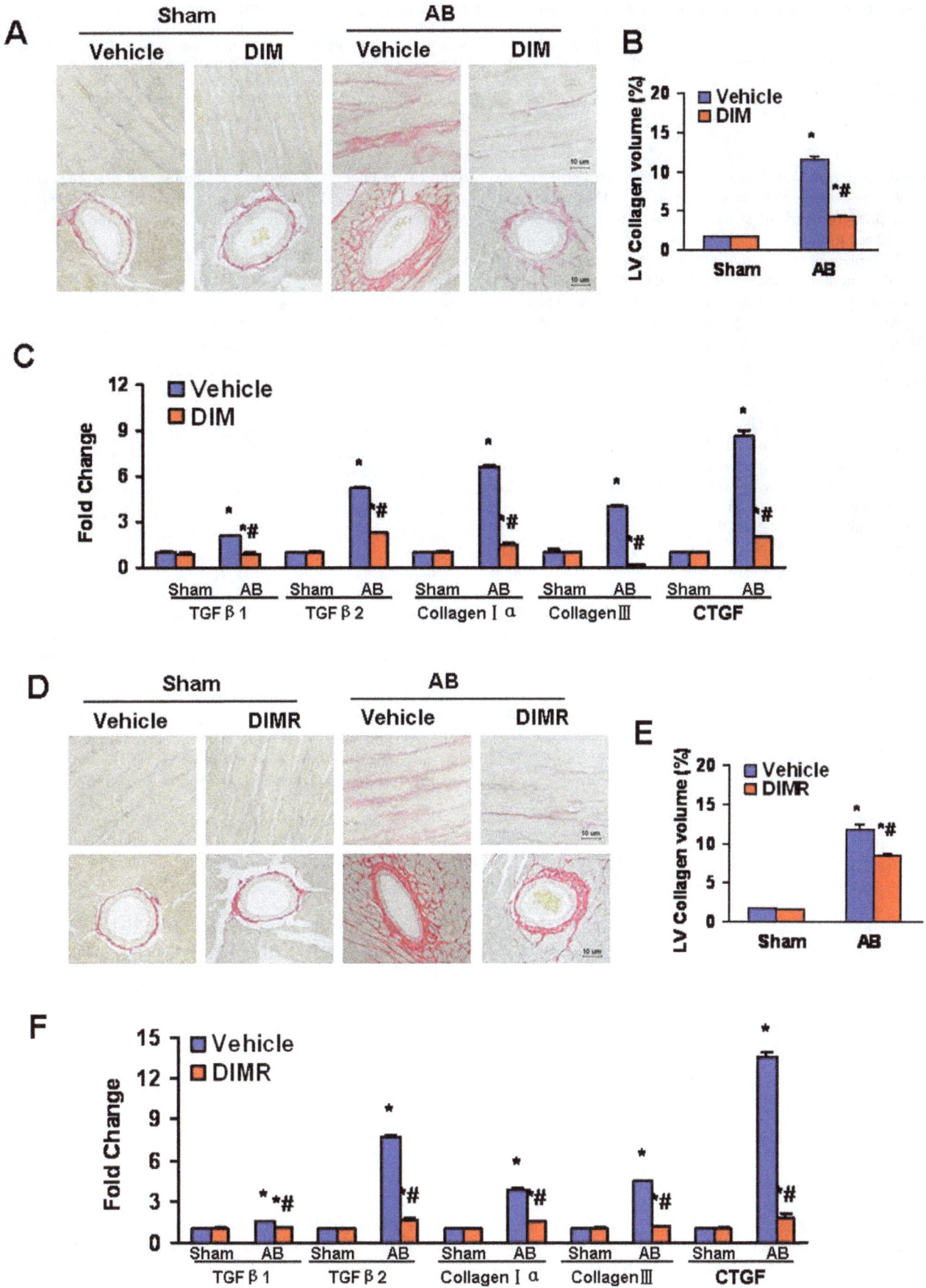

Figure 3. DIM blocked the fibrosis induced by pressure overload. (A) Representative images of PSR staining form indicated groups. (B) Quantitative analysis of left ventricle interstitial collagen volume fraction in indicated groups (n = 6). (C) Real-time PCR analysis of the mRNA expression of TGF-β1, TGF-β2, collagen Iα, collagen β and CTGF in the myocardium obtained from indicated groups (n = 6). (D) Representative images of PSR staining form indicated groups. (E) Quantitative analysis of left ventricle interstitial collagen volume fraction in indicated groups in reverse experiments (n = 6). (F) Real-time PCR analysis of the mRNA expression of TGF-β1, TGF-β2, collagen Iα, collagen β and CTGF in the myocardium obtained from indicated groups in reverse experiments (n = 6). The results were reproducible in three separate experiments. Values are expressed as mean±SEM. *P<0.05 compared with the corresponding sham group. #P<0.05 vs Vehicle+AB group.

overload. In former and reverse experiments, echocardiographic and pressure-volume (PV) loop analyses of DIM-treated mice showed pressure overload significantly increased LV mass and poor cardiac function in the vehicle-treated group that was limited by DIM replacement. Pressure overload led to increases in left ventricular enddiastole diameter (LVEDD), left ventricular end-systole diameter (LVESD) and decreased fractional shortening (FS) in vehicle-treated mice. LV systolic pressures were similar in the DIM- treated and vehicle-treated mice after 8 weeks of AB, being statistically greater than shams. In the vehicle group, pressure overload significantly decreased maximal LV dP/dt (dp/dt max) and minimum LV dP/dt (dp/dt min, absolute value), both of which were improved by DIM replacement (Figure 1A, B, F, G). DIM replacement normalized these parameters. DIM-treated mice showed attenuated cardiac hypertrophy after 8 weeks of AB with improvements in heart weight/body weight, heartweight/tibia length, and cardiomyocyte cross sectional area (Figure 1C, H). The inhibitory effect of DIM on cardiac hypertrophy was confirmed by the morphology of the gross hearts, hematoxylin-eosin (H&E) staining, and wheat germ agglutinin (WGA) staining (Figure 1D, I).

Quantitative increases in cardiac mass after pressure overload are always accompanied by the re-expression of a fetal gene program. Under baseline conditions, atrial natriuretic peptide (ANP), B-type natriuretic peptide (BNP), and β-myosin heavy chain (β-MHC) was strikingly suppressed in DIM-treated after pressure overload, accompanied by the upregulation of α-myosin heavy chain (α-MHC). (Figure 1E, J). Collectively, these data suggested DIM that impaired cardiac hypertrophy and protected cardiac function after pressure overload.

DIM Promoted the Phosphorylation of AMPKα and Attenuated mTOR Signaling Activation Induced by Pressure Overload

To explore the molecular mechanisms of the antihypertrophic actions of DIM, we analyzed protein extracts by Western blotting. In vehicle-treated mice, pressure overload significantly increased the cardiac amounts of p-AMPKα, increases that were promoted after DIM-treated. Phosphorylation of mTOR, p70S6K, S6, eIF4e and 4E-BP1, the known downstream targets of AMPKα, were also increased after 8 weeks of AB. However, they were blocked in DIM-treated hearts (Figure 2A, B, C, D). Collectively, these data suggest that DIM significantly inhibits cardiac hypertrophy through directly stimulating p-AMPKα activity and inhibiting the mTOR/p70S6K signaling pathway.

DIM Inhibited the Fibrosis Induced by Pressure Overload in WT Mice

To determine the extent of left ventricular interstitial fibrosis in the heart, in both former and reverse experiments, paraffin-embedded slides were stained with picrosirius red (PSR). Perivascular and interstitial fibrosis was detected in both vehicle-treated and DIM-treated mice, but the extent of cardiac fibrosis was markedly reduced in DIM treated mice (Figure 3A, B, D, E). Subsequent analysis of mRNA expression levels of

known mediators of fibrosis, including transforming growth factor β1 (TGF-β1), transforming growth factor β2 (TGF-β2), procollagen type Iα (collagen Iα), procollagen type β (collagen β) and connective tissue growth factor (CTGF), demonstrated a blunted response in DIM-treated mice after 8 weeks of AB (Figure 3C, F).

DIM had no Protective Effect on Cardiac Hypertrophy Induced by Pressure Overload in AMPKα2 Knockout Mice

The above data, which shows the ability of DIM to inhibit cardiac hypertrophy, suggest that synaptic activity may be modulated by AMPKα. To examine whether AMPK was critical for the effect of DIM in the hypertrophic response to pressure overload, AMPKα2 knockout (KO) mice were subjected to AB surgery or sham surgery. After 4 weeks of AB, AMPKα2 deficiency significantly more impairment of cardiac function, as demonstrated by a significant increase in LVEDD and LVESD, and a greater reduction of systolic fractional shortening as compared with Sham mice. Pressure-volume loop analysis further revealed that AMPKα2 deficiency worsened hemodynamic dysfunction in response to AB. Moreover, DIM treatment did not prevent the development of adverse cardiac remodeling or ventricular dysfunction in AMPKα2 KO mice (Figure 4A, B). Pressure overload-induced increased HW/BW, HW/TL and myocyte cross-sectional (Figure 4C), according with the morphology of the gross hearts, hematoxylin-eosin staining, and wheat germ agglutinin staining (Figure 4D) However, these measures were not improved after DIM-treated. In addition, the mRNA levels of ANP, BNP and β-MHC, which were the induction of hypertrophic markers, were greatly escalated and α-MHC was decreased in both DIM-treated and vehicle-treated KO mice in response to AB (Figure 4E). These results suggest that DIM could negatively regulate the extent of cardiac hypertrophy through AMPKα2 in response to pressure overload.

DIM Lost Protective Property against the Fibrosis Induced by Pressure Overload in AMPKα2 Knockout Mice

Paraffin-embedded slides were stained with picrosirius red (PSR) to explore whether AMPK was also critical for the effect of DIM on fibrosis in the heart. Perivascular and interstitial fibrosis was detected in both DIM-treated and vehicle-treated KO mice subjected to AB or sham surgery, but the extent of cardiac fibrosis was markedly enhanced in both AB group and no difference between them (Figure 5A, B). Subsequent analysis of mRNA expression levels of TGF-β1, TGF-β2, collagen Iα, collagen β and CTGF, which are responsible for cardiac fibrosis, showed the similar results (Figure 5C).

Role of DIM in the Regulation of Cardiac Oxidative Stress after Pathological Pressure Overload

Resent studies shown that DIM induces the transactivation of Nrf2 in cultured murine fibroblasts [19], while AMPKα2 regulates expression of estrogen-related receptor-alpha (ERRα, a transcriptional factor often affects mitochondrial antioxidants and energy

A

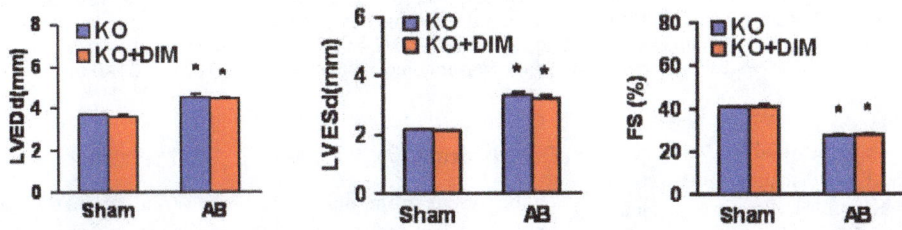

B

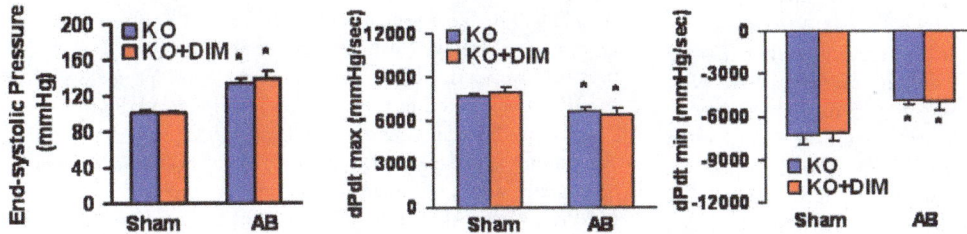

C

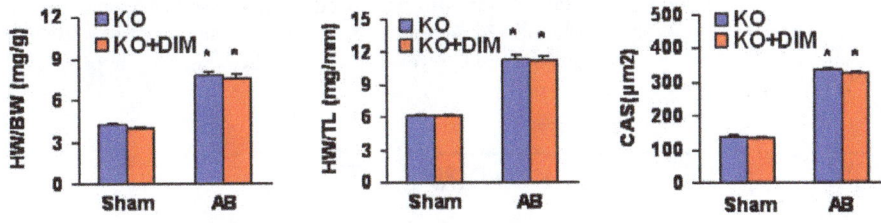

D

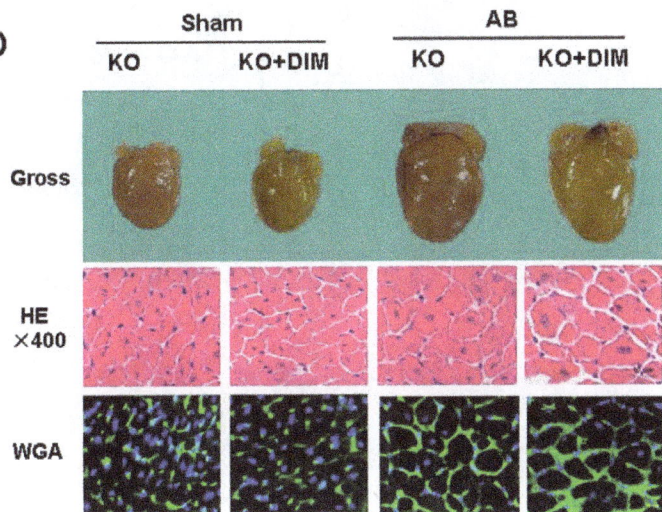

E

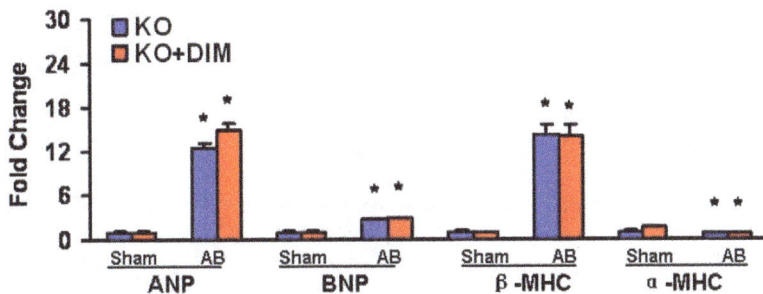

Figure 4. DIM inhibited cardiac hypertrophy by targeting AMPKα2. (A and B) Echocardiography and pressure volume results from four groups of mice at 4 weeks after AB or sham surgery. (C) Statistical results of the HW/BW ratio, HW/TL ratio (n = 12) and myocyte cross-sectional areas (n = 100 cells per section) at 4 weeks after AB or sham surgery. (D) Histology: representative gross hearts (top), H&E staining (middle) and WGA–FITC staining (bottom). (E) Real-time PCR analysis of hypertrophic markers including ANP, BNP, α-MHC and β-MHC, from hearts of mice in the indicated groups (n = 6). Values are expressed as mean±SEM. *P<0.05 compared with the corresponding sham group. #P<0.05 vs KO+AB group.

metabolism) [20]. Thus, we detect the myocardial oxidative stress markers and expression of NRF2 and ERRα etc after DIM-treated in both wild type and AMPKα2 KO mice. Pressure overload increased myocardial expression of ERRα, Nrf2 and its downstream genes, including glutathione peroxidase (GPx), heme oxygenase 1 (HO-1), thioredoxin-1 (Txn-1), thioredoxin reductase (Txnrd-1), superoxide dismutase (SOD)-1, SOD-2, and SOD-3 mRNAs in DIM-treated WT mice (Figure 6A) but not in AMPKα2 KO mice (Figure 6B). Nuclear translocation of Nrf2 proteins was dramatically enhanced in the cardiomyocytes of DIM-treated WT hypertrophied hearts (Figure 6C) but not in AMPKα2 KO hearts after AB (Figure 6D). The protein expression of Nrf2 and ERRα were consistent with the mRNAs expreesion (Figure 6E, F). These results indicate that Nrf2 and ERRα expression and activity are enhanced by DIM partly through AMPKα2 in the process of maladaptive responses to the sustained hemodynamic stress.

Discussion

The results from our study demonstrate that DIM protects against cardiac hypertrophy both in former and reverse experiments. The protective role of DIM in cardiac hypertrophy is mediated by direct interruption of AMPK-dependent mTOR signaling. The biological effects of DIM are also robust enough to reverse established cardiac hypertrophy induced by chronic pressure overload. More importantly, the cardioprotective effects of DIM ameliorated in mice lacking functional AMPKα2.

As a traditional Chinese medicine, DIM is widely used in combating against various diseases, such as anti-cancer, anti-angiogenic and anti-inflammatory effects, involved in affecting MAPKs, PI3K/Akt and the NF-κB signaling pathway [7,8]. In the present study, we have demonstrated that DIM not only attenuated cardiac hypertrophy in response to hypertrophic stimuli but also improved cardiac performance and reduced chamber dimensions. Another main finding of this study is that DIM could reverse pre-established cardiac hypertrophy and

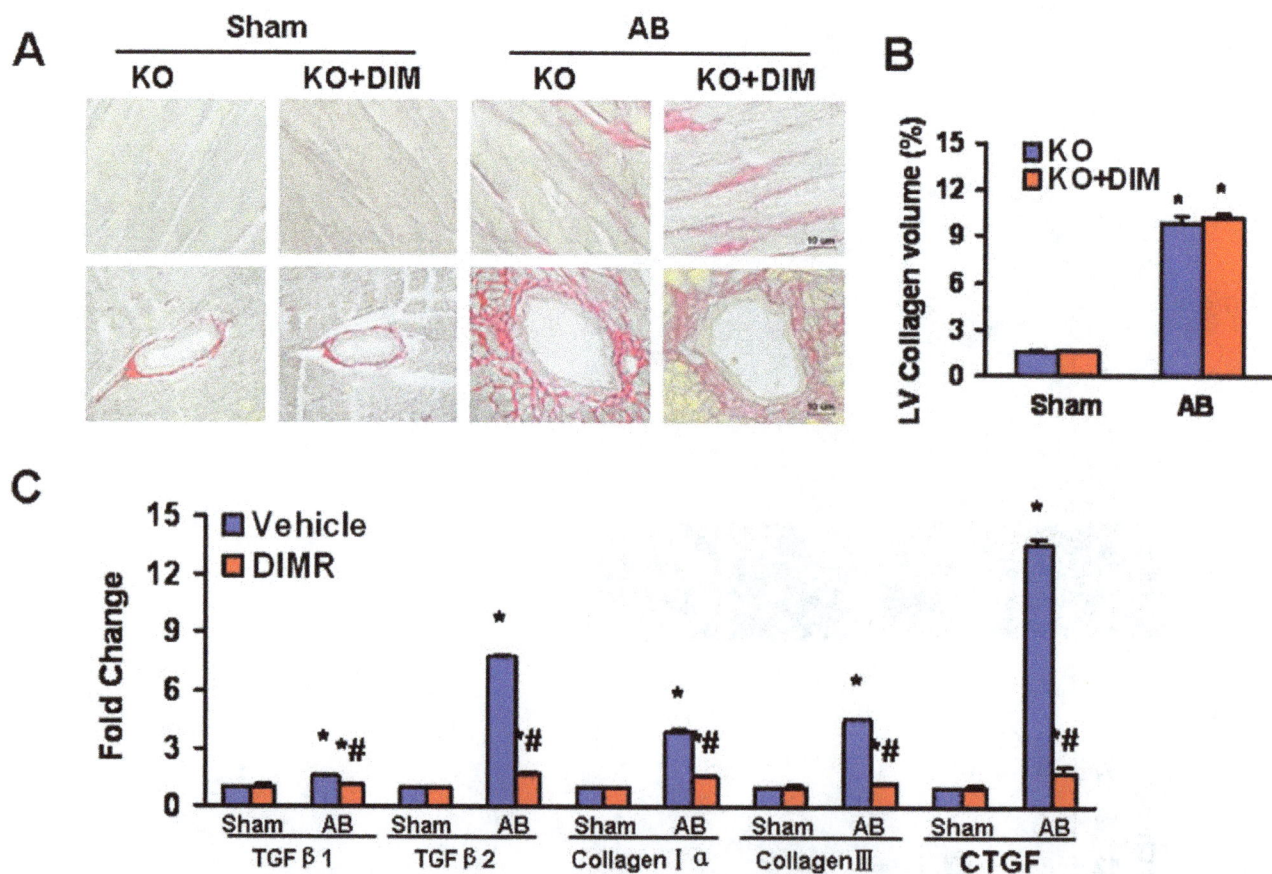

Figure 5. AMPKα2 is necessary in the anti-fibrotic effect of DIM. (A) Representative images of PSR staining form indicated groups. (B) Quantitative analysis of left ventricle interstitial collagen volume fraction in indicated groups (n = 6). (C) Real-time PCR analysis of the mRNA expression of TGF-β1, TGF-β2, collagen Iα, collagen β and CTGF in the myocardium obtained from indicated groups (n = 6). The results were reproducible in three separated experiments. Data are expressed as means±SEM. *P<0.05 compared with the corresponding sham group. #P<0.05 vs KO+AB group.

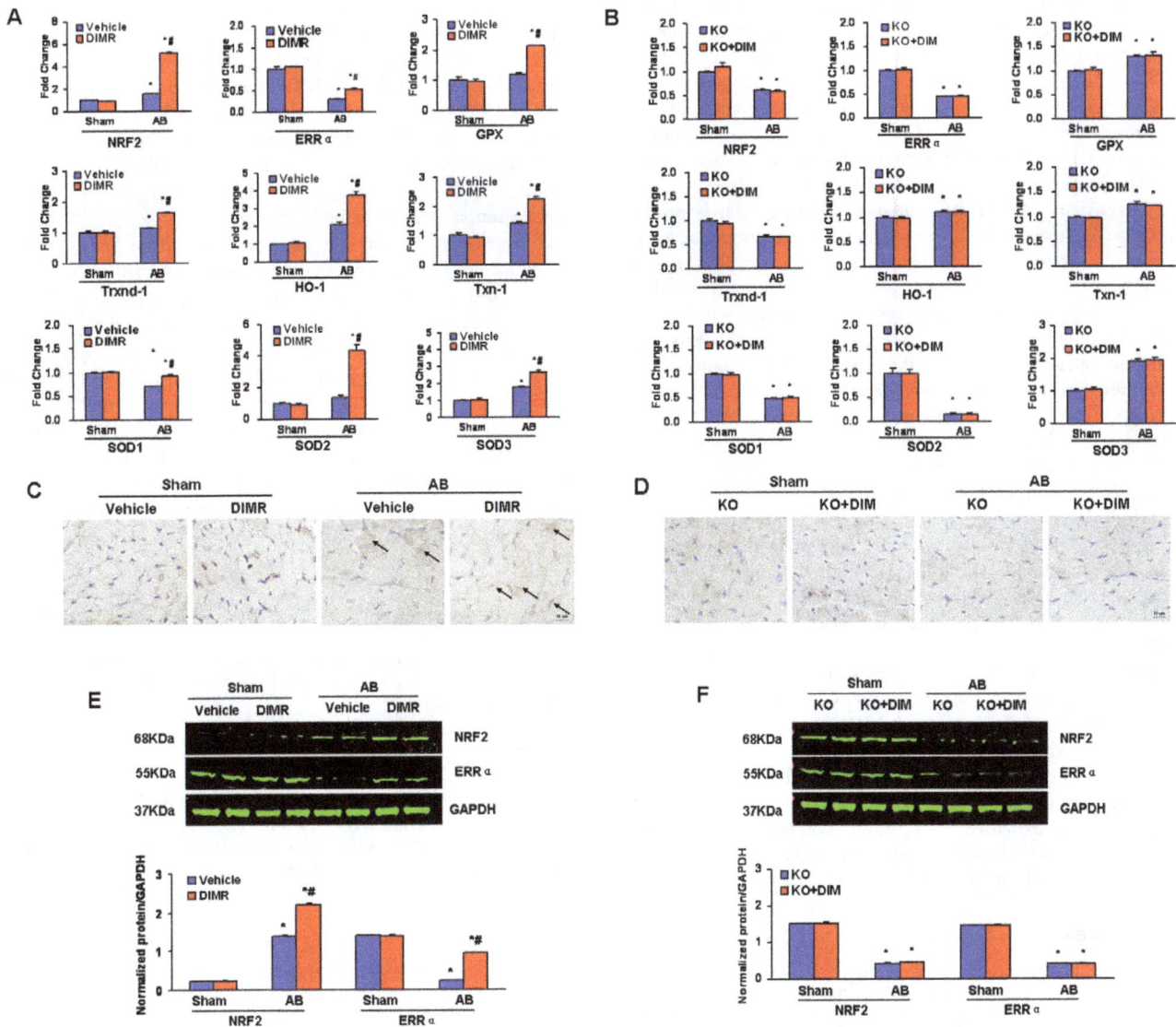

Figure 6. DIM inhibited Cardiac Oxidative Stress through AMPKα2. (A and B) Real-time PCR analysis of the mRNA expression of ERRα, Nrf2 and its downstream genes including GPx, HO-1, Txn-1, Txnrd-1, SOD1, SOD-2 and SOD-3 in the myocardium obtained from indicated groups (n = 6). A, in WT mice and B, in AMPKα2 KO mice. (C and D) Representative immunohistochemial staining of Nrf2 protein expression in WT mice and AMPKα2 KO mice after AB. (E and F) The protein levels of the cardiac expression of Nrf2 and ERRα in the myocardium obtained from indicated groups (n = 6). E, in WT mice and F, in AMPKα2 KO mice. Top, Representative Western blots; bottom, Quantitative results. *$P < 0.05$ compared with the corresponding sham group. #$P < 0.05$ vs Vehicle+AB/KO+AB group.

dysfunction induced by chronic pressure overload, which is of markedly clinical relevance.

The biochemical mechanism by which DIM mediates its antihypertrophic effects remains elusive. AMPK is an important regulator of cardiac metabolism [21]. AMPK signaling appears to have comprehensive effects in cardiovascular health and disease [22]. Previous study has demonstrated that *in vitro* AMPK activation is a key mediator of the changes in substrate utilization during cardiac ischemia and functions to maintain energy homeostasis, cardiac function and myocardial viability [10]. *In vivo* studies have shown that AMPKα2 plays a significant role in regulating pressure-overload induced LV remodeling [12].Our data demonstrate that DIM increases AMPKα phosphorylation. However, the cardioprotective actions of DIM ameliorated in AMPKα2 deficiency mice. AMPKα2 disruption aggravated cardiac hypertrophy, fibrosis, and dysfunction after AB in both

vehicle-treated and DIM-treated groups. These results suggest that the chronic activation of AMPKα2 during the development of cardiac hypertrophy is a primary mechanism mediating the beneficial actions of DIM.

We first found DIM interferes with the activation of AMPKα phosphorylation. Although AMPK activation is generally linked to degrading processes, this action seems to be largely indirect via mammalian target of rapamycin (mTOR) inhibition [23]. mTOR plays a significant role in the development of cardiovascular disease [24]. It is well known that the main downstream targets of mTOR are the S6 kinases (p70/85 and p54/56), the translation initiation factor binding protein (4E-BP1) [25,26], which is a repressor of eukaryotic translation initiation factor 4E (eIF4E) [27,28]. Importantly, previous studies have shown mTOR or its target(s) plays an important role in cardiac hypertrophy [29] and mTOR is required for the development of cardiac hypertrophy induced by rising blood pressure in spontaneously hypertensive rats [30]. In line with results from previous studies, we observed a significant increase in the phosphorylated levels of mTOR, p70S6K, S6, 4E-BP1 and eIF4E in the hypertrophic hearts of AB mice. When DIM was administered, the phosphorylation of them were markedly blocked. These findings indicate that the inhibitory effects of DIM on cardiac hypertrophy are mediated through mTOR signaling.

Fibrosis is another classical feature of pathological hypertrophy, which is characterized by the expansion of the extracellular matrix due to the accumulation of collagen [31]. Cardiac fibrosis plays a major role in the development of abnormal myocardial stiffness and ventricular dysfunction in response to pathological stimuli [32]. Thus, it is important to explore the mechanisms that stimulate collagen deposition in the heart and define approaches to limit these processes. As shown here, DIM-treated significantly attenuated cardiac fibrosis after pressure overload in WT mice and AMPKα2 deficiency mice. In current study, we found that DIM could downregulate mRNA expression levels of known mediators of fibrosis including TGF-β1, TGF-β2, collagen Iα, collagen β and CTGF were blunted in WT mice after AB. However, the mRNA expression levels of fibrosis mediators were markedly enhanced in both AMPKα2 KO AB groups and no difference was found between them. These results show that DIM could inhibit the fibrosis induced by pressure overload, primarily through AMPKα2.

Oxidative stress has been identified as one of the key contributing factors in the development of cardiac hypertrophy [33]. Recent research has suggested DIM induced Nrf2 transactivation [19], which is a protective regulator that prevents the maladaptive cardiac remodeling and heart failure associated with a sustained pathological hemodynamic stress via at least partly the suppressing of oxidative stress [32]. Loss of Nrf2 sensitizes cardiomyocytes and cardiac fibroblasts to oxidative stress-mediated cell death [34]. In present study, we found DIM increased myocardial expression of Nrf2 and its downstream genes in WT mice but not in AMPKα2 KO mice after AB. In addition, we detected DIM-treated resulted in a significant increase of myocardial ERRα at both mRNA and protein levels in WT mice but not in AMPKα2 KO mice after AB. Similar to our observations in AMPKα2 KO mice, previous study found that the reduced ERRα expression in the AMPKα2 KO mice contributed to the dysregulation of only some of the energy metabolism related genes [20].

In conclusion, our present study showed for the first time that DIM can not only prevent the development of cardiac hypertrophy but also reverse established cardiac hypertrophy by regulating the AMPKα and mTOR. The cardioprotective effects of DIM were ameliorated in mice lacking functional AMPKα2. This study is highly relevant to the understanding of the inhibitory effect of DIM on cardiac hypertrophy and related molecular mechanisms. Our observations revealed new insight into the pathogenesis of cardiac remodeling and may have considerable implications for the development of strategies for the treatment of cardiac hypertrophy and heart failure through the application of DIM. Additional studies are necessary to elucidate the potential clinical use of DIM.

Acknowledgments

We thank Professor Lianfeng Zhang from Institute of Laboratory Animal Science, Chinese Academy of Medical Sciences for providing the AMPKα2 knockout mice.

Author Contributions

Conceived and designed the experiments: QT J. Zong WD HL. Performed the experiments: J. Zong WD HZ ZB RZ JD YZ J. Zhang. Analyzed the data: J. Zong WD YY QW HG. Contributed reagents/materials/analysis tools: QT HL. Wrote the paper: J. Zong WD HL QT.

References

1. Gupta S, Das B, Sen S (2007) Cardiac hypertrophy: mechanisms and therapeutic opportunities. Antioxid Redox Signal 9: 623–652.
2. Barry SP, Davidson SM, Townsend PA (2008) Molecular regulation of cardiac hypertrophy. Int J Biochem Cell Biol 40: 2023–2039.
3. Balakumar P, Singh AP, Singh M (2007) Rodent models of heart failure. J Pharmacol Toxicol Methods 56: 1–10.
4. Azmi AS, Ahmad A, Banerjee S, Rangnekar VM, Mohammad RM, et al. (2008) Chemoprevention of pancreatic cancer: characterization of Par-4 and its modulation by 3,3′ diindolylmethane (DIM). Pharm Res 25: 2117–2124.
5. Li Y, Wang Z, Kong D, Murthy S, Dou QP, et al. (2007) Regulation of FOXO3a/beta-catenin/GSK-3beta signaling by 3,3′-diindolylmethane contributes to inhibition of cell proliferation and induction of apoptosis in prostate cancer cells. J Biol Chem 282: 21542–21550.
6. Xue L, Firestone GL, Bjeldanes LF (2005) DIM stimulates IFNgamma gene expression in human breast cancer cells via the specific activation of JNK and p38 pathways. Oncogene 24: 2343–2353.
7. Kunimasa K, Kobayashi T, Kaji K, Ohta T (2010) Antiangiogenic effects of indole-3-carbinol and 3,3′-diindolylmethane are associated with their differential regulation of ERK1/2 and Akt in tube-forming HUVEC. J Nutr 140: 1–6.
8. Cho HJ, Seon MR, Lee YM, Kim J, Kim JK, et al. (2008) 3,3′-Diindolylmethane suppresses the inflammatory response to lipopolysaccharide in murine macrophages. J Nutr 138: 17–23.
9. Shirwany NA, Zou MH (2010) AMPK in cardiovascular health and disease. Acta Pharmacol Sin 31: 1075–1084.
10. Russell RR, 3rd, Li J, Coven DL, Pypaert M, Zechner C, et al. (2004) AMP-activated protein kinase mediates ischemic glucose uptake and prevents postischemic cardiac dysfunction, apoptosis, and injury. J Clin Invest 114: 495–503.
11. Hwang JT, Kwon DY, Park OJ, Kim MS (2008) Resveratrol protects ROS-induced cell death by activating AMPK in H9c2 cardiac muscle cells. Genes Nutr 2: 323–326.
12. Zhang P, Hu X, Xu X, Fassett J, Zhu G, et al. (2008) AMP activated protein kinase-alpha2 deficiency exacerbates pressure-overload-induced left ventricular hypertrophy and dysfunction in mice. Hypertension 52: 918–924.
13. Tian R, Musi N, D'Agostino J, Hirshman MF, Goodyear LJ (2001) Increased adenosine monophosphate-activated protein kinase activity in rat hearts with pressure-overload hypertrophy. Circulation 104: 1664–1669.
14. Chen DZ, Qi M, Auborn KJ, Carter TH (2001) Indole-3-carbinol and diindolylmethane induce apoptosis of human cervical cancer cells and in murine HPV16-transgenic preneoplastic cervical epithelium. J Nutr 131: 3294–3302.
15. Khwaja FS, Wynne S, Posey I, Djakiew D (2009) 3,3′-diindolylmethane induction of p75NTR-dependent cell death via the p38 mitogen-activated protein kinase pathway in prostate cancer cells. Cancer Prev Res (Phila) 2: 566–571.
16. Li H, He C, Feng J, Zhang Y, Tang Q, et al. (2010) Regulator of G protein signaling 5 protects against cardiac hypertrophy and fibrosis during biomechanical stress of pressure overload. Proc Natl Acad Sci U S A 107: 13818–13823.
17. Bian ZY, Huang H, Jiang H, Shen DF, Yan L, et al. (2010) LIM and cysteine-rich domains 1 regulates cardiac hypertrophy by targeting calcineurin/nuclear factor of activated T cells signaling. Hypertension 55: 257–263.
18. Zhou H, Shen DF, Bian ZY, Zong J, Deng W, et al. (2011) Activating transcription factor 3 deficiency promotes cardiac hypertrophy, dysfunction, and fibrosis induced by pressure overload. PLoS One 6: e26744.
19. Ernst IM, Schuemann C, Wagner AE, Rimbach G (2011) 3,3′-Diindolylmethane but not indole-3-carbinol activates Nrf2 and induces Nrf2 target gene expression in cultured murine fibroblasts. Free Radic Res 45: 941–949.
20. Hu X, Xu X, Lu Z, Zhang P, Fassett J, et al. (2011) AMP activated protein kinase-alpha2 regulates expression of estrogen-related receptor-alpha, a metabolic transcription factor related to heart failure development. Hypertension 58: 696–703.
21. Heidrich F, Schotola H, Popov AF, Sohns C, Schuenemann J, et al. (2010) AMPK - Activated Protein Kinase and its Role in Energy Metabolism of the Heart. Curr Cardiol Rev 6: 337–342.
22. Viollet B, Horman S, Leclerc J, Lantier L, Foretz M, et al. (2010) AMPK inhibition in health and disease. Crit Rev Biochem Mol Biol 45: 276–295.
23. Jensen TE, Wojtaszewski JF, Richter EA (2009) AMP-activated protein kinase in contraction regulation of skeletal muscle metabolism: necessary and/or sufficient? Acta Physiol (Oxf) 196: 155–174.

24. Finckenberg P, Mervaala E (2010) Novel regulators and drug targets of cardiac hypertrophy. J Hypertens 28 Suppl 1: S33–38.

25. Tee AR, Blenis J (2005) mTOR, translational control and human disease. Semin Cell Dev Biol 16: 29–37.

26. Ojamaa K (2010) Signaling mechanisms in thyroid hormone-induced cardiac hypertrophy. Vascul Pharmacol 52: 113–119.

27. Inoki K, Corradetti MN, Guan KL (2005) Dysregulation of the TSC-mTOR pathway in human disease. Nat Genet 37: 19–24.

28. McKinsey TA, Kass DA (2007) Small-molecule therapies for cardiac hypertrophy: moving beneath the cell surface. Nat Rev Drug Discov 6: 617–635.

29. Proud CG (2004) Ras, PI3-kinase and mTOR signaling in cardiac hypertrophy. Cardiovasc Res 63: 403–413.

30. Soesanto W, Lin HY, Hu E, Lefler S, Litwin SE, et al. (2009) Mammalian target of rapamycin is a critical regulator of cardiac hypertrophy in spontaneously hypertensive rats. Hypertension 54: 1321–1327.

31. Berk BC, Fujiwara K, Lehoux S (2007) ECM remodeling in hypertensive heart disease. J Clin Invest 117: 568–575.

32. Li J, Ichikawa T, Villacorta L, Janicki JS, Brower GL, et al. (2009) Nrf2 protects against maladaptive cardiac responses to hemodynamic stress. Arterioscler Thromb Vasc Biol 29: 1843–1850.

33. Maulik SK, Kumar S (2012) Oxidative stress and cardiac hypertrophy: a review. Toxicol Mech Methods 22: 359–366.

34. Zhu H, Jia Z, Misra BR, Zhang L, Cao Z, et al. (2008) Nuclear factor E2-related factor 2-dependent myocardiac cytoprotection against oxidative and electrophilic stress. Cardiovasc Toxicol 8: 71–85.

5

TNNI3K, a Cardiac-Specific Kinase, Promotes Physiological Cardiac Hypertrophy in Transgenic Mice

Xiaojian Wang[1⦾], **Jizheng Wang**[1⦾], **Ming Su**[1], **Changxin Wang**[1], **Jingzhou Chen**[1], **Hu Wang**[1], **Lei Song**[2], **Yubao Zou**[2], **Lianfeng Zhang**[3], **Youyi Zhang**[4], **Rutai Hui**[1*]

1 Sino-German Laboratory for Molecular Medicine, State Key Laboratory of Cardiovascular Disease, FuWai Hospital & Cardiovascular Institute, Chinese Academy of Medical Sciences, Peking Union Medical College, Beijing, People's Republic of China, 2 Department of Cardiology, State Key Laboratory of Cardiovascular Disease, FuWai Hospital & Cardiovascular Institute, Chinese Academy of Medical Sciences, Peking Union Medical College, Beijing, People's Republic of China, 3 Key Laboratory of Human Disease Comparative Medicine, Ministry of Health, Institute of Laboratory Animal Science, Chinese Academy of Medical Sciences and Comparative Medical Center, Peking Union Medical College, Beijing, People's Republic of China, 4 Institute of Vascular Medicine, Peking University Third Hospital, Beijing, People's Republic of China

Abstract

Purpose: Protein kinase plays an essential role in controlling cardiac growth and hypertrophic remodeling. The cardiac troponin I-interacting kinase (TNNI3K), a novel cardiac specific kinase, is associated with cardiomyocyte hypertrophy. However, the precise function of TNNI3K in regulating cardiac remodeling has remained controversial.

Methods and Results: In a rat model of cardiac hypertrophy generated by transverse aortic constriction, myocardial TNNI3K expression was significantly increased by 1.62 folds ($P<0.05$) after constriction for 15 days. To investigate the role of TNNI3K in cardiac hypertrophy, we generated transgenic mouse lines with overexpression of human TNNI3K specifically in the heart. At the age of 3 months, the high-copy-number TNNI3K transgenic mice demonstrated a phenotype of concentric hypertrophy with increased heart weight normalized to body weight (1.31 fold, $P<0.01$). Echocardiography and non-invasive hemodynamic assessments showed enhanced cardiac function. No necrosis or myocyte disarray was observed in the heart of TNNI3K transgenic mice. This concentric hypertrophy maintained up to 12 months of age without cardiac dysfunction. The phospho amino acid analysis revealed that TNNI3K is a protein-tyrosine kinase. The yeast two-hybrid screen and co-immunoprecipitation assay identified cTnI as a target for TNNI3K. Moreover, TNNI3K overexpression induced cTnI phosphorylation at Ser22/Ser23 *in vivo* and *in vitro*, suggesting that TNNI3K is a novel upstream regulator for cTnI phosphorylation.

Conclusion: TNNI3K promotes a concentric hypertrophy with enhancement of cardiac function via regulating the phosphorylation of cTnI. TNNI3K could be a potential therapeutic target for preventing from heart failure.

Editor: Tohru Fukai, University of Illinois at Chicago, United States of America

Funding: This work was supported by Ministry of Science and Technology of China (2007DFC30340 to RTH); National Science and Technology Major Projects (2009ZX09501-026 to RTH); and the National Natural Science Foundation of China (30840041 to XJW, 30700322 to JZW). The funders had no role in study design, data collection and analysis, decision to publish, or preparation of the manuscript.

Competing Interests: The authors have declared that no competing interests exist.

* E-mail: huirutai@sglab.org

⦾ These authors contributed equally to this work.

Introduction

In response to increased workload, the heart undergoes hypertrophic enlargement, which is characterized by an increase in the size of individual cardiac myocyte.[1] This hypertrophic response can be traditionally classified as either physiological or pathological. Physiological stimuli such as exercise lead to compensatory growth of the cardiomyocyte, accompanied by normal cardiac structure, preserved or improved cardiac function, and minimal alteration in cardiac gene expression pattern.[2] In contrast, the pathological hypertrophy, which is induced by persistent pressure or volume overload at various disease conditions, is associated with reactivation of fetal gene program, interstitial fibrosis, cardiac dysfunction and eventual heart failure.[3] As heart failure is almost invariably associated with cardiac hypertrophy, the elucidation of signaling cascades involved in these two forms of hypertrophy will be of critical importance for the design of specific therapy against heart failure.[4,5]

Protein kinase plays an essential role in regulating cardiac growth and hypertrophic response. Various kinases transmit hypertrophic signals from membrane bound receptors and change the phosphorylation status of functionally significant proteins.[6] Cardiac myofilament, the ultimate determinant in the control of cardiac contractility, is a central feature of kinase signal transduction. Levels of contractile protein phosphorylation are associated with stretch of the myocardium, the myofilament response to Ca^{2+} and the progression of cardiac remodeling.[7–9] Despite considerable progress has been made in elucidating the roles of various kinases in regulating myofilament during the past decades, understanding the molecular mechanism underlying myofilament phosphorylation and cardiac hypertrophy remains limited. This is due to, at least in part, lack of knowledge for the function of novel protein kinases in the heart. In this regard, it is crucial to identify novel genes potential involved in cardiac hypertrophy.

The cardiac troponin I-interacting kinase (TNNI3K), also known as CARK, is a novel cardiac-specific kinase. It contains a central kinase domain, flanking by an ankyrin repeat domain in the amino terminus and a serine-rich domain in the carboxyl terminus. TNNI3K is a functional kinase and directly interacts with cardiac troponin I (cTnI). [10] It has been suggested as a factor that moderates electrocardiographic parameters and the susceptibility for viral myocarditis. [11,12] Our group has verified that Mef2c, an important determinant for cardiac hypertrophy, play a critical role in regulating basal TNNI3K transcription activity.[13] The precise function of TNNI3K in regulating cardiac remodeling, however, has remained elusive and controversial. Some studies have shown that TNNI3K induces cardiomyocyte hypertrophy in vitro [14] and enhances cardiac performance and protects the myocardium from ischemic injury in vivo, [15] while others have shown that overexpression of TNNI3K can accelerate disease progression in mouse models of heart failure. [16]

To better understand the role of TNNI3K in cardiac remodeling, we generated transgenic mice overexpressing TNNI3K specifically in the heart. Our data demonstrated that increasing basal TNNI3K expression resulted in enhancement of cardiac function and adaptive hypertrophy. Furthermore, TNNI3K directly interacts with cTnI and induced cTnI phosphorylation at Ser22/Ser23 in vivo and in vitro. These data suggest that TNNI3K promotes cardiac remodeling via regulating the phosphorylation of cTnI.

Materials and Methods

2.1. Ethics Statement

All animal experiments were approved by the FuWai Administrative Panel for Laboratory Animal Care and were consistent with the Guide for the Care and Use of Laboratory animals published by the United States National Institutes of Health. Rats and Mice were housed in an AAALAC-accredited facility with a 12-hour light-dark cycle and allowed water and food ad libitum. All surgery was performed under anesthesia, and all efforts were made to minimize suffering.

2.2. Transverse aortic constriction (TAC) surgery

Male Sprague-Dawley rats (200–250 g) were anesthetized with 2% isoflurane. Adequacy of anesthesia was assessed by monitoring the respiratory rate as well as the loss of response to toe pinch. The rats were then intubated and ventilated using a rodent ventilator (Model 683, Harvard Apparatus, South Natick, MA, USA). Midline sternotomy was performed, and the transverse aorta was exposed. The aorta was ligated between the innominate and left common carotid arteries by tying a 7–0 silk suture around a tapered 22-gauge needle placed on top of the aorta. Sham-operated controls underwent an identical surgical procedure including isolation of the aorta, only without placement of the suture. At different time points (day 1 to day 15) after surgery, animals (n = 4 to 5 for each time point) were euthanized by overdose anesthesia (pentobarbital sodium 150 mg/kg, i.p.) and cervical dislocation. The hearts were removed; left ventricles were weighed and quickly frozen in liquid nitrogen for total RNA extraction.

2.3. Quantitative real-time PCR analysis

Total RNA was isolated from left ventricular tissue using Trizol and reverse transcribed with Superscript III transcript kit (Invitrogen, Carlsbad, CA, USA). SYBR green-based quantitative real-time PCR was carried out with the DNA Engine Opticon 2 real-time PCR Detector (BIO-RAD, Richmond, CA, USA) as previous described.[13] Melting curve analysis was used to confirm amplification specificity. GAPDH gene was used as internal control. The primers are listed in Table S1. All experiments were repeated at least twice in triplicate.

2.4. Plasmid Constructs and Generation of Transgenic Mice

A human wild-type TNNI3K cDNA (2508 bp, NM_015978) was subcloned into the SalI/HindIII site of between the 5.5-kb murine α-myosin heavy chain promoter (α−MHC) and the 0.6-kb human growth hormone (hGH) polyadenylation sequence, carried in the pBluescriptII-SK+ vector (Stratagene). The transgenic mice were generated in the key laboratory of Human Disease Comparative Medicines as previously described[17]. Briefly, an 8.7-kb DNA fragment was isolated, purified from transgenic vector after digestion with NotI, and microinjected into fertilized oocytes from C57BL/6J mice. The surviving eggs were surgically transferred into pseudopregnant females. The resulting pups were screened by diagnostic PCR using the primers for TNNI3K, 5′-ATG GCA AGA GCA TTG ACC TAG TC-3′ and 5′-GGA TGA TTG AGC TGG CAG AGA-3′. The Fabpi gene was amplified as internal control using the primers, 5′-TGG ACA GGA CTG GAC CTC TGC TTT CCT AGA-3′ and 5′-TAG AGC TTT GCC ACA TCA CAG GTC ATT CAG-3′. To determine the transgene copy number, Southern blot analysis was performed on tail genomic DNA digested with EcoRI and probed with a ^{32}P-labeled 0.6 kb HindIII/NotI hGH fragment. The purified transgene insert DNA was added into the EcoRI digested wild-type mouse DNA to yield the equivalent of 1, 5, and 10 copies of the gene per haploid genome (based on 3×10^9 base pairs per haploid genome). The signals were quantified using ImageJ, and the copy number was determined from the standard curve. Three independent founder lines were identified and mated to C57BL/6J wild-type mice. Transgenic hemizygous mice were born, studied, and compared with their wild-type counterparts.

2.5. Northern Blot Analysis

Transgenic mice and their wild-type counterparts were sacrificed by cervical dislocation at the age of 3 months. Total RNAs were isolated using Trizol (Invitrogen, Carlsbad, CA, USA) from multiple organs, including heart, liver, spleen, lung, and kidney. Aliquots (20 μg) of total RNA were separated on 1% agarose gels containing 2.2 M formaldehyde and were blotted on Hybond N+ membrane (Amersham Pharmacia, Piscataway, NJ, USA). The probe was a 611 bp TNNI3K cDNA fragment amplified from the transgenic vector using the following primers, 5′-AAA GAT TAG AAG ATG ACC TGC-3′ and 5′-ATC TTG AGC ATT CAC ATC TG-3′. The probe was labeled with ^{32}P using a Random Primer DNA Labeling Kit (TaKaRa, Dalian, China) based on supplier's protocol. After hybridization, the membranes were washed, and exposed to films (Kodak). The signal was detected using ImageJ software.

2.6. Echocardiography

Mice were weighted and anesthetized with 2.5% avertin (0.018 mL/g) given i.p. Adequacy of anesthesia was monitored by lack of reflex response to toe pinch. Two-dimensional short-

and long-axis views of the left ventricule (LV) were obtained by transthoracic echocardiography with the Vevo 770 Imaging System and a 30-MHz probe (VisualSonics, Toronto, Canada). M-mode tracings were recorded and used to determine LV end-diastolic diameter (LVEDD), LV end-systolic diameter (LVESD), and LV posterior wall thickness (LVPWT) and interventricular septum (IVS) in diastole over three cardiac cycles. LV fractional shortening (FS) was calculated with the formula %FS = (LVEDD−LVESD)/LVEDD. After echocardiography examination, the mice were sacrificed by cervical dislocation. The hearts were excised, rinsed in ice-cold saline, weighed, dissected into left and right ventricles, frozen in liquid nitrogen and stored at −80 °C.

2.7. In Vivo Hemodynamics Analysis in Transgenic Mouse

Non-invasive hemodynamic analysis was performed in 3-month-old TNNI3K transgenic mice and age-matched littermate controls as previous described.[18] Mice were anesthetized with an intraperitoneal injection of 2.5% avertin (0.018 mL/g). Adequacy of anesthesia was monitored by lack of reflex response to toe pinch. A 1.4 French Millar catheter-tip micromanometer catheter (SPR-719, Millar Instruments Inc, Houston, Texas) was inserted through the right carotid artery into the left ventricular. After stabilization for 10 min, the pressure signal was continuously recorded on a computer. The peak LV systolic pressure and LV end-diastolic pressure were measured, and the maximal slopes of systolic pressure increment (dP/dt$_{max}$) and diastolic pressure decrement (dP/dt$_{min}$), indexes of contractility and relaxation, respectively, were analyzed.

2.8. Histological and Morphometric Analysis

Hearts from transgenic mice and nontransgenic littermate controls were collected and fixed in 4% paraformaldehyde buffered with PBS, routinely dehydrated, and paraffin embedded. Hearts were sectioned at 4 μm and stained with hematoxylin and eosin, and Masson's Trichrome. Mean myocyte size was calculated by measuring 150 cells from sections stained with hematoxylin and eosin.

2.9. Cell Culture and Recombinant Adenovirus

Adenovirus encoding full-length human TNNI3K (Ad-TNNI3K) was constructed using AdEasy Adenoviral Vector System. The 1- to 2-day-old neonates were sacrificed by cervical dislocation and the primary ventricular cardiomyocyte was isolated by enzyme digestion as we previously described.[19] The cardiomyocytes were planted onto 35-mm-diameter wells (six well plates) at a density of $\approx 2 \times 10^5$ cells per square centimeter and cultured in DMEM supplemented with 10% fetal bovine serum, 100 units/ml penicillin/streptomycin and 0.1 mM bromodeoxyuridine (BrDu). The following day the cells were washed in phosphate-buffer saline and cultured in serum-free DMEM, containing penicillin/streptomycin (100 units/ml). For adenoviral infection, cardiomyocytes were incubated for 2 hours with Ad-TNNI3K and Ad-GFP at an approximate multiplicity of infection of 50. Forty-eight hours following infection, >95% of the cells were GFP positive. The cells were harvested at basal level or after isoproterenol-stimulation for 10 min (10 nmol/l). The protein kinase activity was assessed by Western Blot.

2.10. Western Blots

Western blots were carried out on extracts from left ventricular or cultured cardiomyocytes. Proteinase inhibitor and phosphatase inhibitor cocktail (Roche, Basel, Switzerland) were added accord-

ing to the supplier's protocol. Protein concentrations were determined by the method of Bradford[20] and thirty micrograms of proteins were loaded on gels. Antibodies to Akt, phospho-Thr-308-Akt, phospho-Ser-473-Akt, ERK, phospho-Thr-202/204-ERK, GAPDH were purchased from Cell Signaling Technology (Beverly, MA), Antibodies to total and phosphorylated cTnI were generous gift from Prof. Xianmin Meng. Proteins were detected by Western blotting and stained with NBT/BCIP (Promega, Madison, WI, USA) or ECL detection reagents (Amersham Pharmacia Biotech).

2.11. Yeast two-hybrid Screen and co-immunoprecipitation

A full-length human TNNI3K cDNA, fused to the GAL4 DNA binding domain, was used as bait in a yeast two-hybrid screen of approximately 3×10^6 clones of a human heart cDNA library (Clontech, California, USA). The interaction domain of TNNI3K to cTnI was determined by protein truncation test using immunoprecipitation techniques. The full-length and truncated TNNI3K cDNA sequence encoding amino acids 1–421, 422–726, 727–835, 1–726, and 422–835 of TNNI3K were cloned into pCMV-Myc vector between *EcoRI* and *XhoI* sites to generate pCMV-Myc-TNNI3K, pCMV-Myc-TNNI3K-ANK, pCMV-Myc-TNNI3K-PK, pCMV-Myc-TNNI3K-SR, pCMV-Myc-TNNI3K-ANK+PK, and pCMV-Myc-TNNI3K-PK+SR, respectively. Full-length human cTnI cDNA was cloned into pCMV-HA vector between *EcoRI* and *KpnI* sites to generate pCMV-HA-cTnI. The integrity of all of the constructs was verified by sequencing.

H9C2 cells were transiently transfected with 2 μg of plasmid DNA using Lipofectamine 2000 (Invitrogen) according to the manufacturer's protocol. Double transfections were carried out with the pCMV-HA-cTnI and empty pCMV-Myc or each of the TNNI3K plasmids. Forty-eight hours after transfection, cells were washed with cold PBS and harvested. Protein to protein interaction was assayed by co-immunoprecipitation using Pro-Found c-Myc-Tag IP/Co-IP Kits (Pierce Biotechnology, Rockford, IL) according to the manufacturer.

2.12. Immunoprecipitation of TNNI3K and Phospho Amino Acid Analysis.

A full-length myc-tagged human TNNI3K DNA was expressed in H9C2 cells. The myc-tagged TNNI3K protein was immunoprecipitated using ProFound Mammalian c-Myc Tag IP/Co-IP kit (Pierce, Rockford, IL) and was analyzed by SDS-PAGE followed by immunoblotting with rabbit anti-phosphoamino acid antibody, anti-phosphotyrosine antibody, anti-phosphothreonine antibody, and anti-phosphoserine antibody, respectively.

2.13. Statistics

All measurement data are expressed as mean±SE. The statistical significance of differences between groups was analyzed by Student's t-test. Differences were considered significant at a P-value<0.05.

Results

3.1. TNNI3K was involved in Cardiac Hypertrophy

To investigate whether TNNI3K is involved in cardiac hypertrophy, the expression of TNNI3K was examined in a rat model of cardiac hypertrophy generated by transverse aortic constriction (TAC). After constriction for 15 days, the heart weight/body weight ratio (HW/BW) and left ventricular weight/body weight ratio (LVW/BW) were increased by 59.2% and

64.3% in TAC rats compared with those of sham operated controls (both p<0.001) (Figure 1A and B). Atrial natriuretic peptide (ANP), a cardiac hypertrophic marker, was upregulated by 40 folds in TAC rats (Figure 1C). TNNI3K was significantly downregulated on day 1 (0.66 fold, P<0.05), return to basal levels on day 7, and then increased on day 15 (1.62 folds, P<0.05) (Figure 1D). This unique expression pattern indicates that TNNI3K is involved in cardiac remodeling.

3.2. Generation of Cardiac-Specific TNNI3K Transgenic Mice

To investigate the role of TNNI3K as a potential regulator of cardiac hypertrophy *in vivo*, transgenic mice overexpressing the human TNNI3K specifically in heart using the mouse αMHC promoter were generated (Figure 2A). By PCR genotyping, three independent transgenic founders were identified from 33 F0 mice (Figure 2B). These founders carried 2, 8, and 44 copies of transgene, and were designated as TG-L (low copy number), TG-M (medium copy number), and TG-H (high copy number), respectively (Figure 2C). The expression of the transgene was restricted to the heart. No expression was detected in the kidneys,

spleen, liver and lung (Fig. 2D). Furthermore, the transgene expression was positively associated with the transgene copy number. TG-H displayed 20-fold higher transgene expression level than TG-L (Figure 2D).

3.3. Overexpression of TNNI3K Induced Cardiac Hypertrophy *in vivo*

In all three lines of transgenic mice, no premature death or sign of heart failure were found after 1 year of observation. Both the TG-L and TG-M lines had no demonstrable cardiac phenotype when compared with their respective littermate controls (Table 1). In contrast, TG-H mice showed a unique profile of increased HW/BW ratio of 31.3% and 43.1% at 3 months and 12 months of age, respectively (P<0.01 and P<0.05).Therefore, further characterization studies of the transgenic phenotype were carried out using male mice from TG-H.

Cardiac size was significantly larger in TG-H mice than in nontransgenic littermates at the age of 3 month (Figure 3A). Macroscopic sections showed a phenotype of concentric ventricular hypertrophy in the transgenic mice, which was characterized with smaller chamber size and thicker ventricular wall (Figure 3B).

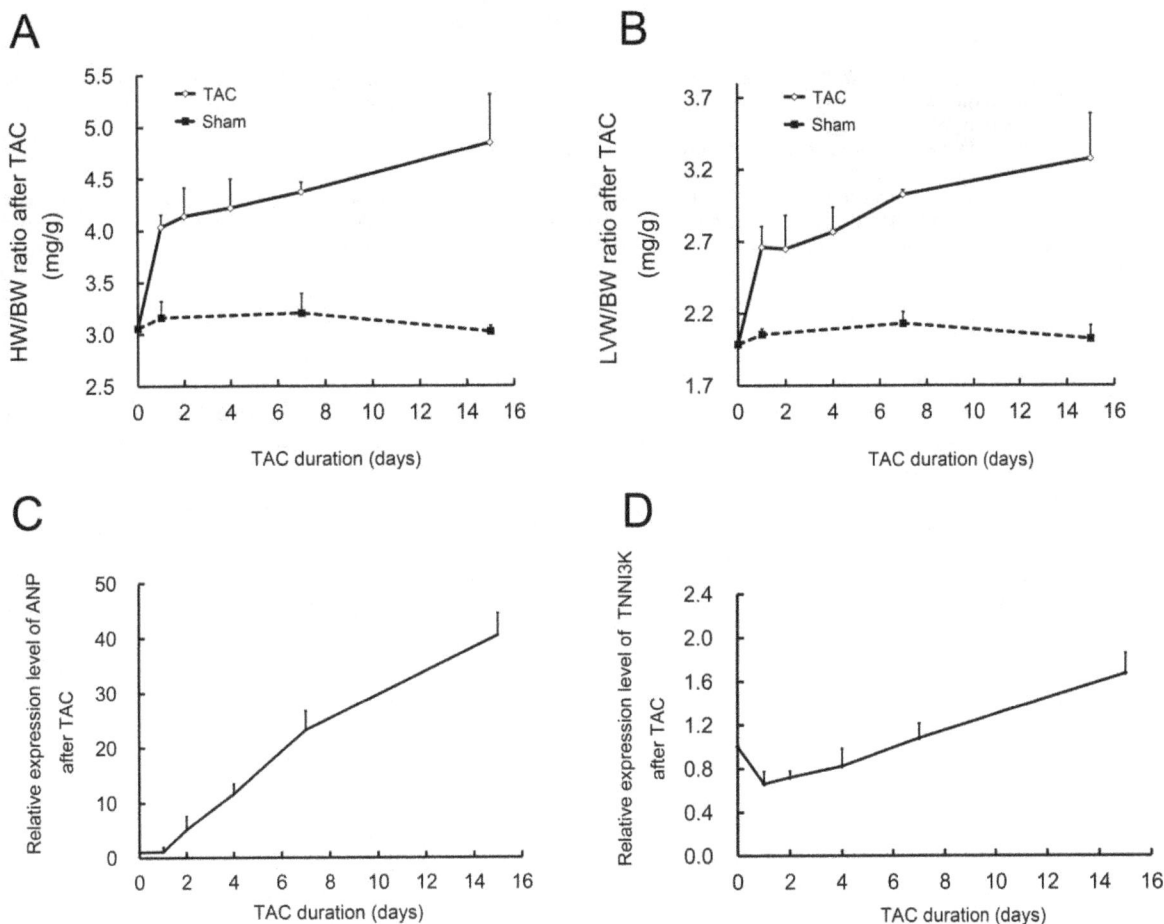

Figure 1. TNNI3K expression was dynamically regulated in the hypertrophic hearts in rats. A and B: the heart weight/body weight (HW/BW) and left ventricular weight/body weight (LVW/BW) were continuously increased after TAC. Five different time points were analyzed for TAC group and 3 different time points for sham operation group. Each time point included 4–5 animals. C and D: The expression of ANP and TNNI3K were detected by real-time PCR analysis. *Gapdh* was used for internal control and data were presented as fold-change compared with that of sham operation controls. Five different time points were analyzed (1, 2, 4, 7, 15 days post-operation, respectively). Each time point contained 4–5 animals.

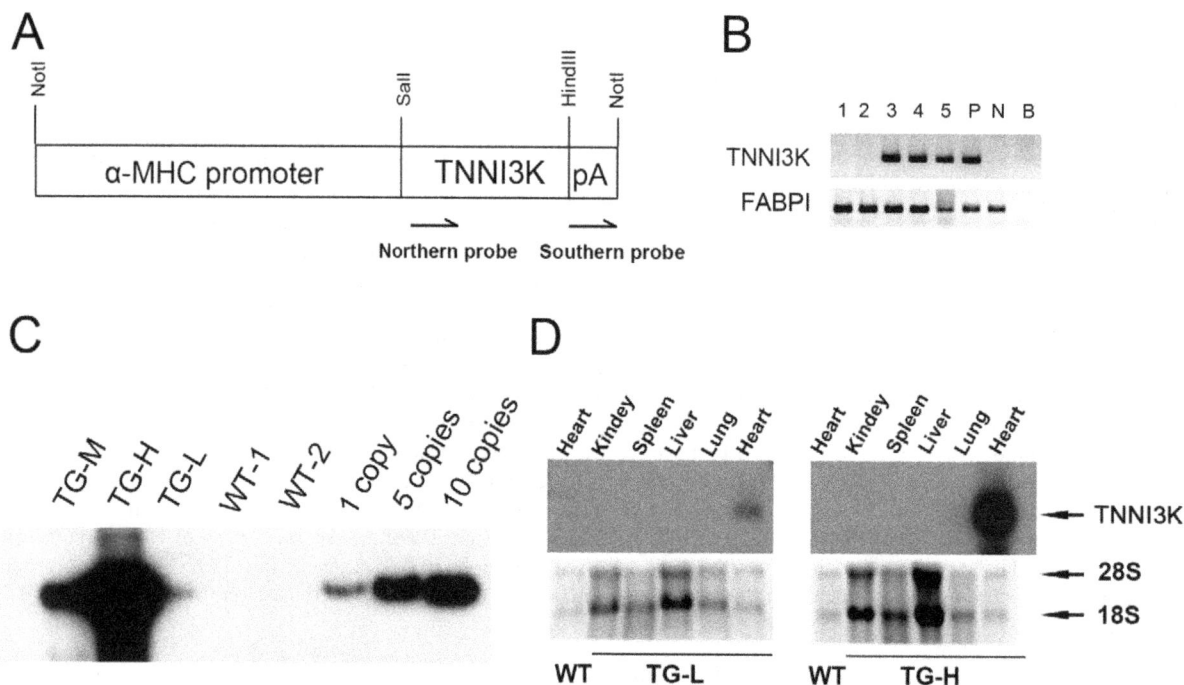

Figure 2. Generation of cardiac-specific *TNNI3K* transgenic mice. (A), Schematic of the TNNI3K transgene that was constructed with the α-MHC mouse promoter. pA: human growth hormone polyA sequences The positions of the Southern probe and northern probe were shown below the construct; (B), PCR genotyping of TNNI3K transgenic mice. 1–5: transgenic mice. P: positive control, wild-type mouse genomic DNA mixed with linearized transgenic fragment. N: negative control, wild-type mouse genomic DNA. B: blank, none DNA template. *FABPI* gene was amplified as internal control. (C), Southern blot analysis of wild-type and *TNNI3K* transgenic mice. Tail genomic DNA was digested with *EcoRI* and probed with *hGH* polyA sequence. Hybridization signals were present only in transgenic positive mice. Transgenic copy number was determined from the gray density against standard curve. 1 copy -10 copies: transgenic copy standards. (D). Northern blot analysis of RNA isolated from multiple tissues of the transgenic TG-L and TG-H lines. Hybridization signals were present only in the heart of transgenic mice. The RNA isolated from the heart of wild-type mouse was used as a negative control.

Upon microscopic observation, necrosis or myocyte disarray was not observed in TG-H mice (Figure 3C, upper panels). Masson-trichrome stain showed no interstitial fibrosis in TG-H mice (Figure 3C, lower panels). To examine whether the increase in cardiac size was due to cellular growth, the cross-section area of myocytes was quantitatively measured on the hematoxylin–eosin-stained LV myocardium of two representative transgenic mice and two controls, respectively. TG-H myocytes were substantially larger with a mean surface area 1.8-fold greater than those seen in littermate controls (Figure 3D).

Table 1. Gravimetric Data for the TNNI3K Transgenic Mouse Heart.

	3 months				12 months	
	NTG	TG-L	TG-M	TG-H	NTG	TG-H
N	11	6	6	6	6	6
BW (g)	24.5±0.5	24.5±0.6	26.2±1.2	26.4±1.0	38.0±0.7	38.1±0.7
HW/BW(mg/g)	5.1±0.2	5.4±0.4	5.5±0.3	6.7±0.2**	5.8±0.5	8.3±0.9*
LVW/BW(mg/g)	3.6±0.4	3.5±0.4	3.6±0.2	4.4±0.3*	3.8±0.5	5.8±0.9*

Heart weight/body weight ratios and left ventricular weight/body weight ratio were calculated from TNNI3K transgenic or non-transgenic mice at the indicated time points. Values given are Mean±SE and P values were calculated by Student's t-test. *: compared with non-transgenic mice, P<0.05, **: compared with non-transgenic mice, P<0.01.

To assess *in vivo* cardiac morphology and function, echocardiography were performed on TG-H and littermate control mice at the age of 3 months and 12 months, respectively. In agreement with the histological analysis, the 3-month-old TG-H mice showed a concentric cardiac hypertrophy. The left ventricular wall thickness was significantly increased (36.6% and 46.9% in IVS and LVPWT, respectively, both P<0.01), accompanied by decreased chamber dimension (19.0% and 10.8% in LVESD and LVESD, respectively, both P<0.01), and increased fraction shortening (Table 2 and Figure S1). Surprisingly, this phenotype of concentric hypertrophy persisted up to the age of 12 months (Table 2). Echocardiography showed increased ventricular wall thickness and decreased chamber dimension in the transgenic heart. More importantly, there is no loss of systolic functional performance between 3 and 12 months of age, indicating that cardiac hypertrophy in TNNI3K transgenic mice was compensated hypertrophy.

To evaluate the effect of overexpressing TNNI3K on cardiac function more accurately, noninvasive hemodynamic assessment was performed using LV catheterization. After anesthesia, there was no significant difference in heart rate and blood pressure between the 3-month-old TG-H mice and non-transgenic littermates. LV pressure was mildly increased both at systolic and diastolic in transgenic heart. In consistent with the echocardiography analysis, LV dP/dt$_{max}$ and LV dP/dt$_{min}$ were increased by 9% and 20% in transgenic mice compared with those in wild-type mice, respectively (Table 3), indicating enhanced contractility and diastolic function for the TG-H mice.

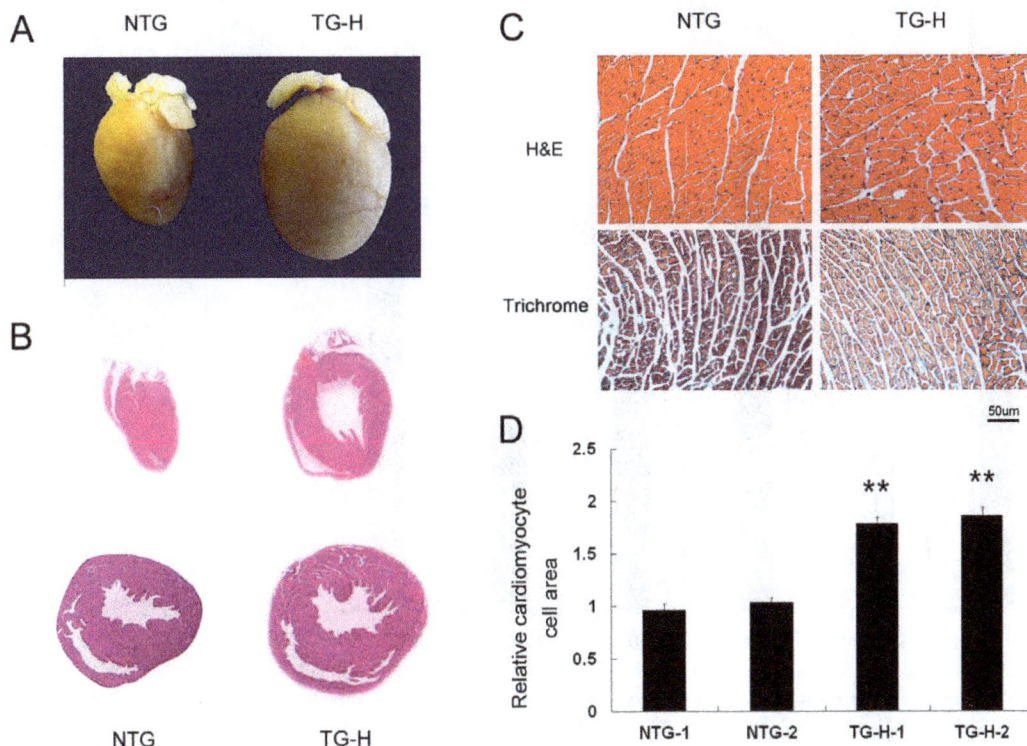

Figure 3. Cardiac histological analysis of TNNI3K transgenic mice at the age of 3 Months. (A) Whole heart, (B) Macroscopic view after hematoxylin–eosin-stained hearts revealed a concentric hypertrophy in TG-H mice. Upper was longitudinally sectioned. Lower was transversely sectioned. (C) Microscopic histological analysis of demonstrated cardiomyocyte hypertrophy without an increase in interstitial fibrosis in TG-H hearts. Upper panel was H&E stained sections. Lower panel was trichrome stained sections. Blue staining represents collagen deposition. Original magnification x200 (D) Cross-sectional areas of cardiomyocyte were quantified from hematoxylin–eosin-stained histological sections. At least 150 myocytes were measured each in two non-transgenic (NTG) hearts and two TG-H transgenic heart. **$P<0.01$ compared with wild-type.

Cardiac hypertrophy is accompanied by reprogramming of cardiac gene expression. To characterize the molecular phenotype of TNNI3K-induced cardiac hypertrophy, we examined the transcriptional levels of a set of hypertrophic markers, including atrial natriuretic peptide (*ANP*), brain natriuretic peptide (*BNP*), skeletal muscle α-actin (*Actc1*), α- and β-myosin heavy chain (*Myh6* and *Myh7*, respectively), phospholamban (*PLN*) and sarcoplasmic reticulum Ca^{2+} ATPase (*SERCA2a*). In 3-month-old TG-H transgenic hearts, the expression of ANP and BNP was increased

($P<0.01$), whereas Actc1 was decreased ($P<0.05$). On the other hand, the expression of β-MHC was mildly increased, whereas α-MHC and SERCA2a mRNA were markedly increased (Figure 4). These discordant changes in gene expression indicate that the fetal gene program is differentially regulated in the TNNI3K transgenic heart.

Table 2. M-mode echocardiograms.

	3 months		12 months	
	NTG	**TG-H**	**NTG**	**TG-H**
N	13	7	6	5
IVS (mm)	0.71±0.03	0.97±0.03**	0.95±0.03	1.40±0.07**
LVPWT (mm)	0.66±0.02	0.97±0.05**	0.93±0.03	1.16±0.07*
LVESD (mm)	2.32±0.06	1.88±0.10**	2.75±0.25	1.83±0.21*
LVEDD (mm)	3.79±0.05	3.38±0.14**	4.23±0.22	3.67±0.15
%FS	38.7±1.4	46.5±2.8**	35.5±3.0	50.4±4.3*

LVEDD, LV end-diastolic diameter; LVESD, LV end-systolic diameter; LVPWT, LV posterior wall thickness, IVS, interventricular septum; %FS, fraction shorting. Values given are Mean±SE and P values were calculated by Student's t-test. *: compared with non-transgenic mice, $P<0.05$, **: compared with non-transgenic mice, $P<0.01$.

Table 3. Hemodynamic Analysis of TNNI3K Transgenic Mice.

	NTG	**TG-H**
N	8	6
HR (beats/min)	388.5±4.8	380.5±5.7
AP systolic (mmHg)	93.0±4.6	98.0±4.2
AP diastolic (mmHg)	62.7±3.4	61.2±2.5
LVP systolic (mmHg)	104.0±3.2	125.4±11.3
LVP diastolic (mmHg)	−17.3±1.0	−13.1±1.8
LVEDP (mmHg)	−3.3±0.5	−2.2±0.3
dP/dt$_{max}$ (mmHg/s)	6311.6±143.6	6881.8±514.6
dP/dt$_{min}$ (mmHg/s)	−6325.3±169.6	−7567.8±720.4

HR: heart rate; AP: arterial pressure; LVP: left ventricular pressure; LVEDP: left ventricular end-diastolic pressure, dP/dt$_{max}$ and dP/dt$_{min}$: average maximum and minimum values, respectively, of first derivative of ventricular pressure wave.

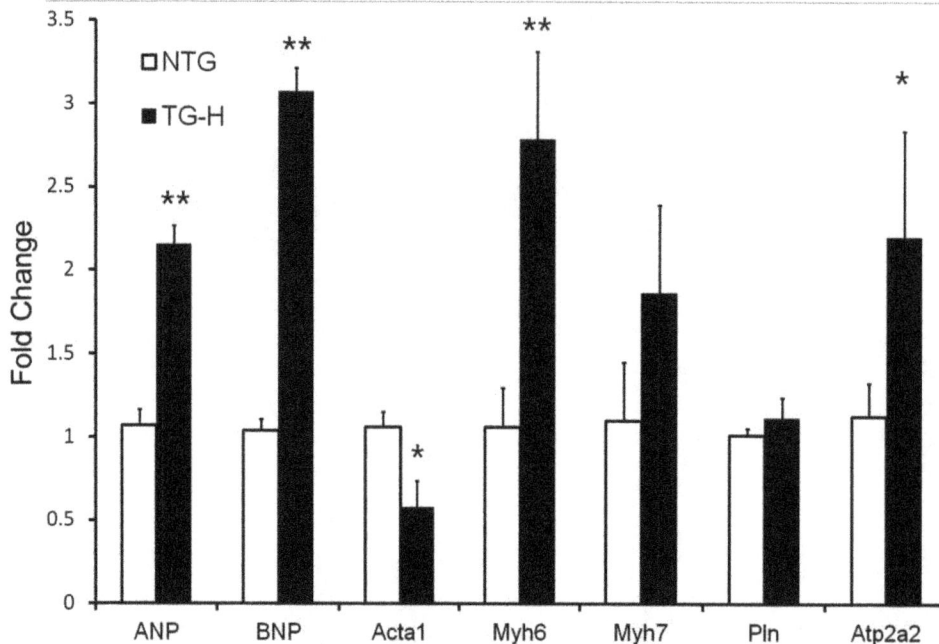

Figure 4. Assessment of hypertrophy marker genes. The mRNA levels were measured in left ventricle by RT-PCR analysis (N = 4 hearts in each group). *Gapdh* was used for internal control. **: $P<0.01$, *: $P<0.05$ vs nontransgenic littermates.

3.4. TNNI3K does not induce the activation of ERK and Akt

Akt and ERK were among the best characterized signaling cascades that induce cardiac hypertrophy. In the left ventricular of TG-H mice at the age of 3 months, however, no significant difference was identified in the amount of total or phosphorylated Akt and ERK (Figure 5A). Consistent with the *in vivo* results, overexpression of TNNI3K in cardiomyocyte with a recombinant adenovirus does not induced activated of Akt or ERK (Figure 5B). Therefore, TNNI3K might not be involved in these two signal pathway.

3.5. TNNI3K interacts with cTnI and induced cTnI phosphorylation at Ser22/Ser23

To gain insight into the proteins those physiologically interact with TNNI3K in the heart, we performed the yeast two-hybrid study using full-length TNNI3K as bait. Screening of human heart cDNA library resulted in the identification of thirteen TNNI3K-interacting factors, one of which was cTnI. Previous data suggest there is a physical interaction between TNNI3K and cTnI[10]. To map the region of TNNI3K that bind cTnI, amino- and carboxyl-terminal truncations of TNNI3K were co-expressed with full-length cTnI, and the TNNI3K protein was immunoprecipitated. As expected, the full-length TNNI3K efficiently immunoprecipitated cTnI (Figure 6B, lane 1). cTnI also binds the truncations of TNNI3K lacking the amino-terminal ANK-repeat domain and/or the central protein kinase domain. However, once the carboxyl-terminal serine-rich domain was truncated, all detectable cTnI binding was lost (Figure 6B). These results indicate that TNNI3K binds to cTnI in its carboxyl-terminal region bound by amino acids 727 and 835, outside the protein kinase domain.

TNNI3K is a functional kinase. To identify the specificity of phosphoamino-acid, TNNI3K was overexpressed in H9C2 cells, immunoprecipitated, and immunoblotted with anti-phosphoamino acid antibodies. As shown in Figure 7, only phosphotyrosine,

but no phosphoserine or phosphothreonine was detectable in TNNI3K, suggesting it is a protein-tyrosine kinase.

As TNNI3K is a functional kinase and it directly interacts of cTnI, we then performed immunoblot analysis to examine the effect of TNNI3K on cTnI phosphorylation. In the TNNI3K transgenic heart, the overexpression of TNNI3K was accompanied by increased cardiac troponin I phosphorylation at Ser22/Ser23 (Figure 8A). In cultured cardiomyocytes, infection with Ad-TNNI3K significantly induced cTnI phosphorylation at Ser22/Ser23 on the basal and isoproterenol-stimulated level, relative to cells infected with Ad-GFP (Figure 8B). Since the phosphorylation of troponin is a highly significant element in the control of cardiac contractility, these data suggested the role of TNNI3K in regulating cTnI phosphorylation and contractile function in the heart.

Discussion

In this study, we found that TNNI3K is associated with cardiac remodeling induced by hemodynamic overload. Overexpression of human TNNI3K specifically in the heart of transgenic mouse lines caused long-standing concentric hypertrophy associated with enhanced cardiac pump function. Furthermore, TNNI3K directly interacts with cTnI and induced cTnI phosphorylation at Ser22/Ser23 *in vivo* and *in vitro*. These data suggest that TNNI3K promotes cardiac remodeling via regulating the phosphorylation of cTnI.

In consistent with previous studies *in vitro*,[14,15] we found that overexpression TNNI3K could induce significantly enlargement of cardiomyocyte *in vivo*. Moreover, the TNNI3K transgene resulted in a concentric hypertrophy that is associated with enhanced cardiac function at the age of 3 months. There was no sign of pathological phenotype such as interstitial fibrosis. More importantly, the concentric hypertrophy remained up to 12 months of age and the left ventricular function was still normal. Therefore,

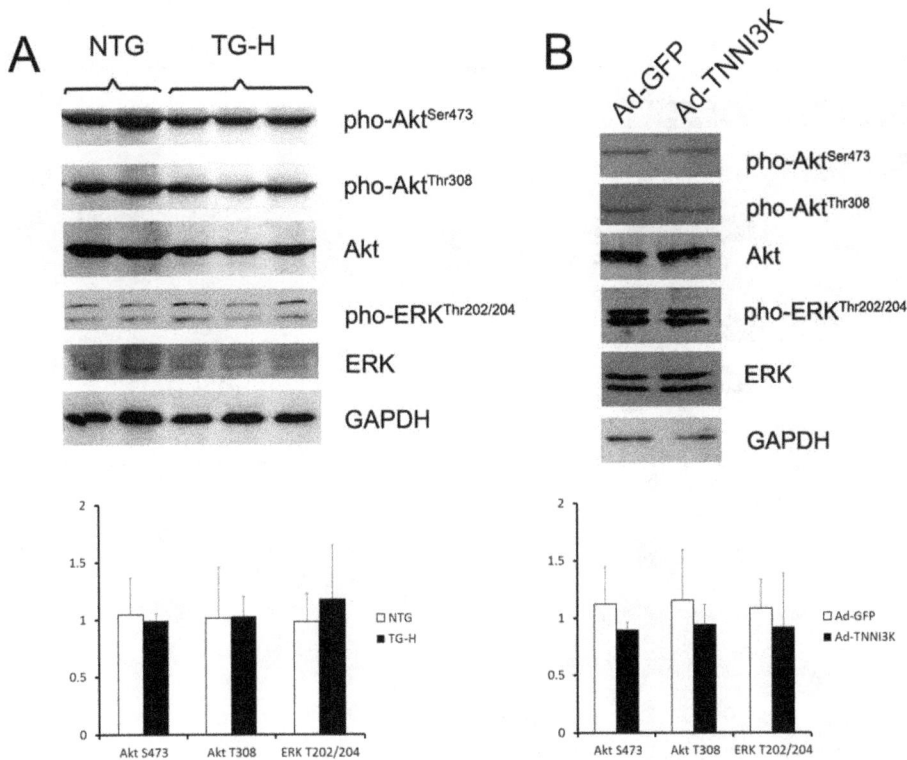

Figure 5. TNNI3K did not induce activation of Akt and ERK *in vivo* and *in vitro*. A: Western blot assessment for phosphorylation of Akt and ERK from transgenic hearts and nontransgenic control hearts at the age of 3 month. B: Cardiomyocytes were infected with Ad-TNNI3K and Ad-GFP for 48 hours and phosphorylation of Akt and ERK were analyzed by western blot. No significant phosphorylation increase was detected for the two effectors *in vivo* and *in vitro*. Each data point is shown as mean±SD.

we believe that the TNNI3K overexpression leads to an adaptive cardiac hypertrophy rather than maladaptive hypertrophy.

Cardiac hypertrophy is associated with alternation of cardiac gene expression.[21,22] For example, physiologic hypertrophy of the heart is generally associated with the induction of α-MHC expression; however, during pathologic hypertrophy, β-MHC is increased at the expense of α-MHC. In TNNI3K transgenic hearts, although β-MHC was mildly up-regulated, the expression of α-MHC was significantly increased. This result is in agreement with the previous report, showing that the adenovirus-mediated TNNI3K overexpression increases the content of α-MHC in cardiomyocytes,[14] Moreover, the expression of SERCA2a is also increased in transgenic heart. As α-MHC-to-β-MHC ratio and SERCA2a-to-phosholamban ratio are positively correlated with left ventricular contractility,[23,24] these molecular changes provide an explanation for the enhanced cardiac function and hyperhemodynamic state of TNNI3K transgenic heart.

To study the function of TNNI3K, we used "gain-of-function" strategy to generate transgenic mice in the C57BL/6J strain. Among the three transgenic lines, only the highest-copy-number transgenic mice developed a significantly cardiac remodeling. We believe the most likely explanation for this phenotype differences between the three lines of mouse is the endogenous counterbalancing mechanism. Firstly, C57BL/6J strain shows robust expression of TNNI3K in the heart at baseline.[16] Secondly, we generated transgenic mice expressing a wild-type CARK rather than a continuous-active CARK mutant. Therefore, lower expression level of exogenous CARK might be well tolerated by an endogenous counterbalancing mechanism.

Our observations with mice expressing TNNI3K are different from the previous report that described an accelerated disease progression in TNNI3K transgenic mice in response to pressure overload and in Csq transgenic mice.[16] This apparent discrepancy may be explained by the difference in the level of activation of TNNI3K signaling in the two mouse models. In Wheeler's study, the expression of TNNI3K in high-copy-number is comparable with that of low-copy-number transgenic lines. In our study, however, the difference in expression level is more than 20 folds. In addition, Wheeler et. al. found no major phenotype in the transgenic at baseline, which is consistent with our findings with the two lines that expresses low and moderate levels of TNNI3K. Hence, it is possible that because of differences in levels of activity of TNNI3K, pathways are less activated in Wheeler's mice than in our mice.

Up to date, little is known about the downstream targets of TNNI3K that are involved in the regulation cardiac hypertrophy. Given the facts that the IGF-1-phosphoinositide 3-kinase (PI3K)-Akt pathway and MEK1-ERK1/2 pathway are mainly advocated to mediate physiological cardiac growth,[2,25] and the physiological hypertrophy demonstrated by TNNI3K transgenic mice is reminiscent of phenotypes displayed in transgenic mice expressing a caPI3K mutant[26] and caMEK1 mutant,[27] we hypothesized that the functional role of TNNI3K may be accomplished through the two signaling pathways. However, the activities of Akt and ERK were not changed by TNNI3K overexpression either *in vivo* or *in vitro*, suggesting TNNI3K promotes cardiac hypertrophy through other signaling pathway.

Previous study reported that TNNI3K directly binds to cTnI.[10] In our study, this interaction was confirmed indepen-

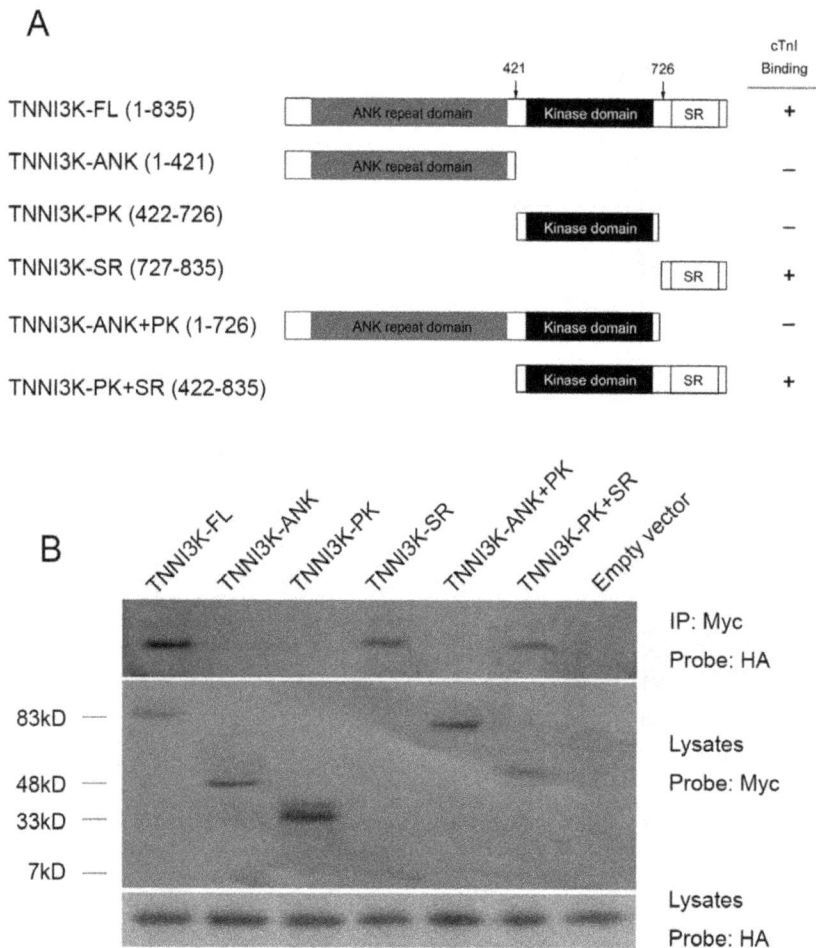

Figure 6. cTnI interacts with the serine-rich domain in the carboxyl terminus of TNNI3K. (A) Schematic representation of cTnI TNNI3K binding results. The selected domains on TNNI3K were indicated by labeled boxes. FL: full length, ANK: ANK repeat domain, PK: protein kinase domain, SR: serine rich domain. (B) H9C2 cells were transiently transfected with plasmids expressing full-length HA-tagged cTnI and the full-length Myc-tagged TNNI3K or the indicated truncations of Myc-tagged TNNI3K. TNNI3K was immunoprecipitated (IP) with anti-Myc antibodies and the presence of cTnI in the immunoprecipitate was assessed by immunoblotting with anti-HA antibodies. The expression of myc-TNNI3K from transfected constructs in the lysates is shown on the middle panel. The abundant of HA-cTnI in the lysates probed with anti-HA was used as an input.

dently both in the two-hybrid screen and in *in vitro* binding experiments. As the unique isoform expressed in heart muscle, cTnI plays a key role in the modulation of cardiac myofilament response to protein phosphorylation. cTnI can be phosphorylated at multiple amino acid residues by various kinases.[28] The phosphorylation level of cTnI at different residues has been proved to be a highly significant element in the control of cardiac contractility and a potential point of vulnerability in the network of

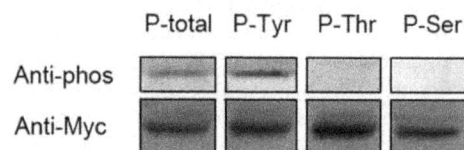

Figure 7. Detection of specificity of phosphoproteins in TNNI3K. Myc-tagged TNNI3K was overexpressed in H9C2 cells. TNNI3K proteins were immunoprecipitated with anti-myc antibody and Western blotted with anti-phosphoamino acid antibody (P-total), anti-phospho-tyrosine antibody (P-Tyr), anti-phosphothreonine antibody (P-Thr), anti-phosphoserine antibody (P-Ser) (top panel) or anti-myc (bottom panel).

signals by which hypertrophy and failure evolve.[29,30] Ser22/Ser23 locates in the cardiac-specific N terminus of cTnI. Phosphorylation at the Ser22/Ser23 sites alters the shape of the cTnI, resulting in accelerated relaxation and augmented contractility[31]. In the present study, we found that TNNI3K overexpression induced cTnI phosphorylation at Ser22/Ser23 *in vivo* and *in vitro*, suggesting that TNNI3K is a novel upstream regulator for cTnI phosphorylation. Moreove, the TNNI3K transgenic mice demonstrate a unique hypertrophic phenotype with enhanced cardiac function and hyperhemodynamic state, which is consistent with the lusitropic effect of cTnI phosphorylation on Ser22/Ser23. Therefore, TNNI3K may promote cardiac remodeling via regulating the phosphorylation of cTnI.

In conclusion, our study shows that upregulation of TNNI3K was characterized by long-standing concentric hypertrophy with enhancement of cardiac function. This prohypertrophic effect of TNNI3K was associated with the increased cTnI phosphorylation on Ser22/Ser23. As the phosphorylation state of Ser22 and/or Ser23 is significantly reduced in end-stage failing hearts[32,33], future studies investigating whether TNNI3K could be a potential therapeutic target for heart failure should be pursued.

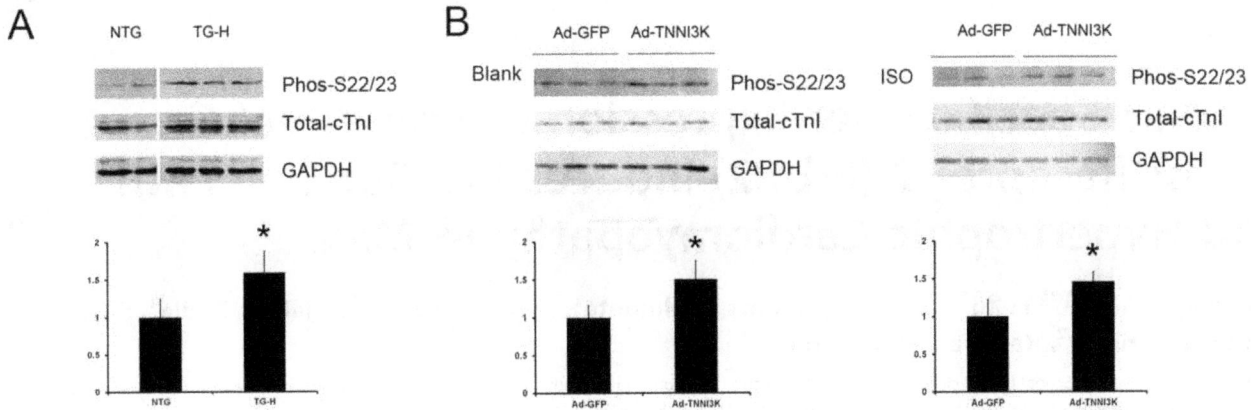

Figure 8. TNNI3K induced cTnI phosphorylation at Ser22/Ser23 *in vivo* and *in vitro*. (A), Heart lysates of TG-H and NTG mice were immunoblotted with antibodies against total and phosphorylated cTnI. TNNI3K induced cardiac troponin I phosphorylation at Ser22/Ser23 *in vivo*. (B), TNNI3K-induced cTnI phosphorylation at Ser22/Ser23 in cardiomyocytes on the basal and isoproterenol-stimulated level. Immunoblots are representative of 3 independent experiments. *: P<0.05 vs control group.

Acknowledgments

We gratefully thank Shan Gao and Wei Dong for their superb assistance in generating and phenotyping transgenic mice. Thanks a lot to Dr. Yusheng Wei and Dr. Han Xiao for their great support in performing experiments.

References

1. Frey N, Olson EN (2003) Cardiac hypertrophy: the good, the bad, and the ugly. Annu Rev Physiol 65: 45–79.
2. Dorn GW, 2nd (2007) The fuzzy logic of physiological cardiac hypertrophy. Hypertension 49: 962–970.
3. Chien KR (1999) Stress pathways and heart failure. Cell 98: 555–558.
4. Frey N, Katus HA, Olson EN, Hill JA (2004) Hypertrophy of the heart: a new therapeutic target? Circulation 109: 1580–1589.
5. Hill JA, Olson EN (2008) Cardiac plasticity. N Engl J Med 358: 1370–1380.
6. Dorn GW, 2nd, Force T (2005) Protein kinase cascades in the regulation of cardiac hypertrophy. J Clin Invest 115: 527–537.
7. Copeland O, Sadayappan S, Messer AE, Steinen GJ, van der Velden J, et al. (2010) Analysis of cardiac myosin binding protein-C phosphorylation in human heart muscle. J Mol Cell Cardiol 49: 1003–1011.
8. Jacques AM, Copeland O, Messer AE, Gallon CE, King K, et al. (2008) Myosin binding protein C phosphorylation in normal, hypertrophic and failing human heart muscle. J Mol Cell Cardiol 45: 209–216.
9. Vorotnikov AV, Risnik VV, Gusev NB (1988) [Phosphorylation of troponin in the heart and skeletal muscle by Ca2+–phospholipid-dependent protein kinase]. Biokhimiia 53: 31–40.
10. Zhao Y, Meng XM, Wei YJ, Zhao XW, Liu DQ, et al. (2003) Cloning and characterization of a novel cardiac-specific kinase that interacts specifically with cardiac troponin I. J Mol Med (Berl) 81: 297–304.
11. Wiltshire SA, Leiva-Torres GA, Vidal SM (2011) Quantitative trait locus analysis, pathway analysis, and consomic mapping show genetic variants of Tnni3k, Fpgt, or H28 control susceptibility to viral myocarditis. J Immunol 186: 6398–6405.
12. Milano A, Lodder EM, Scicluna BP, Sun AY, Tang H, et al. (2011) Tnni3k is a Novel Modulator of Cardiac Conduction. Circulation 124: A16031.
13. Wang H, Chen C, Song X, Chen J, Zhen Y, et al. (2008) Mef2c is an essential regulatory element required for unique expression of the cardiac-specific CARK gene. J Cell Mol Med 12: 304–315.
14. Wang L, Wang H, Ye J, Xu RX, Song L, et al. (2011) Adenovirus-mediated overexpression of cardiac troponin I-interacting kinase promotes cardiomyocyte hypertrophy. Clin Exp Pharmacol Physiol 38: 278–284.
15. Lai ZF, Chen YZ, Feng LP, Meng XM, Ding JF, et al. (2008) Overexpression of TNNI3K, a cardiac-specific MAP kinase, promotes P19CL6-derived cardiac myogenesis and prevents myocardial infarction-induced injury. Am J Physiol Heart Circ Physiol 295: H708–716.
16. Wheeler FC, Tang H, Marks OA, Hadnott TN, Chu PL, et al. (2009) Tnni3k modifies disease progression in murine models of cardiomyopathy. PLoS Genet 5: e1000647.
17. Juan F, Wei D, Xiongzhi Q, Ran D, Chunmei M, et al. (2008) The changes of the cardiac structure and function in cTnTR141W transgenic mice. Int J Cardiol 128: 83–90.

Author Contributions

Conceived and designed the experiments: XJW JZW RTH. Performed the experiments: XJW JZW MS CXW JZC HW. Analyzed the data: XJW MS LS YBZ. Contributed reagents/materials/analysis tools: LFZ YYZ. Wrote the paper: XJW RTH.

18. Wang J, Xu N, Feng X, Hou N, Zhang J, et al. (2005) Targeted disruption of Smad4 in cardiomyocytes results in cardiac hypertrophy and heart failure. Circ Res 97: 821–828.
19. Wang X, Yang X, Sun K, Chen J, Song X, et al. (2010) The haplotype of the growth-differentiation factor 15 gene is associated with left ventricular hypertrophy in human essential hypertension. Clin Sci (Lond) 118: 137–145.
20. Bradford MM (1976) A rapid and sensitive method for the quantitation of microgram quantities of protein utilizing the principle of protein-dye binding. Anal Biochem 72: 248–254.
21. Izumo S, Lompre AM, Matsuoka R, Koren G, Schwartz K, et al. (1987) Myosin heavy chain messenger RNA and protein isoform transitions during cardiac hypertrophy. Interaction between hemodynamic and thyroid hormone-induced signals. J Clin Invest 79: 970–977.
22. Izumo S, Nadal-Ginard B, Mahdavi V (1988) Protooncogene induction and reprogramming of cardiac gene expression produced by pressure overload. Proc Natl Acad Sci U S A 85: 339–343.
23. Gupta MP (2007) Factors controlling cardiac myosin-isoform shift during hypertrophy and heart failure. J Mol Cell Cardiol 43: 388–403.
24. Catalucci D, Latronico MV, Ceci M, Rusconi F, Young HS, et al. (2009) Akt increases sarcoplasmic reticulum Ca2+ cycling by direct phosphorylation of phospholamban at Thr17. J Biol Chem 284: 28180–28187.
25. Weeks KL, McMullen JR (2011) The athlete's heart vs. the failing heart: can signaling explain the two distinct outcomes? Physiology (Bethesda) 26: 97–105.
26. Shioi T, Kang PM, Douglas PS, Hampe J, Yballe CM, et al. (2000) The conserved phosphoinositide 3-kinase pathway determines heart size in mice. EMBO J 19: 2537–2548.
27. Bueno OF, De Windt LJ, Tymitz KM, Witt SA, Kimball TR, et al. (2000) The MEK1-ERK1/2 signaling pathway promotes compensated cardiac hypertrophy in transgenic mice. EMBO J 19: 6341–6350.
28. Sumandea MP, Burkart EM, Kobayashi T, De Tombe PP, Solaro RJ (2004) Molecular and integrated biology of thin filament protein phosphorylation in heart muscle. Ann N Y Acad Sci 1015: 39–52.
29. Layland J, Solaro RJ, Shah AM (2005) Regulation of cardiac contractile function by troponin I phosphorylation. Cardiovasc Res 66: 12–21.
30. Scruggs SB, Solaro RJ (2011) The significance of regulatory light chain phosphorylation in cardiac physiology. Arch Biochem Biophys 510: 129–134.
31. van der Velden J, de Jong JW, Owen VJ, Burton PB, Stienen GJ (2000) Effect of protein kinase A on calcium sensitivity of force and its sarcomere length dependence in human cardiomyocytes. Cardiovasc Res 46: 487–495.
32. Bodor GS, Oakeley AE, Allen PD, Crimmins DL, Ladenson JH, et al. (1997) Troponin I phosphorylation in the normal and failing adult human heart. Circulation 96: 1495–1500.
33. Kooij V, Saes M, Jaquet K, Zaremba R, Foster DB, et al. (2010) Effect of troponin I Ser23/24 phosphorylation on Ca2+–sensitivity in human myocardium depends on the phosphorylation background. J Mol Cell Cardiol 48: 954–963.

6

Cardiac-Specific Over-Expression of Epidermal Growth Factor Receptor 2 (ErbB2) Induces Pro-Survival Pathways and Hypertrophic Cardiomyopathy in Mice

Polina Sysa-Shah[1,9], Yi Xu[1,9], Xin Guo[1], Frances Belmonte[1], Byunghak Kang[1], Djahida Bedja[1], Scott Pin[1], Noriko Tsuchiya[1,2], Kathleen Gabrielson[1]*

1 Johns Hopkins University, School of Medicine, Department of Molecular and Comparative Pathobiology, Baltimore, Maryland, United States of America, 2 Drug Safety Evaluation, Drug Developmental Research Laboratories, Shionogi & Co., Ltd., Osaka, Japan

Abstract

Background: Emerging evidence shows that ErbB2 signaling has a critical role in cardiomyocyte physiology, based mainly on findings that blocking ErbB2 for cancer therapy is toxic to cardiac cells. However, consequences of high levels of ErbB2 activity in the heart have not been previously explored.

Methodology/Principal Findings: We investigated consequences of cardiac-restricted over-expression of ErbB2 in two novel lines of transgenic mice. Both lines develop striking concentric cardiac hypertrophy, without heart failure or decreased life span. ErbB2 transgenic mice display electrocardiographic characteristics similar to those found in patients with Hypertrophic Cardiomyopathy, with susceptibility to adrenergic-induced arrhythmias. The hypertrophic hearts, which are 2–3 times larger than those of control littermates, express increased atrial natriuretic peptide and β-myosin heavy chain mRNA, consistent with a hypertrophic phenotype. Cardiomyocytes in these hearts are significantly larger than wild type cardiomyocytes, with enlarged nuclei and distinctive myocardial disarray. Interestingly, the over-expression of ErbB2 induces a concurrent up-regulation of multiple proteins associated with this signaling pathway, including EGFR, ErbB3, ErbB4, PI3K subunits p110 and p85, bcl-2 and multiple protective heat shock proteins. Additionally, ErbB2 up-regulation leads to an anti-apoptotic shift in the ratio of bcl-xS/xL in the heart. Finally, ErbB2 over-expression results in increased activation of the translation machinery involving S6, 4E-BP1 and eIF4E. The dependence of this hypertrophic phenotype on ErbB family signaling is confirmed by reduction in heart mass and cardiomyocyte size, and inactivation of pro-hypertrophic signaling in transgenic animals treated with the ErbB1/2 inhibitor, lapatinib.

Conclusions/Significance: These studies are the first to demonstrate that increased ErbB2 over-expression in the heart can activate protective signaling pathways and induce a phenotype consistent with Hypertrophic Cardiomyopathy. Furthermore, our work suggests that in the situation where ErbB2 signaling contributes to cardiac hypertrophy, inhibition of this pathway may reverse this process.

Editor: Ferenc Gallyas, University of Pecs Medical School, Hungary

Funding: This work was supported by NIH grant RO1 HL088649. The funder had no role in study design, data collection and analysis, decision to publish, or preparation of the manuscript.

Competing Interests: Noriko Tsuchiya is affiliated with Drug Safety Evaluation, Drug Developmental Research Laboratories, Shionogi & Co., Ltd., Osaka, Japan.

* E-mail: kgabriel@jhmi.edu

9 These authors contributed equally to this work.

Introduction

ErbB2 (HER2/neu), a member of the EGFR family of receptor tyrosine kinases, first attracted attention after the discovery that this gene is amplified and over-expressed in a high percentage of breast cancers. The importance of ErbB2 signaling in cardiac physiology soon became evident by a discovery that some breast cancer patients treated with Trastuzumab (Herceptin, anti-ErbB2), an inhibitor of HER2 signaling, develop synergistic cardiac dysfunction, particularly when Trastuzumab is combined with doxorubicin [1], [2], [3]. A variety of transgenic mouse studies have extended our awareness of the role of ErbB2 in the

heart. For example, ErbB2 knockout mice die in utero at E10.5 due to the defective cardiac trabeculation [4], [5], [6]. In conditional deletion models, adult mice develop heart failure [7], [8], and isolated cardiomyocytes from these mice are more sensitive to doxorubicin [7].

While the studies on ErbB2 in the heart have focused on consequences of blocking activity of this kinase, there is also clinical evidence that, in humans, ErbB2 is expressed at variable levels in cardiomyocytes. One of the most illuminating studies used SPECT imaging and identified differences in cardiac anti-ErbB2 binding to human hearts [9]. This research group originally planned to image the binding of radiolabeled anti-ErbB2

(Herceptin) to breast cancers but unexpectedly found that anti-ErbB2 also bound to the hearts of some patients. Since only the patients that showed anti-ErbB2 cardiac binding subsequently developed cardiac toxicity, it has been suggested that variable levels of ErbB2 expression among individuals might be an important determinant of susceptibility to doxorubicin and Herceptin toxicity.

In previous studies of cardiac toxicity of doxorubicin in the rat, we noted that doxorubicin treatment results in induction of ErbB2 expression [10]. While it appears that an up-regulation of ErbB2 in hearts in cancer patients might initially offer protection from toxic effects of doxorubicin, long-term effects of ErbB2 over-expression, particularly when not induced as a response to doxorubicin treatment, are unknown. We therefore generated two transgenic lines of mice with cardiomyocyte-specific ErbB2 over-expression to investigate consequences of long-term over-expression of ErbB2 in the heart.

Methods

Animals

This study was performed in strict accordance with the recommendations in the Guide for the Care and Use of Laboratory Animals of the National Institutes of Health. The protocol was approved by the Committee on the Ethics of Animal Experiments of the Johns Hopkins Medical Institutions (Animal Welfare Assurance # A-3273-01).

Transgenic Constructs and Mouse Lines

Rat ErbB2 mRNA was isolated and converted to cDNA. The 5 kb cDNA fragment was then subcloned into the BamHI-SalI site of the cardiac specific expression vector, α-myosin heavy chain promoter construct (kindly provided by Dr. Jeffrey Robbins), followed by polyadenylation signal from human growth hormone (hGH), located downstream of the insert. The B6SJLF1/J strain was used for pronuclear microinjection of the received fragment and production of the transgenic mice by Johns Hopkins Transgenic Core Facility. Founder animals were identified by PCR and Southern blotting. Two founders were used to develop two transgenic lines. All the wild type and transgenic mice were housed under a 12 hours light-dark cycle with free access to food and water.

Necropsy

Mice were euthanized and weighed, and tibia lengths measured. Hearts were excised, weighed, and sectioned at mid-papillary level. In selected mice, left ventricle, right ventricle and septum were snap frozen and saved for the further molecular studies. The basal to mid-papillary level of the heart was fixed in 10% formalin and paraffin-embedded for the histological evaluation. Five micron sections were stained with hematoxylin and eosin (H&E) for the morphological evaluation, with Masson's trichrome for detection of fibrosis, or wheat germ agglutinin for cardiomyocyte morphology.

Chest Radiography

Faxitron X-ray MX-20 Specimen Radiography system (Faxitron Bioptics, LLC, Tuscan, AZ) was used to perform chest radiography. The mice (8–10 weeks old, 2 mice per genotype) were euthanized and anterio-posterior radiography was immediately performed. Voltage and integration time were adjusted to visualize the heart shadow. Following the chest radiography, the mice were euthanised, skin and anterior portion of ribs with the sternum were cut and raised to open the thoracic cavity and expose the heart and lungs, and photos of the opened chest cavity with exposed heart and lungs were taken to match the gross pathology with radiograph.

Real-time PCR and Primers Design

Total RNA was isolated from the hearts of the wild type and ErbB2 transgenic mice (8–10 weeks old, 3 mice per genotype) as described [10]. Hypertrophy molecular markers atrial natriuretic peptide ANP (NPPA) and β-myosin heavy chain (MYH) were evaluated by quantitative real-time reverse transcriptase-polymerase chain reaction (qRT-PCR). The primers are listed in Table S1. Peptidylprolylisomerase A (PPIA) was used for RNA normalization [11]. The quantitative RT-PCR results were calculated by delta-delta Ct method using the mean of the delta Ct value of wild type mice as a normalization factor.

Immunoblotting

Both lines of mice were evaluated by Western blotting for protein expression and pathway activation. 8–10 week old male mice for each genotype were evaluated (n = 7); for lapatinib studies 3–6 animals per group were used. Frozen left ventricle (40 mg) was rapidly homogenized in 200–300 μL of RIPA buffer (Table S2), and standard gel electrophoresis and immunoblotting were performed. The antibodies used are listed in Table S3. After incubation in anti-rabbit, anti-mouse (1:5000; GE Healthcare, Piscataway, NJ) or anti-rat (1:5000, Cell Signaling Technology, Danvers, MA) horseradish peroxidase-linked secondary antibody, blots were exposed to chemiluminescent substrate (Pierce, Rockford, IL) and exposed to CL-Xposure film (Pierce, Rockford, IL). Levels of AKT protein were measured to normalize protein quantities across samples.

Immunoprecipitation

Lysates were prepared from the hearts of wild type and ErbB2 transgenic mice (8–10 weeks old, 7 mice per genotype; for lapatinib experiments, 12.5 or 31 days old mice were used, 3–4 mice per group). Total protein quantification was performed prior to immunoprecipitation. Lysates were incubated with anti-ErbB2 or anti-EGFR antibody (3 μg of antibody per 1000 μg of total protein) at 4°C for 2 hours.

IgA beads were washed with ice cold lysis buffer (Table S2) and centrifuged (3000RPM, 1 min), buffer was aspirated, and beads were mixed with antibody-treated lysates and incubated at 4°C overnight. Subsequently, beads were washed 3 times and centrifuged (3000RPM, 1 min), the supernatant was aspirated, urea sample buffer (Table S2) was added to beads, and the suspension was heated at 95°C for 5 minutes, followed by centrifugation (3000RPM, 1 min). Supernatant was then loaded on SDS running gel, and the standard immunoblotting protocol was followed. The resulting membrane was probed with anti-phospho-tyrosine, anti-ErbB2 or EGFR antibodies.

WGA Staining

Unstained sections of formalin-fixed, paraffin-embedded heart tissues were de-parafinized in xylene and rehydrated in decreasing concentrations of ethanol (100%, 95%, 70%). Antigen retrieval was performed with Dako S1700 Target Retrieval solution (Dako North America, Carpinteria, CA) in a steamer. Nonspecific background was quenched and active aldehyde was blocked by 10 minutes incubation of the slides in 1 mg/ml NaBH4 (Sigma-Aldrich, St. Louis, MO) in PBS. The slides were stained with wheat germ agglutinin conjugated to Alexa Fluor 488 (Life Technologies (Invitrogen), Grand Island, NY) overnight and coverslipped with DAPI-containing anti-fading media (Vectashield

(Vector Technologies, Burlingame, CA)). The resulting sections were visualized with Nikon Eclipse E600 microscope and micrographs were obtained. 8–10 week old male mice for each genotype were evaluated (n = 5–6); for lapatinib study 31 days old animals were used (n = 3–4).

Adult Cardiomyocytes Isolation and Measurements

Cardiomyocytes were isolated from hearts of 8–10 weeks old wild type and ErbB2 transgenic mice (3–4 mice per genotype). The hearts were quickly removed from the chest after euthanasia and the aorta was retroperfused at $100 \, cmH_2O$ and 37°C for 3 min with a Ca_{2+}−free bicarbonate-based buffer, gassed with 95% O2–5% CO_2 (Table S2). Enzymatic digestion was initiated by addition of 0.9 mg/ml collagenase type 2 (Worthington Biochemical Co., 299 U/mg) and 0.05 mg/ml protease type XIV (Sigma Chemical Co.) to the perfusion solution (6–7 min). Dispersed myocytes were filtered through a 150 μm mesh and gently centrifuged at 500 rpm for 30 seconds. Longitudinal surface areas of isolated cardiomyocytes were visualized with Nikon Eclipse 90 microscope, measured and calculated from the digitized micrographs with NIS Elements 3.10 Imaging Software.

Echocardiography

Trans-thoracic echocardiography was performed on conscious mice using Acuson Sequoia C256 ultrasound machine (Siemens Corps, Mountain View, CA) equipped with the 15 MHz linear array transducer. The mouse heart was imaged by two-dimensional and M-mode approaches using the parasternal short axis view at a sweep speed of 200 mm/sec. Measurements were acquired using the leading-edge method, according to the American Echocardiography Society guidelines [11]. Left ventricle wall thickness and left ventricle chamber dimensions were acquired during the end diastolic and end systolic phase including: inter-ventricular septum (IVSD), left ventricular posterior wall thickness (PWTED), left ventricular end diastolic dimension (LVEDD) and left ventricular end systolic dimension (LVESD). Three to five values for each measurement were acquired and averaged for evaluation. The LVEDD and LVESD were used to derive fractional shortening (FS) to measure left ventricular performance by the following equation: FS (%) = [(LVEDD − LVESD)/LVEDD] ×100.

For quantifying left ventricular geometrical changes and phenotype, relative wall thickness (RWT) and left ventricular mass (LV mass) were measured, and the RWT ratio was used to define left ventricle wall thickness in proportion to left ventricle cavity size using the following equation: (RWT) = 2×PWTD/ LVEDD. Left Ventricular mass (LV mass) was calculated with the following equation: LV mass (mg) = 1.055[(IVST + LVEDD + PWTD)3 − (LVEDD)3], where 1.055 is the specific gravity of the cardiac muscle. 8–10 week old male mice for each genotype were evaluated (n = 15–18). Cardiac output (CO) was calculated using the following equations: CO = SV×HR; SV = VTI×CSA, where: SV = stroke volume; HR = heart rate; CSA = cross sectional area of aortic root; VTI = the velocity time integral. Four to five animals per group (wild type and ErbB2 transgenic mice, 8–10 weeks old) were used with 8–10 peaks measured for each VTI measurement per mouse.

Blood Pressure

Blood pressure was obtained using tail-cuff plethysmography (CODA2, Kent Scientific, Torrington, CT, USA) as previously described [12]. Conscious mice were placed in a restrainer on a warming pad and allowed to rest inside the cage for 10–15 min before the measurements were taken. Mouse tails were placed in a tail

cuff, which was inflated and released several times to allow the mouse to be accustomed to the procedure. Four to five animals per group (wild type and ErbB2 transgenic mice, 8–10 weeks old) were used.

Electrocardiography (EKG)

Electrocardiography recordings were performed in 14 conscious mice per genotype (8–10 weeks old). Surface probes were inserted subcutaneously and EKG signal (Standard lead II) was obtained for five to ten seconds using a PowerLab data acquisition system (ML866) and Animal Bio Amp (ML136; AD Instruments, Colorado Springs, CO, USA). LabChart Pro 7.2 software (AD Instruments, Colorado Springs, CO, USA) was used for automated EKG tracing analysis.

Isoproterenol Administration for EKG Studies

At eight weeks of age, male or female mice (3–4 animals per genotype) were anesthetized with intraperitoneal injection of ketamine HCl (90 mg/kg) and xylazine HCl solution (10 mg/kg). Anesthetized mice were placed in a supine position on a temperature controlled heating pad. Isoproterenol (0.1 mg/kg, 0.5 mg/ kg or 100 mg/kg) was administered with an intraperitoneal injection to wild type and ErbB2 transgenic mice. Body temperature was monitored with rectal probe and maintained at 37–38°C. 5 minutes of EKG signal were recorded prior to the isoproterenol injection, followed by 30 minutes of recording after the injection.

Lapatinib Treatment

Wild type or ErbB2 transgenic mice male and female mice (P4.5) were treated with oral lapatinib (160 mg/kg) of lapatinib PO daily, (n = 4–7/group). 24G-1″ Gavage needles (Braintree Scientific, Inc., Braintree, MA) were used. Lapatinib (LC Laboratories, Woburn, MA) suspension was made fresh before each treatment. Lapatinib was diluted with a buffer containing 0.5% carboxymethylcellulose, 1.8% sodium chloride, and 0.4% Tween-80in dH_2O. Because a percentage of unchanged lapatinib is excreted with feces, we assigned entire separately caged litters to either vehicle or lapatinib group. Animals were treated daily for 8 days and euthanized 2 hours following final treatments. Hearts were excised, weighed, and sectioned, with the apical part immediately frozen for further molecular studies and the basal part with the atria fixed in 10% formalin for histopathology. Tails were saved for genotyping.

In a separate dosing experiment, 10.5 days old pups (n = 5–12) were treated daily with 100 mg/kg of lapatinib, following the same scheme. The pups were euthanized 21 days after the treatment initiation.

Statistical Methods

GraphPad Prism software (GraphPad, La Jolla, CA) was used to perform statistical analysis.

After determining means and standard deviations, the Student unpaired T-test was used to determine significance of differences between groups, with a P-value of <0.05 accepted as a significant difference. For survival statistics Log-rank (Mantel-Cox) test was used.

Results

ErbB2 Over-expression Induces Concentric Cardiac Hypertrophy in Novel Transgenic Mouse Lines

Our laboratory developed two ErbB2-over-expressing transgenic (TG) mouse lines, using an ErbB2construct driven by the

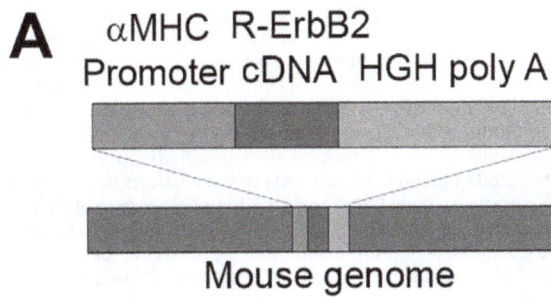

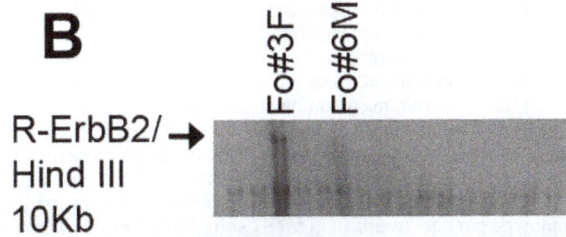

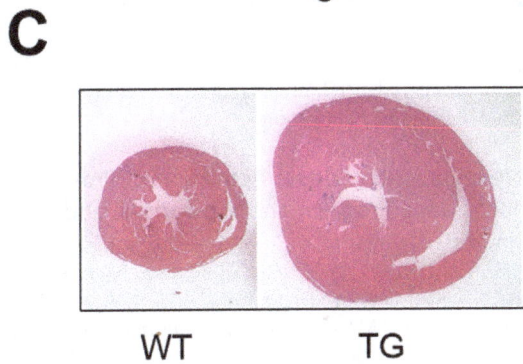

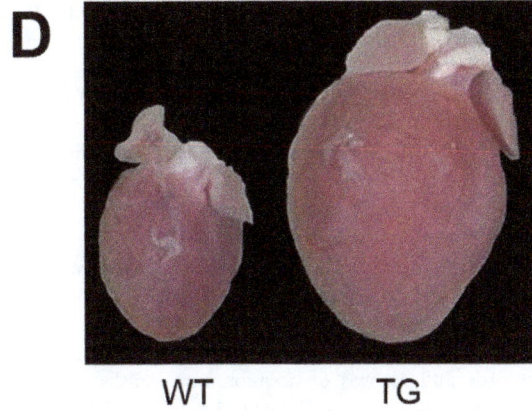

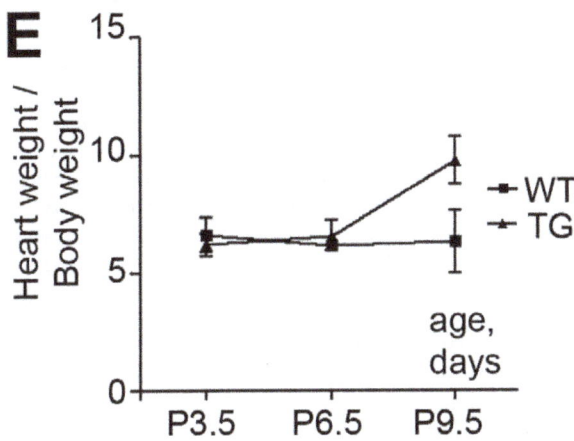

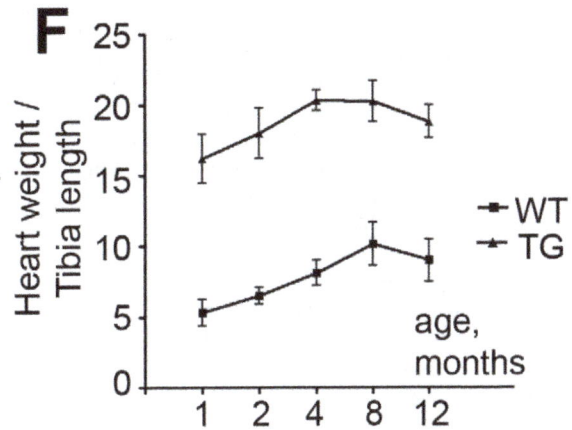

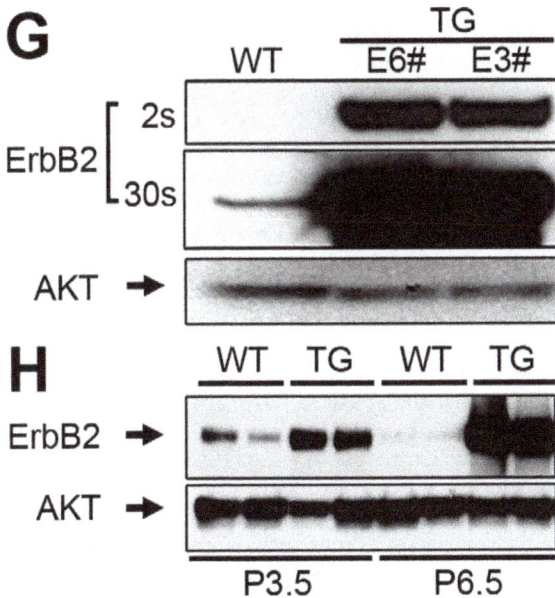

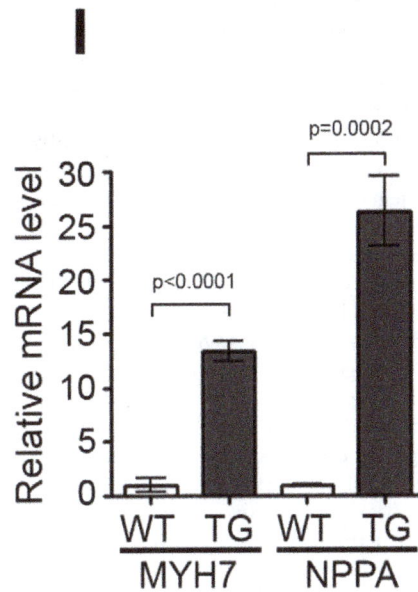

Figure 1. Concentric cardiac hypertrophy in ErbB2 transgenic mice. (A) Schematic illustration of DNA construct, consisting of cardiac-specific alpha-myosin heavy chain (αMHC) promoter, rat ErbB2 cDNA and polyadenylation signal from human growth hormone (HGH); (B) Identification of ErbB2 transgenic founder mice by southern blotting (tail DNA from 16 potential founders was used, two animals were found to have the transgene); (C) Hematoxylin-eosin staining (H&E) of transverse cross sections of the wild type and ErbB2 transgenic hearts. (D) Gross pathology of enlarged atria and ventricles in ErbB2 transgenic mice compared to wild type littermates. (E) Heart weight-to-body weight ratios of the wild type and ErbB2 transgenic mice at P3.5 (postnatal day 3.5), P6.5, P9.5 (n = 5–22 per genotype per age group). The data are presented as the mean ± SD. (F) Heart weight-to-tibia length ratios in adult mice. The transgenic-to-wild type heart weight ratio of 2.5–3 is maintained into adulthood (n = 4–27 per genotype per age group). The data are presented as the mean ± SD. (G) Western blot of ErbB2 protein in left ventricle protein extracts from wild type and ErbB2 transgenic mice. (H) Western blot of ErbB2 protein in left ventricle protein extracts from wild type and ErbB2 transgenic mice at P3.5 and P6.5 (n = 2 per genotype per age group). (I) m-MYH7 and m-NPPA expression was evaluated by quantitative RT-PCR in triplicates with mRNA isolated from the left ventricles of wild type and ErbB2 transgenic (n = 3 per genotype). The quantitative RT-PCR results were calculated by delta-delta Ct method using the mean of the delta Ct value of wild type mice as a normalization factor. The data are presented as the mean ± SD. The studies were performed on 8–10 weeks old mice, unless different age is specified.

αMHC promoter for cardiac restricted expression [Figure 1a]. Two founder animals (#3 and #6) selected by screening of 16 mice [Figure 1b] were used to establish two separate breeding colonies. Heterozygotes have been continuously bred to maintain wild type controls and over-expressing littermates.

Body weights at birth were not different between the mice genotypes or ErbB2 mouse lines, and we noted no significant differences in survival rates of transgenic mice compared to wild-type littermates within the breeding colony over 20 months of observation (Figure S1). This data was obtained from colony management records and records of occasion rare deaths that occurred during ultrasound handling. We consider these mortality differences to be stress-related, with transgenic mice being more susceptible to adrenergic stress and associated mortality. In addition, we noticed increased mortality in older transgenic dams, which may be explained by multiple pregnancies-related cardiac remodeling, exaggerating the existing cardiac hypertrophy.

Transgenic mice from both lines (E6#, Figure 1c and d, Figure S2 and E3#, data not shown) exhibit marked cardiac hypertrophy as evident from gross pathology and radiographs. Heart weight-to-body weight ratios were comparable in transgenic and wild type mice up to postnatal day 6.5, with a significant 54% increase at P9.5 [Figure 1e]. Heart weight-to-tibia length ratio differences reached a maximum of about a 2.5-fold difference at 10–12 weeks of age [Figure S3b], after which slight, age-related parallel increases in the heart weight-to-tibia length ratio were observed in both transgenic and wild type mice [Figure 1f].

Protein levels of ErbB2 in hearts of transgenic mice were measured by Western blot analysis [Figure 1g], and comparable levels of ErbB2 protein were observed in both lines (E3# and E6#). Lysates from the left ventricles of 8 weeks old transgenic mice and wild type littermates were compared. The ErbB2 protein levels were approximately 40 times higher in left ventricles of transgenic animals compared to wild type littermates, while ErbB2 levels in other organs were not changed (data not shown). There were no differences in protein expression between male and female mice or between E3# and E6# lines, thus E6# males were used for the majority of subsequent experiments.

We evaluated ErbB2 protein expression in wild type and ErbB2 transgenic mice at days P3.5 and P6.5 [Figure 1h]. Wild type mice have higher ErbB2 expression at P3.5 compared to wild type mice at P6.5 days. In ErbB2 transgenic mice due to the transgene promoter activation, ErbB2 expression dramatically increases between P3.5 and P6.5 days. At P3.5, heart weights are not different between wild type and ErbB2 transgenic mice, yet at P9.5 the difference becomes significant. At P3.5, ErbB2 protein expression in transgenic hearts is increased compared to wild type hearts before the hypertrophy becomes obvious, yet the relative ErbB2 protein expression between wild type and ErbB2 transgenic mice is much higher in P6.5 and in adult animals

[Figure 1g, h] compared to P3.5 mice reflective of α-myosin heavy chain promoter transgene activation.

ErbB2 Over-expression Causes Activation of Pro-hypertrophic Gene Program and Pro-survival and Translational Pathways

We confirmed by qRT-PCR that adult mice have increased levels of mRNA encoding for atrial natriuretic peptide(NPPA) and β-myosin heavy chain (MYH7), two characteristic mRNAs and proteins that increase in cardiac hypertrophy [Figure 1i].

To explore signaling pathways affected by ErbB2 over-expression, we conducted a series of experiments to evaluate levels of proteins and levels of protein phosphorylation for key components of the ErbB2 pathway. Left ventricles from the two lines of ErbB2 transgenic mice showed highly similar patterns of protein expression or pathway activation. As expected, total phospho-ErbB2 is elevated in hearts of transgenic mice [Figure 2a], but surprisingly, ErbB2 over-expression induced a unique expression profile suggestive of a signal amplification effect. Specifically, we noted increased levels of proteins within the ErbB2 pathway that could be expected to facilitate and amplify pathway effects in the cell [Figure 2c]. ErbB2 over-expression activates and up-regulates cardiac pro-survival signaling and hypertrophic pathways, including PI3K/AKT pathway, a well-known pathway involved in increasing cardiomyocyte survival and protein translation during cardiac hypertrophy [13], [14], [15]. Both regulatory (p85) and catalytic (p110) PI3K subunits were markedly increased in hearts of ErbB2 transgenic mice. ErbB2 over-expression also induced a modest increase in AKT phosphorylation in transgenic hearts compared to wild type littermates, while total AKT levels remained unchanged. Total PTEN levels, as well as phospho-PTEN levels, were slightly increased in the ErbB2 transgenic hearts.

The EGFR family is represented in the heart by four proteins, EGFR, ErbB2, ErbB3 and ErbB4 receptor tyrosine kinases. We were surprised to see that total phospho-EGFR, and total EGFR, ErbB3 and ErbB4 levels were all elevated in ErbB2 transgenic hearts [Figure 2b,c].

We also explored signal transduction pathways that activate translation in ErbB2 transgenic hearts. Cardiac protein translation and cardiomyocyte hypertrophy is regulated through activation of p70S6K, subsequent S6 phosphorylation [16] and activation of translational regulators, such as eIF4E/4E-BP1 system [17]. Active p70S6K is required for hypertrophic transformation of neonatal rat cardiomyocytes in vitro [18], [19] and pressure overload-induced cardiac hypertrophy in rats in vivo [20]. These key proteins in the translational machinery were activated in ErbB2 transgenic hearts, as confirmed by increased phosphorylation of p70S6K, ribosomal S6 protein, eIF4E and 4E-BP1 [Figure 2c].

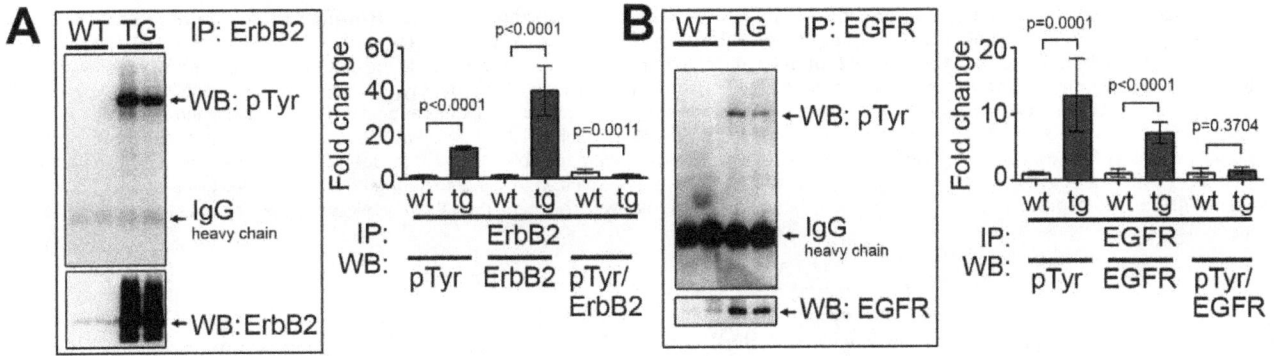

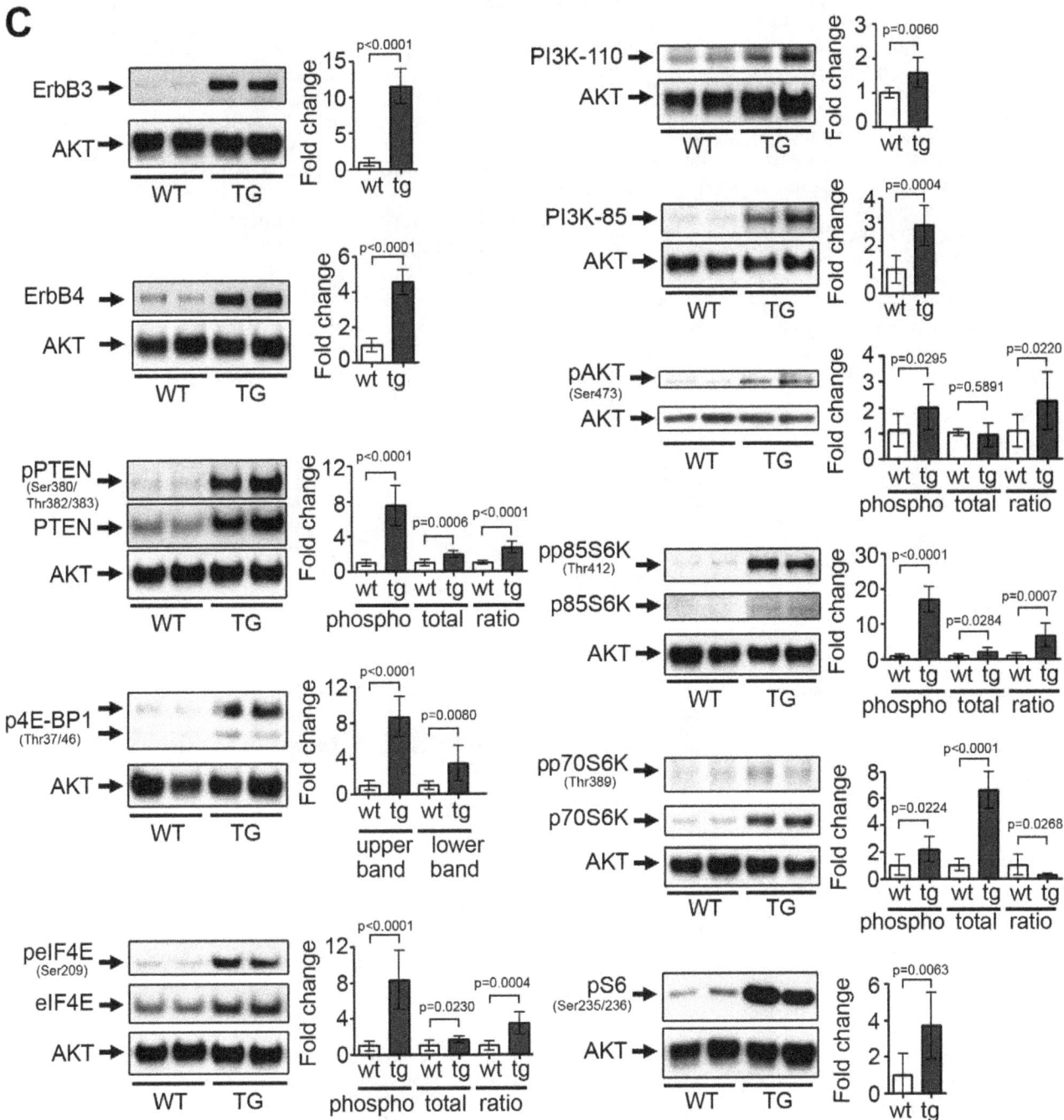

Figure 2. Up-regulation and activation of ErbB family proteins and downstream pro-hypertrophic proteins in the hearts of ErbB2 transgenic mice. (A) Total phosphorylation of ErbB2 and total ErbB2 levels (A), as well as total EGFR phosphorylation and total EGFR levels (B) were assessed by immunoprecipitation of ErbB2 or EGFR from the total left ventricle lysates and subsequent blotting with anti-phospho-tyrosine, anti-ErbB2 and anti-EGFR antibodies. Densitometry was performed using ImageJ software (n = 7 per genotype). The data are presented as the mean ± SD. (C) Representative western blots demonstrate activation of pro-survival, hypertrophic and translational signaling in the left ventricles of ErbB2 transgenic mice. Two bands of p4E-BP1 represent different levels of 4E-BP1 phosphorylation. AKT was used as loading control, since other proteins traditionally used as loading controls (GAPDH, tubulin, α-actin and β-actin) were variable in ErbB2 transgenic hearts. Densitometry was performed using ImageJ software (n = 7 per genotype). Phosphorylated proteins were normalized to the corresponding total proteins levels and AKT; phospho-protein-to-AKT and total protein-to-AKT ratios are also shown. All the studies were performed on 8–10 weeks old mice. The data are presented as the mean ± SD.

Next, we evaluated balance of pro- and anti-apoptotic Bcl-2 proteins. Bcl-2 family is comprised of anti-apoptotic (bcl-xL and bcl-2), and pro-apoptotic (bcl-xS, BAK, BAX) proteins. Correlation of cardiac ErbB2 expression and the balance of pro-survival bcl-xL and apoptotic bcl-xS proteins have been described [21], [22]. We found the same ratio pattern in hearts of ErbB2 transgenic mice, such as we noted a shift in the balance of bcl-x forms from predominantly the bcl-xS form (pro-apoptotic) to predominantly the bcl-xL form (anti-apoptotic) [Figure 3a], supporting the mechanism of ErbB2 in cardioprotection. In heart failure, the down-regulation of ErbB2 and ErbB4 receptors has also been correlated with decreased bcl-xL/xS ratios [23]. Additionally, we found that Bcl-2 levels were increased in ErbB2 transgenic hearts, supporting another mechanism of cardioprotection induced by ErbB2 [Figure 3a].

Another potential protective mechanism of ErbB2 over-expression in transgenic hearts, not previously associated with ErbB2 expression, is up-regulation of the transcription factor Heat shock factor 1 (HSF-1) and concomitant up-regulation of heat shock protein family, including HSP72, HSP25 and HSP90 [Figure 3b], all considered protective proteins. For example, HSP90 is a chaperone of both ErbB2 and EGFR and thus may be partially responsible for stability of these proteins in ErbB2 transgenic mice cardiac hypertrophy. HSF1 and its target HSP genes were shown to be induced in exercise-induced adaptive hypertrophy, but not pressure-overload maladaptive hypertrophy [24]. Supporting our finding in the heart, HSF1 protein levels and activation were shown to be induced by ErbB2 over-expression in a breast cancer cell line, while the mechanism of this ErbB2 connection to HSF1 is still unknown [25].

ErbB2 Over-expression Induces Cardiomyocyte Hypertrophy with Myocardial Disarray

Remarkably, ErbB2 over-expressing hearts have diffuse myocardial hypertrophy extending throughout the entire myocardium, with strikingly enlarged nuclei [Figure 4a, Figure 5a–f]. Masson's Trichrome staining did not reveal obvious differences in fibrosis

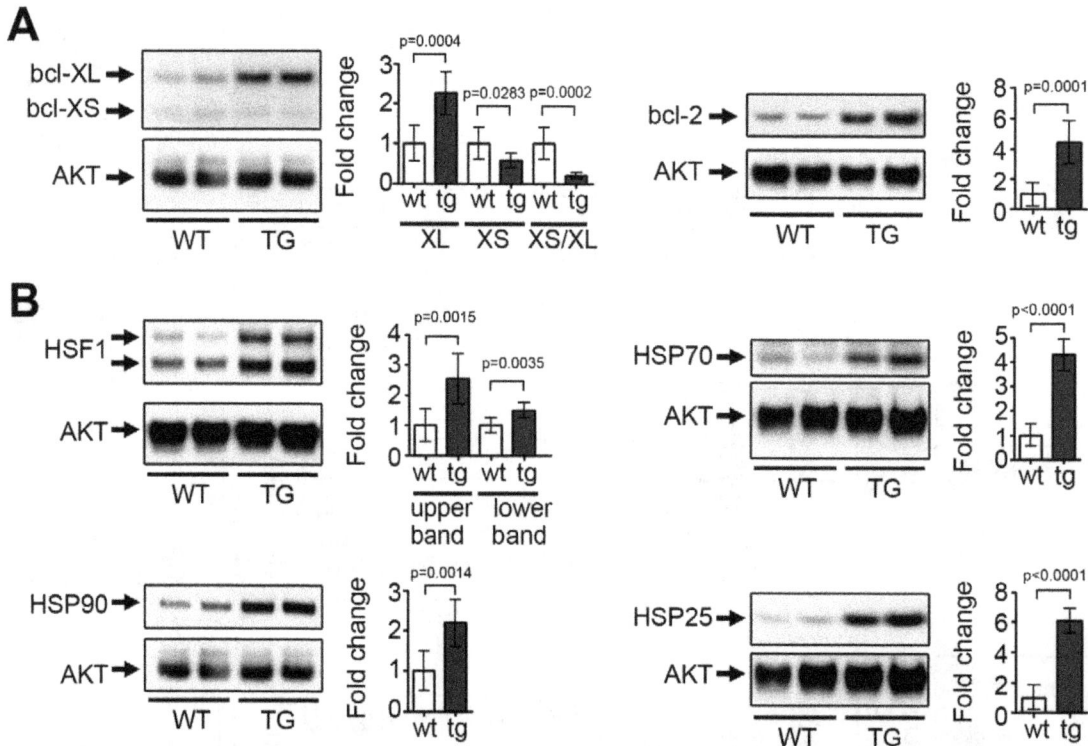

Figure 3. Up-regulation of pro-survival proteins and heat shock proteins in the hearts of ErbB2 transgenic mice. (A) Bcl-2 and Bcl-xL levels are increased, Bcl-xS levels are decreased and bcl-xS/XL ratio is reduced in left ventricles of ErbB2 transgenic mice. (B) Heat shock factor 1 (HSF1) and Heat shock proteins 25 (HSP25), 70 (HSP70) and 90 (HSP90) are elevated in left ventricles of ErbB2 transgenic mice. Two bands of HSF1 represent differentially phosphorylated HSF1 forms. Densitometry was performed using ImageJ software (n = 7 per genotype). All the studies were performed on 8–10 weeks old mice. The data are presented as the mean ± SD.

between transgenic and wild type mice at 8 weeks, but interstitial, perivascular and endocardial fibrosis did increase with age, as seen in the hearts of 6 months old transgenic mice compared to the age-matched littermates [Figure 4b and c]. Fibrosis continued to increase with age, as seen in 12 month- old ErbB2 transgenic mice compared to wild type mice [Figure S4]. Mineral deposits in fibrotic tissue were also observed in the left ventricular subendocardium in ErbB2 over-expressing hearts in mice as young as 4 weeks of age, without having deleterious effects on life span.

Microscopic studies confirmed that hypertrophy is related to increase in the size of individual cardiomyocytes. Cross sectional diameters of the cardiomyocytes were found to be increased in ErbB2 mice compared to the wild type mice, upon review of mid-papillary level transverse sections of hearts [Figure 4d]. In separate *in vitro* experiments, cardiomyocyte surface area was also measured in isolated cardiomyocytes; and ErbB2 over-expressing cardiomyocytes were found to be substantially larger than those of wild-type littermates, with a mean increase of surface area of 1.8 fold [Figure 4e and f].

A distinctive morphological feature of hypertrophic cardiomyocytes in ErbB2 transgenic mice is myocardial disarray, defined as disordered arrangement of cardiomyocytes with respect to one another. Disarray is more prominent in the septum but also was observed to a lesser degree throughout both ventricular walls of ErbB2 transgenic mice [Figure 5a–f] compared to wild type mice [Figure 5g, h]. The disarray in ErbB2 transgenic mice is characterized by a herring-bone, sometimes haphazard pattern of cardiomyocytes, with markedly enlarged cardiomyocytes and nuclei [black arrows] compared to the wild-type hearts [Figure 5a–h].

ErbB2 Over-expression Induces Concentric Cardiac Hypertrophy, but does not Lead to Heart Failure

Cardiac hypertrophy can lead to a decrease of cardiac function with subsequent heart failure and death. We performed echocardiographic studies to compare functional performance and morphology in the transgenic mice and wild type littermates by examining male mice at 8 weeks of age (n = 15–18/group). Gross pathological specimens of longitudinal cross sections of heart demonstrate concentric hypertrophy in ErbB2 transgenic mice [Figure 6a]. Additionally, M-mode comparisons of echocardiograms highlight marked concentric cardiac hypertrophy.

Table 1 summarizes cardiac function and morphology. Comparing ErbB2 transgenic mice to wild type mice, we noted left ventricle wall thickness parameters (IVSD: 2.23±0.15 vs. 0.98±0.07 mm; PWTED: 2.24±0.13 vs. 0.91±0.08 mm; RWT: 2.12±0.34 vs. 0.63±0.1; and LV mass: 299.8±54.49 vs. 91.86±12.32 mg) consistent with the concentric hypertrophy observed at necropsy. The left ventricle cavity (LVEDD 2.16±0.33 vs. 2.91±0.28 mm) was significantly smaller during diastole in ErbB2 transgenic mice, suggesting concentric left ventricular hypertrophy as shown in representative M-mode [Figure 6b]. These changes are age-dependent, and at 2 months of age, the increase in LVESD (1.09±0.09 vs. 0.94±0.17 mm) and small decline in FS (56.31±2.35% vs. 62.51±2.41%) are still within the limits of normal function and morphology. Cardiac output and blood pressure were significantly reduced in transgenic mice, compared to wild type littermates [Figure 6e,f] but not to a degree which would be reflective of heart failure. Remarkably, the hypertrophy induced by ErbB2 over-expression does not progress to overt heart failure. At 12 months, FS is 61.20+/−2.63% versus 43.71+/−11.11% (wild type vs. transgenic). At 17–18 months, the fractional shortening in ErbB2 transgenic mice

did not decline further and was maintained at 45.8+/−8.68% (n = 4).

ErbB2 Transgenic Mice Possess Electrophysiological Features of Cardiac Hypertrophy

Cardiac hypertrophy in humans is characterized by a number of specific electrocardiographic features. To evaluate electrophysiological parameters of ErbB2 over-expressing hearts, we evaluated a total of 28 mice (14 per genotype), aged 8–10 weeks, by electrocardiography. Representative EKG tracings for each genotype are shown in [Figure 6c]. The EKG parameters of wild type and transgenic mice were compared. Heart rate was similar between wild type and ErbB2 transgenic mice [Figure 6d]. The P wave represents a depolarization of atria. P wave duration varied among transgenic mice, being increased in the most of them; biphasic, two-peaked and tall P waves were also common, corresponding to the left and right atria hypertrophy. PR interval was shortened in transgenic mice, which, although is not common, but may occur in cardiac hypertrophy. Other features, characteristic of cardiac hypertrophy, were also observed including significantly increased QRS complex voltage and duration, left axis deviation, and repolarization abnormalities (electrocardiographic strain pattern) [26], [27]. The distinctive differences observed between genotypes allowed EKGs to be routinely used to phenotype litters into wild type or ErbB2 genotypes for longitudinal *in vivo* experiments.

Isoproterenol Induces Cardiac Arrhythmias and Death in ErbB2 Transgenic Mice

Although ErbB2 transgenic mice show cardiac hypertrophy-specific EKG changes, in general we did not note any arrhythmias during routine EKG recording. However, after recognizing the sudden death of several transgenic animals with routine handling, we further explored a possible increased tendency for transgenic animals to develop arrhythmias with adrenergic stimulation. Under ketamine and xylazine anesthesia, wild-type and ErbB2 transgenic mice responded to the standard dose of isoproterenol (0.1 mg/kg, 0.5 mg/kg or 100 mg/kg) administration with comparable increases in heart rate, at 6–9 seconds after the injection. However, ErbB2 transgenic mice developed progressive electrocardiographic changes, including decreased R wave amplitude, widened QRS complex, and complex arrhythmias, followed by asystole and eventually death 5 to 8 minutes after isoproterenol administration. These arrhythmias included atrio-ventricular blocks, and in some cases ventricular tachycardia [Figure 7b,c]. In ErbB2 transgenic mice, 100% mortality was observed with isoproterenol with dosages as low as 0.1 mg/kg, 1/1000of the standard dosage (100 mg/kg) routinely tolerated by wild type littermates. Wild-type littermates maintained increased heart rate until the end of the 30-minute period of recording [Figure 7a]; in some mice, heart rate slowed, followed by sinus bradycardia, but heart rates in all wild type animals normalized with time.

In a separate experiment, 4–5 conscious mice per genotype were injected with 0.1 mg/kg isoproterenol, and in this setting, transgenic mice had fewer arrhythmias than the group of mice that were anesthetized. However, when these mice were returned to cages for monitoring, 100% of ErbB2 transgenic mice died, usually within several hours, after isoproterenol injection.

Lapatinib Treatment Reduces both Cardiac Hypertrophy and ErbB2activation

Next, we used lapatinib, a pharmacological inhibitor of ErbB2 phosphorylation to induce pathway inactivation and determine

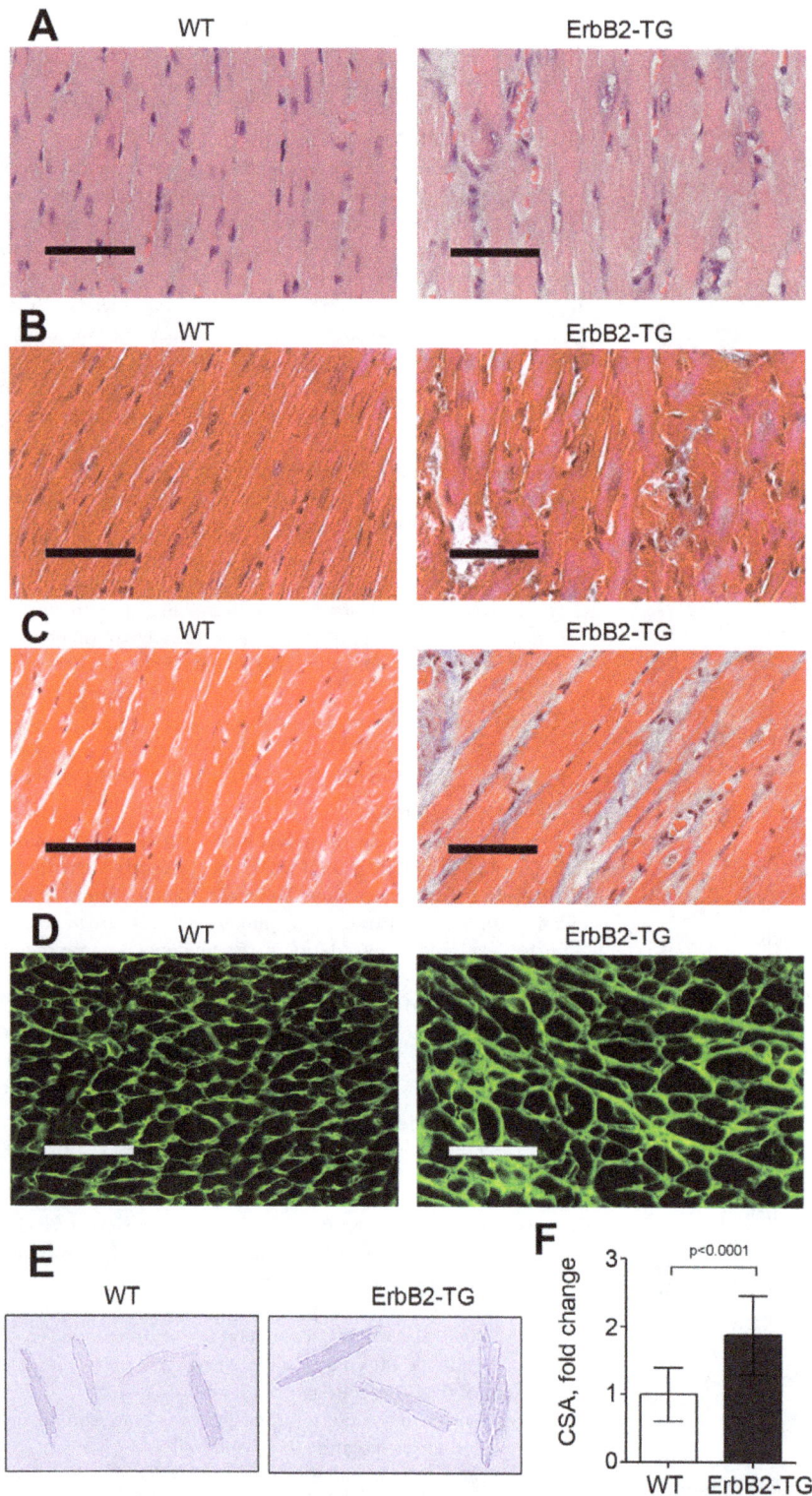

Figure 4. Cardiomyocyte hypertrophy and age-related interstitial fibrosis in ErbB2 transgenic mice. (A) H&E staining shows hypertrophied cardiomyocytes with enlarged nuclei in ErbB2 transgenic mice compared to wild type mice. Bar = 50 um. Masson trichrome staining was used to evaluate fibrosis in the hearts of 2 months (B) and 6 months old (C) wild type and ErbB2 transgenic mice. Bar = 50 um. (D) Representative images of WGA (wheat germ agglutinin) staining of left ventricle sections of wild type and ErbB2 transgenic mice hearts. (E) Isolated unstained cardiomyocytes from wild type and ErbB2 transgenic mice hearts. (F) Measurement of area of cardiomyocytes, isolated from wild type and ErbB2 transgenic hearts. 12–25 cardiomyocytes (3–4 mice per genotype) were used for calculations. The data are presented as the mean ± SD. All the studies were performed on 8–10 weeks old mice, unless different age is specified.

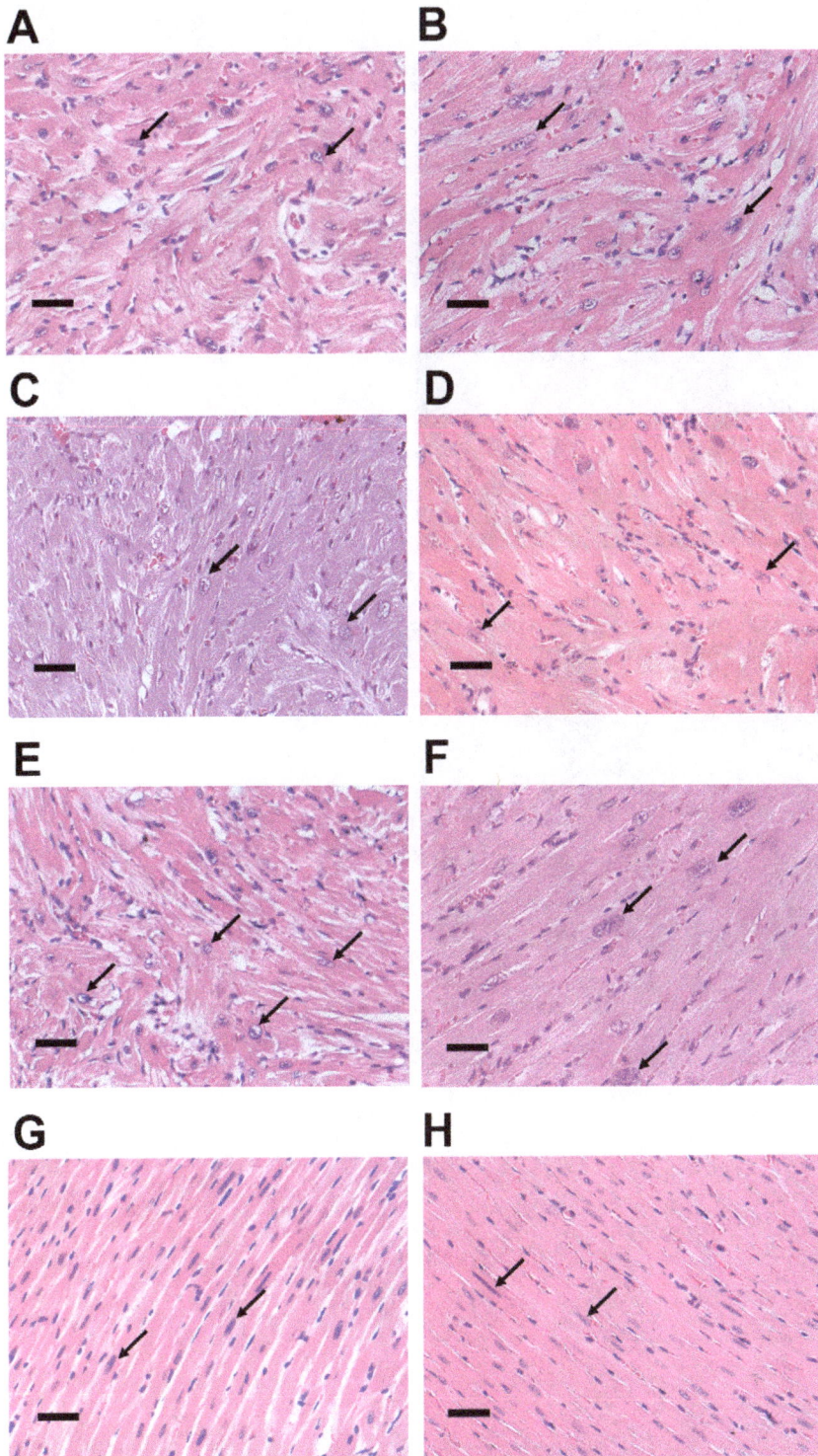

Figure 5. Histopathological evaluation of myocardial disarray in left ventricles and septa in ErbB2 transgenic mice. H&E staining of the heart sections of wild type and ErbB2 transgenic hearts. Left ventricles and septa of wild type and ErbB2 transgenic mice were evaluated for cardiomyocytes alignment and cell size. Enlarged nuclei are shown with arrows. Representative H&E stained sections from different heart regions are compared. Bar = 25 um. All the studies were performed on 8–10 weeks old mice. (A,C) ErbB2 transgenic mouse septum. (B,D,F) ErbB2 transgenic mouse left ventricle. (E) ErbB2 transgenic mouse junction of septum and left ventricle. (G) Wild type septum. (H) Wild type left ventricle.

whether cardiac hypertrophy in ErbB2 transgenic mice is dependent on translation pathway activation. Lapatinib is a small molecule reversible inhibitor of EGFR ($IC_{50} = 11$ nM) and ErbB2 ($IC_{50} = 9$ nM) tyrosine kinases. We chose lapatinib in our studies because it is commonly used in cancer patients and evaluating any potential toxicity would be also beneficial to uncover. Un-

A

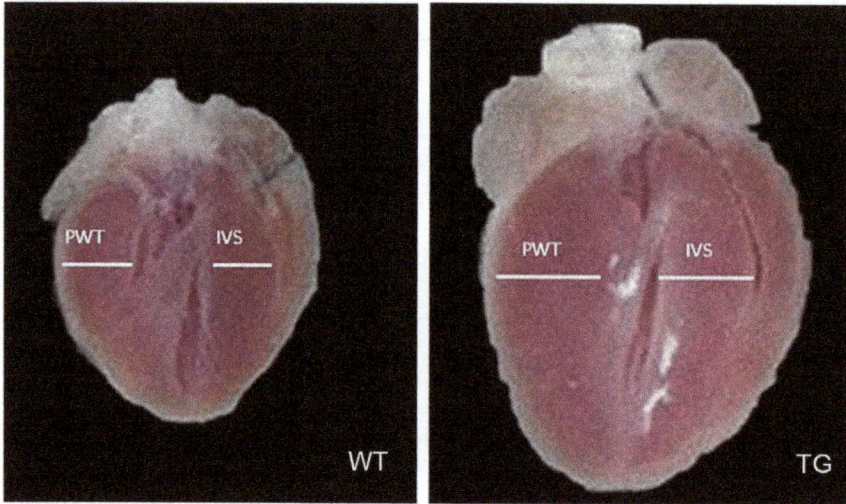

B

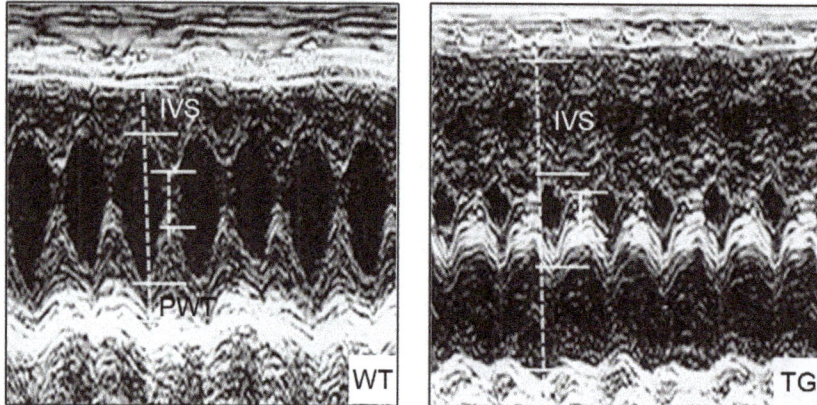

C

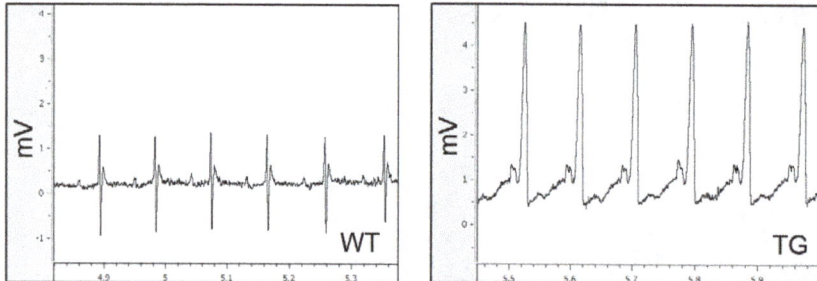

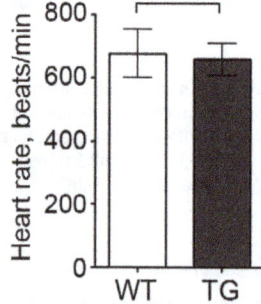

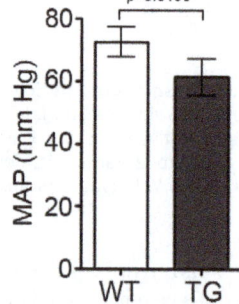

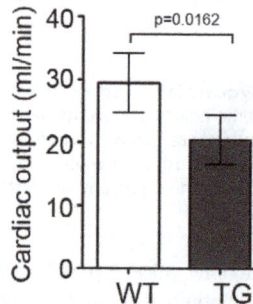

Figure 6. Gross pathology, echocardiography and electrocardiography of wild type and ErbB2 transgenic hearts. The wild type mice representative images are on the left and ErbB2 transgenic mice images are on the right of the panel. (A) Gross pathology reveals significant cardiac hypertrophy in ErbB2 transgenic mice. Longitudinal sections demonstrate hypertrophy of the heart walls and smaller left ventricle and right ventricle chambers in ErbB2 transgenic mouse. (B) M-mode produced by echocardiographic imaging demonstrates marked hypertrophy of the heart walls and reduction of left ventricle chamber in ErbB2 transgenic mice. IVS - interventricular septum, PWT – left ventricle posterior wall. 8–10 weeks old mice were used. (C) EKG was recorded in awake wild type and ErbB2 transgenic mice. Representative EKG tracings for each genotype are shown. (D) EKG was used for calculating the heart rate in wild type and ErbB2 transgenic mice (n = 14 per genotype). The data are presented as the mean ± SD. (E) Blood pressure was recorded in wild type and ErbB2 transgenic mice (n = 4–5 per genotype). The data are presented as the mean ± SD. MAP – mean arterial pressure. (F) Cardiac output was quantified in wild type and ErbB2 transgenic mice (n = 4–5 per genotype). The data are presented as the mean ± SD. All the studies were performed on 8–10 weeks old mice.

fortunately, there were no substitute compounds that are specific inhibitors of only ErbB2. Lapatinib binds to cytoplasmic ATP-binding site of the ErbB2 and EGFR and blocks its phosphorylation and activation, with subsequent inhibition of downstream pathways. Lapatinib peak plasma levels occur 3–6 hours (in humans) [28], 1–2 hours (in mice) [29], [30] after oral administration.

We hypothesized that ErbB pathway inhibition would block or blunt cardiac hypertrophy initiation in mice with constitutive over-expression of ErbB2. We performed two separate experiments, varying the dose and the age when the study began. In one study, we began lapatinib treatment at P4.5 and in another study we began treatment at P10.5.

In general, the molecular findings were similar in the two lapatinib dosing schemes, although starting the treatment before significant transgene activation and hypertrophy onset, induces a more substantial result in heart weight to body weight reduction in the younger group treated. In the 4–5 day old mice, treatment was given orally by gavage with 160 mg/kg of lapatinib for 8 days to test whether lapatinib can prevent the development of cardiac hypertrophy before it commences. Lapatinib administration successfully prevented hypertrophy development in ErbB2 transgenic mice, both in males (p<0.0001) and females (p<0.0001) while not affecting wild type littermates [Figure 8a]. Lapatinib treatment also reduces ErbB2 protein expression and significantly reduces levels of pAKT, and pS6 compared to wild type littermates resulting in abolishment of activation of ErbB2-dependent pathways and hypertrophic phenotype [Figure 8b]. A pathologist blinded to the treatment and genotypes reviewed the slides from this study. There was no evidence of cell death in the vehicle or lapatinib treated transgenic or wild type mice seen by histopathology or in TUNEL staining (data not shown).

Table 1. Cardiac function and morphology in wild type and ErbB2 transgenic mice.

Parameters	WT (n = 15)	TG (n = 18)	t-test (p)
LVEDD (mm)	2.91±0.28	2.16±0.33	0.0001***
LVESD (mm)	0.94±0.17	1.09±0.09	0.007**
IVSD (mm)	0.98±0.07	2.23±0.15	0.0001***
PWTED (mm)	0.91±0.08	2.24±0.13	0.0001***
FS (%)	62.51±2.41	56.31±2.35	0.0001***
LV mass (mg)	91.86±12.32	299.8±54.49	0.0001***
RWT	0.63±0.1	2.12±0.34	0.0001***

Echocardiographic parameters of ErbB2 transgenic mice confirm concentric hypertrophy consistent with necropsy results. Trans-thoracic echocardiography was performed on conscious 8–10 weeks old wild type (WT) and ErbB2 transgenic (TG) mice. Two-tailed t-test with **p<0.001, ***p<0.0001, Mean±SD.

Lapatinib also reduced the heart weights when given to older ErbB2 transgenic mice. Ten day old transgenic mice already have significant cardiac hypertrophy, which can be detected morphologically, on the necropsy, or electrophysiologically by EKG. At P9.5 the transgenic hearts are on average 1.5 times larger than the wild type hearts [Figure 1 and Figure S3a]. We hypothesized that lapatinib may delay further increase in cardiac mass in older ErbB2 transgenic mice. The mice were treated orally by gavage with lapatinib at 100 mg/kg, starting at P10.5 for 21 days. A lower dose was used in this study due to the extended period of dosing. Additionally, this dose is the most common dose used in the literature for chronic cancer studies.

We were able to perform immunoprecipitation and echocardiography studies in the older mice study since the hearts were large enough in 31 day old mice at euthanasia versus at 12 days old mice. ErbB2 cytosolic domain contains multiple sites of phosphorylation and partner factors binding sites. For complete estimate of ErbB2 activity, it is important to evaluate the total phosphorylation status of ErbB2, rather than phosphorylation of individual tyrosine residues. For this purpose, we performed immunoprecipitation of ErbB2 and the precipitate was probed for the total phospho-tyrosine. Mice were euthanized 2 hours after the lapatinib dose to evaluate ErbB2 status by immunoprecipitation and phospho-tyrosine immunoblotting. In vehicle treated group, transgenic mice had significantly higher phospho-tyrosine levels than wild types. Lapatinib administration decreased total ErbB2 phosphorylation in transgenic mice. In wild type mice the pTyr signal of ErbB2 was too low to detect with vehicle or lapatinib treatment. Surprisingly, total ErbB2 level in ErbB2 transgenic mice was decreased by lapatinib (occurred in both dosing models). A significant reduction in heart-to-body weight ratio in both genders of transgenic mice was observed (p = 0.0309 in males, and 0.0002 in females) [Figure 9a]. The heart function, assessed by echocardiography, was not altered significantly in either wild type or transgenic mice after lapatinib treatment [Figure 9b]. In parallel with the modest but significant reduction of HW/BW, phosphorylation of AKT and pS6 was reduced [Figure 9d], similar to the other dosing model (figure 8b).

Lapatinib treatment only reduced the HW/BW in the mice with ErbB2 over-expression, not the wild type mice. Correspondingly, the extent of hypertrophy and numbers of hypertrophic cells were reduced by lapatinib treatment in transgenic hearts [figure 9c]. In general, ErbB2 over-expression induces an extensive variation of cardiomyocyte size with a mixture of hypertrophic cells, normal-sized cardiomyocytes, and even some unusually small cardiomyocytes. Lapatinib reduced the number of large cells in the ErbB2 transgenic mice and did not appear to have an effect on cardiomyocyte sizes in control littermate's hearts. There was no evidence of cell death in the vehicle or lapatinib treated mice. TUNEL staining revealed no evidence of cell death in this experiment (data not shown), supporting our echocardiography studies that demonstrated normal function in mice treated with lapatinib for 21 days.

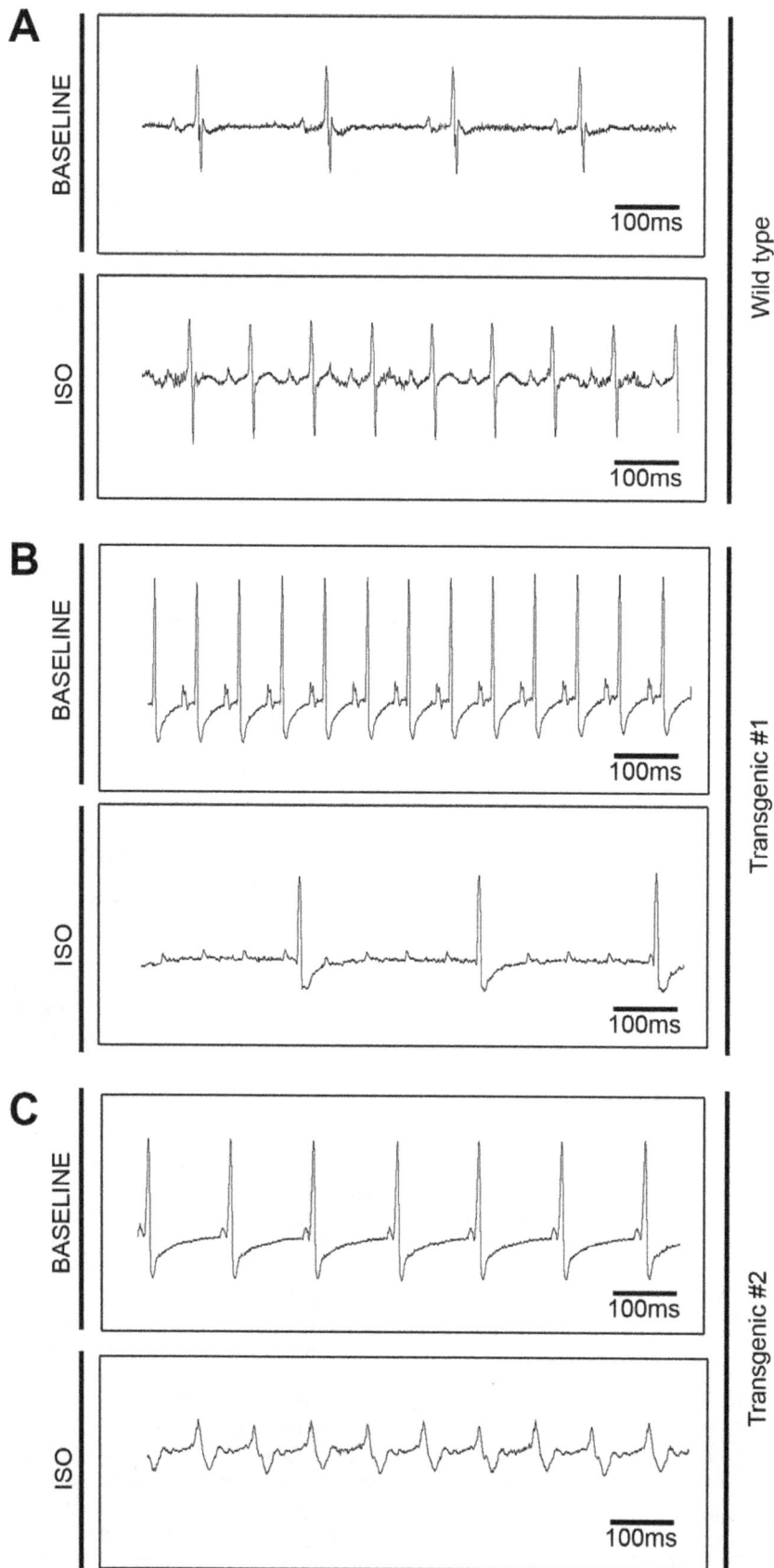

Figure 7. Isoproterenol treatment induces increased incidence of arrhythmias and sudden death in ErbB2 transgenic mice. Wild type (A) and ErbB2 transgenic (B) mice (n = 3–4 per genotype per treatment group) were anesthetized, and baseline EKG was recorded for 5 minutes.

Isoproterenol (0.1 mg/kg, 0.5 mg/kg or 100 mg/kg) was injected intraperitoneally and EKG was recorded for 30 minutes. EKG tracings from 2 different ErbB2 transgenic mice are displayed to present 2 different types of arrhythmias. All the studies were performed on 8–10 weeks old mice.

Discussion

ErbB2 over-expression in the mouse heart leads to concentric hypertrophy with significant increase in sizes of individual cardiomyocytes. Remarkably, animals with ErbB2-induced cardiac hypertrophy do not develop heart failure. But mice with hypertrophic hearts are susceptible to arrhythmias, which are readily triggered by isoproterenol, and occasionally experience sudden death caused by routine handling of animals. ErbB2 over-expression activates cardiac pro-survival signaling and hypertrophic pathways in cardiomyocytes, including the PI3K/AKT pathway, which regulates cardiomyocyte survival and protein translation. ErbB2 over-expression also leads to up-regulation of the pro-survival bcl-2 family of proteins in the heart, with an anti-apoptotic shift in the balance of pro-survival bcl-xL and apoptotic bcl-xS proteins. Thus, the hypertrophic effects of ErbB2 are likely related to the role of this protein as a key regulator of protein translation and the balance between survival and apoptosis of cardiomyocytes.

By defining a role for ErbB2 in inducing cardiac hypertrophy, our results reveal new insights into previously recognized phenomena in human heart patients. In humans, ErbB2 protein was shown to increase early in the development of the heart failure from multiple etiologies, while ErbB2 protein decreases in patients with terminal heart failure [23]. Previous studies and the work we present here, suggest that, although ErbB2 may drive hypertrophy in an attempt to improve heart function, ErbB2 expression is not maintained and heart failure ensues. Mechanisms that induce ErbB2 expression in the human heart are not currently known, but clues to these mechanisms could possibly be revealed by investigating pathways activated after unloading the heart subsequent to left ventricular assist device (LVAD) implantation. In limited investigations into these pathways, ErbB2 mRNA was found to be increased following unloading in 36 patients with severe heart failure (NYHA class IV) due to ischemic and non-ischemic cardiomyopathy [31], but ErbB2 protein levels were not evaluated in this study. Other investigators found that ErbB2 protein is shed into serum when patients are in heart failure and this correlates inversely with left ventricular ejection fraction [32], providing additional circumstantial evidence that ErbB2 protein and its signaling could be increased at some phases of development of human heart failure.

Clues to the down-regulation of ErbB2 in terminal heart failure may be related to mechanisms involving miRNA. For example, an inverse relationship of ErbB2 and miR7 was found in humans with dilated cardiomyopathy [33] in a setting where ErbB2 appears to have an important role in cardiomyocytes of humans approaching heart failure. It is possible that, in this situation, stressed cardiomyocytes transiently develop hypertrophy, driven by ErbB2 expression and activity. Based on human evidence noted above, induction (and then loss) of ErbB2 expression and signaling is likely important in the transition from hypertrophy to heart failure. While molecular inducers and molecular inhibitors of ErbB2 are

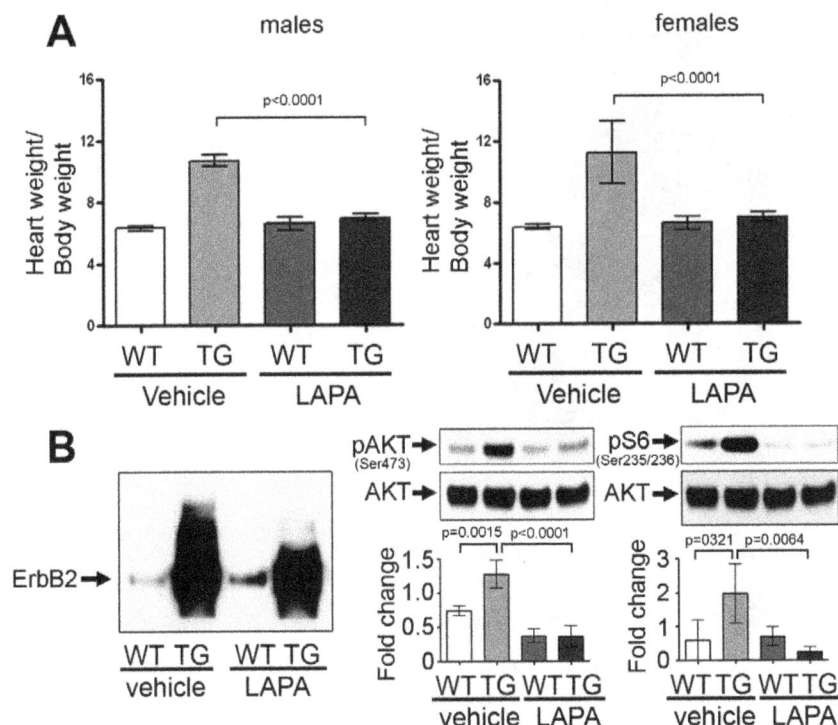

Figure 8. Lapatinib blocks hypertrophy development in ErbB2 transgenic mice. P4.5 male and female mice were treated with lapatinib via gavage for 8 days until P12.5 (n = 4–7 per genotype per treatment group per sex). (A) Increased heart weight to body weight ratio in ErbB2 transgenic mice at P12.5. Lapatinib treatment significantly reduces this ratio both in males and females. The data are presented as the mean ± SD. (B) Representative western blots of total ErbB2, phospho-AKT and phospho-S6 proteins in wild type and ErbB2 transgenic mice, treated with vehicle or lapatinib. Densitometry was performed using ImageJ (n = 4–6 per genotype per treatment group per sex). The data are presented as the mean ± SD.

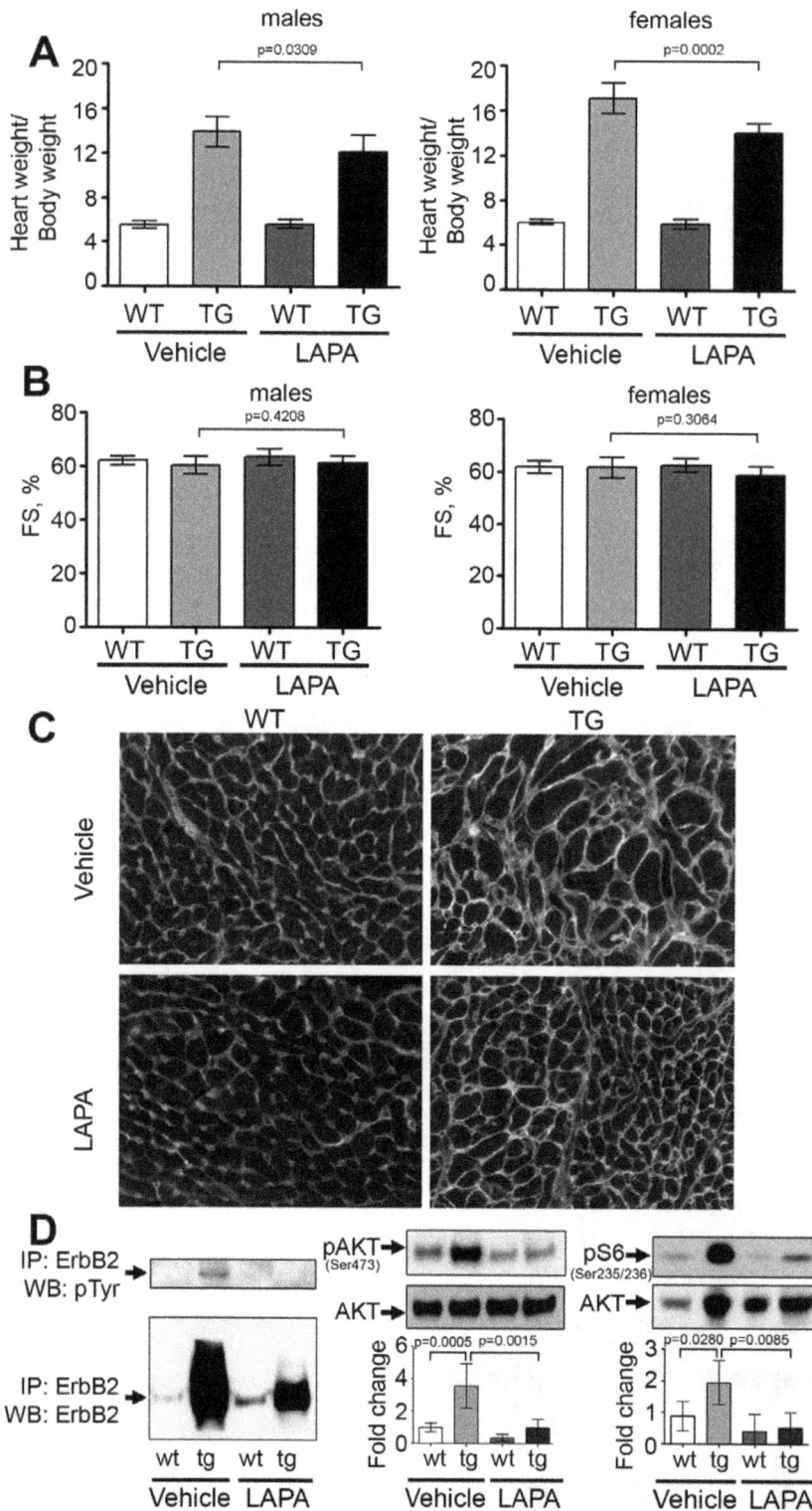

Figure 9. Lapatinib reduces hypertrophy in ErbB2 transgenic mice. Wild type and ErbB2 transgenic male and female mice were treated with lapatinib via gavage for 3 weeks, starting at P10.5 (n = 5–12 per genotype per treatment group per sex). (A) Increased heart weight to body weight ratio in ErbB2 transgenic mice compared to wild type mice, which is reduced with lapatinib treatment (n = 5–12 per genotype per treatment group per sex). The data are presented as the mean ± SD. (B) Fractional shortening was evaluated in wild type and ErbB2 transgenic mice, treated with vehicle or lapatinib (n = 5–12 per genotype per treatment group per sex). The data are presented as the mean ± SD. (C) WGA staining reveals cell size variation in the hearts of ErbB2 transgenic mice, compared to wild type littermates, including large, medium and small-sized cells. Lapatinib reduces the size of cardiomyocytes in the ErbB2 hypertrophied cells. (n = 3–4 per genotype per treatment group). (D) Total ErbB2 phosphorylation was evaluated by immunoprecipitation in wild type and ErbB2 transgenic mice, treated with vehicle or lapatinib. Densitometry was performed using ImageJ software (n = 3–6 per genotype per treatment group). The data are presented as the mean ± SD.

not well understood, our animal model unequivocally for the first time establishes that activation of ErbB2 induces cardiac hypertrophy.

Decline in ErbB2 protein expression temporally correlating with transition to heart failure is also seen in animal models. In various experimental models of heart failure in animals, ErbB2 pathway is activated in early stages of heart failure but subsequently becomes inactivated in later stages of heart failure. For example, ErbB2 is up-regulated initially following doxorubicin induced damage before there is a systolic dysfunction in rats [10]. Yet in later stages of doxorubicin toxicity, in a mouse model, miR146 is responsible for reducing ErbB pathway activation by decreasing cardiac ErbB4 protein levels, hence decreasing protective signaling [34]. In a canine cardiac stress model, ventricular pacing induces ErbB2 phosphorylation, apparently (and surprisingly) without activation of AKT or ERK pathways [35]. Lastly, in an aortic stenosis model of hypertrophy in rats, with progression to heart failure, ErbB2 levels are maintained in hypertrophic hearts but decrease as heart failure develops [36], suggesting that ErbB2 pathway activity is important in preventing heart failure progression under conditions of stress. We recognize that in many situations of cardiac stress, up-regulation of ErbB2 as a protective response might occur only in the most stressed cells requiring a hypertrophic response, and not uniformly among all cardiomyocytes. If so, a significant up-regulation in ErbB2 protein may not always be appreciated by Western blotting techniques.

Since other models of hypertrophy lead to heart failure, our finding of a lack of heart failure in the ErbB2 mouse model is particularly remarkable. The propensity to cause hypertrophy without heart failure is also seen with over-expression of insulin-like growth factor 1 (IGF-1) [37] and insulin-like growth factor 1 receptor (IGF1R) [38]. Both ErbB2 and IGF1R share downstream proteins that are pro-survival in nature, explaining why heart failure is not seen with over-expression of these proteins. In another example, PI3K over-expression in the heart induces hypertrophy without heart failure [14], [39]. Multiple cardiac AKT over-expression models have been described, with various degrees of cardiac hypertrophy, which resulted in heart failure in some models, but not in others [13], [15], [40], [41]. A few factors can modulate the phenotypes between different AKT over-expression models, including fold increase in the transgene expression and different signaling pathways activated by constitutive versus inducible AKT over-expression. Concerning the comparison of AKT- and ErbB2-over-expressing mice, activation of survival pathways by ErbB2 aside of PI3K/AKT pathway, such as HSPs and bcl-2 family proteins, may contribute to a sustained survival of ErbB2 transgenic mice versus AKT transgenic mice with resulting heart failure. Also, increased total AKT levels in AKT over-expression models may provide additional signaling changes, while in ErbB2 over-expressing model AKT phosphorylation was modestly increased, without an increase in total AKT.

ErbB4 is another protein in the ErbB family that has been over-expressed experimentally in the heart, but surprisingly this over-expression does not result in hypertrophy. Tidcombe and colleagues over-expressed human ErbB4 in hearts of erbB4 knock-out mice to determine whether this over-expression could rescue hearts from the trabeculation defect seen in erbB4 complete knock outs [42]. While this over-expression of ErbB4 did rescue the trabeculation defect phenotype, neither the degree of erbB4 over-expression level, nor the hypertrophic phenotype, was reported in these mice. Phenotypic differences between our model and the erbB4 over-expression model may be explained by comparing signaling differences between these two mouse models, since multiple ligand and receptor combinations [43] could offer

a plethora of cellular phenotypes [44], [45], [46]. Notably, each receptor tyrosine kinase possesses a set of -phosphorylation sites, activation of which may also define unique downstream activation patterns [47] As an example, NRG-induced ErbB2 heterodimerization with ErbB4 can activate Stat5, but both ErbB2-ErbB2 and ErbB4-ErbB4 homodimers lack this ability [48]. Differential activation of pro-hypertrophic versus proliferative pathways may explain why ErbB4 over-expression led to a proliferative response in cardiac myocytes, but not to hypertrophy [49].

A far as we can determine, this study is the first to demonstrate that ErbB2 over-expression regulates the expression of EGFR, ErbB3 and ErbB4, as well as both PI3K subunits. These findings may have relevance, not only to cardiac studies, but also for understanding the role of ErbB2 role in cancer biology. We suggest that ErbB2 is a major regulator of ErbB receptors family and its downstream signaling [Figure 10], and it is possible that ErbB2 controls a subset of proteins that drive cardiac hypertrophy either through receptor signaling or through ErbB2 effects in the nucleus, where ErbB2 translocates in cleaved [50] or intact [51] forms and has been linked to the trans-activation of the COX-2 promoter [51].

Comparing animal models with cardiac expression of signaling proteins, ErbB2 over-expression induces myocardial disarray, while PI3K, AKT and IGF1R over-expression do not induce myocardial disarray. Additionally, compared to Hypertrophic Cardiomyopathy mouse models [52], [53], [54], ErbB2 transgenic mice have a much greater degree of disarray, and thus may be useful in dissecting molecular mechanisms of disarray and the effects of myocardial disarray on cardiomyocyte physiology. Notably, myocardial disarray is commonly seen in human heart disease, including HCM, and it is linked to arrhythmias, syncope and sudden death [55], [56]. Currently, there is controversy on whether myocardial disarray induces arrhythmias. In some experiments, changes in myofiber direction were shown to interfere with conduction [57], [58], and the presence of disarray is a risk factor for arrhythmias development in some animal models [59]. Conversely, other studies show that occurrence of cardiac arrhythmias is not related to amount and distribution of the disarray [60]. In humans, a direct association between the disarray and sudden death has been accepted [61], [62], with ventricular tachycardia and fibrillation considered to be primary causes of sudden cardiac death in HCM patients. Defining molecular determinants of cardiomyocyte interaction with its cellular environment, including cells and extracellular matrix, in the ErbB2 transgenic mouse may uncover new insights into myocardial disarray and mechanisms of cardiac arrhythmias.

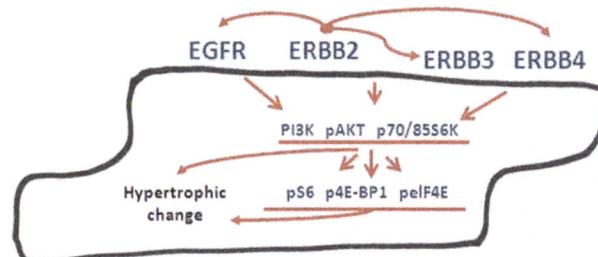

Figure 10. Schematic representation of the pathways involved in cardiac hypertrophy in ErbB2 transgenic mice. ErbB2 over-expression results in increased levels of other ErbB family members, EGFR, ErbB3 and ErbB4. ErbB family signals to downstream PI3K, AKT and p70/85S6K proteins, which leads to activation of translational machinery and hypertrophic phenotype.

Thus, our finding that ErbB2 expression in the heart induces both myocardial disarray and arrhythmias is potentially important for understanding the relationship between these phenomena in human disease.

Support for the use of this model for investigating the role of myocardial disarray in cardiac rhythm disturbances come from our findings that hearts of ErbB2 transgenic mice share distinctive electrophysiological features with human HCM patients, including increased QRS voltage and duration, ST segment and T wave abnormalities, as well as shortened PQ interval. Shortened PQ interval is observed in some patients with HCM, particularly in those without contractile proteins mutations, such as PRKAG2 mutations [63], [64], Danon disease [65], [66], Pompe disease [67] and Fabry disease [68], [69]. The electrophysiological disorder of ErbB2 transgenic mice heart physiology was also reflected in a particularly high sensitivity to the non-specific beta-adrenergic agonist, isoproterenol. Transgenic mice treated with modest doses of isoproterenol developed electrocardiographic changes and died shortly after isoproterenol injection, similar to the response seen in other HCM mouse models [70], [71]. This is consistent with humans with HCM and their heightened sensitivity to adrenergic stimulation and arrhythmias.

We propose that this novel model of ErbB2 over-expression in cardiomyocytes meets the criteria for the model of hypertrophic cardiomyopathy (HCM), which is characterized by cardiomyocyte hypertrophy, myocardial disarray and interstitial fibrosis [56]. Most of the HCM cases that have been genetically evaluated have mutated sarcomeric contractile proteins, but not all are associated with sarcomeric proteins (reviewed here) [55]. In humans with HCM, cardiac hypertrophy of a similar degree (as erbB2 transgenic mice) is not observed. Yet the similarities in the disease course, histopathology and functional changes between our model and human HCM allowed us to suggest our model as a potential model for human HCM, and particularly HCM not induced by contractile proteins mutations. Our model has distinctive cardiomyocyte disarray and chamber restriction/constriction consistent with HCM. Interstitial, subendocardial and perivascular fibrosis is minimal in 2 month old mice but does increase with age contributing to the stiffness of the heart, a feature shared with other mouse models and human HCM cases. Reduced cardiac output and decreased blood pressure, seen in ErbB2 transgenic mice, are other features often observed in HCM human patients particularly during exercise tests [72] and hypertrophic cardiomyopathy mouse models [73], [74].

The lapatinib studies were initiated to confirm the role of ErbB2 in cardiac hypertrophy. We assessed whether pathway activation, hypertrophy and heart weight/body weight would be affected by lapatinib or the age during treatment. We treated 2 groups of mice, one from 4.5 to 12.5 days of age, and another from 10.5 to 31 days of age. In the younger group, although we gave a higher dose of lapatinib, we did observe a much more robust reduction in heart weights/body weights, while lapatinib inhibited translation activation markers similarly in each model. Comparison of our two dosing models and the subsequent heart weight/body weight results may uncover novel mechanisms of hypertrophy or novel mechanisms related to ErbB2 biology.

It is tempting to speculate that the timing of lapatinib initiation is crucial and these two treatment schemes should be studied for novel ways by which ErbB2 could affect cell size or cell number. It is possible that ErbB2 transgene expression, we see dramatically induced via αMHC induction in the first week of postnatal life, has an effect on chromatin remodeling, thus influencing hypertrophy or possibly hyperplasia. When ErbB2 (and EGFR) are pharmacologically inhibited after transgene activation, potential chromatin remodeling

changes may have already taken place, and may not be so easily or rapidly reversed in the 3 weeks of treatment. Future studies will be necessary to mechanistically link ErbB2 to chromatin remodeling. Yet a more plausible suggestion relates to cardiomyocyte proliferation. https://jhem.johnshopkins.edu/iframe.html - _mso-com_1 ErbB2 expression in the first week of life may extend the length of time cardiomyocytes divide, thus inhibiting ErbB2 signaling at this stage may both inhibit proliferative and hypertrophic ErbB2 effects. Later in life, ErbB2's effect on hyperplasia may not be as dominant as in neonatal period, although, recently it was found that NRG/ErbB4 pathway does induce hyperplasia in adult cardiomyocytes [49]. This hypothesis has to be tested but cardiomyocyte proliferation may explain the differences in HW/BW changes in the two lapatinib dosing models.

Furthermore, and most importantly, the present study may shed some light on why synergistic toxicity occurs in some cancer therapy patients treated with ErbB2 inhibitors (Herceptin) and doxorubicin [10]. We suggest that some patients with various stages of cardiac hypertrophy, including sub-clinical stages of disease, have dependence on ErbB2 to maintain cardiac function, and loss of ErbB2 activity (which can occur as a result of cancer therapy) results in heart failure.

Supporting Information

Figure S1 Kaplan-Meyer survival curves of wild type and ErbB2 transgenic mice. Kaplan-Meyer survival curves for males (A) and females (B) of wild type (square - ■) and ErbB2 transgenic (diamond - ♦) mouse lines. n = 142 (wild type males), n = 154 (transgenic males), n = 59 (wild type females), n = 58 (transgenic females).

Figure S2 Chest radiography and gross morphology of the heart display significant cardiac hypertrophy in ErbB2 transgenic mice. Chest anterio-posterior radiography reveals enlarged cardiac silhouette in ErbB2 transgenic mouse (B), compared to a normal size of the cardiac silhouette in wild type mouse (A). Bone structures, liver and clear lung fields are also visible in both wild type and ErbB2 transgenic mice radiographs. Wild type (C) and ErbB2 transgenic (D) hearts *in situ*. ErbB2 transgenic mouse present with enlarged heart with enlargement of both atria and ventricles. 8–10 weeks old mice were used, n = 2 per genotype.

Figure S3 Heart weight and heart weight-to-body weight ratios are increased in ErbB2 transgenic mice. Heart weights (A) and body weights (C) were measured in wild type and ErbB2 transgenic mice at P3.5, 6.5, 9.5 (n = 5–22 per genotype per age group). The data are presented as the mean ± SD. Heart weights (B), body weights (D) and heart weight-to-body weight ratios (E) were measured in wild type and ErbB2 transgenic mice at 1, 2, 4, 8, 12 months (n = 4–27 per genotype per age group). The data are presented as the mean ± SD.

Figure S4 Age-related cardiac fibrosis in ErbB2 transgenic mice. Wild type and ErbB2 transgenic hearts were examined by Masson's trichrome staining. 2 months old wild type (A) or ErbB2 transgenic (B) mice hearts, 6 months old wild type (C) or ErbB2 transgenic (D) mice hearts, and 12 months old wild type (E) or ErbB2 transgenic (F) mice hearts were evaluated.

Table S1 Primers used for quantitative RT-PCR.

Table S2 Buffers composition.

Table S3 Antibodies used for immunoprecipitation and western blotting.

Acknowledgments

We are grateful to Dr. Dan Judge, Dr. Charles Steenbergen, Dr. David Kass, Dr. Nazareno Paolocci and Dr. Anne Murphy for critical conversations and review of the figures and to Dr. Dan Berkowitz for providing us with CODA2 Tail-Cuff System for blood pressure measurements.

Author Contributions

Conceived and designed the experiments: PSS YX KG. Performed the experiments: PSS YX XG FB BK DB SP NT KG. Analyzed the data: PSS YX XG FB BK DB SP NT KG. Contributed reagents/materials/analysis tools: KG. Wrote the paper: PSS YX XG FB BK DB SP NT KG.

References

1. Baselga J (2001) Clinical trials of Herceptin(R) (trastuzumab). Eur J Cancer 37 Suppl 1: 18–24.
2. Baselga J, Tripathy D, Mendelsohn J, Baughman S, Benz CC, et al. (1996) Phase II study of weekly intravenous recombinant humanized anti-p185HER2 monoclonal antibody in patients with HER2/neu-overexpressing metastatic breast cancer. J Clin Oncol 14(3): 737–744.
3. McKeage K, Perry CM (2002) Trastuzumab: a review of its use in the treatment of metastatic breast cancer overexpressing HER2. Drugs 62(1): 209–243.
4. Negro A, Brar BK, Lee KF (2004) Essential roles of Her2/erbB2 in cardiac development and function. Recent Prog Horm Res 59: 1–12.
5. Lee KF, Simon H, Chen H, Bates B, Hung MC, et al. (1995) Requirement for neuregulin receptor erbB2 in neural and cardiac development. Nature 378(6555): 394–398.
6. Camenisch TD, Schroeder JA, Bradley J, Klewer SE, McDonald JA (2002) Heart-valve mesenchyme formation is dependent on hyaluronan-augmented activation of ErbB2-ErbB3 receptors. Nat Med 8(8): 850–855.
7. Crone SA, Zhao YY, Fan L, Gu Y, Minamisawa S, et al. (2002) ErbB2 is essential in the prevention of dilated cardiomyopathy. Nat Med 8(5): 459–465.
8. Ozcelik C, Erdmann B, Pilz B, Wettschureck N, Britsch S, et al. (2002) Conditional mutation of the ErbB2 (HER2) receptor in cardiomyocytes leads to dilated cardiomyopathy. Proc Natl Acad Sci U S A 99(13): 8880–8885.
9. Behr TM, Behe M, Wormann B (2001) Trastuzumab and breast cancer. N Engl J Med 345(13): 995–996.
10. Gabrielson K, Bedja D, Pin S, Tsao A, Gama L, et al. (2007) Heat shock protein 90 and ErbB2 in the cardiac response to doxorubicin injury. Cancer Res 67(4): 1436–1441.
11. Sahn DJ, DeMaria A, Kisslo J, Weyman A (1978) Recommendations regarding quantitation in M-mode echocardiography: results of a survey of echocardiographic measurements. Circulation 58(6): 1072–1083.
12. Daugherty A, Rateri D, Hong L, Balakrishnan A (2009) Measuring blood pressure in mice using volume pressure recording, a tail-cuff method. J Vis Exp(27).
13. Matsui T, Li L, Wu JC, Cook SA, Nagoshi T, et al. (2002) Phenotypic spectrum caused by transgenic overexpression of activated Akt in the heart. J Biol Chem 277(25): 22896–22901.
14. Shioi T, Kang PM, Douglas PS, Hampe J, Yballe CM, et al. (2000) The conserved phosphoinositide 3-kinase pathway determines heart size in mice. Embo Journal 19(11): 2537–2548.
15. Shioi T, McMullen JR, Kang PM, Douglas PS, Obata T, et al. (2002) Akt/protein kinase B promotes organ growth in transgenic mice. Mol Cell Biol 22(8): 2799–2809.
16. Fenton TR, Gout IT (2011) Functions and regulation of the 70kDa ribosomal S6 kinases. Int J Biochem Cell Biol 43(1): 47–59.
17. Pause A, Belsham GJ, Gingras AC, Donze O, Lin TA, et al. (1994) Insulin-dependent stimulation of protein synthesis by phosphorylation of a regulator of 5'-cap function. Nature 371(6500): 762–767.
18. Sadoshima J, Izumo S (1995) Rapamycin selectively inhibits angiotensin II-induced increase in protein synthesis in cardiac myocytes in vitro. Potential role of 70-kD S6 kinase in angiotensin II-induced cardiac hypertrophy. Circ Res 77(6): 1040–1052.
19. Boluyt MO, Zheng JS, Younes A, Long X, O'Neill L, et al. (1997) Rapamycin inhibits alpha 1-adrenergic receptor-stimulated cardiac myocyte hypertrophy but not activation of hypertrophy-associated genes. Evidence for involvement of p70 S6 kinase. Circ Res 81(2): 176–186.
20. Boluyt MO, Li ZB, Loyd AM, Scalia AF, Cirrincione GM, et al. (2004) The mTOR/p70S6K signal transduction pathway plays a role in cardiac hypertrophy and influences expression of myosin heavy chain genes in vivo. Cardiovasc Drugs Ther 18(4): 257–267.
21. Rohrbach S, Muller-Werdan U, Werdan K, Koch S, Gellerich NF, et al. (2005) Apoptosis-modulating interaction of the neuregulin/erbB pathway with anthracyclines in regulating Bcl-xS and Bcl-xL in cardiomyocytes. J Mol Cell Cardiol 38(3): 485–493.
22. Grazette LP, Boecker W, Matsui T, Semigran M, Force TL, et al. (2004) Inhibition of ErbB2 causes mitochondrial dysfunction in cardiomyocytes: implications for herceptin-induced cardiomyopathy. J Am Coll Cardiol 44(11): 2231–2238.
23. Rohrbach S, Niemann B, Silber RE, Holtz J (2005) Neuregulin receptors erbB2 and erbB4 in failing human myocardium – depressed expression and attenuated activation. Basic Res Cardiol 100(3): 240–249.
24. Sakamoto M, Minamino T, Toko H, Kayama Y, Zou Y, et al. (2006) Upregulation of heat shock transcription factor 1 plays a critical role in adaptive cardiac hypertrophy. Circ Res 99(12): 1411–1418.
25. Zhao YH, Zhou M, Liu H, Ding Y, Khong HT, et al. (2009) Upregulation of lactate dehydrogenase A by ErbB2 through heat shock factor 1 promotes breast cancer cell glycolysis and growth. Oncogene 28(42): 3689–3701.
26. Romhilt DW, Estes EH Jr (1968) A point-score system for the ECG diagnosis of left ventricular hypertrophy. Am Heart J 75(6): 752–758.
27. Okin PM, Devereux RB, Fabsitz RR, Lee ET, Galloway JM, et al. (2002) Quantitative assessment of electrocardiographic strain predicts increased left ventricular mass: the Strong Heart Study. J Am Coll Cardiol 40(8): 1395–1400.
28. Martens UM (2009). Small Molecules in Oncology, Springer.
29. Emanuel SL, Hughes TV, Adams M, Rugg CA, Fuentes-Pesquera A, et al. (2008) Cellular and in vivo activity of JNJ-28871063, a nonquinazoline pan-ErbB kinase inhibitor that crosses the blood-brain barrier and displays efficacy against intracranial tumors. Mol Pharmacol 73(2): 338–348.
30. Gorlick R, Kolb EA, Houghton PJ, Morton CL, Phelps D, et al. (2009) Initial testing (stage 1) of lapatinib by the pediatric preclinical testing program. Pediatr Blood Cancer 53(4): 594–598.
31. Uray IP, Connelly JH, Frazier O, Taegtmeyer H, Davies PJ (2001) Altered expression of tyrosine kinase receptors Her2/neu and GP130 following left ventricular assist device (LVAD) placement in patients with heart failure. J Heart Lung Transplant 20(2): 210.
32. Perik PJ, de Vries EG, Gietema JA, van der Graaf WT, Smilde TD, et al. (2007) Serum HER2 levels are increased in patients with chronic heart failure. Eur J Heart Fail 9(2): 173–177.
33. Naga Prasad SV, Duan ZH, Gupta MK, Surampudi VS, Volinia S, et al. (2009) Unique microRNA profile in end-stage heart failure indicates alterations in specific cardiovascular signaling networks. J Biol Chem 284(40): 27487–27499.
34. Horie T, Ono K, Nishi H, Nagao K, Kinoshita M, et al. (2010) Acute doxorubicin cardiotoxicity is associated with miR-146a-induced inhibition of the neuregulin-ErbB signaling. Cardiovasc Res 87(4): 656–664.
35. Doggen K, Ray L, Mathieu M, Mc Entee K, Lemmens K, et al. (2009) Ventricular ErbB2/ErbB4 activation and downstream signaling in pacing-induced heart failure. J Mol Cell Cardiol 46(1): 33–38.
36. Rohrbach S, Yan X, Weinberg EO, Hasan F, Bartunek J, et al. (1999) Neuregulin in cardiac hypertrophy in rats with aortic stenosis. Differential expression of erbB2 and erbB4 receptors. Circulation 100(4): 407–412.
37. Reiss K, Cheng W, Ferber A, Kajstura J, Li P, et al. (1996) Overexpression of insulin-like growth factor-1 in the heart is coupled with myocyte proliferation in transgenic mice. Proc Natl Acad Sci U S A 93(16): 8630–8635.
38. McMullen JR, Shioi T, Huang WY, Zhang L, Tarnavski O, et al. (2004) The insulin-like growth factor 1 receptor induces physiological heart growth via the phosphoinositide 3-kinase(p110alpha) pathway. J Biol Chem 279(6): 4782–4793.
39. McMullen JR, Shioi T, Zhang L, Tarnavski O, Sherwood MC, et al. (2003) Phosphoinositide 3-kinase(p110alpha) plays a critical role for the induction of physiological, but not pathological, cardiac hypertrophy. Proc Natl Acad Sci U S A 100(21): 12355–12360.
40. Shiojima I, Sato K, Izumiya Y, Schiekofer S, Ito M, et al. (2005) Disruption of coordinated cardiac hypertrophy and angiogenesis contributes to the transition to heart failure. J Clin Invest 115(8): 2108–2118.
41. Taniyama Y, Ito M, Sato K, Kuester C, Veit K, et al. (2005) Akt3 overexpression in the heart results in progression from adaptive to maladaptive hypertrophy. J Mol Cell Cardiol 38(2): 375–385.
42. Tidcombe H, Jackson-Fisher A, Mathers K, Stern DF, Gassmann M, et al. (2003) Neural and mammary gland defects in ErbB4 knockout mice genetically rescued from embryonic lethality. Proc Natl Acad Sci U S A 100(14): 8281–8286.
43. Olayioye MA, Graus-Porta D, Beerli RR, Rohrer J, Gay B, et al. (1998) ErbB-1 and ErbB-2 acquire distinct signaling properties dependent upon their dimerization partner. Mol Cell Biol 18(9): 5042–5051.
44. Yarden Y, Sliwkowski MX (2001) Untangling the ErbB signalling network. Nat Rev Mol Cell Biol 2(2): 127–137.

45. Olayioye MA, Neve RM, Lane HA, Hynes NE (2000) The ErbB signaling network: receptor heterodimerization in development and cancer. Embo J 19(13): 3159–3167.

46. Sweeney C, Fambrough D, Huard C, Diamonti AJ, Lander ES, et al. (2001) Growth factor-specific signaling pathway stimulation and gene expression mediated by ErbB receptors. J Biol Chem 276(25): 22685–22698.

47. Sweeney C, Carraway KL 3rd (2000) Ligand discrimination by ErbB receptors: differential signaling through differential phosphorylation site usage. Oncogene 19(49): 5568–5573.

48. Olayioye MA, Beuvink I, Horsch K, Daly JM, Hynes NE (1999) ErbB receptor-induced activation of stat transcription factors is mediated by Src tyrosine kinases. J Biol Chem 274(24): 17209–17218.

49. Bersell K, Arab S, Haring B, Kuhn B (2009) Neuregulin1/ErbB4 signaling induces cardiomyocyte proliferation and repair of heart injury. Cell 138(2): 257–270.

50. Esparis-Ogando A, Diaz-Rodriguez E, Pandiella A (1999) Signalling-competent truncated forms of ErbB2 in breast cancer cells: differential regulation by protein kinase C and phosphatidylinositol 3-kinase. Biochem J 344 Pt 2: 339–348.

51. Wang SC, Lien HC, Xia W, Chen IF, Lo HW, et al. (2004) Binding at and transactivation of the COX-2 promoter by nuclear tyrosine kinase receptor ErbB-2. Cancer Cell 6(3): 251–261.

52. McConnell BK, Fatkin D, Semsarian C, Jones KA, Georgakopoulos D, et al. (2001) Comparison of two murine models of familial hypertrophic cardiomyopathy. Circ Res 88(4): 383–389.

53. Muthuchamy M, Pieples K, Rethinasamy P, Hoit B, Grupp IL, et al. (1999) Mouse model of a familial hypertrophic cardiomyopathy mutation in alpha-tropomyosin manifests cardiac dysfunction. Circ Res 85(1): 47–56.

54. Prabhakar R, Petrashevskaya N, Schwartz A, Aronow B, Boivin GP, et al. (2003) A mouse model of familial hypertrophic cardiomyopathy caused by a alpha-tropomyosin mutation. Mol Cell Biochem 251(1–2): 33–42.

55. Hershberger RE, Cowan J, Morales A, Siegfried JD (2009) Progress with genetic cardiomyopathies: screening, counseling, and testing in dilated, hypertrophic, and arrhythmogenic right ventricular dysplasia/cardiomyopathy. Circ Heart Fail 2(3): 253–261.

56. Ho CY (2010) Hypertrophic cardiomyopathy. Heart Fail Clin 6(2): 141–159.

57. de Bakker JM, van Rijen HM (2006) Continuous and discontinuous propagation in heart muscle. J Cardiovasc Electrophysiol 17(5): 567–573.

58. Uzzaman M, Honjo H, Takagishi Y, Emdad L, Magee AI, et al. (2000) Remodeling of gap junctional coupling in hypertrophied right ventricles of rats with monocrotaline-induced pulmonary hypertension. Circ Res 86(8): 871–878.

59. Ripplinger CM, Li W, Hadley J, Chen J, Rothenberg F, et al. (2007) Enhanced transmural fiber rotation and connexin 43 heterogeneity are associated with an increased upper limit of vulnerability in a transgenic rabbit model of human hypertrophic cardiomyopathy. Circ Res 101(10): 1049–1057.

60. Wolf CM, Moskowitz IP, Arno S, Branco DM, Semsarian C, et al. (2005) Somatic events modify hypertrophic cardiomyopathy pathology and link hypertrophy to arrhythmia. Proc Natl Acad Sci U S A 102(50): 18123–18128.

61. Fineschi V, Silver MD, Karch SB, Parolini M, Turillazzi E, et al. (2005) Myocardial disarray: an architectural disorganization linked with adrenergic stress? Int J Cardiol 99(2): 277–282.

62. Varnava AM, Elliott PM, Baboonian C, Davison F, Davies MJ, et al. (2001) Hypertrophic cardiomyopathy: histopathological features of sudden death in cardiac troponin T disease. Circulation 104(12): 1380–1384.

63. Gollob MH, Green MS, Tang AS, Gollob T, Karibe A, et al. (2001) Identification of a gene responsible for familial Wolff-Parkinson-White syndrome. N Engl J Med 344(24): 1823–1831.

64. Oliveira SM, Ehtisham J, Redwood CS, Ostman-Smith I, Blair EM, et al. (2003) Mutation analysis of AMP-activated protein kinase subunits in inherited cardiomyopathies: implications for kinase function and disease pathogenesis. J Mol Cell Cardiol 35(10): 1251–1255.

65. Di Mauro S, Tanji K, Hirano M (2007) LAMP-2 deficiency (Danon disease). Acta Myol 26(1): 79–82.

66. Yang Z, Funke BH, Cripe LH, Vick GW 3rd, Mancini-Dinardo D, et al. (2010) LAMP2 microdeletions in patients with Danon disease. Circ Cardiovasc Genet 3(2): 129–137.

67. Forsha D, Li JS, Smith PB, van der Ploeg AT, Kishnani P, et al. (2011) Cardiovascular abnormalities in late-onset Pompe disease and response to enzyme replacement therapy. Genet Med 13(7): 625–631.

68. Efthimiou J, McLelland J, Betteridge DJ (1986) Short PR intervals and tachyarrhythmias in Fabry's disease. Postgrad Med J 62(726): 285–287.

69. Yokoyama A, Yamazoe M, Shibata A (1987) A case of heterozygous Fabry's disease with a short PR interval and giant negative T waves. Br Heart J 57(3): 296–299.

70. Jimenez J, Tardiff JC (2011) Abnormal heart rate regulation in murine hearts with familial hypertrophic cardiomyopathy-related cardiac troponin T mutations. Am J Physiol Heart Circ Physiol 300(2): H627–635.

71. Knollmann BC, Blatt SA, Horton K, de Freitas F, Miller T, et al. (2001) Inotropic stimulation induces cardiac dysfunction in transgenic mice expressing a troponin T (I79N) mutation linked to familial hypertrophic cardiomyopathy. J Biol Chem 276(13): 10039–10048.

72. Ciampi Q, Betocchi S, Lombardi R, Manganelli F, Storto G, et al. (2002) Hemodynamic determinants of exercise-induced abnormal blood pressure response in hypertrophic cardiomyopathy. Journal of the American College of Cardiology 40(2): 278–284.

73. Abraham TP, Jones M, Kazmierczak K, Liang HY, Pinheiro AC, et al. (2009) Diastolic dysfunction in familial hypertrophic cardiomyopathy transgenic model mice. Cardiovasc Res 82(1): 84–92.

74. Georgakopoulos D, Christe ME, Giewat M, Seidman CM, Seidman JG, et al. (1999) The pathogenesis of familial hypertrophic cardiomyopathy: early and evolving effects from an alpha-cardiac myosin heavy chain missense mutation. Nat Med 5(3): 327–330.

7

The Complex Regulation of Tanshinone IIA in Rats with Hypertension-Induced Left Ventricular Hypertrophy

Hui Pang[1]*, Bing Han[1], Tao Yu[1], Zhen Peng[2]

1 Department of Cardiovascular Medicine, Central Hospital of Xuzhou, Xuzhou Clinical School of Xuzhou Medical College, Affiliated Hospital of Southeast University, Xuzhou, Jiangsu, China, **2** Department of Ultrasonography, Central Hospital of Xuzhou, Xuzhou Clinical School of Xuzhou Medical College, Affiliated Hospital of Southeast University, Xuzhou, Jiangsu, China

Abstract

Tanshinone IIA has definite protective effects on various cardiovascular diseases. However, in hypertension-induced left ventricular hypertrophy (H-LVH), the signaling pathways of tanshinone IIA in inhibition of remodeling and cardiac dysfunction remain unclear. Two-kidney, one-clip induced hypertensive rats (n = 32) were randomized to receive tanshinone IIA (5, 10, 15 mg/kg per day) or 5% glucose injection (GS). Sham-operated rats (n = 8) received 5%GS as control. Cardiac function and dimensions were assessed by using an echocardiography system. Histological determination of the fibrosis and apoptosis was performed using hematoxylin eosin, Masson's trichrome and TUNEL staining. Matrix metalloproteinase 2 (MMP2) and tissue inhibitor of matrix metalloproteinases type 2 (TIMP2) protein expressions in rat myocardial tissues were detected by immunohistochemistry. Rat cardiomyocytes were isolated by a Langendorff perfusion method. After 48 h culture, the supernatant and cardiomyocytes were collected to determine the potential related proteins impact on cardiac fibrosis and apoptosis. Compared with the sham rats, the heart tissues of H-LVH (5%GS) group suffered severely from the oxidative damage, apoptosis of cardiomyocytes and extracellular matrix (ECM) deposition. In the H-LVH group, tanshinone IIA treated decreased malondialdehyde (MDA) content and increased superoxide dismutase (SOD) activity. Tanshinone IIA inhibited cardiomyocytes apoptosis as confirmed by the reduction of TUNEL positive cardiomyocytes and the down-regulation of Caspase-3 activity and Bax/Bcl-2 ratio. Meanwhile, plasma apelin level increased with down-regulation of APJ receptor. Tanshinone IIA suppressed cardiac fibrosis through regulating the paracrine factors released by cardiomyocytes and the TGF-β/Smads signaling pathway activity. In conclusion, our *in vivo* study showed that tanshinone IIA could improve heart function by enhancing myocardial contractility, inhibiting ECM deposition, and limiting apoptosis of cardiomyocytes and oxidative damage.

Editor: Alessandra Rossini, University of Milano, Italy

Funding: This research was supported by the Xuzhou Municipal Bureau of Science and Technology (No. XZZD1020) and Xuzhou Municipal Health Bureau (No. XWJ2011030). The funders had no role in study design, data collection and analysis, decision to publish, or preparation of the manuscript.

Competing Interests: The authors have declared that no competing interests exist.

* E-mail: phui81@126.com

Introduction

Hypertension is a progressive vascular syndrome characterized by continuous increase in arterial blood pressure. It is one of the major risk factors for cardiovascular diseases, and is always complicated with multiple risk factors, impairments in target organs or clinical diseases [1]. In response to the elevated pressure load, the left ventricular (LV) wall thickens as a compensatory mechanism to minimize wall stress. The mechanisms responsible for different grades of severity of left ventricular hypertrophy (LVH) involve not only the pressure load itself, whether it be the severity, duration, or rate of increase of the blood pressure, but also the influences of neurohormones [2], growth factors, cytokines [3] and genetic factors. There is widespread agreement that LVH is defined as an increase in LV mass attributable to wall thickening or chamber dilation [4]. Pathologic features of LVH include an increase in cardiomyocyte size, LV hypertrophy and cardiac fibrosis, which is marked by changes in the quality and quantity of the extracellular matrix (ECM) [5,6]. LVH one of the most important risk factors results in a worse cardiovascular prognosis. Thus, we suggest that additional clinical benefit from the inhibition of LVH as a potential therapeutic target is as important as the blood pressure control.

Danshen is a crude herbal drug extracted from the dry root and rhizome of Salvia miltiorrhiza Bge (Labiatae) [7]. Tanshinone IIA is one of the main components isolated from Danshen for the treatment of cardiovascular diseases including hypertension [8], cardiac hypertrophy [9], heart failure [10], and myocardial ischemia-reperfusion injury [11]. It can improve heart function [12] by limiting oxidative stress [13], attenuating cardiac fibrosis [14], and inhibiting the hypertrophy and apoptosis of cardiomyocytes. Tanshinone IIA, an ideal cardio-protective agent, can regulate numerous molecular targets including transcription factors, scavenger receptors, ion channels, kinases, pro- and anti-apoptotic proteins, growth factors, inflammatory mediators, microRNA, and others [15]. However, in hypertension-induced hypertrophy, the signaling pathways of tanshinone IIA in inhibition of remodeling and cardiac dysfunction are not fully understood. Our in vivo study was to determine the protective molecular mechanisms from three major respects, reducing apoptosis, inhibiting cardiac fibrosis and decreasing oxidative stress. The molecular mechanisms in apoptosis involve initiator cysteinyl-aspartate proteases (caspases) activation, apoptotic body formation, and cell fragmentation [16]. Some of the paracrine factors released by cardiomyocytes may influence ECM regulation through multiple synergistic paracrine mechanisms [17]. Therefore, we explored the roles of transforming growth factor β1 (TGF-β1) [18] and basic fibroblast growth factor (bFGF) as possible paracrine molecular regulators of this remodeling response.

Materials and Methods

Animals and Reagents

The experimental protocol was approved by the Animal Care and Use Committee of Xuzhou Medical College. Rats were housed in a climate-controlled room. Sterile water and standard chow diet were available ad libitum. Six-week-old male Sprague-Dawley (SD) rats were provided by the Animal Department, Xuzhou Medical College. All of the antibodies, including anti-forkhead box H1 (Foxh1) antibody, anti-c-Myc antibody, anti-p-Smad3 antibody, anti-matrix metalloproteinase 2 (MMP2) antibody, anti-tissue inhibitor of matrix metalloproteinases type 2 (TIMP2) antibody, anti-Bax antibody, anti-Bcl-2 antibody, anti-Caspase-3 antibody and anti-APJ antibody, were purchased from Santa Cruz Biotechnology (Santa Cruz, CA, USA). All other reagent-grade chemicals were purchased from the Sigma- Aldrich Chemical Co. (St. Louis, MO, USA).

Experimental Designs

Male SD rats (200~220 g) were subjected to hypertension as described previously [19]. Briefly, a U-shaped silver clip having internal diameter of 0.2 mm was placed around the left renal artery after the rats under 10% chloral hydrate anesthesia. Sham-operated rats underwent a similar procedure without clip of the left renal artery. We performed our analysis on systolic blood pressure (SBP) in unanesthetized rats via noninvasive tail cuff. Four weeks after clipping, if SBP was higher than 160 mmHg, the animals were considered hypertensive. Then the hypertensive rats (n = 32) were randomized to receive tanshinone IIA (5, 10, 15 mg/ kg per day) or 5% glucose injection (GS) in a dose matched design. Blood pressure was observed at two weeks intervals following tanshinone IIA therapy. Sham-operated rats (n = 8) received 5% GS as control. Eight weeks later, the animals' plasma was extracted and heart was removed for use.

Determination of Cardiac Function

Cardiac function and dimensions were assessed by using an echocardiography system (GE Healthcare Ultrasound, Horten, Norway; 11.5 MHz linear transducer). All measurements were made with the animals under full anesthesia and the body temperature maintained at 36–37°C with the ST-1 homeothermic blanket system. The echocardiography parameters measured were: the left ventricular internal dimension at end diastole (LVIDd), interventricular septal thickness at end diastole (IVSd), left ventricular posterior wall thickness at end diastole (LVPWd), LV fractional shortening (FS%) and ejection fraction (EF%). All parameters were measured five times by the same observer in a blinded method, with the final result the average of the five.

Histological Determination of Fibrosis and Apoptosis

Fresh heart ventricles were fixed using 4% paraformaldehyde, dehydrated with alcohol, embedded in paraffin, and cut into 5 mm slices (RM2016, Leica, Wetzlar, Germany). All hearts were embedded in a cross section orientation, and all slices were taken from the cross section at the papillary muscle level of the left ventricles. Three cross sections of each heart were analyzed. From each section, eight areas of hematoxylin eosin and Masson's trichrome stained slices were randomly selected across the wall thickness to assess the relative fibrosis area (expressed as a percentage of total heart area). Each field was taken at 200 magnification (IX71, Olympus, Tokyo, Japan) and then analyzed using the Adobe ImageReady 7.0.1 software (Adobe Systems, San Jose, CA).

Apoptosis assays were carried out using the terminal deoxynu-cleotidyl transferase dUTP nick- end labeling (TUNEL) kit (ZSGB-BIO, Beijing, China) and the protocol recommended by the manufacturer. The TUNEL index (%) was calculated as the ratio of the number of TUNEL- positive cells divided by the total number of cells. At least eight representative fields were evaluated for each experimental group, from which an average value was calculated.

Immunohistochemistry

Nonspecific binding was blocked with 5% normal goat serum. Then the slices were incubated overnight with anti - MMP2 antibody and anti - TIMP2 antibody. Staining was visualized with the streptavidin - perosidase reaction using diaminobenzidine

Table 1. General characteristics and cardiac function and remodeling.

Parameter	Sham (n = 8)	H-LVH 5%GS (n = 8)	Tan (5) (n = 8)	Tan (10) (n = 8)	Tan (15) (n = 8)
HR (bpm)	386.4±40.8	410.7±42.5	403.9±38.9	421.5±35.1	411.0±43.6
LV Mass/BW (mg/g)	2.15±0.24	2.93±0.31#	2.84±0.25	2.69±0.27	2.36±0.34*
mSP (mmHg)	105.2±2.7	215.2±4.2#	207.5±3.8	212.8±4.5	216.6±4.1
IVSd (mm)	2.1±0.06	2.8±0.04#	2.7±0.04	2.5±0.05	2.3±0.06*
FS (%)	36.9±2.0	37.7±2.8	37.1±2.4	38.9±2.5	40.0±3.4
LVIDd (mm)	7.1±0.5	6.8±0.4	7.0±0.6	7.3±0.4	7.1±0.6
LVPWd (mm)	1.7±0.04	2.7±0.06#	2.5±0.06	2.1±0.05*	2.0±0.04*
EF (%)	74.7±4.2	72.8±4.5	74.5±5.1	78.0±3.7	77.9±3.9

#P<0.05 compared with sham group.
*P<0.05 compared with 5%GS group.

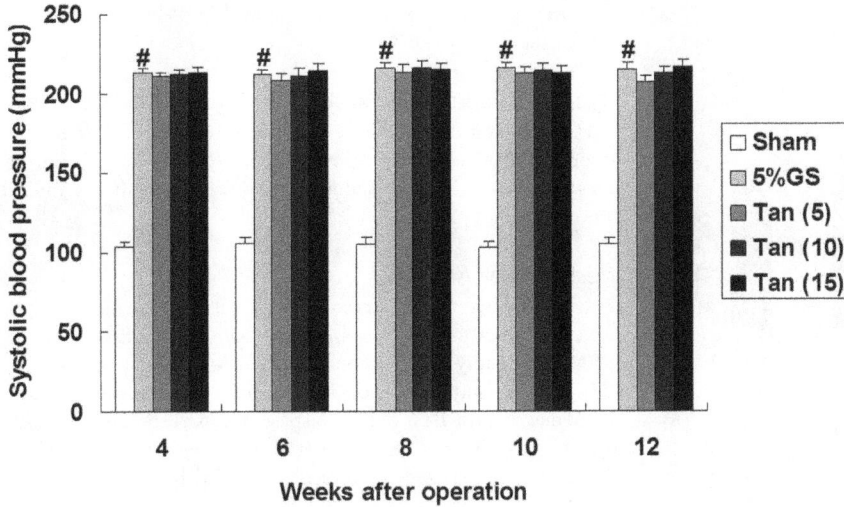

Figure 1. Systolic blood pressure in sham-operated rats (Sham) and hypertension-induced left ventricular hypertrophy (H-LVH) rats treated with 5% glucose injection (GS) or tanshinone IIA (Tan) was observed via noninvasive tail cuff (N = 8 per group). Four weeks after clipping, blood pressure was observed at two weeks intervals for eight weeks. #P<0.05 compared with sham group.

(Boster Bio - engineering Limited Company, Wuhan, China) and the images were analyzed by staining densitometry using Adobe ImageReady 7.0.1 software (Adobe Systems, San Jose, CA).

Plasma Concentration of Apelin

Apelin concentration was determined using the apelin-12 ELISA assay kit (Phoenix Pharmaceuticals INC, Belmont, CA, USA), following the manufacturer's instructions. The antibody

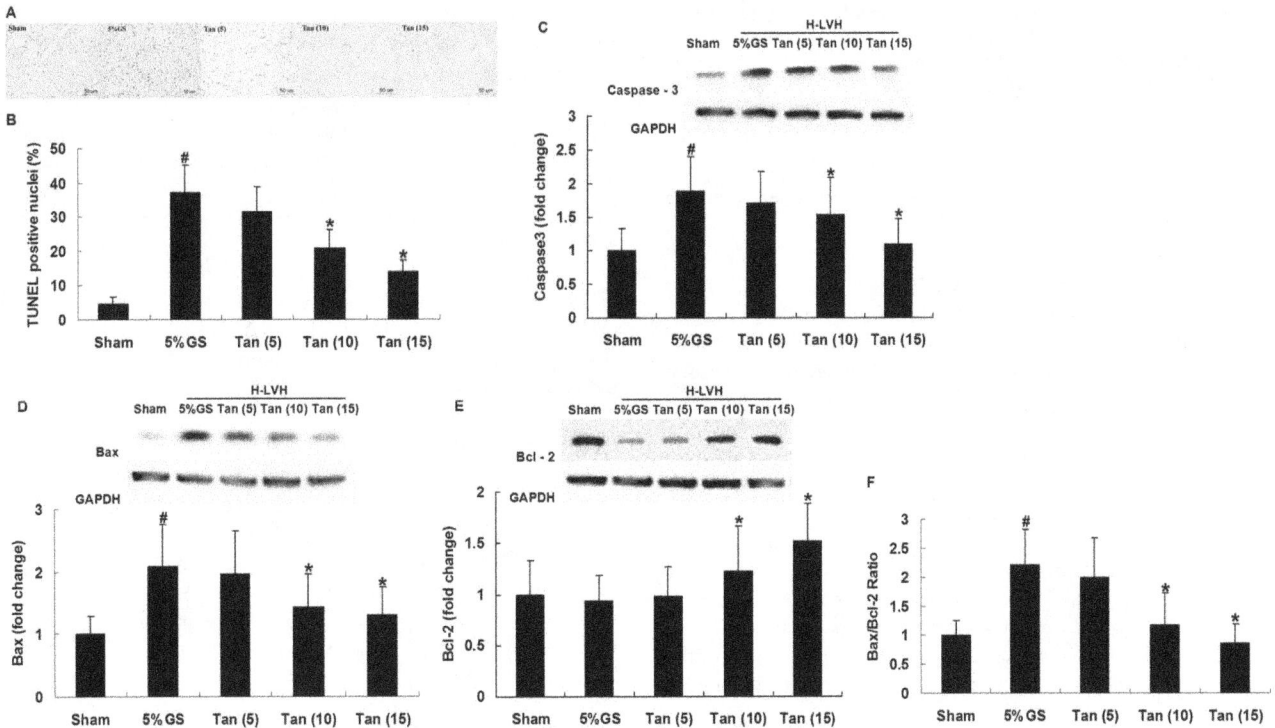

Figure 2. Effects of Tanshinone IIA on cardiomyocyte apoptosis. (A) Representative photographs of TUNEL-stained heart sections from different groups at 12 weeks after operation (N = 8 per group). Apoptotic nuclei were identified by TUNEL staining (buffy) and normal nuclei by hematoxylin staining (blue). (B) The percentage of TUNEL-positive nuclei was calculated. For each sample, eight randomly selected areas of TUNEL-stained slices were counted. (C) Caspase-3, (D) Bax, (E) Bcl-2 protein expression and (F) Bax/Bcl-2 ratio in isolated left ventricular cardiomyocytes of sham-operated rats (Sham) and hypertension-induced left ventricular hypertrophy (H-LVH) rats treated with 5% glucose injection (GS) or tanshinone IIA (Tan) was observed by western blot (N = 8 per group). #P<0.05 compared with sham group. *P<0.05 compared with 5%GS group.

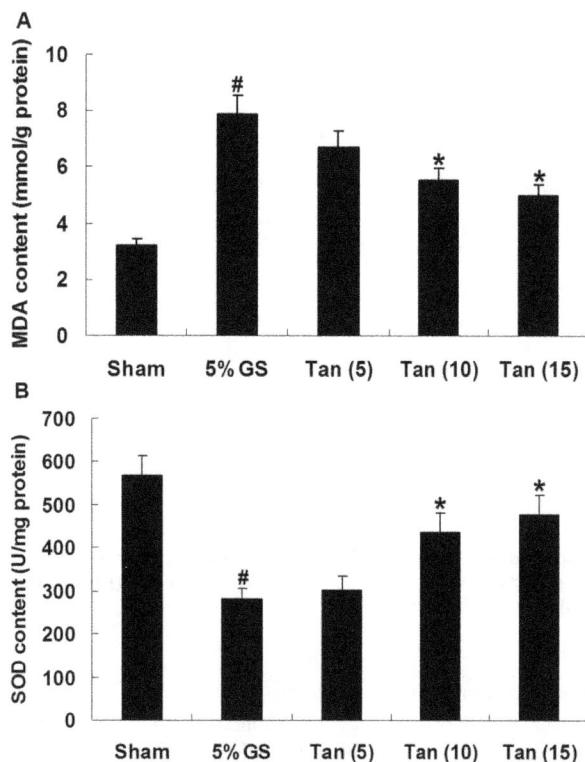

Figure 3. Cardiomyocytes content of malondialdehyde (MDA) and superoxide dismutase (SOD) in sham-operated rats (Sham) and hypertension-induced left ventricular hypertrophy (H-LVH) rats treated with 5% glucose injection (GS) or tanshinone IIA (Tan) was observed (N = 8 per group). (A) MDA contents in rats cultured cardiomyocytes; (B) SOD activities in rats cultured cardiomyocytes. #P<0.05 compared with sham group. *P<0.05 compared with 5%GS group.

used in this apelin assay cross-reactivity 100% with rat apelin-13 and apelin-36.

Cardiomyocyte Isolation and Culture

A Langendorff perfusion method according to the criteria adapted as previously described [20]. The heart was rapidly cannulated via the aorta attached to a Langendorff perfusion apparatus and perfused with Krebs Henseleit (KH) buffer containing 1 mM Ca^{2+} for 5 minutes in a retrograde manner. Then a low-Ca^{2+} solution was changed to perfuse 5 minutes followed by 1 mg/ml collagenase buffer for 10 minutes. The temperature remained 37°C unchanged throughout the perfusion. The heart ventricles were cut into small sections and incubated with collagenase buffer in a thermostat water bath tank for 3 minutes at 35°C. The cardiomyocytes were collected by centrifuging with 400 rpm at room temperature for 1 minute and then cultured as previously described [21]. After 48 hours culture, the supernatant and cardiomyocytes were collected by centrifuging for use.

Assessment of Oxidative Stress

The activity of malondialdehyde (MDA) and superoxide dismutase (SOD) in cultured cardiomyocytes was measured by use of the commercial kit (Jian-Cheng Biochemical Engineering, Nanjing, China). The absorbance was detected at 532 nm and 550 nm with use of a spectrophotometer (UV-2450, Shimadzu, Kyoto, Japan) separately.

Myocyte Supernatant Markers of Cardiac Fibrosis

TGF-β1 and bFGF were measured with ELISA kits used according to manufacturer's instructions (R&D systems, Minneapolis, Minnesota, USA). Values were normalized to a standard curve.

Western Blot Analysis

The proteins were extracted from cultured cardiomyocytes, using the Micro BCA Protein Assay Kit (Pierce, Rockford, IL, USA) to quantify protein concentrations as previously described [22]. Protein was then used for Western blotting with primary antibodies against Bax, Bcl-2, Caspase-3, Foxh1, c-Myc, p-Smad3 and APJ. All images were captured and analyzed by the Gene Genius system (Syngene, Cambridge, United Kingdom).

Statistical Analysis

All the data were presented as mean ± standard deviation. SPSS 13.0 Software was used for the data analysis. Student's t-test was applied for the statistical significance between the sham and H-LVH (5%GS) group. A repeated measure ANOVA with Bonferroni's post test was used for comparison among four groups of H-LVH rats. P<0.05 demonstrated statistical difference.

Results

General Characteristics and Echocardiography Parameters

Twelve weeks after operation, remarkable increase was noted in LV Mass, LV Mass/BW, mSP, IVSd and LVPWd in the H-LVH (5%GS) group compared with those in the sham group (P<0.05). For the above parameters except mSP, significant decrease was observed after treatment of tanshinone IIA in H-LVH rats than those of the 5%GS group (P<0.05, Table 1). Blood pressure was observed at two weeks intervals following tanshinone IIA therapy. But tanshinone IIA had no significant effect on pressure compared with control group (P>0.05, Fig. 1). At last, we selected the pressure before the animals sacrificed to illuminate that the inhibition of tanshinone IIA on myocardial hypertrophy was blood pressure independent. HR, FS (%), LVIDd and EF (%) in both sham and H-LVH rats were not significantly different throughout the entire experiment.

Effects of Tanshinone IIA on Cardiomyocyte Apoptosis

The percentage of TUNEL-positive cells of left ventricular tissues in the H-LVH (5%GS) group was significantly increased compared with the sham group (P<0.05). However, the percentage of TUNEL-positive cells was significantly reduced after treatment of tanshinone IIA (P<0.05, Fig. 2A and B).

H-LVH induced cultured left ventricular cardiomyocytes protein expressions of Caspase-3 and Bax and Bax/Bcl-2 ratio significantly increased compared with control (P<0.05). Bcl-2 protein expression was slightly decreased, but did not reach statistical significance (P>0.05). After treatment of tanshinone IIA for eight weeks, we found protein expressions of Caspase-3 and Bax and Bax/Bcl-2 ratio were all reduced (P<0.05). Only Bcl-2 protein expression was enhanced compared with the 5%GS group (P<0.05, Fig. 2C–F).

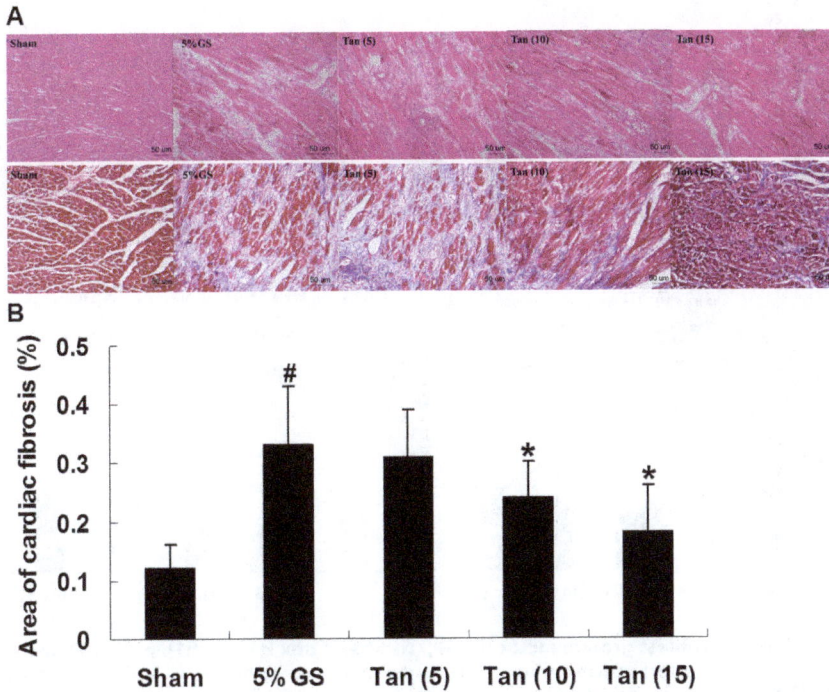

Figure 4. Collagen content was observed in rat left ventricular tissues of sham-operated rats (Sham) and hypertension-induced left ventricular hypertrophy (H-LVH) rats treated with 5% glucose injection (GS) or tanshinone IIA (Tan). (A) Upper panels were stained with hematoxylin eosin. Lower panels were stained with Masson's trichrome. They were all taken at 200×magnification; (B) Quantitative analysis of blue stained area to the total area was used to assess the cardiac fibrosis (N=8 per group). #P<0.05 compared with sham group. *P<0.05 compared with 5%GS group.

Effects of Tanshinone IIA on Oxidative Stress

H-LVH increased MDA content and reduced SOD content in rat cultured cardiomyocytes (P<0.05). MDA levels were significantly lower in the tanshinone IIA-treated group than in the 5%GS group (P<0.05). Furthermore, tanshinone IIA treated ameliorated the inhibited SOD activity induced by H-LVH (P< 0.05, Fig. 3).

Effects of Tanshinone IIA on Cardiac Fibrosis

In the left ventricle, an increase in the interstitial myocardial collagen content was observed in the H-LVH (5%GS) group as compared with sham groups (P<0.05). However, tanshinone IIA-treated H-LVH rats exhibited a lower interstitial myocardial collagen content than the 5%GS group (P<0.05, Fig. 4).

Immunohistochemical assay showed that compared with the sham group, left ventricular tissues MMP2 and TIMP2 protein expressions of the H-LVH (5%GS) group significantly rose (P< 0.05). However, tanshinone IIA reduced MMP2 protein expression and increased TIMP2 protein expression in the H-LVH left ventricular tissues (P<0.05, Fig. 5A–D). MMP2/TIMP2 ratio was higher in the H-LVH (5%GS) group than that detected in the sham group (P<0.05). Interestingly, MMP2/TIMP2 ratio was reduced in tanshinone IIA-treated H-LVH rats compared to 5%GS rats (P<0.05, Fig. 5E).

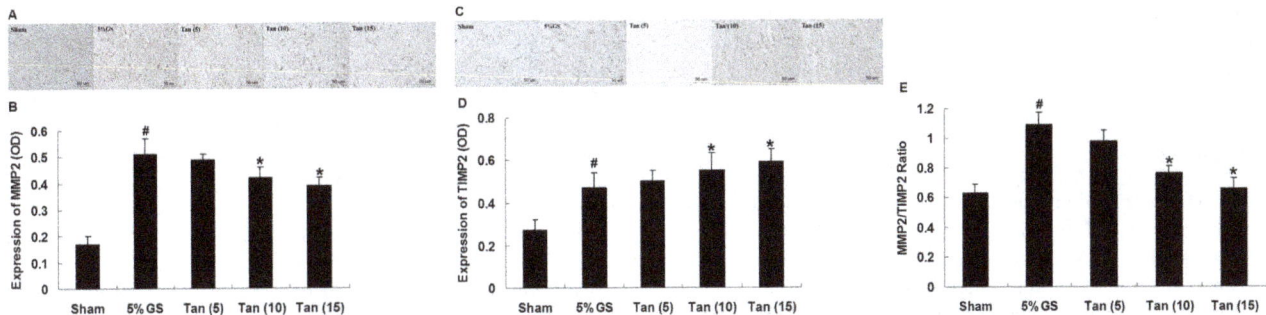

Figure 5. Matrix metalloproteinase 2 (MMP2, A and B), tissue inhibitor of matrix metalloproteinases type 2 (TIMP2, C and D) protein expression and MMP2/TIMP2 ratio (E) in rat left ventricular tissues of sham-operated rats (Sham) and hypertension-induced left ventricular hypertrophy (H-LVH) rats treated with 5% glucose injection (GS) or tanshinone IIA (Tan) was detected by immunohistochemistry (N=8 per group). #P<0.05 compared with sham group. *P<0.05 compared with 5%GS group.

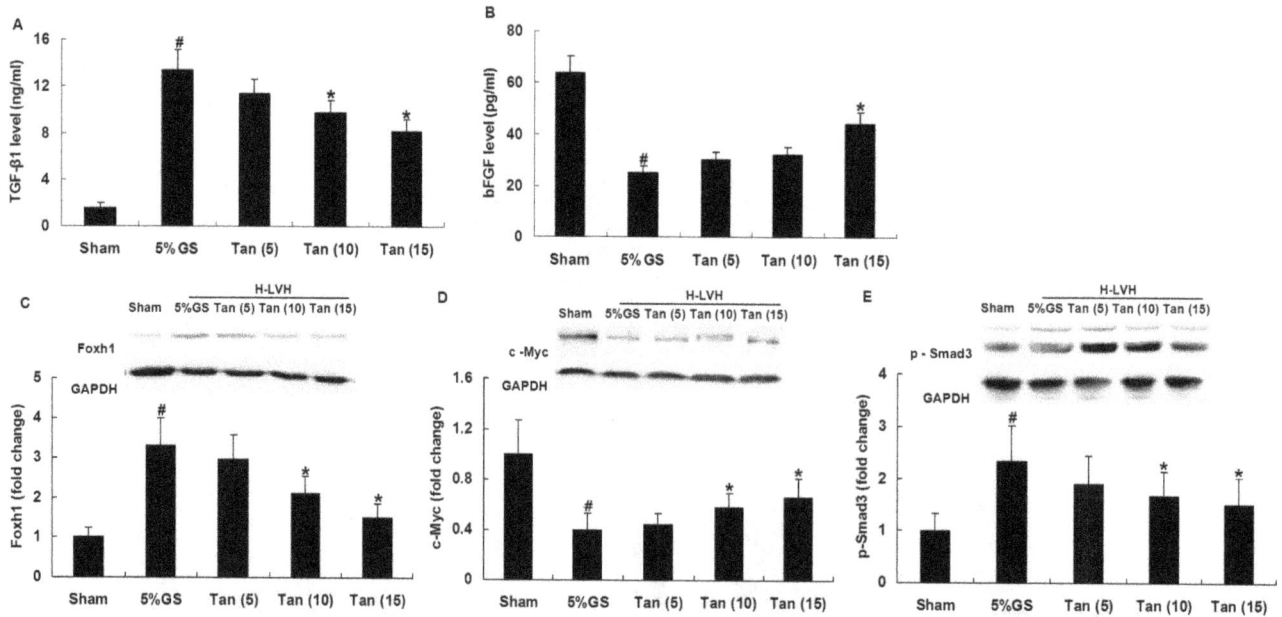

Figure 6. Transforming growth factor β1 (TGF-β1), basic fibroblast growth factor (bFGF), forkhead box H1 (Foxh1), p-Smad3 and c-Myc protein expression in sham-operated rats (Sham) and hypertension-induced left ventricular hypertrophy (H-LVH) rats treated with 5% glucose injection (GS) or tanshinone IIA (Tan) was observed (N = 8 per group). (A) TGF-β1 and (B) bFGF protein expression of the supernatant in rat isolated left ventricular cardiomyocytes after 48 hours culture was detected by ELISA; (C) Foxh1, (D) p-Smad3 and (E) c-Myc protein expression in rat isolated left ventricular cardiomyocytes was detected by western blot. #P<0.05 compared with sham group. *P<0.05 compared with 5%GS group.

In response to pressure overload, increased TGF-β1 protein and decreased bFGF protein were secreted by cardiomyocytes after 48 hours culture to activate cardiac fibrosis in H-LVH (5%GS) rats (P<0.05). After tanshinone IIA treated, TGF-β1 secretion was decreased and bFGF secretion was increased significantly than 5%GS group (P<0.05, Fig. 6A and B). Our data indicated that the levels of Foxh1 and p-Smad3 were significantly increased in cultured left ventricular cardiomyocytes of H-LVH (5%GS) group (P<0.05). Compared with the sham group, c-Myc protein expression of the rats in the H-LVH (5%GS) group was significantly reduced (P<0.05). After tanshinone IIA treated, lower expression of p-Smad3 and Foxh1 and higher expression of c-Myc than that detected in the 5%GS group (P<0.05, Fig. 6C–E).

Effects of Tanshinone IIA on Apelin-APJ System

In H-LVH (5%GS) group, our data showed that plasma apelin level decreased and APJ protein expression increased significantly than the sham group (P<0.05). Tanshinone IIA enhanced plasma apelin level and reduced APJ protein expression in H-LVH rats (P<0.05, Fig. 7).

Discussion

The classic paradigm of hypertensive heart disease is from asymptomatic LVH to clinical heart failure. The transition is associated with ECM remodeling [23] and elevated LV filling pressures [24,25]. The mechanisms include not only pressure overload but also the influences of neurohormones, growth factors, and cytokines consistent with a progressive remodeling process [26,27]. In this study, rat models of experimental hypertension were induced using the two-kidney and one clip method. This model is one the widely-used models for the study of antihypertensive effects of various drugs or medicinal plants. After the

clipping of the left renal artery, this is also a model of renovascular hypertension that has a high activation of the renin-angiotensin-aldosterone system. Angiotensin II (Ang II), the effector peptide of the renin-angiotensin- aldosterone system, is a critical mediator in neurohormonal activation in hypertension [14]. It is well known that Ang II induces cardiac myocyte hypertrophy, fibroblast proliferation, collagen formation and stimulates reactive oxygen species (ROS). These variations in the multi-factorial aetiology are involved in cardiac remodeling during the development of hypertension. Previous studies, performed in vivo and in vitro, prove that tanshinone II A can prevent Ang II - induced cardiac remodeling process by several molecular biological mechanisms, such as depressing cardiac fibroblast proliferation, inhibiting angiotensin I type 1 receptor (AT1R) gene expression [28], ameliorating cardiomyocytes hypertrophy [29] and apoptosis [30]. Moreover, tanshinone II A can also down-regulate genes related to aldosterone synthesis CYP11B1 and CYP11B2 mRNA expression and inhibit aldosterone synthesis in hypertensive left ventricular hypertrophy rats [31]. Therefore, we hypothesized that tanshinone II A could ameliorate the cardiac remodeling due to its direct or indirect effects on the AngII system. The primary goal of our study was to identify the complex regulation of tanshinone IIA in rats with hypertension-induced left ventricular hypertrophy, including myocardial contractility, ECM deposition, apoptosis of cardiomyocytes and oxidative damage. The secondary goal was to investigate the paracrine factors released by cardiomyocytes to explain the cause of cardiac fibrosis from the cellular level. The cardiomyocytes of adult hypertensive rats were isolated using a Langendorff perfusion method. Because the TGF-β1 alone could not take an effect on cardiac fibrosis. Subsequently, we explored the expressions of downstream TGF-β1 pathway components.

Four weeks after clipping, if SBP was higher than 160 mmHg, the animals were considered hypertensive. Then tanshinone IIA was intraperitoneal administrated daily, 5% GS as the control.

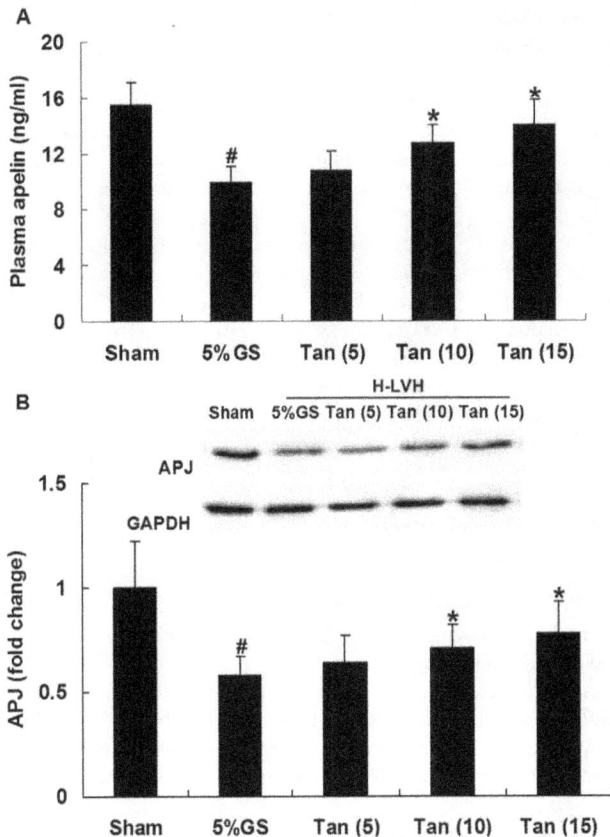

Figure 7. Plasma concentration of apelin and cardiomyocytes protein expression of APJ in sham-operated rats (Sham) and hypertension-induced left ventricular hypertrophy (H-LVH) rats treated with 5% glucose injection (GS) or tanshinone IIA (Tan) was observed (N = 8 per group). (A) Plasma concentration of apelin was detected by ELISA; (B) APJ protein expression in rat isolated left ventricular cardiomyocytes was detected by western blot. #P<0.05 compared with sham group. *P<0.05 compared with 5%GS group.

Blood pressure was observed at two weeks intervals following tanshinone IIA therapy. Eight weeks later, cardiac function and dimensions were assessed by using an echocardiography system. In this study, twelve weeks after operation, remarkable increase was noted in LV Mass, LV Mass/BW, mSP, IVSd and LVPWd in the H-LVH (5%GS) group compared with those in the sham group. For the above parameters except mSP, significant decrease was observed after treatment of tanshinone IIA in H-LVH rats than those of the 5%GS group. These changes of cardiac structure and function were associated with myocardial hypertrophy inhibition effect of tanshinone IIA with blood pressure independent.

Apoptosis, or programmed cell death, playd an important role in myocardial stress, including ventricular remodeling [32]. Thus, interfering with the cardiomyocytes apoptosis was considered as a key therapy target of myocardial injury [33]. Numerous signaling pathways were implicated in mediating the process of hypertrophy-induced apoptosis, such as Bcl-2 family proteins [34] and caspases. The Bcl-2 family proteins consist of pro- and anti-apoptotic members. The balance between Bax (pro-apoptotic) and Bcl-2 (anti-apoptotic) plays an important role in determination the possibility of cells to either survive or undergo apoptosis after a certain stimulus or injury [35]. Our in vivo study showed that tanshinone IIA could inhibit cardiomyocytes apoptosis as confirmed by the reduction of TUNEL positive cardiomyocytes.

Activated intrinsic signal pathways might directly trigger cardiomyocytes apoptosis in H-LVH, including the up-regulation of caspase-3 activity and ratio of Bax/Bcl-2. But tanshinone IIA modified the apoptosis signal pathway in H-LVH which down-regulated the caspase-3 activity and ratio of Bax/Bcl-2. Furthermore, our study confirmed that tanshinone IIA had protective effect on cardiomyocytes through limitation oxidative stress to change the redox state.

Oxidative stress is defined as an imbalance between ROS production and removal of excess ROS [36]. The changed redox state causes contractile dysfunction and structural damage in the myocardium, leading to apoptosis at the subcellular level [37]. Oxidative stress interaction with apoptosis represents an integral part in the pathophysiology of myocardial damage. Our study revealed that tanshinone IIA decreased MDA content and increased SOD activity in cardiomyocytes of the H-LVH group. Thus, both the activation of oxidative stress and the impaired antioxidant capacity were responsible for myocardial damage together.

Apelin peptide, its C-terminal fragments could bind with high affinity to apelin receptor (APJ) and exert biological activities [38]. The orphan seven transmembrane receptor APJ, composed of 380 amino acids, is a class A G-protein-coupled receptor (GPCR) [39]. In H-LVH (5%GS) group, our data showed that plasma apelin level decreased and APJ protein expression increased significantly than the sham group. Tanshinone IIA enhanced plasma apelin level and reduced APJ protein expression in H-LVH rats. Receptor level can vary in response to different concentration of the agonist and is sorted between recycling and degradative pathways. Thus, we suggested that tanshinone IIA was capable of reducing APJ protein expression in H-LVH rats via a direct action and an indirect action on the plasma apelin level. After activated by apelin, APJ receptor had definite protective effects on relaxing blood vessels [40], enhancing myocardial contractility and inhibiting the hypertrophy [41].

The dynamic balance between degradation and accumulation of ECM proteins is a physiological process that takes place in heart normally [42]. ECM in H-LVH has a profound effect on the formation of fibrotic lesions by altering its abundance, composition, and spatial organization [43]. Myocardial fibrosis is a common cause of LV remodeling, which leads to diastolic dysfunction and dilated cardiac failure. MMPs are proteolytic enzymes, whereas their activity is regulated by TIMPs as their endogenous inhibitors. Thus, the balance of MMPs/TIMPs expression is emerging as critical regulator of myocardial remodeling [44,45]. MMP2 is a gelatinase and a collagenase [46], however, the function of TIMP2 is to inhibit a number of MMPs except MMP9 [47,48]. Fang et al. reported that tanshinone IIA treated improved cardiac function and prevented cardiac fibrosis by regulation the MMPs/TIMPs balance in a rat model of two-kidney two-clip hypertension [49]. Our study found that compared with the sham group, left ventricular tissues MMP2 and TIMP2 protein expressions of the H-LVH (5%GS) group significantly rose. However, tanshinone IIA reduced MMP2 protein expression and increased TIMP2 protein expression in the H-LVH left ventricular tissues. MMP2/TIMP2 ratio was higher in the H-LVH (5%GS) group than that detected in the sham group. Interestingly, MMP2/TIMP2 ratio was reduced in tanshinone IIA-treated H-LVH rats compared to 5%GS rats. But our echocardiographic data indicated that the cardiac function of sham and H-LVH rats was not significantly different throughout the experimental period. Thus, our data suggested that tanshinone IIA played an important role on inhibiting ECM deposition and improving cardiac remodeling.

Profibrotic cytokine TGF-β has been reported to play a central role in regulating the composition of the ECM in many tissues [18]. In the cardiovascular system, TGF-β1 has been implicated in the development of heart hypertrophy and heart failure, associated with increasing in both cardiomyocyte growth and intercellular fibrosis [50]. bFGF induces endothelial and smooth muscle cell migration and proliferation [51], and linkage to the development of heart hypertrophy [52]. To further assess the influence of ECM-dependent paracrine mechanisms, we determinated the supernatant levels of TGF-β1 and bFGF 48 hours after cardiomyocytes cultured. As performed in this study, in response to pressure overload, increased TGF-β1 protein and decreased bFGF protein were secreted by cardiomyocytes to activate cardiac fibrosis in H-LVH rats. But after tanshinone IIA treated, TGF-β1 secretion was decreased and bFGF secretion was increased significantly than 5%GS group. bFGF is capable of suppressing TGF-β1-induced fibroblast differentiation [53] and limiting progressive fibrosis [54]. TGF-β1, after binding to its receptors, activated downstream mediators that leaded to classic Smads signaling pathways. Afterwards, phosphorylated complex of Smad 2/3 formed a higher-order complex with Smad4 which was subsequently transported into the nucleus. Smad-partner combination targeted a particular subset of genes and recruited transcriptional co-repressor c-Myc, by association with Foxh1 participated as a Smads cofactor which made Smads reach target gene specificity and target specificity [55]. Other investigations have suggested that tanshinone IIA could inhibit myocardial hypertrophy in LVH rats. The underlying mechanism might be the down-regulated expression of AT1R mRNA and Smad-3, increased production of Smad-7, and blocking TGF beta1/Smads signal pathway [56]. Our data indicated that the level of p-Smad3, a downstream receptor-regulated Smad (R-Smad) of TGF-β1 signaling, was significantly increased in the hearts of H-LVH rats. Higher expression of Foxh1 and lower expression of c-Myc resulted in higher activity of the transcription of Smads dependent genes. After tanshinone IIA treated, lower expression of p-Smad3 and Foxh1 and higher expression of c-Myc inhibited Smads induced transcriptional activation. Thus, we suggested that tanshinone IIA might provide additional beneficial effects on suppressing structural remodeling through regulating the paracrine factors released by cardiomyocytes and the TGF-β/Smads signaling pathway activity.

In conclusion, LVH is associated with high risk of clinical events including cardiovascular death, myocardial infarction, and stroke. However, the pathway from hypertension to LVH is not unidirectional. In search of an ideal cardio-protective agent to reduce remodeling and improve LV dilatation and systolic dysfunction, tanshinone IIA emerged as powerful candidate. Our in vivo study showed that tanshinone IIA could improve heart function by enhancing myocardial contractility, inhibiting ECM deposition, and limiting apoptosis of cardiomyocyte and oxidative damage.

Perspectives

This study investigates tanshinone IIA as a definite protective agent for improving cardiac function in hypertension rats. The molecular mechanisms responsible for cardio-protective effects of tanshinone IIA mainly contained four balance systems, MDA/SOD, Bax/Bcl-2, MMP 2/TIMP 2 and TGF-β 1/bFGF, which may be new specific biological targets for the treatment and control of progressive cardiac dysfunction.

Author Contributions

Conceived and designed the experiments: HP. Performed the experiments: ZP. Analyzed the data: TY. Contributed reagents/materials/analysis tools: BH. Wrote the paper: HP.

References

1. Wei-Chuan Tsai (2011) Treatment options for hypertension in high-risk patients. Vascular Health and Risk Management 7: 137–141. doi: 10.2147/VHRM.S11235. PubMed: 21468174.
2. Hill JA, Olson EN (2008) Cardiac plasticity. N Engl J Med 358: 1370–1380. doi: 10.1056/NEJMra072139. PubMed: 18367740.
3. Díez J, Frohlich ED (2010) A translational approach to hypertensive heart disease. Hypertension 55:1–8. doi:10.1161/HYPERTENSIONAHA.109.141887. PubMed: 19933923.
4. Khouri MG, Peshock RM, Ayers CR, de Lemos JA, Drazner MH (2010) 4-Tiered Classification of Left Ventricular Hypertrophy Based on Left Ventricular Geometry The Dallas Heart Study. Circ Cardiovasc Imaging 3: 164–171. doi: 10.1161/CIRCIMAGING.109. 883652. PubMed: 20061518.
5. Berk BC, Fujiwara K, Lehoux S (2007) ECM remodeling in hypertensive heart disease. J Clin Invest 117: 568–575. doi: 10.1172/JCI31044. PubMed: 17332884.
6. Spinale FG (2007) Myocardial matrix remodeling and the matrix metalloproteinases: influence on cardiac form and function. Physiol Rev 87: 1285–1342. doi: 10.1152/physrev.00012.2007. PubMed: 17928585.
7. Si Gao, Zhiping Liu, Hong Li, Peter J Little, Peiqing Liu et al. (2012) Cardiovascular actions and therapeutic potential of tanshinone IIA. Atherosclerosis 220: 3–10. doi: 10.1016/j.atherosclerosis.2011.06.041. PubMed: 21774934.
8. Wang P, Wu X, Bao Y, Fang J, Zhou S et al. (2011) Tanshinone IIA prevents cardiac remodeling through attenuating NAD (P) H oxidase-derived reactive oxygen species production in hypertensive rats. Pharmazie 66: 517–524. PubMed: 21812327.
9. Tan X, Li J, Wang X, Chen N, Cai B et al. (2011) Tanshinone IIA Protects Against Cardiac Hypertrophy via Inhibiting Cal-cineurin/Nfatc3 Pathway. Int J Biol Sci 7: 383–389. PubMed: 21494433.
10. Feng J, Li SS, Liang QS (2012) Effects of Tanshinone II A on the myocardial apoptosis and the miR-133 levels in rats with heart failure. Zhongguo Zhong Xi Yi Jie He Za Zhi 32: 930–933. PubMed: 23019950.
11. Qiao Z, Ma J, Liu H (2011) Evaluation of the antioxidant potential of Salvia miltiorrhiza ethanol extract in a rat model of ischemia-reperfusion injury. Molecules 16: 10002–10012. doi: 10.3390/molecules161210002. PubMed: 22138858.
12. Zhang Y, Zhang L, Chu W, Wang B, Zhang J et al. (2010) Tanshinone IIA Inhibits miR-1 Expression through p38 MAPK Signal Pathway in Post-infarction Rat Cardiomyocytes. Cell Physiol Biochem 26: 991–998. doi: 10.1159/000324012. PubMed: 21220930.
13. Yang P, Jia YH, Li J, Li LJ, Zhou FH (2010) Study of anti-myocardial cell oxidative stress action and effect of tanshinone IIA on prohibitin expression. J Tradit Chin Med 30: 259–264. PubMed: 21287782.
14. Chan P, Liu JC, Lin LJ, Chen PY, Cheng TH et al. (2011) Tanshinone IIA Inhibits Angiotensin II-Induced Cell Proliferation in Rat Cardiac Fibroblasts. Am J Chin Med 39: 381–394. doi: 10.1142/S0192415X11008890. PubMed: 21476213.
15. Xu S, Liu P (2013) Tanshinone IIA: new perspectives for old remedies. Expert Opin Ther Pat 23: 149–153. doi: 10.1517/13543776.2013.743995. PubMed: 23231009.
16. Crow MT, Mani K, Mani K, Mani K, Kitsis RN (2004) The mitochondrial death pathway and cardiac myocyte apoptosis. Circ Res 95: 957–970. doi: 10.1161/01.RES.0000148632. 35500.d9. PubMed: 15539639.
17. Fedak PW (2008) Paracrine effects of cell transplantation: modifying ventricular remodeling in the failing heart. Semin Thorac Cardiovasc Surg 20: 87–93. doi: 10.1053/j.semtcvs.2008. 04.001. PubMed: 18707639.
18. Dobaczewski M, Chen W, Frangogiannis NG (2011) Transforming growth factor (TGF)-beta signaling in cardiac remodeling. J Mol Cell Cardiol 51: 600–606. doi: 10.1016/j. yjmcc.2010.10.033. PubMed: 21059352.
19. Amin Shah, Young-Bin Oh, Sun Hwa Lee, Jung Min Lim, Suhn Hee Kim (2012) Angiotensin- (1–7) attenuates hypertension in exercise-trained renal hypertensive rats. Am J Physiol Heart Circ Physiol 302: H2372–H2380. doi: 10.1152/ajpheart.00846.2011. PubMed: 22467306.
20. Lewis CJ, Gong H, Brown MJ, Harding SE (2004) Overexpression of beta 1-adrenoceptors in adult rat ventricular myocytes enhances CGP 12177A cardiostimulation: implications for 'putative' beta 4-adrenoceptor pharmacology. Br J Pharmacol 141: 813–824. doi: 10.1038/sj. bjp.0705668. PubMed: 14757703.
21. Davia K, Hajjar RJ, Terracciano CM, Kent NS, Ranu HK et al. (1999) Functional alterations in adulate rat myocytes after overexpression of phospholamban using adenovirus. Physiol Genomics 1: 41–50. PubMed: 11015560.

22. Xiang Jun Zeng, Li Ke Zhang, Hong Xia Wang, Ling Qiao Lu, Li Quan Ma et al. (2009) Apelin protects heart against ischemia/reperfusion injury in rat. Peptides 30: 1144–1152. doi: 10.1016/j.peptides.2009.02.010. PubMed: 19463748.

23. Martos R, Baugh J, Ledwidge M, O'Loughlin C, Murphy NF et al. (2009) Diagnosis of heart failure with preserved ejection fraction: improved accuracy with the use of markers of collagen turnover. Eur J Heart Fail 11: 191–197. doi: 10.1093/eurjhf/hfn036. PubMed: 19168518.

24. Zile MR, Bennett TD, St John Sutton M, Cho YK, Adamson PB et al. (2008) Transition from chronic compensated to acute decompensated heart failure: pathophysiological insights obtained from continuous monitoring of intracardiac pressures. Circulation 118: 1433–1441. doi: 10.1161/CIRCULATIO-NAHA.108.783910. PubMed: 18794390.

25. Lam CS, Roger VL, Rodeheffer RJ, Borlaug BA, Enders FT et al. (2009) Pulmonary hypertension in heart failure with preserved ejection fraction: a community-based study. J Am Coll Cardiol 53: 1119–1126. doi: 10.1016/j.jacc.2008.11.051. PubMed: 19324256.

26. Drazner MH (2011) The progression of hypertensive heart disease. Circulation 123: 327–334. doi: 10.1161/CIRCULATIONAHA.108.845792. PubMed: 21263005.

27. Ahmed SH, Clark LL, Pennington WR, Webb CS, Bonnema DD et al. (2006) Matrix metalloproteinases/tissue inhibitors of metalloproteinases: relationship between changes in proteolytic determinants of matrix composition and structural, functional, and clinical manifestations of hypertensive heart disease. Circulation 113: 2089–2096. doi: 10.1161/CIRCULATIONAHA.105.573865. PubMed: 16636176.

28. Li YS, Yan L, Yong YQ (2010) Effect of tanshinone II A on the transforming growth factor beta1/Smads signal pathway in rats with hypertensive myocardial hypertrophy. Zhongguo Zhong Xi Yi Jie He Za Zhi 30: 499–503. PubMed: 20681280.

29. Zhou DX, Liang QS, He XX, Zhan CY (2008) Changes of c-fos, c-jun mRNA expressions in cardiomyocyte hypertrophy induced by angiotensin II and effects of tanshinone II A. Zhongguo Zhong Yao Za Zhi 33: 936–939. PubMed: 18619357.

30. HONG HJ, LIU JC, CHENG TH, CHAN P (2010) Tanshinone IIA attenuates angiotensin II-induced apoptosis via Akt pathway in neonatal rat cardiomyocytes. Acta Pharmacol Sin 31: 1569–1575. doi: 10.1038/aps.2010.176. PubMed: 21102479.

31. Wang ZH,Liang QS,Zheng Z (2009) The Effect of Tanshinone on Myocardial Hypertrophy Induced by High Salt Diet. Acta Med Univ Sci Technol Huazhong 38: 500–503.

32. Santos CX, Anilkumar N, Zhang M, Brewer AC, Shah AM (2011) Redox signaling in cardiac myocytes. Free Radic Biol Med 50: 777–793. doi: 10.1016/j.freeradbiomed. 2011.01. 003. PubMed: 21236334.

33. Sadoshima J (2006) Redox regulation of growth and death in cardiac myocytes. Antioxid Redox Signal 8: 1621–1624. doi:10.1089/ars.2006.8.1621. PubMed: 16987016.

34. Ekhterae D, Hinmon R, Matsuzaki K, Noma M, Zhu W et al. (2011) Infarction induced myocardial apoptosis and ARC activation. J Surgical Res 166: 59–67. doi: 10.1016/j.jss. 2009.05.002. PubMed: 19815236.

35. Whelan RS, Kaplinskiy V, Kitsis RN (2010) Cell death in the pathogenesis of heart disease: Mechanisms and significance. Annu Rev Physiol 72: 19–44. doi: 10.1146/annurev. physiol. 010908.163111. PubMed: 20148665.

36. Brunelle JK, Letai A (2009) Control of mitochondrial apoptosis by the Bcl-2 family. J Cell Sci 122: 437–441. doi: 10.1242/jcs.031682. PubMed: 19193868.

37. Liao YH, Xia N, Zhou SF, Tang TT, Yan XX et al. (2012) Interleukin-17A Contributes to Myocardial Ischemia/Reperfusion Injury by Regulating Cardiomyocyte Apoptosis and Neutrophil Infiltration. J Am Coll Cardiol 59: 420–429. doi: 10.1016/j.jacc.2011.10.863. PubMed: 22261166.

38. Iturrioz X, El Messari S, De Mota N, Fassot C, Alvear-Perez R et al. (2007) Functional dissociation between apelin receptor signaling and endocytosis: implications for the effects of apelin on arterial blood pressure. Archives des maladies du coeur et des vaisseaux 100: 704–708.doi: AMCV-08-2007-100-8-0003-9683-101019-200600023. PubMed: 17928781.

39. Langelaan DN, Reddy T, Banks AW, Dellaire G, Dupre DJ et al. (2013) Structural features of the apelin receptor N-terminal tail and first transmem-brane segment implicated in ligand binding and receptor trafficking. Biochimica et biophysica acta 1828: 1471–1483. doi: 10. 1016/j.bbamem.2013.02.005. PubMed: 23438363.

40. Iturrioz X, Alvear-Perez R, De Mota N, Franchet C, Guillier F et al. (2010) Identification and pharmacological properties of E339-3D6, the first nonpeptidic apelin receptor agonist. Faseb J 24: 1506–1517. doi: 10.1096/fj.09-140715. PubMed: 20040517.

41. Zhang Z, Yu B, Tao GZ (2009) Apelin protects against cardiomyocyte apoptosis induced by glucose deprivation. Chinese medical journal 122: 2360–2365. doi: 10.3760/cma.j.issn.0366-6999.2009.19.031. PubMed: 20079140.

42. Creemers EE, Pinto YM (2011) Molecular mechanisms that control interstitial fibrosis in the pressure-overloaded heart. Cardiovasc Res 89: 265–272. doi: 10.1093/cvr/cvq308. PubMed: 20880837.

43. Gradman AH, Wilson JT (2009) Hypertension and diastolic heart failure. Curr Cardiol Rep 11: 422–429. doi: 10.1007/s11886-009-0061-5. PubMed: 19863866.

44. Heymans S, Schroen B, Vermeersch P, Milting H, Gao F et al. (2005) Increased cardiac expression of tissue inhibitor of metalloproteinase-1 and tissue inhibitor of metalloproteinase-2 is related to cardiac fibrosis and dysfunction in the chronic pressure- overloaded human heart. Circulation 112: 1136–1144. doi: 10.1161/CIRCULATIONAHA. 104.516963. PubMed: 16103240.

45. Dixon JA, Spinale FG (2011) Myocardial remodeling: cellular and extracellular events and targets. Annu Rev Physiol 73: 47–68. doi: 10.1146/annurev-physiol-012110-142230. PubMed: 21314431.

46. Spinale FG, Koval CN, Deschamps AM, Stroud RE, Ikonomidis JS (2008) Dynamic changes in matrix metalloproteinase activity within the human myocardial interstitium during myocardial arrest and reperfusion. Circulation 118: S16–S23. doi: 10.1161/CIRCULATIONAHA.108.786640. PubMed: 18824748.

47. Kandalam V, Basu R, Abraham T, Wang X, Soloway PD et al. (2010) TIMP2 deficiency accelerates adverse postmyocardial infarction remodeling because of enhanced MT1-MMP activity despite lack of MMP2 activation. Circ Res 106: 796–808. doi: 10.1161/CIRCRESAHA.109.209189. PubMed: 20056917.

48. Brew K, Nagase H (2010) The tissue inhibitors of metalloproteinases (TIMPs): an ancient family with structural and functional diversity. Biochim Biophys Acta 1803: 55–71. doi: 10. 1016/j.bbamcr.2010.01.003. PubMed: 20080133.

49. Fang J, Xu SW, Wang P, Tang FT, Zhou SG et al. (2010) Tanshinone II-A attenuates cardiac fibrosis and modulates collagen metabolism in rats with renovascular hypertension. Phytomedicine 18: 58–64. doi: 10.1016/j.phymed.2010.06.002. PubMed: 20638255.

50. Song Y, Xu J, Li Y, Jia C, Ma X et al. (2012) Cardiac Ankyrin Repeat Protein Attenuates Cardiac Hypertrophy by Inhibition of ERK1/2 and TGF-β Signaling Pathways. PLOS ONE 7: e50436. doi: 10.1371/journal.pone.0050436. PubMed: 23227174.

51. Carmeliet P (2000) Mechanisms of angiogenesis and arteriogenesis. Nat Med 6: 389–395. doi: 10.1038/74651. PubMed: 10742145.

52. Chen CH, Poucher SM, Lu J, Henry PD (2004) Fibroblast growth factor 2: from laboratory evidence to clinical application. Curr Vasc Pharmacol 2: 33–43. doi: 10.2174/1570161043476500. PubMed: 15320831.

53. Narine K, De Wever O, Van Valckenborgh D, Francois K, Bracke M et al. (2006) Growth factor modulation of fibroblast proliferation, differentiation, and invasion: implications for tissue valve engineering. Tissue Eng 12: 2707–2716. doi:10.1089/ten.2006.12.2707. PubMed: 17518640.

54. Suzuki T, Akasaka Y, Namiki A, Ito K, Ishikawa Y et al. (2008) Basic fibroblast growth factor inhibits ventricular remodeling in Dahl salt-sensitive hypertensive rats. J Hypertens 26: 2436–2444. doi: 10.1097/HJH.0b013e328312c889. PubMed: 19008723.

55. Kubiczkova L, Sedlarikova L, Hajek R, Sevcikova S (2012) TGF-β - an excellent servant but a bad master. J Transl Med 10: 183. doi: 10.1186/1479-5876-10-183. PubMed: 22943793.

56. Li Y, Yang Y, Yu D, Liang Q (2009) The effect of tanshinone IIA upon the TGF-beta1/Smads signaling pathway in hypertrophic myocardium of hypertensive rats. J Huazhong Univ Sci Technolog Med Sci 29: 476–480. doi: 10.1007/s11596-009-0417-5. PubMed: 19662366.

8

Cardiomyocyte Specific Deletion of Crif1 Causes Mitochondrial Cardiomyopathy in Mice

Juhee Shin[1,2], Seok Hong Lee[3], Min-Chul Kwon[1], Dong Kwon Yang[4], Ha-Rim Seo[1], Jaetaek Kim[3], Yoon-Young Kim[1,2], Sun-Kyoung Im[1,2], Evan Dale Abel[5], Kyong-Tai Kim[2], Woo Jin Park[4], Young-Yun Kong[1]*

1 Department of Biological Sciences, Seoul National University, Gwanak-gu, Seoul, Republic of Korea, 2 Department of Life Sciences, Pohang University of Science and Technology, Pohang, Kyungbuk, Republic of Korea, 3 Division of Endocrinology and Metabolism, Department of Internal Medicine, College of Medicine, Chung-Ang University, Dongjak-gu, Seoul, Republic of Korea, 4 Global Research Laboratory and Department of Life Science, Gwangju Institute of Science and Technology, Gwangju, Republic of Korea, 5 Program in Molecular Medicine, University of Utah School of Medicine, Salt Lake City, Utah, United States of America

Abstract

Mitochondria are key organelles dedicated to energy production. Crif1, which interacts with the large subunit of the mitochondrial ribosome, is indispensable for the mitochondrial translation and membrane insertion of respiratory subunits. To explore the physiological function of Crif1 in the heart, $Crif1^{f/f}$ mice were crossed with *Myh6-cre/Esr1* transgenic mice, which harbor cardiomyocyte-specific Cre activity in a tamoxifen-dependent manner. The tamoxifen injections were given at six weeks postnatal, and the mutant mice survived only five months due to hypertrophic heart failure. In the mutant cardiac muscles, mitochondrial mass dramatically increased, while the inner structure was altered with lack of cristae. Mutant cardiac muscles showed decreased rates of oxygen consumption and ATP production, suggesting that Crif1 plays a critical role in the maintenance of both mitochondrial structure and respiration in cardiac muscles.

Editor: Valdur Saks, Université Joseph Fourier, France

Funding: This work was supported by grants from the Basic Science Research Program through the National Research Foundation of Korea (2012-0000121); the Bio and Medical Technology Development Program (2011-0019269) of National Research Foundation funded by the Korean Government; and the National Research Foundation of Korea Grant funded by the Korean Government (NRF-M1AXA002-2011-0028413). The funders had no role in study design, data collection and analysis, decision to publish, or preparation of the manuscript.

Competing Interests: The authors have declared that no competing interests exist.

* E-mail: ykong@snu.ac.kr

Introduction

Mitochondria are dynamic organelles performing various cellular functions, such as energy production, fatty acid/amino acid oxidation, iron metabolism and apoptosis [1]. According to a recently defined mitochondrial protein inventory, MitoCarta, there are 1098 mitochondrial proteins in mouse [2]. Only thirteen subunits of the respiratory chain complexes are encoded in the mitochondrial genome (MtDNA), and the rest of the mitochondrial proteins are encoded in the nuclear genome (NuDNA) [3,4]. MtDNA encoded proteins are synthesized in the mitochondria by using its own transcriptional and translational machineries, whereas the NuDNA encoded precursor proteins are synthesized in the cytosol, imported into mitochondria, and processed into mature proteins [1,4]. About 600 mitochondrial proteins remain without known function or only with domain predictions based on sequence homology [2,3]. Thus, further investigations are necessary to identify the function of individual proteins constituting the mitochondrial proteome.

Crif1 had been recognized as a nuclear protein acting as a coactivator of transcriptional factors such as STAT3 and Elf3 [5,6,7,8,9], until it was identified as one of the MitoCarta genes [2]. Former studies used N-term tagged Crif1 for experiments, and the exogenous Crif1 was observed exclusively in the nucleus [5,6,7,8,9]. However, it was recently discovered that Crif1 has a signal peptide at the N terminus, and endogenous Crif1 is mostly located in the mitochondria. As a novel interacting factor of the mitoribosomal large subunit, Crif1 is indispensable for mitochondrial translation and membrane insertion of mtDNA encoded respiratory chain subunits. The targeted loss of Crif1 in mouse fibroblasts impaired energy generation and caused cell death. In addition, Crif1 loss in mouse forebrain induces neurodegeneration associated with mitochondrial abnormalities [10]. Crif1 is detected in the mitochondria of diverse mouse organs including cardiac and skeletal muscle, brain, kidney, liver, stomach and intestines [2]. Taken together, Crif1 appears to be a potential target for tissue-specific gene ablation to generate animal models of mitochondrial dysfunction.

Mitochondrial alterations have been implicated in a wide variety of disorders. Especially, defective mitochondrial respiration or oxidative phosphorylation causes mitochondrial respiratory disorders, which have an estimated occurrence of 1:5000 live births, but yet with no curable treatments [11,12,13,14]. Genetic mutations in the mitochondrial as well as the nuclear genome cause the mitochondrial respiratory disorder, and more than 100 causal genes have been reported [15]. The range of clinical manifestations is extensively broad concerning the affected organs, onset age, symptoms, and severity. Multiple defects in different organs are common, and most vulnerable tissues include the nervous, muscle and cardiac tissues, of which cell types require high energy metabolism [12,14]. Mitochondrial cardiomyopathy (MCM), a common manifestation of mitochondrial respiratory disorders, involves the development of cardiac hypertrophy and heart failure [16,17]. The age of onset for MCM is variable, as it can be detected in infants, children or adults [16,18]. In children with mitochondrial respiratory disorders in the central nervous system and neuromuscular tissues, high mortality and poor prognosis are pronounced when MCM is accompanied [19,20]. Researches using mouse models harboring genetic mutations of mitochondrial proteins has provided insights to understand the molecular basis, progression and diversity of mitochondrial respiratory disorders [21].

The cardiac muscle, which shows the highest mitochondrial abundance across tissues [3], is an excellent system to study the physiological role of a mitochondrial protein. To investigate the function of Crif1 in mouse heart, $Crif1^{f/f}$ mice were crossed with $Myh6$-$cre/Esr1$ and $Ckmm$-cre transgenic mice [22,23]. In $Myh6$-$cre/Esr1;Crif1^{f/f}$ mice, Crif1 was deleted in adult cardiomyocytes in a tamoxifen dependent manner, and these mice suffered from progressive hypertrophy and died from heart failure. Oxygen consumption and ATP production rates, COX/SDH activities and electron microscopy demonstrated that Crif1 loss affects both mitochondrial respiration and structure. In $Ckmm$-$cre;Crif1^{f/f}$ mice, Crif1 was undetectable in cardiac muscle at postnatal day 10, and the mutant mice died in two weeks postnatal, showing cardiac hypertrophy associated with mitochondrial dysfunction. We suggest these two cardiac muscle-specific Crif1 deletion mice, $Ckmm$-$cre;Crif1^{f/f}$ and $Myh6$-$cre/Esr1;Crif1^{f/f}$ mice, as animal models for early and late onset MCM, respectively.

Materials and Methods

Ethics Statement

This research is approved by the Seoul National University Institutional Animal Care and Use Committees (Approval number: SNU 081002-2). All animal experiments were performed according to the guidelines from the SNU IACUC and the NIH principles for the Care and Use of Laboratory Animals.

Mice

$Myh6$-$cre/Esr1$ and $Ckmm$-cre mice were purchased from Jackson Laboratories. $Crif1^{f/f}$ mice were previously generated in our laboratory [6] and backcrossed for 8 generations to C57BL/6 mice. Mice were maintained in our animal colony under institutional guidelines. $Crif1^{f/f}$ mice were crossed with $Myh6$-$cre/Esr1$ to generate $Myh6$-$cre/Esr1; Crif1^{f/f}$ and $Crif1^{f/f}$ for the littermate control. Tamoxifen was dissolved in corn oil and administered to each mouse at 20 mg/kg by intraperitoneal injections once a day, for 4 days/round, for total 2 rounds. The 4 day interval between the rounds was to avoid the accumulation of tamoxifen inside the body from prolonged treatment. Tamoxifen injection started when mice reached 6 weeks postnatal. $Ckmm$-$cre;Crif1^{+/f}$ mice were crossed with $Crif1^{f/f}$ to generate $Ckmm$-$cre;Crif1^{f/f}$ and the littermate controls.

Heart Histology, SDH and COX Activity Stains

Mouse hearts were arrested with 1 M KCl, fixed in 3.7% formalin, paraffin-embedded, and sectioned at 4 µm. The sections were subjected to hematoxylin and eosin (H&E) staining. For succinic dehydrogenase (SDH) and cytochrome c oxidase (COX) stain, excised heart were snap frozen in OCT compound (Sakura) and sectioned at 10 µm. Subsequent staining procedure was performed by standard protocols [24]. The staining intensity was quantified using ImageJ program. Microscope images were converted to grayscale and then inverted. Pixels between the threshold 95~255 were selected to avoid the background signal, and the integrated densities were measured.

Western Blot

Protein samples were prepared from excised hearts, and Western blot was performed by standard protocols. Primary antibodies used were: anti-Crif1 [6], and anti-actin (Sigma).

Ecocardia

Echocardiographic measurements were performed as described previously [25]. Briefly, mice were anesthetized and echocardiographed using a Powervision 6000 (TOSHIBA) instrument with a 12-MHz microprobe (PLM-1204AT, TOSHIBA). Hearts were scanned using the M-mode guided by a short-axis view of the 2-dimensional mode.

Mitochondrial Respiration and ATP Measurements

Cardiac muscle fibers were saponin-permeablized [26], and respiratory parameters were measured according to previously published procedures [26,27]. Briefly, 2–3 mg of the wet tissue was transferred into Oxygraph chamber (Ocean Optics Instruments) containing mitochondrial respiration buffer to measure the oxygen concentration. Respiratory rates were expressed as nmol of O_2/min/mg dry fiber weight. Substrates used were: 10 mmol/l pyruvate and 5 mmol/l malate; 0.02 mmol/l palmitoyl-carnitine and 2 mmol/l malate; or 5 mmol/l glutamate and 2 mmol/l malate. 1 mmol/l ADP was included to stimulate state 3 respirations. Subsequently, 8 mmol/L cytochrome c was added, and finally 1 ug/mL oligomycin were added to evaluate state 4 respirations. ATP concentrations were determined using the ATP assay kit (BioVision).

Transmission Electron Microscopy

Cardiac tissue was fixed overnight in 2% paraformaldehyde and 2% glutaraldehyde in 0.05 M sodium cacodylate buffer (pH 7.2) at 4°C. Samples were rinsed with sodium cacodylate buffer, postfixed with 1% osmium tetroxide at 4°C for 2 hrs. After rinsing with distilled water, samples were en bloc stained with 0.5% uranyl acetate at 4°C for overnight. After the dehydration process with ethanol series, samples were transferred to propylene oxide, and embedded in Spurr's resin. After polymerization, ultrathin sections were prepared with an ultramicrotome (MT-X, RMC, Tucson, AZ, USA). Images were captured using LIBRA 120 (Carl Zeiss, Germany). All process was performed at the EM facility of NICEM at Seoul National University.

Cell Culture

E13.5 embryos of $Crif1^{+/+}$ and $Crif1^{f/f}$ were digested with trypsin/EDTA to isolate $Crif1^{+/+}$ and $Crif1^{f/f}$ MEFs. SV40 large T antigen was transfected into MEFs for immortalization. Cells were grown in DMEM (Hyclone) supplemented with 10% FBS (Hyclone) and antibiotic-antimycotic (Gibco) in a humidified incubator with 5% CO_2. For Cre-retrovirus production, PT67 packaging cell line containing the retrovirus construct expressing Cre recombinase was established and maintained in standard culture medium with puromycin (3 µg/ml). When the cells become confluent, medium was changed with non-puromycin containing medium, and incubated for 24 hrs. To induce Cre mediated recombination of the floxed alleles, MEFs were incubated in Cre-retrovirus containing medium mixed with polybrene (6 µg/ml) for 24 hrs. After virus infection, cells were incubated for 36 hrs in standard medium. Virus infected MEFs were selected with puromycin (3 µg/ml) for 60 hrs until uninfected cells are fully eliminated. Chloramphenicol (Sigma) was treated at a final concentration of 100 µg/ul for 48 hrs.

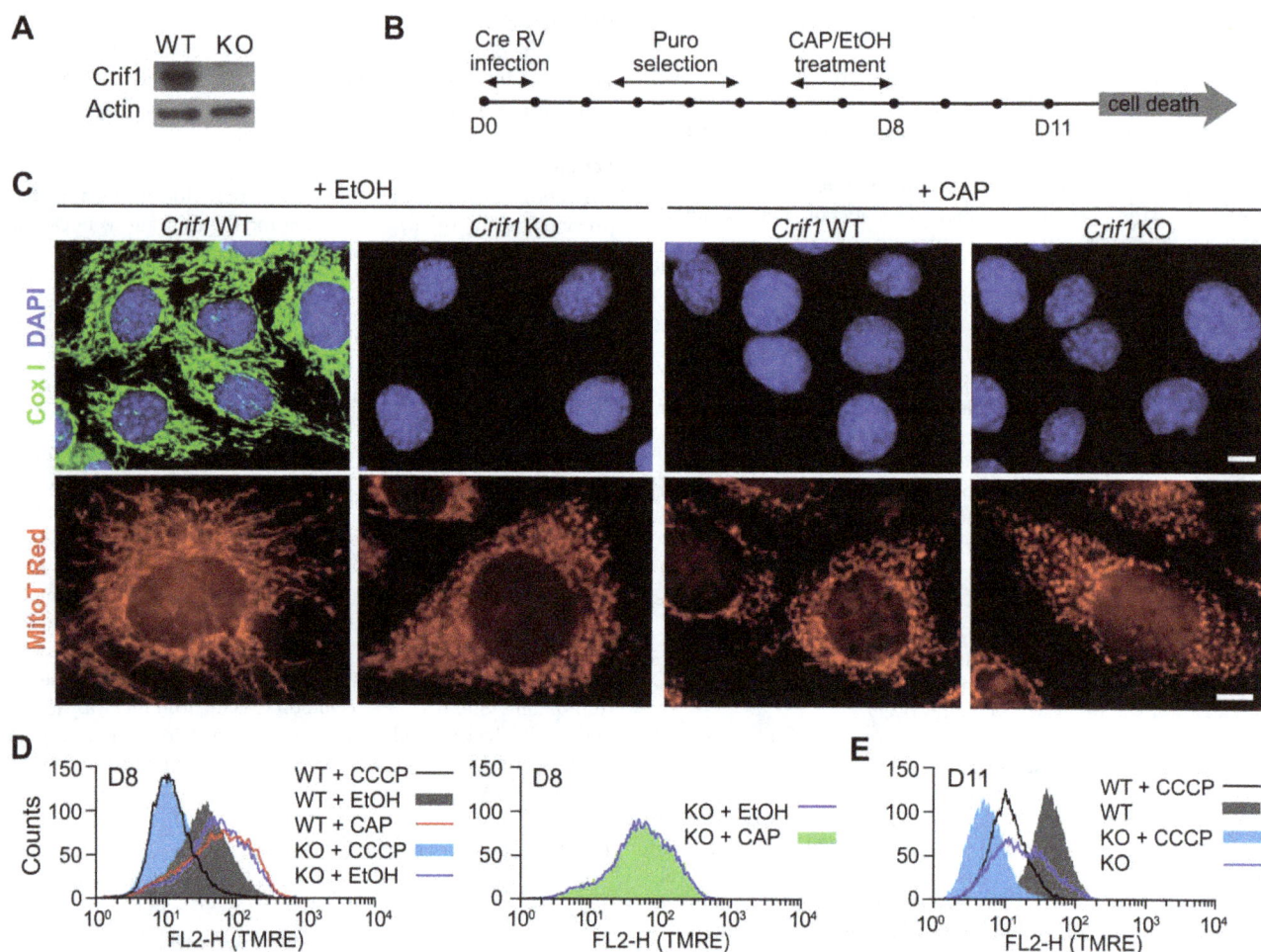

Figure 1. *Crif1^{Δ/Δ}* and CAP treated *Crif1^{+/+}* MEFs show mitochondrial abnormalities. (A) Western blot analysis of Crif1 expression in *Crif1^{+/+}* and *Crif1^{Δ/Δ}* MEFs. (B) Schematic presentation of experimental procedures. At day 0 (D0), MEFs were infected with retrovirus that expresses Cre recombinase. After puromycin selection, mitochondrial characteristics were analyzed after the treatment of either ethanol (EtOH) vehicle or chloramphenicol (CAP). (C) At day 8, cells were immunostained with Cox I antibody (in green) and DAPI (in blue) (upper panel), or stained with Mitotracker Red (bottom panel). Scale bars, 10 μm. (D, E) To measure mitochondrial membrane potential (MMP), MEFs were stained with tetramethylrhodamine ethyl ester (TMRE), a cationic fluorescent dye sensitive to MMP, and analyzed by flow cytometry on the FL2 channel at day 8 (D) and day 11 (E). Carbonyl cyanide *m*-chlorophenyl hydrazone (CCCP), a proton ionophore that disrupts proton gradient, was treated to gain the control peak of MMP decrease.

Immunofluorescence

MEFs were fixed with 3.7% formalin diluted in culture medium for 15 minutes at 37°C. After washing and blocking, cells were incubated with anti-Cox I antibody (Molecular probes), followed by incubation with anti-mouse secondary antibody. For mitochondrial stain, cells were incubated with culture medium containing 400 nM MitoTracker Red (Molecular probes) for 30 minutes at 37°C prior to fixation.

Mitochondrial Membrane Potential

MEFs were collected by trypsinization, and resuspended in PBS containing 1% FBS and 20 mM HEPES. Fluorochrome tetramethylrhodamine ethyl ester (TMRE, Molecular probes, T669) was added to the final concentration of 100 nM for the 30 minute incubation at room temperature. For the controls of disrupted mitochondrial membrane potential, 20 μM CCCP was included in the staining solution. The fluorescence intensity was monitored in FL-2 channel and analyzed using CellQuest software (Becton Dickinson).

Statistical Analyses

Data are presented as the mean ± SD or mean ± SE. Significance ($P<0.05$) was evaluated by a two tailed, unpaired Student's t test.

Results

Mitochondrial Abnormalities in *Crif1^{Δ/Δ}* MEFs

Crif1, which associates with the large subunit of mitochondrial ribosome, is essential for the protein synthesis of mtDNA encoded genes [10]. To demonstrate that the mitochondrial alterations in Crif1-deleted cells are caused by impaired mitochondrial translation, the mitochondria of Crif1 knockout cells were compared to that of wild type cells treated with chloramphenicol (CAP), which inhibits peptide bond formation on mitoribosomes. Immortalized *Crif1^{+/+}* and *Crif1^{f/f}* mouse fibroblasts were infected with Cre retrovirus and selected with puromycin to generate *Crif1^{+/+}* and *Crif1^{Δ/Δ}* cells, respectively. Crif1 deletion was confirmed by Western blot analysis (Fig. 1A). Changes in mitochondria were assessed in *Crif1^{+/+}* and *Crif1^{Δ/Δ}* cells after treating either ethanol

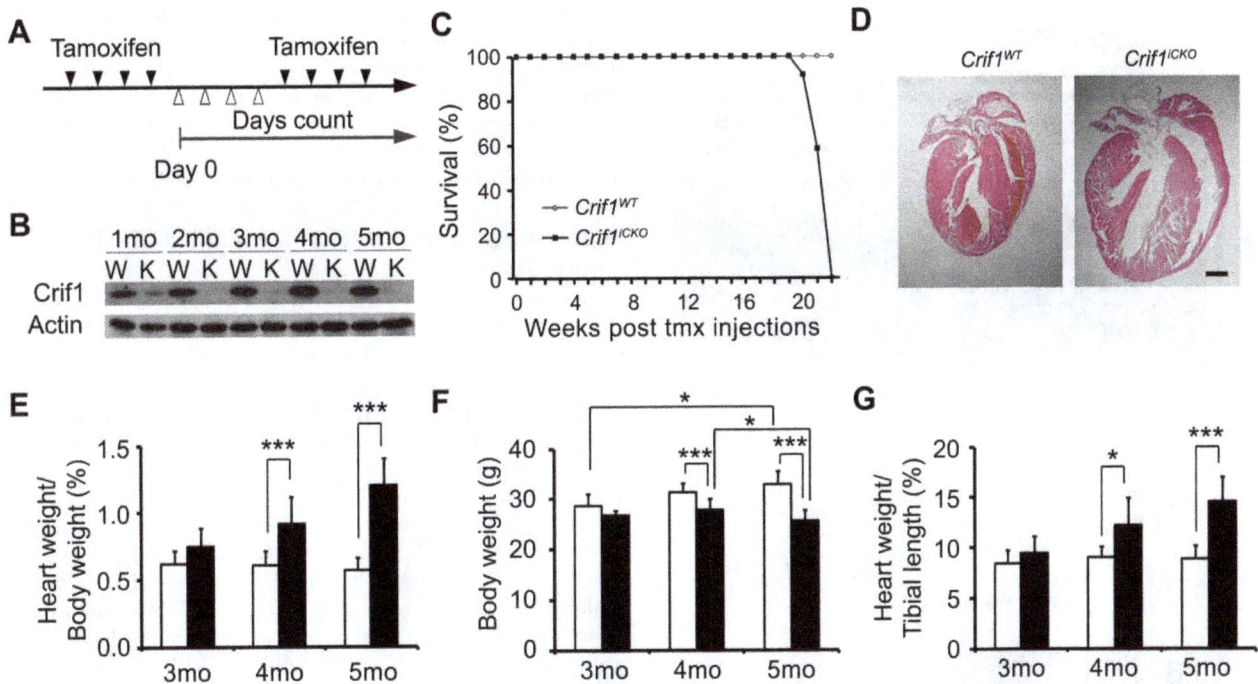

Figure 2. Inducible excision of Crif1 in adult cardiac myocytes causes cardiac hypertrophy. (A) Scheme of tamoxifen injections. 6 week old *Crif*$^{f/f}$ (*Crif1*^{WT}) and *Myh6-cre/Esr1;Crif*$^{f/f}$ (*Crif1*^{iCKO}) mice were administrated with tamoxifen intraperitoneally at a dose of 20 mg/kg/day, for 8 days. Black arrows, days with injections. White arrows, days without injections. Day 0, start of days counted. (B) Western blot analysis of Crif1 expression in *Crif1*^{WT} and *Crif1*^{iCKO} hearts at 1~5 months post tamoxifen injections (C) The survival graph of *Crif1*^{WT} and *Crif1*^{iCKO} mice. Survivality were checked every week after tamoxifen (txm) injections. n = 12 for both groups. (D) H&E staining of the heart sections from *Crif1*^{WT} and *Crif1*^{iCKO} mice at 5 months post tamoxifen injections. Scale bar, 1 mm. (E) heart weight per body weight ratio, (F) body weight and (G) heart weight per tibia length ratio of *Crif1*^{WT} and *Crif1*^{iCKO} mice at 3 ~ 5 months. The tibia length of *Crif1*^{iCKO} mice was not different from that of *Crif1*^{WT} mice. n = 5 for each genotype at 3 months, n = 7 for *Crif1*^{WT} at 4 months, n = 9 for *Crif1*^{iCKO} at 4 months, n = 10 for *Crif1*^{WT} at 5 months, n = 12 for *Crif1*^{WT} at 5 months. Error bars show SD. $^*P<0.05$, $^{***}P<0.005$.

vehicle or CAP (Fig. 1B). Immunofluorescence of Cox I, a mtDNA encoded subunit consisting respiratory chain complex IV, revealed filamentous structure of mitochondria in ethanol-treated *Crif1*$^{+/+}$ cells. The Cox I expression was completely diminished by CAP treatment, showing that CAP effectively prevents mitochondrial translation. As expected, *Crif1*$^{Δ/Δ}$ cells exhibited loss of Cox I expression regardless of CAP treatment (Fig. 1C, top panel). When the mitochondrial network was visualized by MitoTracker Red staining, *Crif1*$^{+/+}$ cells showed filamentous structure. However, the mitochondria of *Crif1*$^{Δ/Δ}$ and CAP-treated *Crif1*$^{+/+}$ cells were fragmented (Fig. 1C, bottom panel).

CAP transiently induces an increase of mitochondrial membrane potential [28]. In accordance with the previous report, *Crif1*$^{+/+}$ cells showed increased mitochondrial membrane potential by CAP treatment (Fig. 1D, red). Interestingly, the mitochondrial membrane potential in *Crif1*$^{Δ/Δ}$ cells increased to a similar extent as that in CAP-treated *Crif1*$^{+/+}$ cells (Fig. 1D, compare the red and blue lines). The increased mitochondrial membrane potential in the *Crif1*$^{Δ/Δ}$ cells was not further increased by CAP treatment (Fig. 1D, right panel) and readily depolarized by the treatment of carbonyl cyanide *m*-chlorophenyl hydrazone (CCCP), a proton ionophore (Fig. 1D). Eventually, 11 days after the gene disruption, *Crif1*$^{Δ/Δ}$ cells exhibited decrease in membrane potential, which is one of the common features of dying cells (Fig. 1E). Taken together, Crif1 loss causes mitochondrial abnormalities comparable to the effect of CAP treatment.

Tamoxifen-inducible Deletion of Crif1 in Adult Cardiac Muscle

To investigate the physiological function of Crif1 in cardiac muscle, *Crif1*$^{f/f}$ mice were bred with *Myh6-cre/Esr1* transgenic line, which has cardiomyocyte-specific Cre recombinase activity in a tamoxifen-dependent manner [22]. *Myh6-cre/Esr1; Crif1*$^{f/f}$ and the littermate control *Crif1*$^{f/f}$ mice were administrated with tamoxifen at 6 weeks postnatal (Fig. 2A), and they are hereafter termed *Crif1*^{iCKO} (Crif1 inducible cardiac KO) and *Crif1*^{WT}, respectively. To verify the ablation of Crif1, we prepared the cardiac lysates from 1~5 months post tamoxifen injections, and performed Western blot analysis using anti-Crif1 antibody. There was a significant reduction of Crif1 at one month, and it was reduced to the undetectable level at two months after the tamoxifen injections (Fig. 2B).

Cardiac Hypertrophy in the *Crif1*^{iCKO} Mice

Five months after tamoxifen treatment, *Crif1*^{iCKO} mice started to die, and none of them survived more than 22 weeks (Fig. 2C). The moribund *Crif1*^{iCKO} mice showed cardiac enlargement (Fig. 2D). To evaluate cardiac hypertrophy in *Crif1*^{WT} and *Crif1*^{iCKO} mice, the ratio of heart weight-to-body weight was measured at each month after the tamoxifen treatment. At 1~3 months, the body weight and the heart weight-to-body weight ratios of *Crif1*^{iCKO} mice appeared normal. However, cardiac hypertrophy became significant at 4 months (Fig. 2E, $^{***}P=0.0016$). The *Crif1*^{iCKO} hearts were severely hypertrophied by a 2.1 fold increase compared to the *Crif1*^{WT} hearts at 5 months.

A

B

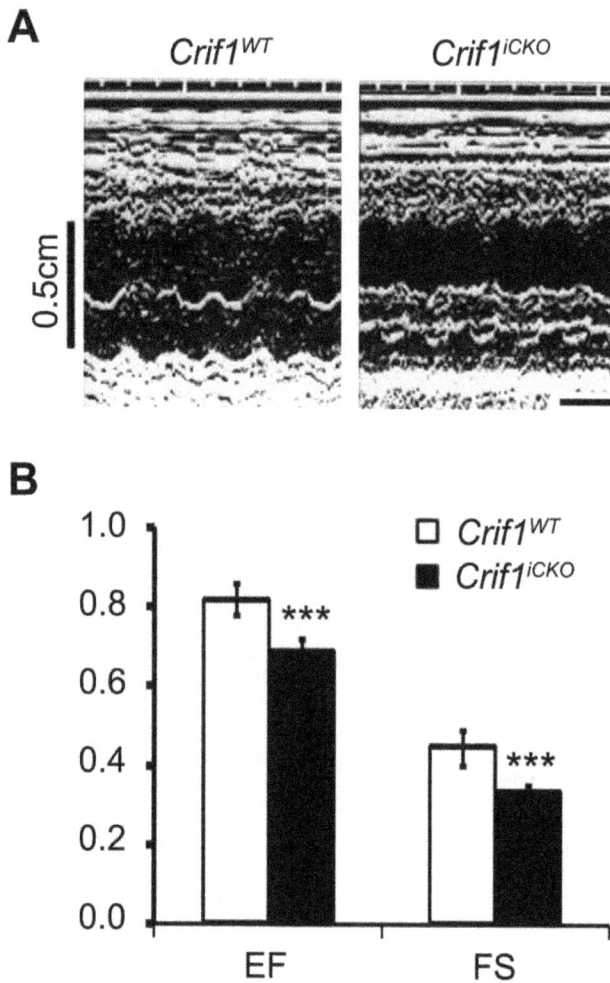

Figure 3. Crif1 loss impairs *in vivo* heart function. (A) Echocardiographic tracings of *Crif1^WT* and *Crif1^iCKO* mice at 4 months post tamoxifen injections. Scale bar = 0.1 sec. (B) Values of ejection fraction (EF) and fractional shortening (FS) obtained from echocardiography. n = 8 for *Crif1^WT* and n = 11 for *Crif1^iCKO* mice. Error bars show SD. ***P<0.0001.

While *Crif1^WT* mice significantly gained weight from 3 to 5 months (*P = 0.016), the body weight of *Crif1^iCKO* mice did not increase; rather, an apparent decrease from 4 to 5 months was observed (*P = 0.029) (Fig. 2F). We also observed a dramatic loss of abdominal and visceral fat in the moribund *Crif1^iCKO* mice (data not shown). Thus, the decrease in heart weight-to-body weight ratios could be due to loss of body weight. To exclude this possibility, the heart weight-to-tibia length ratios were also calculated. As shown in Fig. 2G, cardiac hypertrophy in the *Crif1^iCKO* mice was significant at 4 months (*P = 0.011), and one month later, the heart weight-to-tibia length ratio was increased by 1.6-fold compared to the *Crif1^WT* ratio. From these results, we conclude that Crif1 deletion in adult cardiac muscle causes progressive cardiac hypertrophy.

Reduced Cardiac Function Caused by Crif1 Loss

As *Crif1^iCKO* mice died with cardiac hypertrophy that is often implicated in heart failure, we examined the cardiac function of *Crif1^iCKO* mice by echocardiography at 4 months after tamoxifen treatment. The *Crif1^iCKO* mice showed abnormal patterns of

cardiac contractions when compared to the controls (Fig. 3A). In addition, the values of ejection fraction (EF) and fractional shortening (FS) were markedly decreased in the mutant mice (Fig. 3B). Hydrothorax, one of the consequences that can be caused by cardiac failure, was occasionally observed in *Crif1^iCKO* mice at 5 months (data not shown). Thus, loss of Crif1 in cardiac muscle results in hypertrophic heart failure that leads to death.

Impaired Mitochondrial Respiration in Crif1 Deficient Cardiac Tissues

Since mtDNA encodes the catalytic core subunits of respiratory chain complexes, its expression is crucial for mitochondrial respiration [29,30,31,32]. To demonstrate that Crif1 is necessary for mitochondrial respiration in cardiac muscles, we measured the rate of oxygen consumption and ATP production using *Crif1^iCKO* and *Crif1^WT* tissues. Saponin-permeablized cardiac fibers were independently incubated with three metabolic substrates: pyruvate, palmitoyl-carnitine (PC) or glutamate. *Crif1^iCKO* tissues incubated with pyruvate showed decreased oxygen uptake compared to *Crif1^WT* tissues (Fig. 4A, state 2, 4.97 ± 1.06 vs. 8.37 ± 0.84, **$P = 0.0086$). When ADP was added in order to stimulate the maximal respiration (state 3), *Crif1^iCKO* cardiac tissues showed significantly reduced oxygen uptake compared to *Crif1^WT* tissues: pyruvate (Fig. 4A, 10.03 ± 1.40 vs. 16.81 ± 2.36, *$P = 0.017$), PC (Fig. 4B, 11.77 ± 0.51 vs. 17.35 ± 1.31, *$P = 0.014$) or glutamate (Fig. 4C, 9.66 ± 1.23 vs. 16.83 ± 2.52, *$P = 0.034$). When oligomycin was added to inhibit the activity of ATP synthase (state 4), the oxygen uptake of *Crif1^iCKO* tissues was not significantly different from that of *Crif1^WT* tissues, indicating that uncoupled respiration is not present in *Crif1^iCKO* tissues.

The ATP production during state 3 respiration was reduced in *Crif1^iCKO* tissues compared to *Crif1^WT* tissues when incubated with pyruvate (Fig. 4D, 28.46 ± 2.47 vs. 51.00 ± 6.16, *$P = 0.025$), PC (Fig. 4E, 17.46 ± 1.29 vs. 39.28 ± 4.17, ***$P = 0.0048$) and glutamate (Fig. 4F, 25.59 ± 5.79 vs. 62.68 ± 9.69, *$P = 0.021$). For all substrates, the ratios of ATP generation to oxygen consumption (ATP/O) in *Crif1^iCKO* tissues were insignificantly different from those of *Crif1^WT* tissues. These data show that Crif1 is indispensible for mitochondrial respiration.

To further analyze the effect of Crif1 loss on mitochondrial respiration, the activities of respiratory chain complexes were examined by histochemical methods [24]. Serial sections of *Crif1^WT* and *Crif1^iCKO* hearts were stained for succinate dehydrogenase (SDH, respiratory chain complex II) and cytochrome oxidase (COX, respiratory chain complex IV) activities. The COX activity in *Crif1^iCKO* sections decreased (68% of the *Crif1^WT* staining intensity) at 3 months and was dramatically reduced (45% of the *Crif1^WT* staining intensity) at 5 months (Fig. 4G and J). In contrast, the SDH activity in *Crif1^iCKO* sections was unaffected at 3 months and showed only a subtle decrease (92% of the *Crif1^WT* staining intensity) at 5 months (Fig. 4H and K). These results indicate that the activity of COX is progressively diminished by Crif1 loss whereas the activity of SDH, the respiratory complex exclusively composed of nuDNA encoded subunits [29,33], is less affected in *Crif1^iCKO* heart.

Crif1^WT and *Crif1^iCKO* heart sections were also stained with hematoxylin/eosin to examine histological abnormalities (Fig. 4I). *Crif1^iCKO* hearts appeared normal at 3 months. However, most of the *Crif1^iCKO* fibers were distinguished by faint eosin staining at 5 months (Fig. 4C). Tunnel staining was performed using the adjacent sections to determine necrotic fibers. However, no dying cells were observed (data not shown), indicating that the loss of mitochondrial respiration and cardiac contractility of *Crif1^iCKO* hearts is not attributed to the death of cardiac myocytes.

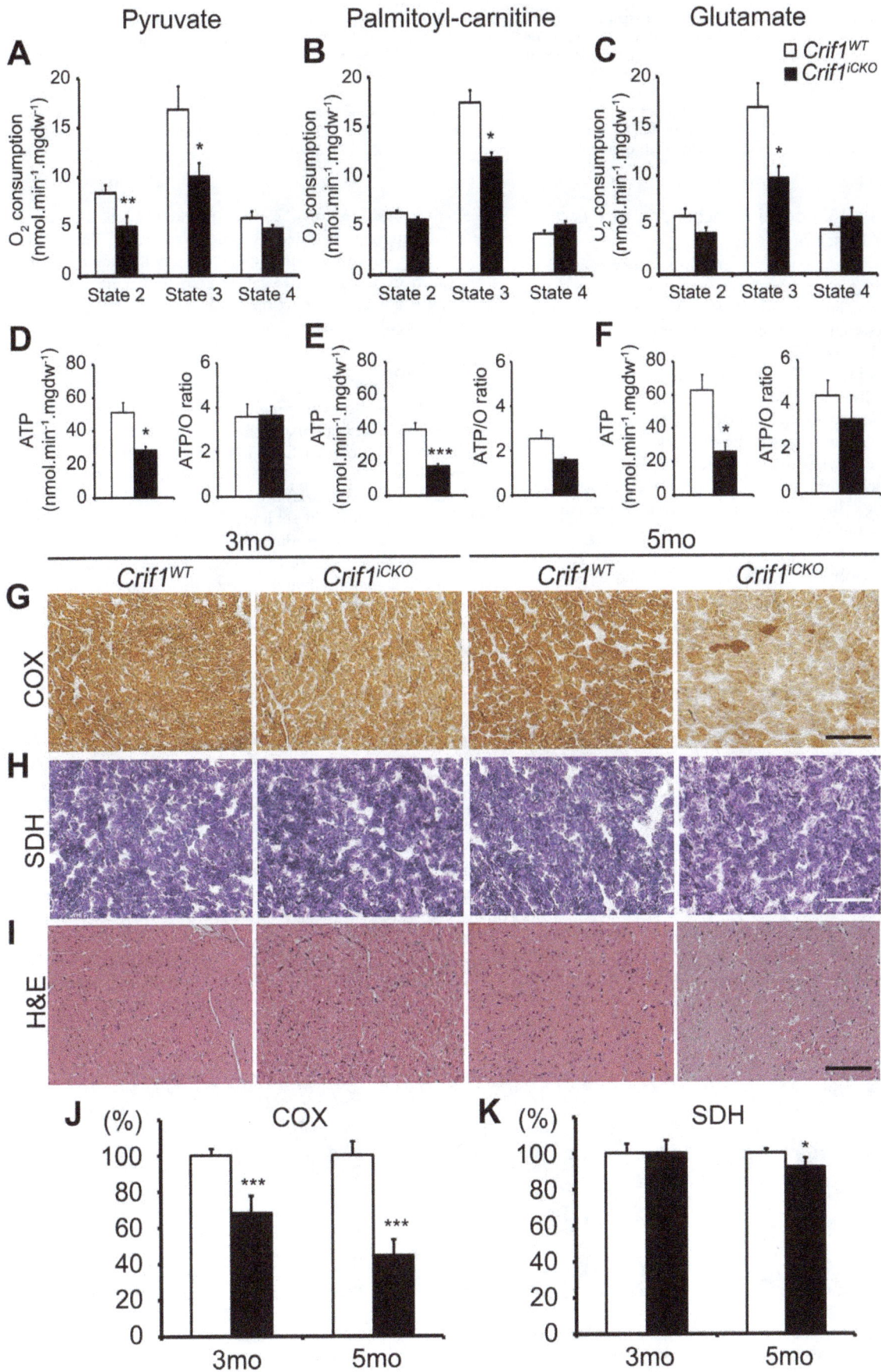

Figure 4. Crif1 is required for mitochondrial respiratory activities in cardiac muscle. (A~C) Oxygen consumption rates and (D~F) ATP synthesis rates using the saponin-permeablized cardiac fibers from $Crif1^{WT}$ and $Crif1^{iCKO}$ mice at 4.5 months post tamoxifen injections. (A, D) Pyruvate-malate respiration. n = 6 for each genotype. (B, E) PC-malate respiration. n = 6 for each genotype. (C, F) Glutamate-malate respiration. n = 5 for $Crif1^{WT}$ and n = 6 for $Crif1^{iCKO}$ mice. Error bars show SE. *$P<0.05$, **$P<0.01$, ***$P<0.005$. No significant changes were observed in ATP/O with all substrates ($P>0.05$). (G) COX, (H) SDH and (I) H&E stain on the cardiac sections of $Crif1^{WT}$ and $Crif1^{iCKO}$ mice at indicated time points. Scale bar, 100 μm. Quantification of (J) COX and (K) SDH staining intensities. Microscope images were analyzed using ImageJ software. The total intensity of the $Crif1^{iCKO}$ heart (black) is shown as the relative ratio to the $Crif1^{WT}$ stain (white). Microscope images were taken from two different sections for each heart sample. Three heart samples were collected for each genotype. Error bars show SE. *$P<0.05$, ***$P<0.005$.

Increased Mass of Abnormal Mitochondria with Lack of Cristae in Crif1 Deficient Hearts

Aberrant mitochondrial structure in cardiomyocytes is one of the characteristic features in MCM patients [19,20,21]. To examine the possibility that Crif1 loss does not only affects mitochondrial respiration but also the structure, cardiac tissues were analyzed by transmission electron microscopy. Several dramatic changes in the ultrastructure were observed: decreased mass of myofibrils, increased number of mitochondria, and abnormal inner structure of mitochondria (Fig. 5A). The $Crif1^{WT}$ tissue exhibited mitochondria with densely packed cristae, which is a distinct characteristic of cardiac muscle. However, the structure of increased mitochondria in $Crif1^{iCKO}$ hearts was significantly with loss of cristae (Fig. 5B). Thus, Crif1 is required to maintain the normal mitochondrial structure.

Cardiac Hypertrophy in *Ckmm-cre; Crif1^f/f* Mice

Crif1 was not only ablated in the adulthood, but was also ablated in neonatal cardiac muscle by using *Ckmm-cre* transgenic line, the promoter of which is active in the cardiac and skeletal muscle since embryonic day 13 [23]. Western blot analysis showed that Crif1 was reduced at P0 and undetectable in hearts at P10. Crif1 was residual in soleus muscles, which is a type of highly oxidative skeletal muscle (Fig. 6A). The mice were born in Mendelian ratios, but *Ckmm-cre; Crif1^f/f* mice all died before postnatal day 14 (P14). We assessed COX and NADH activity of P10 *Ckmm-cre; Crif1^f/f* soleus muscle by histochemical staining, but no decrease in these activities was observed compared to the wild type mice (data not shown). In contrast, the *Ckmm-cre;Crif1^f/f* mouse hearts displayed morphological changes: thickened interventricular septum wall and enlarged right ventricle (Fig. 6B). The heart weight per body weight ratio of *Ckmm-cre;Crif1^f/f* mice was higher than that of the control mice by 37.4%, showing significant hypertrophy (Fig. 6C). To test the mitochondrial respiratory activities in the young cardiac tissues, COX and SDH staining were performed (Fig. 6D and E). The decrease in COX

activity in *Ckmm-cre;Crif1^f/f* cardiac muscles (69% of the wild type staining intensity) revealed mitochondrial dysfunction in those tissues. In conclusion, the Crif1 conditional knockout mice generated by using the two different *cre* transgenic lines, *Ckmm-cre* and *Myh6-cre/Esr1*, develop cardiomyopathy due to impaired mitochondrial respiration.

Discussion

Crif1 has been shown to regulate the function of diverse nuclear proteins and transcriptional factors [5,6,7,8,9]. However, a recent study demonstrated that Crif1 is a novel interacting factor of the mitochondrial ribosome [10]. According to this report, Crif1 is essential for mitochondrial translation and membrane integration of the respiratory chain subunits. The protein levels of mtDNA encoded proteins were diminished in Crif1 null MEFs, thus decreasing the amount of respiratory chain complexes. It seems that the mitochondrial function of Crif1 is independent of its nuclear function, as the previous report demonstrates the mitochondrial translation defect of Crif1 null MEFs is only rescued by over-expressing the C-terminal tagged construct, and not by the nuclear-localized construct, of which the signal peptide is masked by N-terminal tagging [10]. In this study, we further investigated the mitochondrial changes in Crif1 null MEFs. Not only reduced expression of Cox I, but also fragmented mitochondrial network and the membrane potential change were observed in Crif1 null MEFs. Intriguingly, these alterations were identically induced in wild type cells by CAP treatment. Furthermore, we observed a dramatic loss of cristae in the Crif1 deleted cardiac tissues. It is well known that CAP treatment reduces the number of cristae in yeast, protozoa, and mammalian cells [34,35,36,37,38]. Our results strongly suggest that the various mitochondrial alterations in Crif1 cells are commonly resulted from impaired mitochondrial translation.

While approximately half of the mitochondrial proteome shows tissue-specific expression [3], Crif1 is one of the mitochondrial proteins that are ubiquitously detected throughout the mouse

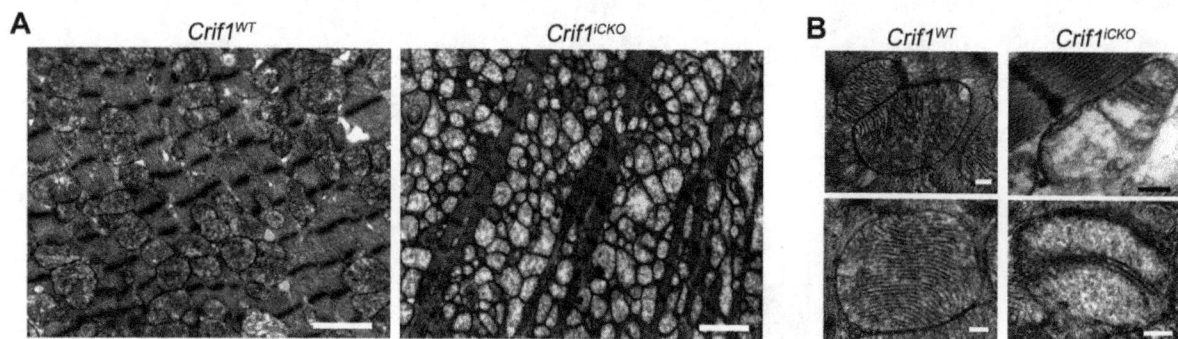

Figure 5. Crif1 loss increases the mass of abnormal mitochondria. (A) Low and (B) high magnification images of transmission electron microscopy. Experiments were performed using the cardiac apex from $Crif1^{WT}$ and $Crif1^{iCKO}$ mice at 5 months post tamoxifen injections. Scale bar, 2 μm (A) and 0.2 μm (B).

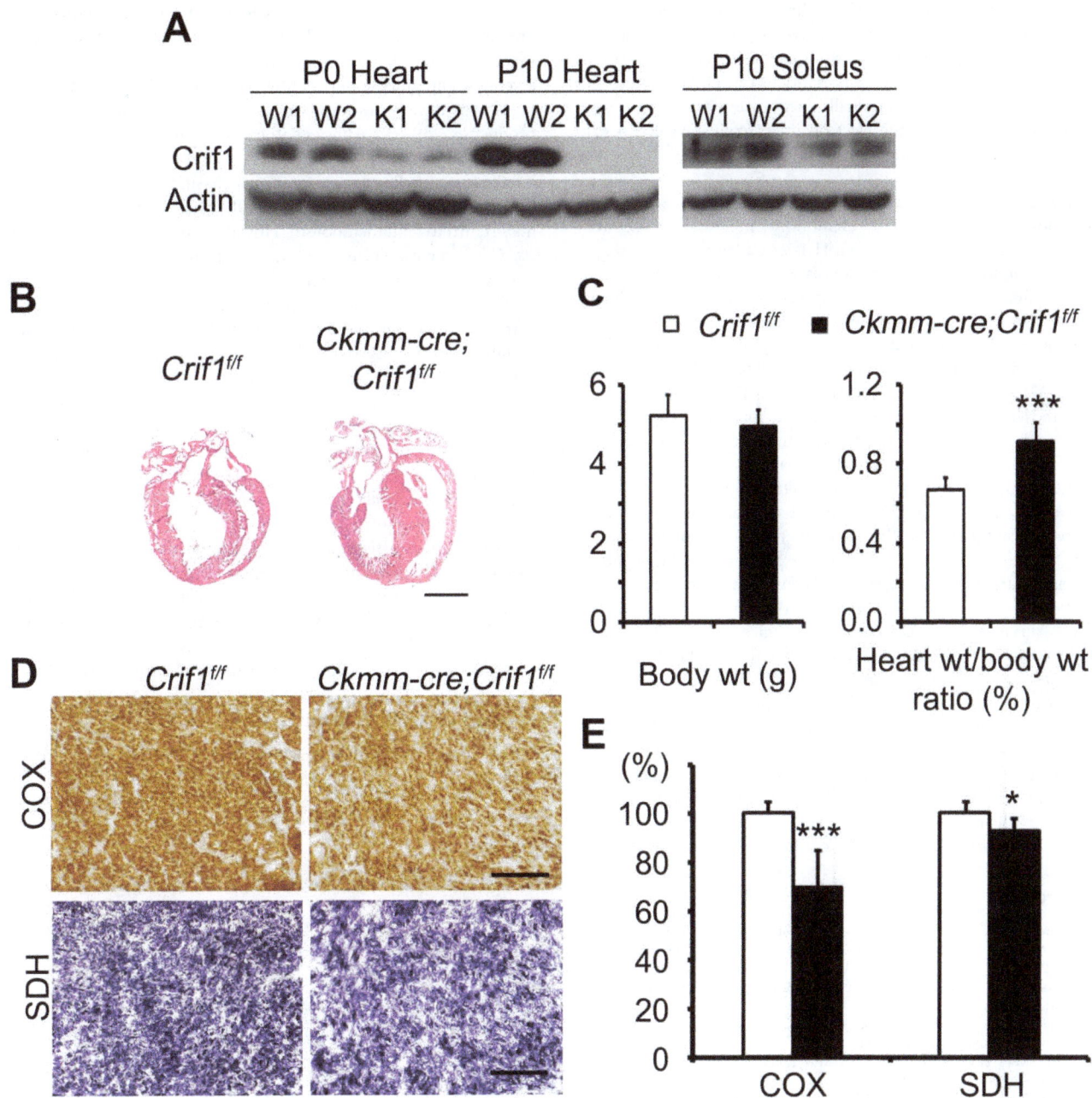

Figure 6. Crif1 deletion in the cardiac muscle using the *Ckmm-cre* transgene leads to cardiac hypertrophy. (A) Western blot analysis of Crif1 expression in isolated hearts and soleus muscles from *Crif1^{f/f}* and *Ckmm-cre;Crif1^{f/f}* mice. Protein lysates were prepared from P0 or P10 mouse tissues. (B) H&E staining of heart sections from *Crif1^{f/f}* (W1 and W2) and *Ckmm-cre;Crif1^{f/f}* mice (K1 and K2) at P10. Scale bar, 1 mm. (C) Heart weight per body weight ratios of P10 mice. n = 7 for each genotype. Error bars show SD. $^{***}P = 0.00001$. (D) COX and SDH stain on snap-frozen P10 heart sections. Scale bars, 100 μm. (E) Quantification of COX and SDH staining intensities using ImageJ. The total intensity of the *Ckmm-cre;Crif1^{f/f}* heart (black) is shown as the relative ratio to the *Crif1^{f/f}* stain (white). Microscope images were taken from two different sections for each heart sample. Three heart samples were collected for each genotype. Error bars show SE. $^{*}P < 0.05$, $^{***}P < 0.005$.

organs [2]. Various conditional knockout mice of Crif1 have been generated to investigate the physiological function of Crif1; however, up to date, there is only one report demonstrating its mitochondrial function *in vivo* [5,6,10]. To further elucidate the mitochondrial function of Crif1, we ablated the gene in the cardiac muscle, where the mitochondrial function is critical for the organ performance. *Myh6-cre/Esr1* transgenic line was crossed with Crif1 conditional knockout mice to generate *Crif1^{iCKO}* mice. The *Crif1^{iCKO}* mice developed severe cardiac hypertrophy, and died

within six months after the tamoxifen injections. Decreased *in vivo* heart function was demonstrated by echocardiography. The heart weight-to-tibia length ratio shows a mild cardiac enlargement (1.3-fold increase) in *Crif1^{iCKO}* mice at 4 months when the echocardiography was performed. Our result suggests that the cardiac function decreases from the early point of hypertrophy in *Crif1^{iCKO}* mice. The rate of substrate-driven respiration using permeablized cardiac tissues revealed no sign of uncoupled respiration in *Crif1^{iCKO}* heart, but the rate of oxygen uptake and ATP generation were significantly reduced. *Crif1^{iCKO}* hearts show a mild decrease in COX activity at 3 months post tamoxifen injections, and it takes two more months to show a dramatic change. These results indicate that the initial mitochondrial defect in Crif1 deleted cells is relatively subtle but gradually aggravates to more severe disruption. In addition, the electron microscopy revealed a dramatic change in mitochondrial morphology in *Crif1^{iCKO}* cardiac tissues.

Our study shows that Crif1 loss brings out a series of mitochondrial damages in membrane potential, respiratory activities and structure. Thus, Crif1 is considered as an essential factor for mitochondrial homeostasis and integrity by playing its primary function in mitochondrial translation. Since each cell type has its own mitochondrial/cytosolic proteome, the progression of mitochondrial dysfunction and secondary alterations of cellular metabolism will differ depending on the cell type of Crif1 deletion. While MEFs are sensitive to Crif1 loss, so that the cell death is triggered in days, adult cardiomyocytes that are specialized in energy production seems to resist against cell death. We speculate that Crif1 loss accumulates mitochondrial alterations until the cells eventually die or fail to perform its cellular function.

We also ablated Crif1 in neonatal cardiac muscle by using *Ckmm-cre* transgenic line. In accordance with the phenotypes of *Crif1^{iCKO}* mice, *Ckmm-cre; Crif1^{f/f}* mice exhibited cardiac hypertrophy associated with mitochondrial dysfunction. The adult cardiac deletion of Crif1 followed a gradual course of hypertrophy and longer survival, while *Ckmm-cre;Crif1^{f/f}* mice showed less severe hypertrophy but early death. We speculate that the heart of *Ckmm-cre; Crif1^{f/f}* mice showed a rapid functional failure in contraction (thus causing early death) before the mitochondria developed prominent pathological defects. Whereas mitochondrial dysfunction is progressively aggravated in *Crif1^{iCKO}* cardiomyocytes, the cardiac function of the young heart seems to be much more vulnerable to early mitochondrial defects caused by Crif1 loss. Here we suggest one possibility how the adult heart is more resistant to Crif1 loss. *Crif1^{iCKO}* cardiomyocytes might activate

glycolytic pathways to compensate for the energy shortage as previously shown in Crif1 deleted MEFs [10]. The energy metabolism of fetal and immediate newborn hearts depends on glycolysis and glucose oxidization, but within 24 hours after birth, the heart rapidly switches to fatty acid oxidization for ATP production [39,40]. Although the precise mechanism is not yet known, redirection toward fetal metabolism is well-documented as a hallmark of failing hearts, and strongly suggested as an adaptive response to increase survival [39,40]. Thus, *Crif1^{iCKO}* heart also may return to fetal metabolism. However, we speculate that *Ckmm-cre; Crif1^{f/f}* hearts fail to reinforce the fetal metabolism when the massive change in gene expression profile is triggered by birth. Crif1 loss is surely a stress for cardiomyocytes, but the ultimate extrinsic signal for the fetal heart is birth [41]. Not only the metabolism, but also other differences between young and adult cardiomyocytes, such as myosin isoform composition [39], may contribute to the phenotypic differences in young and adult cardiac deletion models of Crif1.

The late onset mitochondrial respiratory disorders tend to follow a chronic course, and the early onset respiratory disorders show more severe clinical presentations [12,14]. How the "age-dependent" molecular context affects the disease progression has not yet been investigated. We suggest the two different cardiac specific Crif1 deletion mouse models, *Ckmm-cre; Crif1^{f/f}* and *Crif1^{iCKO}* mice, as early (young) onset and late (adult) onset MCM models, respectively. Further comparative analysis using *Ckmm-cre; Crif1^{f/f}* and *Crif1^{iCKO}* mice may provide insights to understand the progression of mitochondrial cardiomyopathy.

Author Contributions

Conceived and designed the experiments: JS Y.Y. Kong. Performed the experiments: JS SHL DKY. Analyzed the data: JS SHL MCK HRS JK DKY Y. Y. Kim SKI EDA KTK Y.Y. Kong. Contributed reagents/materials/analysis tools: WJP JK. Wrote the paper: JS Y.Y. Kong.

References

1. Schmidt O, Pfanner N, Meisinger C (2010) Mitochondrial protein import: from proteomics to functional mechanisms. Nat Rev Mol Cell Biol 11: 655–667.
2. Pagliarini DJ, Calvo SE, Chang B, Sheth SA, Vafai SB, et al. (2008) A mitochondrial protein compendium elucidates complex I disease biology. Cell 134: 112–123.
3. Calvo SE, Mootha VK (2010) The mitochondrial proteome and human disease. Annu Rev Genomics Hum Genet 11: 25–44.
4. Ryan MT, Hoogenraad NJ (2007) Mitochondrial-nuclear communications. Annu Rev Biochem 76: 701–722.
5. Kwon MC, Koo BK, Kim YY, Lee SH, Kim NS, et al. (2009) Essential role of CR6-interacting factor 1 (Crif1) in E74-like factor 3 (ELF3)-mediated intestinal development. J Biol Chem 284: 33634–33641.
6. Kwon MC, Koo BK, Moon JS, Kim YY, Park KC, et al. (2008) Crif1 is a novel transcriptional coactivator of STAT3. EMBO J 27: 642–653.
7. Chung HK, Yi YW, Jung NC, Kim D, Suh JM, et al. (2003) CR6-interacting factor 1 interacts with Gadd45 family proteins and modulates the cell cycle. J Biol Chem 278: 28079–28088.
8. Park KC, Song KH, Chung HK, Kim H, Kim DW, et al. (2005) CR6-interacting factor 1 interacts with orphan nuclear receptor Nur77 and inhibits its transactivation. Mol Endocrinol 19: 12–24.
9. Suh JH, Shong M, Choi HS, Lee K (2008) CR6-interacting factor 1 represses the transactivation of androgen receptor by direct interaction. Mol Endocrinol 22: 33–46.
10. Kim SJ, Kwon MC, Ryu MJ, Chung HK, Tadi S, et al. (2012) CRIF1 Is Essential for the Synthesis and Insertion of Oxidative Phosphorylation Polypeptides in the Mammalian Mitochondrial Membrane. Cell Metab 16: 274–283.
11. Skladal D, Halliday J, Thorburn DR (2003) Minimum birth prevalence of mitochondrial respiratory chain disorders in children. Brain 126: 1905–1912.
12. Pfeffer G, Chinnery PF (2011) Diagnosis and treatment of mitochondrial myopathies. Ann Med.
13. Wallace DC, Fan W, Procaccio V (2010) Mitochondrial energetics and therapeutics. Annu Rev Pathol 5: 297–348.

14. Haas RH, Parikh S, Falk MJ, Saneto RP, Wolf NI, et al. (2007) Mitochondrial disease: a practical approach for primary care physicians. Pediatrics 120: 1326–1333.
15. Kirby DM, Thorburn DR (2008) Approaches to finding the molecular basis of mitochondrial oxidative phosphorylation disorders. Twin Res Hum Genet 11: 395–411.
16. Antozzi C, Zeviani M (1997) Cardiomyopathies in disorders of oxidative metabolism. Cardiovasc Res 35: 184–199.
17. Marin-Garcia J, Goldenthal MJ (1997) Mitochondrial cardiomyopathy: molecular and biochemical analysis. Pediatr Cardiol 18: 251–260.
18. Lev D, Nissenkorn A, Leshinsky-Silver E, Sadeh M, Zeharia A, et al. (2004) Clinical presentations of mitochondrial cardiomyopathies. Pediatr Cardiol 25: 443–449.
19. Holmgren D, Wahlander H, Eriksson BO, Oldfors A, Holme E, et al. (2003) Cardiomyopathy in children with mitochondrial disease; clinical course and cardiological findings. Eur Heart J 24: 280–288.
20. Scaglia F, Towbin JA, Craigen WJ, Belmont JW, Smith EO, et al. (2004) Clinical spectrum, morbidity, and mortality in 113 pediatric patients with mitochondrial disease. Pediatrics 114: 925–931.
21. Wallace DC, Fan W (2009) The pathophysiology of mitochondrial disease as modeled in the mouse. Genes Dev 23: 1714–1736.
22. Sohal DS, Nghiem M, Crackower MA, Witt SA, Kimball TR, et al. (2001) Temporally regulated and tissue-specific gene manipulations in the adult and embryonic heart using a tamoxifen-inducible Cre protein. Circ Res 89: 20–25.
23. Bruning JC, Michael MD, Winnay JN, Hayashi T, Horsch D, et al. (1998) A muscle-specific insulin receptor knockout exhibits features of the metabolic syndrome of NIDDM without altering glucose tolerance. Mol Cell 2: 559–569.
24. Sciacco M, Bonilla E (1996) Cytochemistry and immunocytochemistry of mitochondria in tissue sections. Methods Enzymol 264: 509–521.
25. Lee SH, Yang DK, Choi BY, Lee YH, Kim SY, et al. (2009) The transcription factor Eya2 prevents pressure overload-induced adverse cardiac remodeling. J Mol Cell Cardiol 46: 596–605.

26. Veksler VI, Kuznetsov AV, Sharov VG, Kapelko VI, Saks VA (1987) Mitochondrial respiratory parameters in cardiac tissue: a novel method of assessment by using saponin-skinned fibers. Biochim Biophys Acta 892: 191–196.

27. Boudina S, Sena S, O'Neill BT, Tathireddy P, Young ME, et al. (2005) Reduced mitochondrial oxidative capacity and increased mitochondrial uncoupling impair myocardial energetics in obesity. Circulation 112: 2686–2695.

28. Li CH, Tzeng SL, Cheng YW, Kang JJ (2005) Chloramphenicol-induced mitochondrial stress increases p21 expression and prevents cell apoptosis through a p21-dependent pathway. J Biol Chem 280: 26193–26199.

29. Barrientos A, Barros MH, Valnot I, Rotig A, Rustin P, et al. (2002) Cytochrome oxidase in health and disease. Gene 286: 53–63.

30. Brandt U (2006) Energy converting NADH:quinone oxidoreductase (complex I). Annu Rev Biochem 75: 69–92.

31. Cramer WA, Zhang H, Yan J, Kurisu G, Smith JL (2006) Transmembrane traffic in the cytochrome b6f complex. Annu Rev Biochem 75: 769–790.

32. Janssen RJ, Nijtmans LG, van den Heuvel LP, Smeitink JA (2006) Mitochondrial complex I: structure, function and pathology. J Inherit Metab Dis 29: 499–515.

33. Cecchini G (2003) Function and structure of complex II of the respiratory chain. Annu Rev Biochem 72: 77–109.

34. Adoutte A, Balmefrezol M, Beisson J, Andre J (1972) The effects of erythromycin and chloramphenicol on the ultrastructure of mitochondria in sensitive and resistant strains of Paramecium. J Cell Biol 54: 8–19.

35. Sumegi B, Freeman DA, Inman L, Srere PA (1988) Studies on a possible molecular basis for the structure of mitochondrial cristae. J Mol Recognit 1: 19–24.

36. Lenk R, Penman S (1971) Morphological studies of cells grown in the absence of mitochondrial-specific protein synthesis. J Cell Biol 49: 541–546.

37. Lipton JH, McMurray WC (1977) Mitochondrial biogenesis in cultured animal cells. I. Effect of chloramphenicol on morphology and mitochondrial respiratory enzymes. Biochim Biophys Acta 477: 264–272.

38. Clark-Walker GD, Linnane AW (1967) The biogenesis of mitochondria in Saccharomyces cerevisiae. A comparison between cytoplasmic respiratory-deficient mutant yeast and chlormaphenicol-inhibited wild type cells. J Cell Biol 34: 1–14.

39. Rajabi M, Kassiotis C, Razeghi P, Taegtmeyer H (2007) Return to the fetal gene program protects the stressed heart: a strong hypothesis. Heart Fail Rev 12: 331–343.

40. Stanley WC, Recchia FA, Lopaschuk GD (2005) Myocardial substrate metabolism in the normal and failing heart. Physiol Rev 85: 1093–1129.

41. Smith R (2007) Parturition. N Engl J Med 356: 271–283.

9

A Transgenic Platform for Testing Drugs Intended for Reversal of Cardiac Remodeling Identifies a Novel 11βHSD1 Inhibitor Rescuing Hypertrophy Independently of Re-Vascularization

Oren Gordon[1][9], Zhiheng He[1][9], Dan Gilon[2], Sabine Gruener[3], Sherrie Pietranico-Cole[3], Amit Oppenheim[2], Eli Keshet[1]*

1 Departments of Developmental Biology and Cancer Research, The Hebrew University–Hadassah University Hospital, Jerusalem, Israel, 2 Department of Cardiology, The Hebrew University–Hadassah University Hospital, Jerusalem, Israel, 3 Department of Metabolic and Vascular Disease, Hoffmann-La Roche Pharmaceuticals, Basel, Switzerland

Abstract

Rationale: Rescuing adverse myocardial remodeling is an unmet clinical goal and, correspondingly, pharmacological means for its intended reversal are urgently needed.

Objectives: To harness a newly-developed experimental model recapitulating progressive heart failure development for the discovery of new drugs capable of reversing adverse remodeling.

Methods and Results: A VEGF-based conditional transgenic system was employed in which an induced perfusion deficit and a resultant compromised cardiac function lead to progressive remodeling and eventually heart failure. Ability of candidate drugs administered at sequential remodeling stages to reverse hypertrophy, enlarged LV size and improve cardiac function was monitored. Arguing for clinical relevance of the experimental system, clinically-used drugs operating on the Renin-Angiotensin-Aldosterone-System (RAAS), namely, the ACE inhibitor Enalapril and the direct renin inhibitor Aliskerin fully reversed remodeling. Remodeling reversal by these drugs was not accompanied by neovascularization and reached a point-of-no-return. Similarly, the PPARγ agonist Pioglitazone was proven capable of reversing all aspects of cardiac remodeling without affecting the vasculature. Extending the arsenal of remodeling-reversing drugs to pathways other than RAAS, a specific inhibitor of 11β-hydroxy-steroid dehydrogenase type 1 (11β HSD1), a key enzyme required for generating active glucocorticoids, fully rescued myocardial hypertrophy. This was associated with mitigating the hypertrophy-associated gene signature, including reversing the myosin heavy chain isoform switch but in a pattern distinguishable from that associated with neovascularization-induced reversal.

Conclusions: A system was developed suitable for identifying novel remodeling-reversing drugs operating in different pathways and for gaining insights into their mechanisms of action, exemplified here by uncoupling their vascular affects.

Editor: Patrick C.H. Hsieh, Institute of Clinical Medicine, National Cheng Kung University, Taiwan

Funding: This study was supported by Israel Science Foundation (ISF) and partly funded by Hoffmann-La Roche Pharmaceuticals. Sabine Gruener, Sherrie Pietranico-Cole and Jacques Himber of Hoffmann-La Roche pharmaceuticals have contributed to the design and interpretation of some of the experiments detailed in this study, in particular for the novel 11HSD1 inhibitor. This does not alter the authors' adherence to PLOS ONE policies on sharing data and materials.

Competing Interests: This study was supported by Israel Science Foundation (ISF) and partly funded by Hoffmann-La Roche pharmaceuticals. Sabine Gruener, Sherrie Pietranico-Cole and Jacques Himber of Hoffmann-La Roche pharmaceuticals have contributed to the design and interpretation of some of the experiments detailed in this study, in particular for the novel 11HSD1 inhibitor.

* E-mail: keshet@cc.huji.ac.il

[9] These authors contributed equally to this work.

Introduction

Cardiac remodeling is a broad term describing the overall functional and structural changes of the myocardium in response to chronic overload or injury [1,2,3]. Remodeling is an adaptive process enabling the heart to withstand increased mechanical stress. Unfortunately, however, at later disease stages this beneficial adaptive process almost always becomes maladaptive and a prognostic determinant of heart failure [4].

Correspondingly, therapeutic approaches to reverse maladaptive remodeling are currently considered a prime clinical goal. In principle, intended reversal can be attained through two different approaches: correcting its underlying cause, e.g. by restoring perfusion to the ischemic myocardium or, alternatively, by a direct pharmacological intervention without necessarily rectifying the underlying cause [5].

On the basis of findings that the renin angiotensin aldosterone system (RAAS) plays a major role in the remodeling pathogenesis [6] RAAS inhibitors were developed and proven useful in alleviating clinical symptoms associated with adverse remodeling, including using Angiotensin converting enzyme inhibitors (ACEIs), Angiotensin receptor blockers (ARBs) and direct renin inhibitors (DRIs) [7]. Unfortunately, however, in most cases currently used drugs come up short in preventing further disease progression [8] thus begging for introduction of new and more efficient drugs. This might require expanding the drug arsenal to include not only drugs belonging to the RAAS family but also drugs affecting other pathways, e.g., cardiac metabolism. The peroxisome proliferator-activated receptor family (PPARα, β/δ, γ) of nuclear receptor transcription factors is an important regulator of cardiac metabolism and was harnessed for targeting cardiac metabolism [9]. A PPARγ agonist was indeed capable of attenuating left ventricular remodeling and failure in a coronary ligation model [10]. Yet, reversing remodeling in heart failure remains a major challenge and new opportunities continue to be sought (for a recent review see #5).

Suitable animal models of heart failure have been instrumental for testing the potential utility of remodeling-reversing drugs and elucidating their mode of action [11,12,13]. In these model systems myocardial insults are inflicted using either a surgical procedure (e.g. ligating the left coronary artery (LAD) [14]) or a pharmacological intervention (e.g., administrating the β1 adren-ergic receptor agonist isoproterenol [13]). To avoid confounding factors associated with these manipulations, genetic systems for inducing cardiac hypertrophy were developed, including trans-genic mice expressing an activated Akt1 [15] gene or transgenic rats over-expressing the renin gene [11]. Yet, a number of large clinical trials prompted by encouraging preclinical studies obtained with the aid of these animal models did not meet expectations [16]. This likely reflects the fact that different insults converging on the common pathway of myocardial remodeling are accompanied by additional processes that might differ between different pathologies not accurately reproduced by the particular animal model. Hence, a complementary animal model displaying gradual progression of ischemic heart disease (IHD) to heart failure and also better amenable to experimental manipulations is highly desired. To this end, we have developed a transgenic system based on conditional (and reversible) blockade of VEGF signaling for the purpose of generating myocardial perfusion deficits of escalating magnitudes. This manipulation leads to development of IHD closely resembling dilated ischemic cardiomyopathy and stepwise development of all hallmarks of cardiac remodeling eventually culminating in heart failure [17]. The system is particularly suitable for studying remodeling reversal as evidenced by complete reversal following VEGF-mediated myocardial re-vascularization [18]. Moreover, because the disruption of coordi-nated cardiac hypertrophy and angiogenesis contribute to transition to heart failure [15], the system provides a unique opportunity to uncouple the beneficial activity of the tested drug on reversing myocardial hypertrophy from its vascular effect. Another advantage of the model for studying remodeling and its reversal is its slow, stepwise development thus allowing attempted reversal at different progressive stages. Indeed, we have previously shown that there is a point-of-no-return beyond which remodeling is no longer reversible via re-vascularization [18] and the question remains whether a similar restriction point also exists for drug-induced reversal.

Here we provide a proof of principle for the general utility of our experimental platform for the discovery of remodeling-reversing drugs by first corroborating the efficacy of known drugs affecting the RAAS pathway, namely, the ACE inhibitor Enalapril and the direct renin inhibitor Aliskiren, as well as of the PPARγ agonist Pioglitazone. Exemplifying the utility of the experimental system for the discovery of new agents capable of reversing cardiac hypertrophy are finding reported here employing a specific 11β-hydroxysteroid dehydrogenase type 1 (11β HSD1) inhibitor. 11β HSD1 catalyses intracellular regeneration of active glucocorticoids (cortisol, corticosterone) from inert 11-keto forms in target tissues, amplifying local action [19]. Transgenic mice overexpressing 11β-HSD1 selectively in adipose tissue faithfully recapitulate metabolic syndrome. Conversely, 11β-HSD1 knockout mice have a 'cardio-protective' phenotype [20,21]. Here, we show that a newly developed inhibitor of 11β-HSD1 (Hoffmann-La Roche) com-pletely reverses cardiac hypertrophy even in the face of persisting compromised perfusion and a compromised cardiac function.

Materials and Methods

Transgenic mice and conditional modulations of VEGF signaling

A bitransgenic system for organ-specific, tetracycline-regulated transgene expression was used. Heart-specific induction was achieved by using a transgenic driver line in which tTA expression is driven by a myosin heavy chain (MHC) heart-specific promoter [22]. The tet–sVEGF-R1 transgenic line encodes a tetracycline-inducible protein composed of an IgG1–Fc tail fused to the extracellular domain of VEGF-R1 (corresponding to amino acid residues 1–631 of human VEGF-R1 containing the ligand-binding domain but lacking the transmembrane and cytoplasmic domains). Induction of sVEGF-R1 in double-transgenic mice was accom-plished by tetracycline withdrawal and the termination of sVEGF-R1 by tetracycline addition (0.5 mg/ml tetracycline and 3% sucrose in the drinking water). Animals were sacrificed using 200 mg/kg pentobarbital IP, followed by removal of the heart. All animal experiments conform to the Guide for the Care and Use of Laboratory Animals published by the US National Institutes of Health and were done under approval of the Hebrew University ethics committee, approval number- MD-10127064.

Drugs

All drugs were administered for 3 weeks. Enalapril (Sigma) was administered in drinking water (50 mg/L). Aliskiren (Novartis) was administered using 2004 Alzet miniosmotic pumps by Durect Corp. (50 mg/kg/d). Pioglitazone (ChemPacific) and the 11β-HSD1 inhibitor, Roche Compound (Cpd)-A (Hoffmann-La Roche) were administered in a food admix (15 mg/kg and 60 mg/kg, respectivly). Isoproterenol (Sigma) was administered to 5–6 weeks old C57BL/6JOLaHsd male mice S.C. (15 mg/kg/ day) for 5 weeks.

Immunohistochemistry

4% paraformaldehyde-fixed paraffin-embedded specimens were used. Sections (5 um) were rehydrated and antigen was retrieved by 0.1% pronase (Sigma) for 20 min at room temperature. Endogenous peroxidase activity was quenched with hydrogen peroxide 3% in PBS for 15 minutes at room temperature. Sections were blocked by incubation in 1% BSA (Amresco) in PBS at room temperature followed by overnight incubation with primary antibody: mouse monoclonal anti-myosin (M8421: skeletal, slow; 1:2000, Sigma). Endothelial cells were visualized by using *Bandeiraea simplicifolia* isolectin B4 staining.

RNA analysis

For real-time PCR analysis, cDNA was generated from 1 µg of total RNA, extracted from the apex of the left ventricle, by using Verso cDNA kit (Thermo scientific) and the respective primers. Samples were normalized according to L19 mRNA levels by SYBR green real-time PCR (StepOnePlus™ Real-Time PCR System, Applied Biosystems).

Echocardiography

Transthoracic echocardiography was performed on shallow anesthetized mice (ketamine and xylazine 200 mg/kg IM and 10 mg/kg IP). For more details please refer to the supplemental information. The high-resolution ultrasound imaging system Vevo 770 (VisualSonics, Toronto, Canada) was used to perform two-dimensional (B-mode) and motion-mode (M-mode) imaging using a mechanical transducer (RMV707B) synchronized to the electrocardiographic signal. The transducer had a central frequency of 40 MHz, a focal length of 6 mm, a frame rate of 30 Hz, and an 8×8 mm field of view with spatial resolution of 30 µm. A 2D-directed M-mode image of the left ventricular short axis was taken just at the level of the papillary muscles, and measurements were performed in triplicate by using the leading-edge convention for myocardial borders, as defined by the American Society of Echocardiography [23]. The following parameters were measured: left ventricular end-diastolic diameter (LVEDD); left ventricular end-systolic diameter (LVESD) and heart rate. The percentage fractional shortening (%SF) was calculated as %SF = [(LVEDD - LVESD)/(LVEDD)] $\times$ 100.

Statistical analysis

Numerical data are the mean $\pm$ standard error. Statistical significance was determined by using student's t-test.

Results

A transgenic system for generating a volume overload-driven cardiac remodeling

Previously, we developed a transgenic system where VEGF blockade led to microvascular insufficiency and resulted in development of an IHD-like phenotype [17,18]. Briefly, because VEGF is indispensable for adjusting the coronary microvasculature to match dynamic changes in oxygen supply and demand, inhibition of myocardial VEGF signaling generates a perfusion deficit the magnitude of which depends on the duration of VEGF blockade [17]. A tetracycline-regulated VEGF decoy receptor (sVEGF-R1) is conditionally induced in the heart (pending on the absence or presence of doxycycline in the drinking water) using a cardiomyocyte-specific promoter driving expression of a trans-activator protein (see Fig 1A for a scheme and "Methods" for experimental details). In agreement with previous studies [17,18], when switched 'on' at an early post-natal age and maintained in the 'on' mode for 9 weeks, sVEGF-R1production in double transgenic (dTg) mice causes microvascular density (MVD) reduction and a markedly reduced as monitored by echocardiography and evidenced by a reduced fractional shortening (left lanes in Figs 1B and 1C). Volume overload resulting from a compromised cardiac function is likely the cause of apparent remodeling manifested by LV enlargement (left lanes in Figs 1D and 1E) and myocardial hypertrophy (left lanes in Figs 1F and 1G).

Harnessing the transgenic system for measuring efficacy of remodeling reversing drugs - feasibility testing using ACE inhibitors

To prove the general utility of our experimental platform to identify pharmaceuticals capable of reversing remodeling, we first tested the performance of a drug already in clinical use for this purpose, namely, the ACE inhibitor Enalapril. To this end we induced LV remodeling as described above. Enalapril was then added and heart retrieved for analysis 3 additional weeks later. Importantly, Enalapril action was tested under condition of ongoing VEGF blockade as indeed reflected by the persistence of the MVD deficit (Fig.1B). Yet, Enalapril treatment led to marked reduction of LV diameter (Figs. 1D&E), fully reversed myocardial hypertrophy (Fig.1F) and partially rectified the compromised contractile function evidenced by improved fractional shortening (Fig.1C).

Reversing cardiac remodeling by the direct renin inhibitor Aliskiren

Direct renin inhibitors have been developed in an attempt to modulate the RAAS more effectively, reasoning that they may provide additional protection over other RAAS inhibitors like ACEIs or ARBs. Aliskiren, a direct renin inhibitor recently introduced (Novartis) as an anti-hypertension drug, was shown to also reverse remodeling in a coronary ligation-induced MI model independently of its effect on blood pressure [24]. To determine whether Aliskiren will have a beneficial effect in our model, we administered Aliskiren to animals in which myocardial remodeling has been pre-induced using an identical protocol to that described above for Enalapril. Results showed that Aliskiren was as effective as Enalapril in reversing remodeling (Fig.1). Interestingly, the combined effect of Enalapril and Aliskiren failed to show an additive effect over that shown for each drug administered alone (Fig.1). Results thus demonstrate the utility of this experimental system for screening new candidate drugs intended for reversing remodeling.

Advanced stages of remodeling are refractory to drug-induced reversal

A major concern in intended rescue of adverse remodeling is that it may reach a refractory stage where it is no longer responsive to remodeling-reversing drugs. We have recently used the system to show that restoring adequate perfusion to the ischemic myocardium via VEGF-induced neovascularization can rescue remodeling at early stages of IHD but fails to do so at an advanced stage distinguished by critical levels of fibrosis [18]. To determine whether a similar point-of-no-return also exists for drug-induced reversal, we have attempted reversal by Enalapril 32 weeks from the onset of VEGF blockade, i.e., a time point during progressive remodeling beyond the point-of-no return for re-vascularization-induced reversal [18]. As shown in Fig.2 and contrary to the earlier time point of 9 weeks post-induction where remodeling was still reversible (Fig.1), Enalapril failed to do so by 32 days post-induction as evidenced by no decrease in LV size and no resolution of hypertrophy. This was further validated through gene expression analysis of remodeling-associated genes (Fig S1 and see below).

Reversing cardiac remodeling by the PPARγ agonist Pioglitazone in an angiogenesis-independent manner

The PPAR system play an important role in regulating myocardial metabolism in health and disease [25]. Its role in heart remodeling is evidenced by findings that mice with a

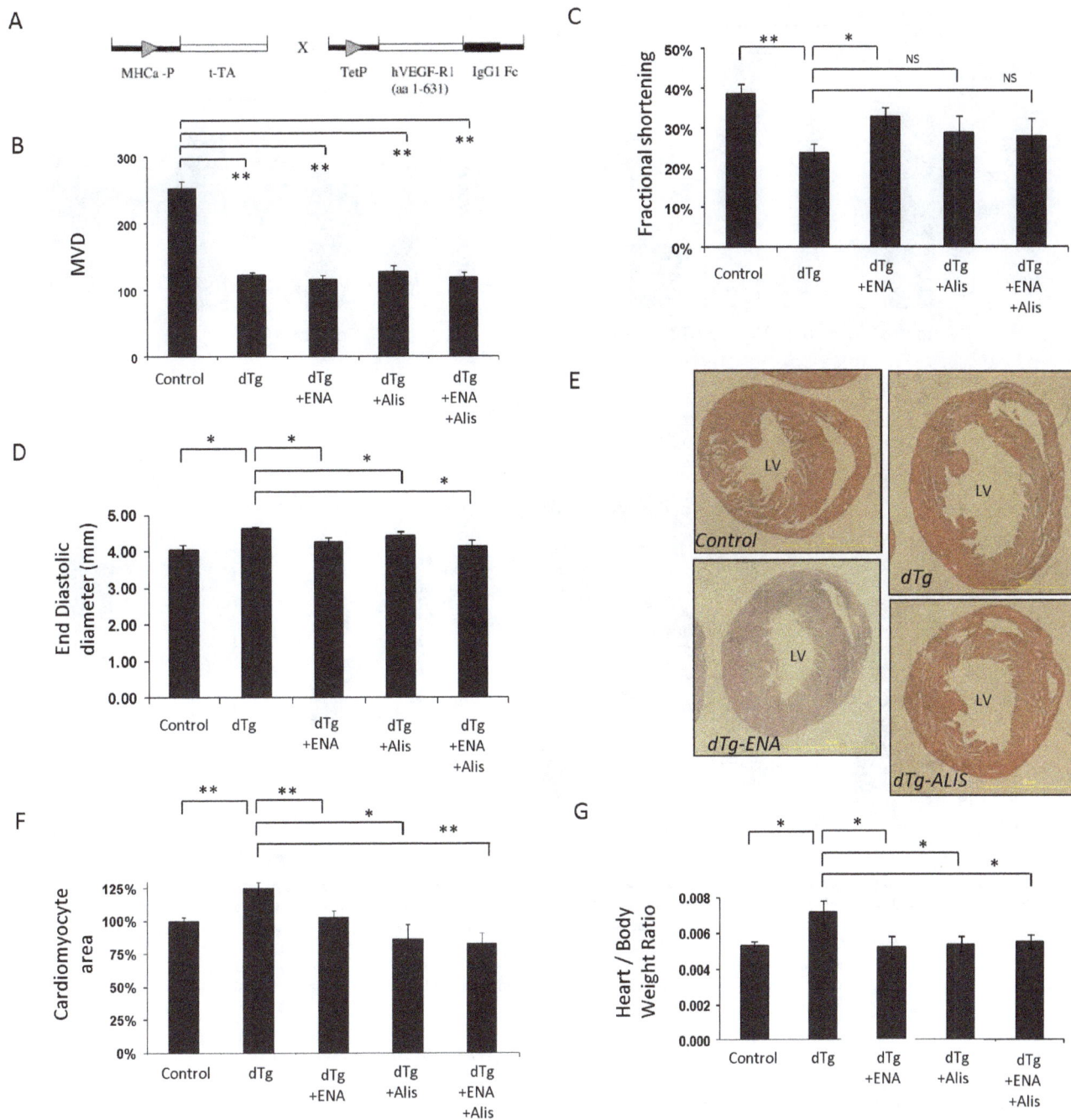

Figure 1. A novel experimental system for testing remodeling reversing drugs shows RAAS inhibition reverses remodeling independently of improving perfusion. (A) Schematic representation of the transgenic lines used in the bi-transgenic inducible system. (B) Quantification of micro-vessels density (MVD), expressed as the number of endothelial cell-specific lectin-positive capillaries per high-power field (HPF). MVD was determined after 12 weeks of sVEGF-R1 induction during the last 3 weeks of which some of the dTg mice were treated with Enalapril (ENA) or Aliskiren (Alis) or both. N = 6–16 mice per treatment group and 3 HPFs were measured for each mouse. (C) Fractional shortening measured by M-mode Echocardiography in mice treated as in B. N = 5 mice. (D) End diastolic LV diameter measured by M-mode Echocardiography. (E) Representative axial sections at the level of the papillary muscle showing drug-induced reduction of LV size. (F) Cardiomyocyte area was measured from H&E-stained sections using Image J software and was standardized to littermate controls. N = 6-12 mice and 25-30 cardiomyocytes were analyzed for each section. (G) Heart to body weight ratio in the same mice shown in F. * $P < 0.05$, ** $P < 0.001$, NS = not statistically significant.

cardiomyocyte-specific knockout of PPARγ develop cardiac hypertrophy [26]. Correspondingly, modulating the PPAR pathway was recognized as an attractive therapeutic avenue for treating cardiac remodeling and Pioglitazone, a PPARγ agonist, was shown to attenuate cardiac remodeling and heart failure after experimental myocardial infarction (MI) [10].

To determine whether the metabolic stress incurred in our experimental model also leads to changes in expression of genes of the PPAR system, we first examined the expression levels of

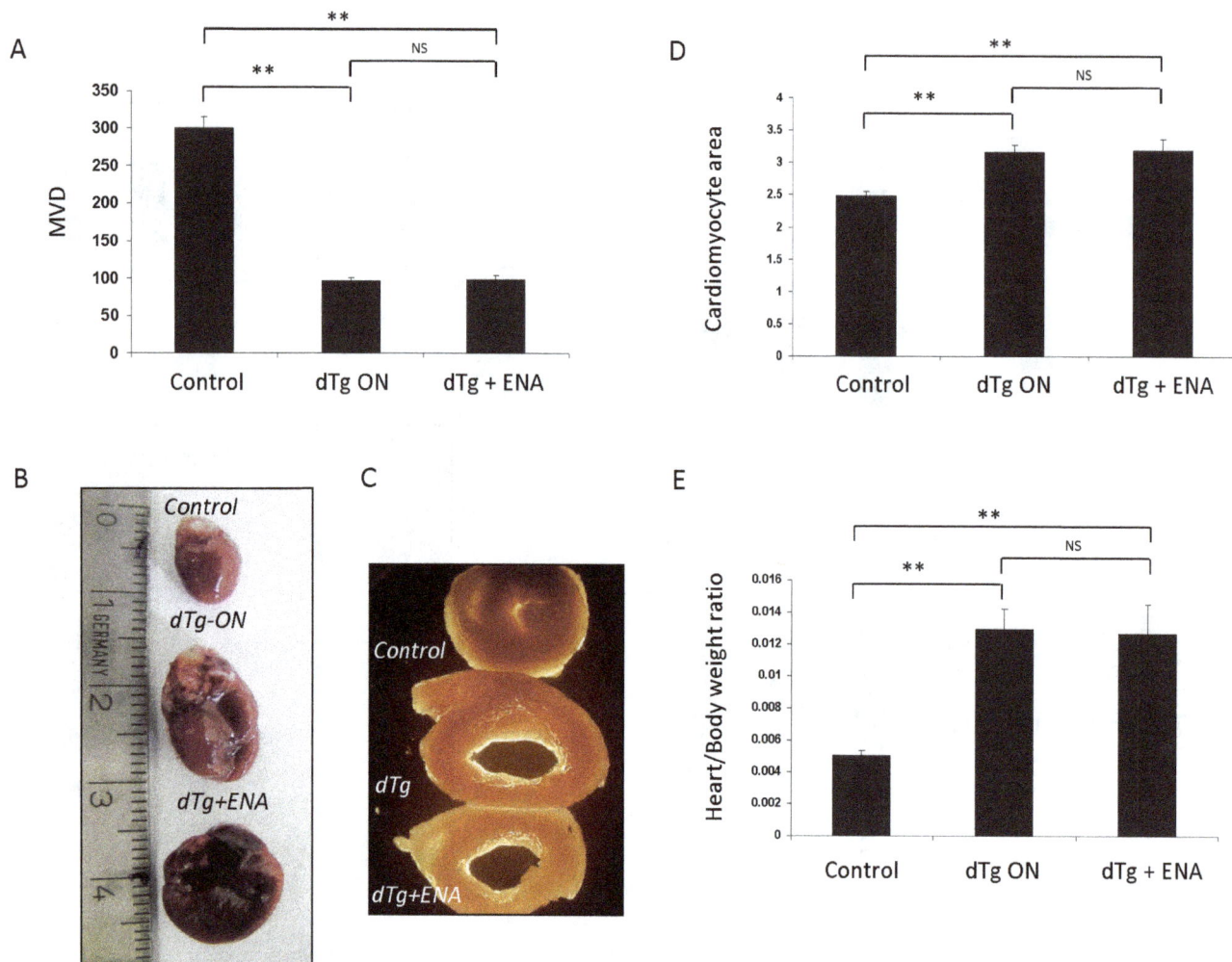

Figure 2. A Point-of-no-return for pharmacological reversal of heart remodeling. (*A*) MVD was determined after 35weeks of sVEGF-R1 induction during the last 3 weeks of which some of the dTg mice were treated with Enalapril (ENA). N = 3 mice per treatment group and 3 HPFs were measured for each mouse. (*B*) Gross examination of cardiac size and comparison between control (upper), dTg at 35 week induction (middle) and dTg after 32 weeks induction and 3 weeks of Enalapril treatment (lower). (*C*) Gross sections at the level of the papillary muscles of control and dTg hearts with and without 3 weeks treatment, as indicated. (*D*) Cardiomyocyte area in control and dTg hearts with or without the indicated treatment. N = 3 mice and 25-30 cardiomyocytes were analyzed for each section. (*E*) Heart to body weight ratio in the same mice shown in D.

PPARγ and PGC1α, a co-activator of the PPARs during heart remodeling and following its reversal. As shown in Fig.3A, both genes were indeed strongly downregulated in the remodeled myocardium and returned to normal expression level upon alleviating the perfusion deficit and the resolution of myocardial remodeling. To examine whether, similarly to its activity in the coronary ligation model, Pioglitazone can reverse remodeling and improve cardiac function in our model as well, we performed similar experiments to those described above for inhibitors of the RAAS pathway. Pioglitazone was found to improve cardiac function evidenced by increased fractional shortening (Fig. 3B) and to resolve cardiac remodeling evidenced by reducing LV size (Fig 3C and D) and reversing myocardial hypertrophy (Figs 3E and F). Notably, these beneficial actions of Pioglitazone took place without improving the vascular deficit (Fig.3G). Note that in accordance to previous reports, Pioglitazone affects cardiac function and end-diastolic diameter in control mice (Fig 3B and C), these differences where statistically insignificant in this study.

Reversing cardiac hypertrophy by 11β-hydroxysteroid dehydrogenase type 1 (11β HSD1) inhibition

11β-HSD1 catalyzes intracellular regeneration of active gluco-corticoids (cortisol, corticosterone) from inert 11-keto forms in target tissues thus amplifying local action on the glucocorticoid receptor and possibly the mineralocorticoid receptor [19]. The possible involvement of 11β-HSD1 in cardiac remodeling was prompted by findings that 11β-HSD1 gene expression was increased in experimentally induced hypertrophy, *in vitro* [27] and findings that 11β-HSD1 knockout mice show enhanced angiogenesis and improved heart function in an MI model [20,21].

To examine in our model whether the level of 11β-HSD1 changes in accordance with the remodeling status, we compared relative levels of expression of the endogenous gene in control and remodeled myocardium, as well as following neovascularization-induced reversal (Fig.4A). Result showed that remodeling is associated with 2-fold increase in 11β-HSD1 expression and that 11β-HSD1 expression returns to normal levels following restora-tion of normal perfusion via VEGF-mediated neovascularization,

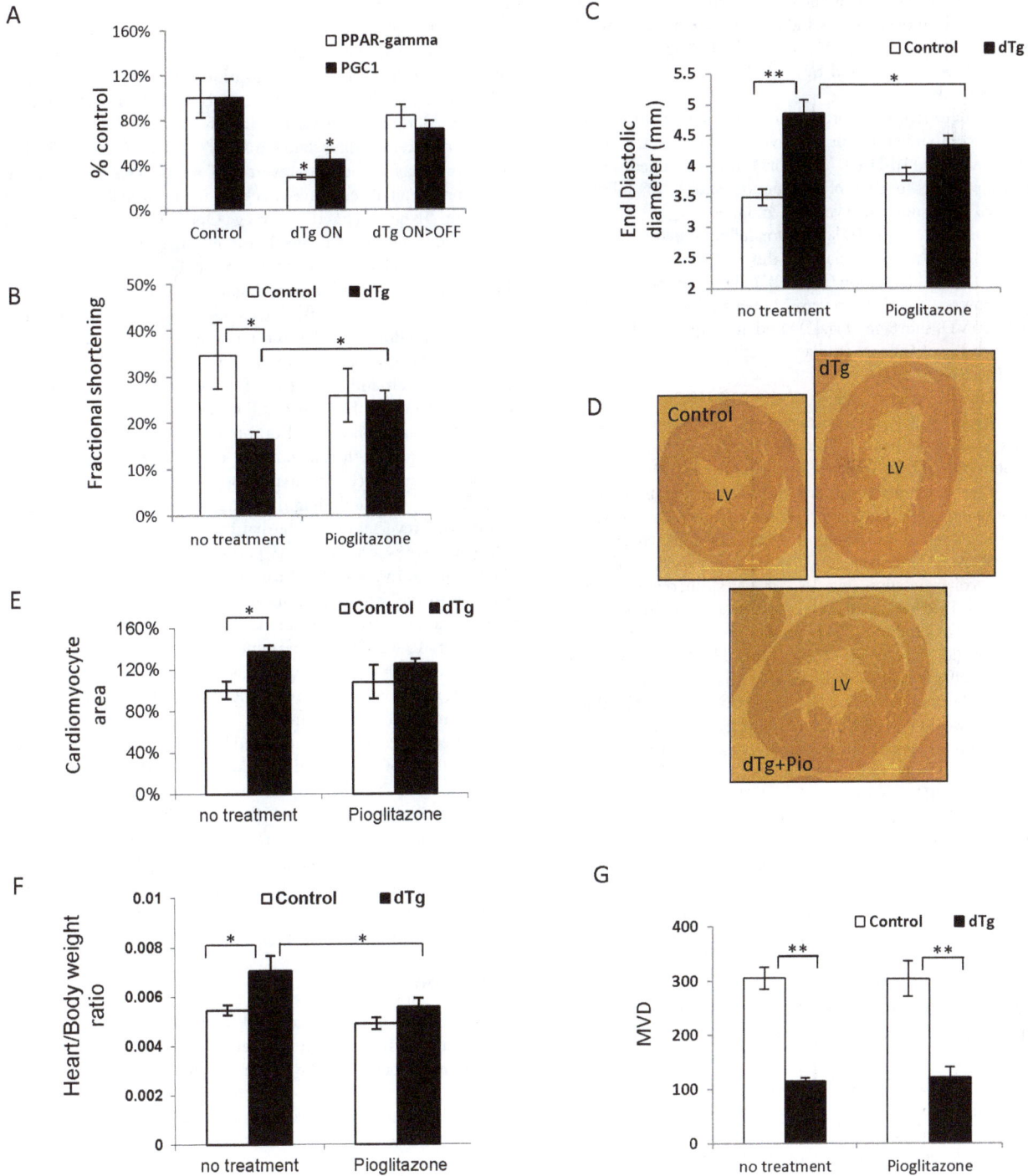

Figure 3. Pioglitazone, a PPARγ agonist, reverses cardiac remodeling without effecting vascular density. (A) Real time PCR results for PPARγ and PGC1α after 12 weeks of sVEGF-R1 induction (dTg-ON), during the last 3 weeks of which in some of the dTg mice, sVEGF-R1 was de-induced (dTg-ON>OFF). (B) Fractional shortening was determined after 12 weeks of sVEGF-R1 induction during the last 3 weeks of which some of the dTg mice were treated with Pioglitazone. N = 4–6 mice. (C) End diastolic LV diameter. (D) Representative axial sections at the level of the papillary muscle showing drug-induced reduction of LV size. (E) Cardiomyocyte area standardized to littermate controls. N = 4–6 mice and 25–30 cardiomyocytes were analyzed for each section. (F) Heart to body weight ratio in the same mice shown in E. (G) MVD. N = 4–6 mice per treatment group and 3 HPFs were measured for each mouse. * P<0.05, ** P<0.001, NS = not statistically significant.

thus prompting the proposition that elevated 11β-might is required to maintain the remodeling state and hence its inhibition might lead to reversion.

To test this proposition, we attempted remodeling reversal by a novel 11β-HSD1 inhibitor, Roche Compound A (Hoffmann-La Roche)(Cpd A for short). Preparatory experiments have exhibited up to 90% inhibition of 11β-HSD1 enzymatic activity when used at the same dose as the dose applied in the experiments described below (Fig.S2). Remodeling was induced as described above for the testing of RAAS inhibitors and a PPARγ agonist (VEGF blockade for 9 weeks) followed by 11β-HSD1 inhibitor administration for 3 weeks.

Usually, progressive deterioration towards heart failure in our system is accompanied by progressive weight loss which was prevented by the 11β-HSD1inhibitor: mice re-gained normal weight comparable to that of littermate controls or following neovascularization-induced reversal (Fig.S3).

Remarkably, the 11β-HSD1 inhibitor fully rescued myocardial hypertrophy and was as efficient in this regard as hypertrophy reversal via neovascularization (Figs. 4B and C). Noteworthy, 11β-HSD1 inhibition acted to reverse hypertrophy in face of a remaining MVD shortage (Fig.4D) and its sequela. 11β-HSD1 inhibition did not affect cardiac function and end-diastolic diameter (Fig.4E-G).

To validate the general utility of the 11β-HSD1 inhibitor in reversing hypertrophy, we examined its performance in an independent model of heart failure, namely the widely-used model of Isoproterenol-induced cardiac hypertrophy and heart failure [11,13,28]. Isoproterenol (ISO), a synthetic catecholamine and a sympathomimetic β-adrenergic receptor agonist, causes severe stress to the myocardium resulting in an infarct-like necrosis of heart muscle. Mice were treated with ISO for 5 weeks resulting in decreased cardiac function (Fig 5A, left lanes), increased cardiac size (Fig 5B and C, left lanes) and significant cardiac hypertrophy (Fig 5D and E, left lanes). When administered together with Isoproterenol (a 'preventive mode'), the 11β-HSD1 inhibitor mitigated the effects of Isoproterenol on cardiac function and size and completely prevented cardiac hypertrophy (Fig 5). When added after 3 weeks of Isoproterenol treatment, i.e., after cardiac function has already been compromised (data not shown), the 11β-HSD1 inhibitor was still capable of completely reversing hypertrophy (Fig 5D and E) even though there was no significant improvement of cardiac function (Fig 5A) or LV end-diastolic diameter (Fig 5B). Likewise, the 11β-HSD1 inhibitor acted to reverse the hypertrophy-associated gene signature in a similar manner to that observed for neovascularization-induced reversal (Fig S3 and see below). Thus, 11β-HSD1 inhibition was proven capable of reversing pathological hypertrophy in two independent experimental models initiated by two different insults.

Rescue of hypertrophy is associated with reversing the hypertrophic gene signature, including of the Myosin heavy chain isoform shift

Cardiac remodeling is associated with extensive alterations in myocardial gene expression and correspondingly, its reversal is likely to be reflected in a return to normal level of expression of genes mediating these pathways. Considering the complex nature of heart remodeling and the different sub-processes involved, different compounds employed for intended reversal and operating on different biochemical pathways are likely to produce differential responses with regard to changes in gene expression. Opportunities provided by the VEGF-based conditional transgenic system to monitor remodeling reversal induced by different treatment modalities (neovascularization vs. pharmacologic intervention) and different drugs has provided a suitable access to this issue.

Among the different pathways implicated in cardiac remodeling outstanding are neuro-hormonal activation, multiple metabolic adaptations, and activation of fibrosis-promoting pathways (e.g. components of the TGF-β pathway) [3]. Here we examined representative genes of these respective pathways, namely BNP, a

clinically used neuro-hormonal marker of heart failure induced by wall stress, the glucose transporter Glut1, an hypoxia-induced gene upregulated in cardiac ischemia[22, 23] and Periostin, a matricellular protein promoting matrix organization following cardiac injury under the regulation of Angiotensin II and TGFβ [29,30]. As expected. All three genes were markedly (5 to15-fold) upregulated during heart remodeling (lanes marked as 'dTg ON' in Fig.6A). Neovascularization-induced reversal of remodeling led to down-regulation of all three genes back to their normal low level of expression (lanes marked as 'dTg ON>OFF' in Fig.6A). In contrast, drug-induced reversal was effective in downregulating some but not all genes. More interestingly, drugs operating on different pathways exhibited a differential response towards the different target genes. Thus, RAAS inhibition by Enalapril led to reduction of Glut1 and Periostin but not of BNP, the PPARγ agonist Pioglitazone led to a reduction of Glut1 and BNP but not of Periostin levels and the 11β-HSD1 inhibitor led to reduction of BNP and Periostin, but not of Glut1 levels (Fig.6A). Analysis of 11β-HSD1 inhibition in the Isoproterenol-induced model yielded similar results by restoring normal levels of expression of ANP (another marker of cardiac hypertrophy and periostin but not of Glut1 (Fig.S4). These finding thus suggest different points of entry for intended reversal of myocardial hypertrophy.

A gene expression change of particular functional significance taking place in hypertrophied cardiomyocytes is a myosin isoform switch from the fast-contracting myosin heavy chain MyHCα to the less energy consuming but slower contracting MyHCβ [31]. We, therefore, wished to determine whether the novel hypertrophy –reversing drug described herein acting through 11β-HSD1 inhibition is also capable of reversing the MyHC isoform shift. As shown in figure 6B, expression of MyHCβ was markedly upregulated in remodeled hearts (dTg-ON) while MyHCα was unchanged. Neovascularization-induced reversal of hypertrophy (dTg ON>OFF) resulted in downregulation of MyHCβ expression back to control levels and 11β-HSD1 inhibition had a similar though smaller effect. These results were corroborated using MyHCβ-specific immune-staining (Fig.6C) thus demonstrating the ability of 11β-HSD1 inhibition to alter myofilament composition within cardiomyocytes as a component of its overall activity in hypertrophy reversal.

Discussion

Meeting the urgent clinical need for means to reverse adverse cardiac remodeling has been hampered by the fact that commonly used animal models employed for testing candidate drugs are confounded by the ramifications of surgical interventions and other confounding factors like massive cell death and inflammation usually associated with these models. More importantly, currently used models do not faithfully recapitulate the slow and progressive nature of heart failure development. These confounding factors are filtered-out in the transgenic system we have developed and, importantly, LV remodeling develops in this system in a slow and progressive manner. These properties provide a unique opportunity to not only examine the efficacy of candidate drugs, in general, but also to compare its potential utility when applied at consecutive stages of progressive remodeling. This is exemplified here by showing that Enalapril is effective in reversing LV remodeling when administered at an early stage but not when administered at a late stage. This finding suggests that there is a restricted time window for an attempted reversal of myocardial remodeling, similarly to the point-of-no-return we have recently demonstrated for neovascularization-induced reversal [18]. A

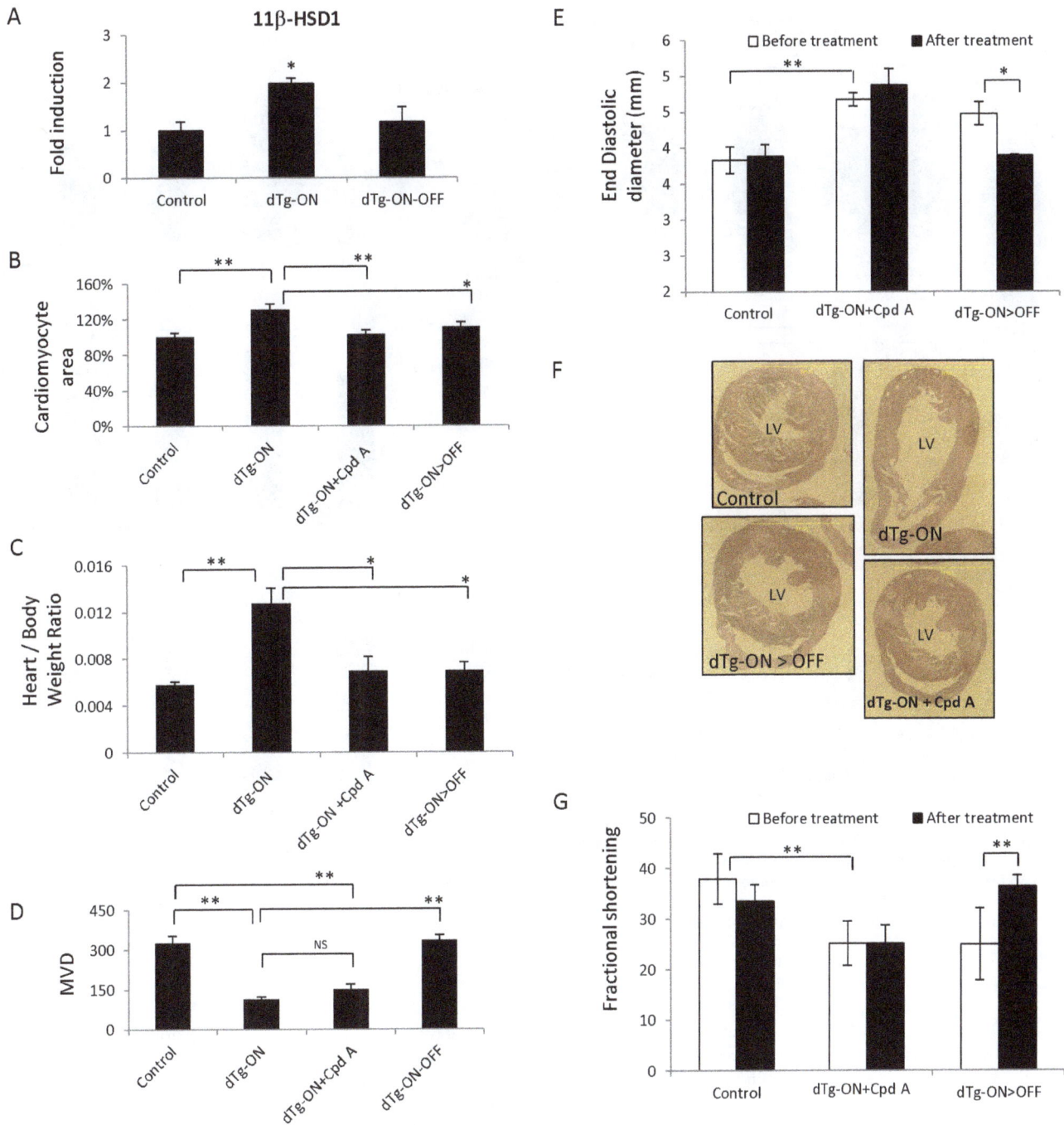

Figure 4. 11β-HSD1 inhibiton reverses cardiac hypertrophy without effecting vascular density and cardiac function. (*A*) Real time PCR results for 11β-HSD1 after 12 weeks of sVEGF-R1 induction (dTg-ON), during the last 3 weeks of which in some of the dTg mice, sVEGF-R1 was de-induced (dTg-ON>OFF). (*B*) Cardiomyocyte area standardized to littermate controls, was determined after 12 weeks of sVEGF-R1 induction during the last 3 weeks of which some of the dTg mice were treated with 11β-HSD1 inhibitor (Roche Cpd A) or de-induced (dTg-ON>OFF). N = 4–5 mice and 25–30 cardiomyocytes were analyzed for each section. (*C*) Heart to body weight ratio in the same mice shown in B (*D*) MVD. N = 4–5 mice per treatment group and 3 HPFs were measured for each mouse. (*E*) End diastolic LV diameter. (*F*) Representative axial sections at the level of the papillary muscle. (*G*) Fractional shortening measured in mice treated as in B. N = 4–5 mice. * $P < 0.05$, ** $P < 0.001$, NS = not statistically significant.

future challenge to be addressed using this experimental platform is to identify drugs effective at the latest stage of remodeling.

An issue to be considered is the potential added value in using two or more drugs together. Here we examined the combined action of Enalapril and Aliskiren, drugs inhibiting two different components of the RAAS pathway, but did not observe any added value over the solitary beneficial effect of each drug. This result might explain the failure of Aliskiren to reveres remodeling after MI in a clinical trial in which Aliskiren was added to standard therapy [32]. Perhaps more advantageous will be an approach of a combined use of drugs operating on different remodeling-promoting pathways. This proposition is supported by our initial

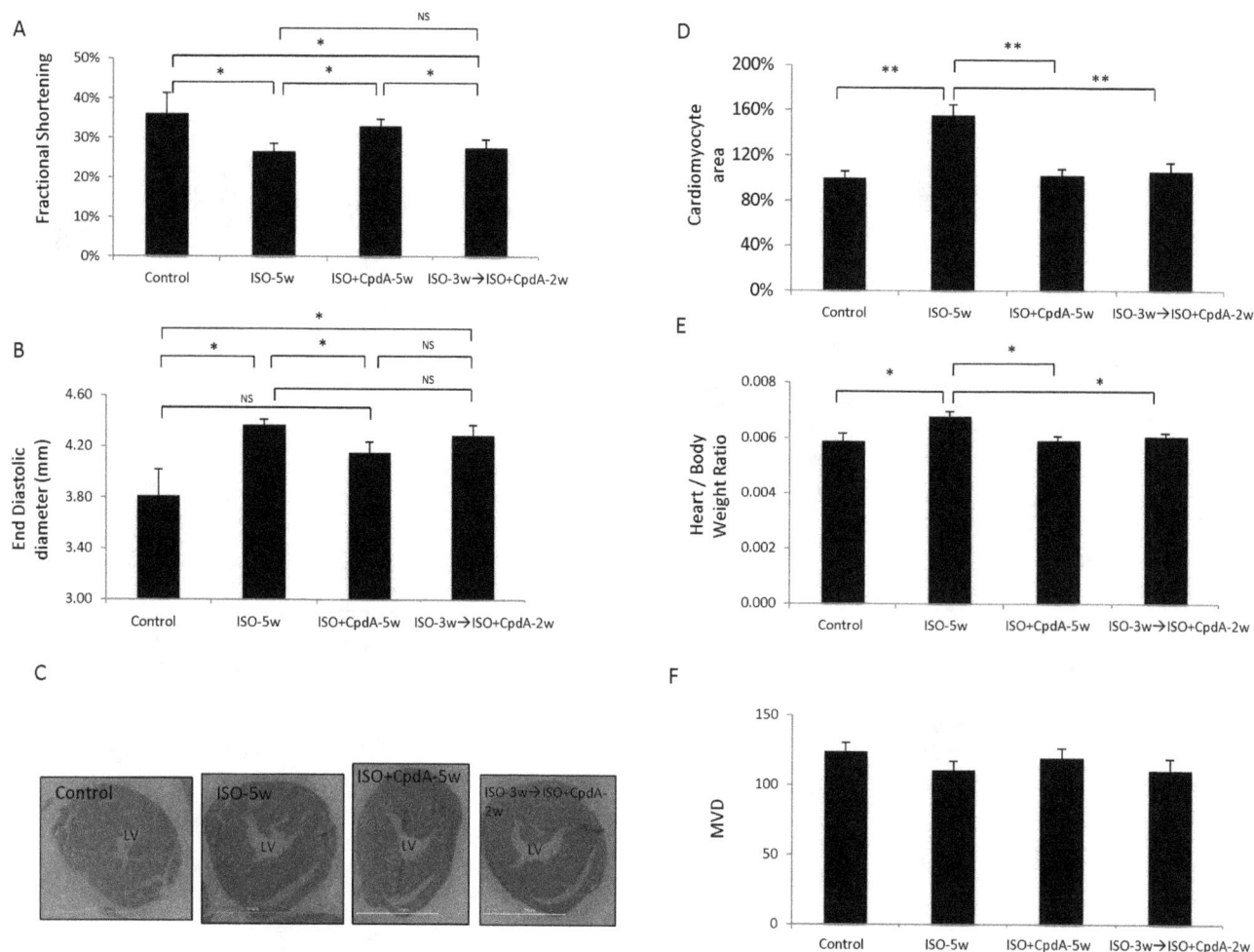

Figure 5. Pharmacological inhibition of 11β HSD1 reverses cardiac hypertrophy in a model of Isoproterenol-induced heart failure.
(*A*) Fractional shortening measured in mice treated for 5 weeks with Isoproterenol(ISO-5w) alone, Isoproterenol together with 11β-HSD1 inhibitor (ISO+CpdA-5w) or treated with Isoproterenol alone for 3 weeks and by Isoproterenol and 11β-HSD1 inhibitor for an additional 2 weeks (ISO-3w→ISO+CpdA-2w). N = 5–7 mice per treatment group. (*B*) End diastolic LV diameter in the same mice as in A. (*C*) Representative axial sections at the level of the papillary muscle. (*D*) Cardiomyocyte area standardized to littermate controls. N = 5–7 mice and 25–30 cardiomyocytes were analyzed for each section. (*E*) Heart to body weight ratio. (*F*) MVD. N = 5–7 mice per treatment group and 3 HPFs were measured for each mouse. * $P<0.05$, ** $P<0.001$, NS = not statistically significant.

gene expression analysis where a successful remodeling reversal induced by drugs operating on three different pathways, namely the RAAS pathway, cardiac metabolism and glucocorticoid biogenesis, was in all cases associated with gene expression changes reflecting the return to a normal state, however, different upregulated genes signifying remodeling where downregulated in each case. A more comprehensive expression analysis may provide better rationales for using particular drug combinations with an additive (or even synergistic) value.

Because remodeling is a natural response secondary to a compromised cardiac output, treatment modalities intended for reversing adverse remodeling can either rectify the primary cause (e.g. perfusion insufficiency) or, alternatively, directly target the remodeling process without necessarily correcting its underlying cause. For RAAS inhibitors, it has been argued that at least some of its effects on heart remodeling and its reversal are mediated by promoting angiogenesis [33]. Here we took advantage of our ability to fully block angiogenesis to demonstrate that contrary to this report complete reversal by Enalapril or Aliskiren could be achieved in the complete absence of angiogenesis. In fact, the

beneficial reversal effect exerted by all four drugs examined in this study was achieved without any angiogenesis response, arguing that drug-induced reversal, at least by these drugs targeting these pathways is feasible even without rectifying the perfusion deficit.

11β-HSD1 inhibition was proved by this study as a novel approach to effectively reverse pathological myocardial hypertrophy. While previous studies have shown that 11β-HSD1 knockout mice have a better post-MI heart function [20,21], this is the first study showing the potential utility of pharmacological inhibition of local glucocorticoid activation, in general and of 11β-HSD1 inhibition, specifically, to efficiently reverse pathological hypertrophy. Our findings that this key enzyme in glucocorticoid activation is strongly upregulated in the course of hypertrophy and, in turn, down regulated upon resolution of hypertrophy via neovascularization has provided incentive to examine a causative role for 11β-HSD1 in the process and for its pharmacologic inhibition. Interestingly, 11β-HSD1 inhibition also led to its reduced expression (Fig S5) suggesting a direct or indirect positive regulation of 11β-HSD1 and intensifying the effect of its inhibition. At the molecular level, 11β-HSD1inhibition resulted

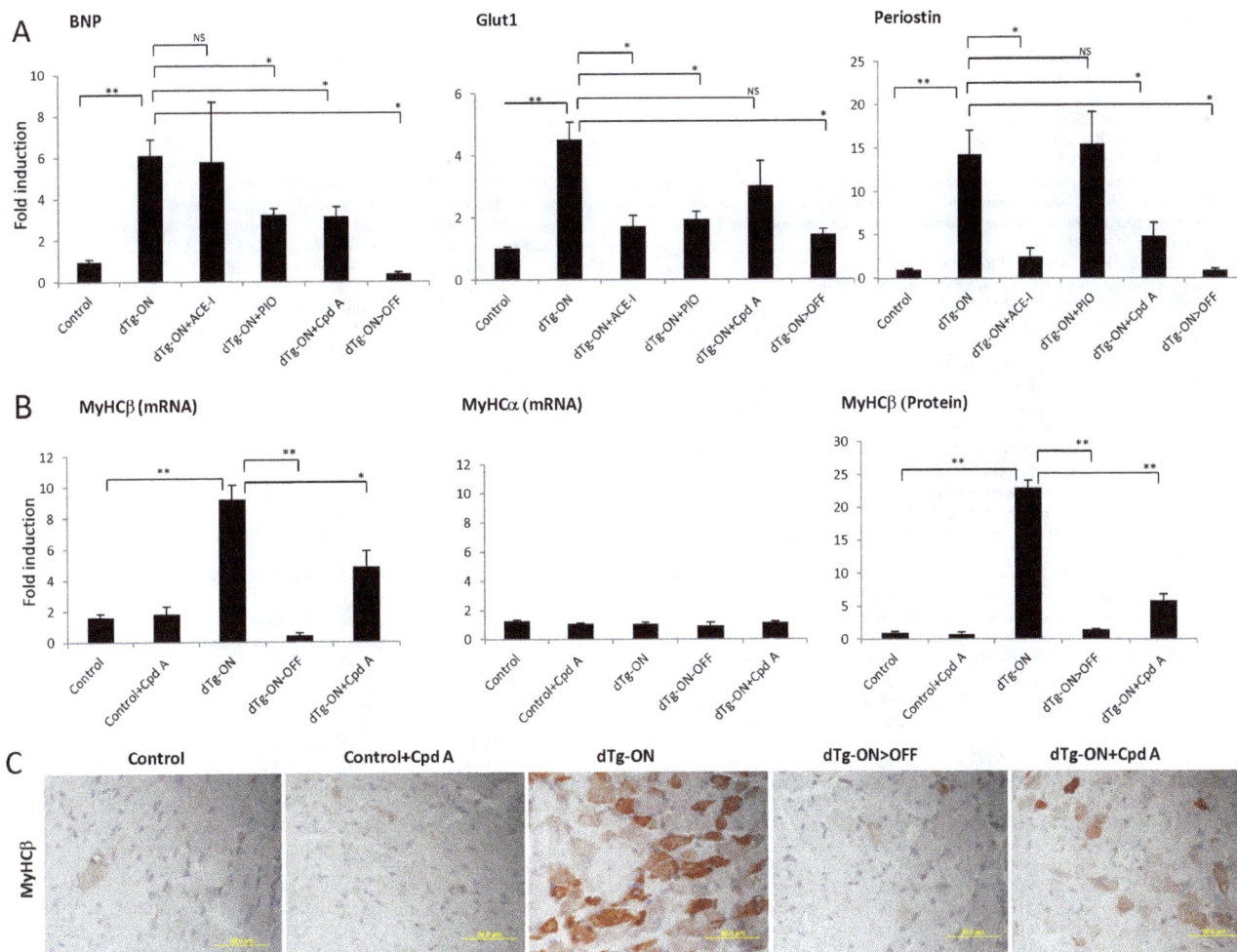

Figure 6. Rescue of hypertrophy is associated with reversing the hypertrophic gene signature, including of the Myosin heavy chain isoform shift. (A) Real time PCR results of selected genes in control and dTg (dTg ON) mice after 12 weeks of sVEGF-R1 induction, with or without treatment in the last 3 weeks. Treatment groups included either 11βHSD1 inhibitor (Roche Cpd A), Enalapril (ACE-I), Pioglitazone (PIO) or VEGF-driven neo-vascularization by sVEGF-R1 withdrawal (dTg ON>OFF). Results are normalized relative to litter-mate controls (designated as 1). N = 4-6 mice. Genes examined: Brain naturetic peptide (BNP). Glucose transporter 1 (Glut1) and Periostin. See text for further elaboration. (B) Real time PCR results of MyHCβ and MyHCα in control and dTg (dTg ON) mice after 12 weeks of sVEGF-R1 induction, with or without treatment in the last 3 weeks. N = 4–6 mice. Quantification (right diagram in B) and representative images (C) of immunohistochemistry for MyHCβ in the same mice as in B, depicting MyHCβ protein level elevation in dTg mice and rescue by both treatments. Scale bars: 50 μm. * $P<0.05$, ** $P<0.001$, NS = not statistically significant.

in a myosin heavy chain isoform shift from the fast-contracting MyHCα to the slow contracting MyHCβ. As marked by reversing the upregulated expression of BNP and periostin (a TGFβ target gene), 11β-HSD1inhibition also acted to relieve wall stress. It is assumed that the failure to restore normal cardiac function via 11β-HSD1inhibition in this system in face of ongoing VEGF blockade is due to persistent ischemia enforced by continued inhibition of angiogenesis. Thus, combining pro-angiogenic therapy with 11β-HSD1inhibition might have an additive effect.

Acknowledgments

We thank Dr. Jacques Himber of Hoffmann-La Roche pharmaceuticals, for his important contribution to this study.

Author Contributions

Conceived and designed the experiments: OG DG SG EK. Performed the experiments: OG ZH AO SPC. Analyzed the data: OG DG EK. Wrote the paper: OG EK.

References

1. Fedak PWM, Verma S, Weisel RD, Li R-K (2005) Cardiac remodeling and failure: From molecules to man (Part I). Cardiovascular Pathology 14: 1–11.
2. Opie LH, Commerford P, Gersh BJ, Pfeffer MA (2006) Controversies in ventricular remodelling. Lancet 367: 356–367.
3. Swynghedauw B (1999) Molecular Mechanisms of Myocardial Remodeling. Physiol Rev 79: 215–262.
4. Cohn JN, Ferrari R, Sharpe N, on Behalf of an International Forum on Cardiac Remodeling (2000) Cardiac remodeling—concepts and clinical implications: a consensus paper from an international forum on cardiac remodeling. J Am Coll Cardiol 35: 569–582.
5. Koitabashi N, Kass DA (2012) Reverse remodeling in heart failure- mechanisms and therapeutic opportunities. Nat Rev Cardiol 9: 147–157.
6. Pfeffer J, Fischer T, Pfeffer M (1995) Angiotensin-converting enzyme inhibition and ventricular remodeling after myocardial infarction. Annu Rev Physiol 57: 805–826.
7. Lopez-Sendon J, Swedberg K, McMurray J, Tamargo J, Maggioni A, et al. (2004) Expert consensus document on angiotensin converting enzyme inhibitors in cardiovascular disease. The Task Force on ACE-inhibitors of the European Society of Cardiology. Eur Heart J 25: 1454–1470.
8. Pfeffer M, Braunwald E, Moye L, Basta L, Brown E Jr, et al. (1992) Effect of captopril on mortality and morbidity in patients with left ventricular dysfunction after myocardial infarction. Results of the survival and ventricular enlargement trial. The SAVE Investigators. N Engl J Med 327: 669–677.
9. Finck BN (2007) The PPAR regulatory system in cardiac physiology and disease. Cardiovasc Res 73: 269–277.
10. Shiomi T, Tsutsui H, Hayashidani S, Suematsu N, Ikeuchi M, et al. (2002) Pioglitazone, a peroxisome proliferator-activated receptor-gamma agonist, attenuates left ventricular remodeling and failure after experimental myocardial infarction. Circulation 106: 3126–3132.
11. Balakumar P, Singh AP, Singh M (2007) Rodent models of heart failure. Journal of Pharmacological and Toxicological Methods 56: 1–10.
12. Zaragoza C, Gomez-Guerrero C, Martin-Ventura JL, Blanco-Colio L, Lavin B, et al. (2011) Animal models of cardiovascular diseases. J Biomed Biotechnol 2011: 497841.
13. Zbinden G, Bagdon RE (1963) Isoproterenol-Induced Heart Necrosis, an Experimental Model for the Study of Angina Pectoris and Myocardial Infarct. Rev Can Biol 22: 257–263.
14. Pfeffer M, Pfeffer J, Fishbein M, Fletcher P, Spadaro J, et al. (1979) Myocardial infarct size and ventricular function in rats. Circ Res 44: 503–512.
15. Shiojima I, Sato K, Izumiya Y, Schiekofer S, Ito M, et al. (2005) Disruption of coordinated cardiac hypertrophy and angiogenesis contributes in the transition to heart failure. The Journal of Clinical Investigation 115: 2108–2118.
16. Tamargo J, Lopez-Sendon J (2011) Novel therapeutic targets for the treatment of heart failure. Nat Rev Drug Discov 10: 536–555.
17. May D, Gilon D, Djonov V, Itin A, Lazarus A, et al. (2008) Transgenic system for conditional induction and rescue of chronic myocardial hibernation provides insights into genomic programs of hibernation. Proceedings of the National Academy of Sciences 105: 282–287.
18. Gordon O, Gilon D, He Z, May D, Lazarus A, et al. (2012) VEGF-induced neovascularization rescues cardiac function but not adverse remodeling at

19. advanced ischemic heart disease Arteriosclerosis, Thrombosis, and Vascular Biology.
19. Wamil M, Seckl J (2007) Inhibition of 11beta-hydroxysteroid dehydrogenase type 1 as a promising therapeutic target. Drug Discov Today 12: 504–520.
20. McSweeney S, Hadoke P, Kozak A, Small G, Khaled H, et al. (2010) Improved heart function follows enhanced inflammatory cell recruitment and angiogenesis in 11betaHSD1-deficient mice post-MI. Cardiovasc Res 88: 159–167.
21. Small G, Hadoke P, Sharif I, Dover A, Armour D, et al. (2005) Preventing local regeneration of glucocorticoids by 11beta-hydroxysteroid dehydrogenase type 1 enhances angiogenesis. Proc Natl Acad Sci U S A 102: 12165–12170.
22. Yu Z, Redfern CS, Fishman GI (1996) Conditional Transgene Expression in the Heart. Circ Res 79: 691–697.
23. Schiller N, Shah PM., Crawford M., DeMaria A., Devereux R., Feigenbaum H., Gutgesell H., Reichek N., Sahn D., Schnittger I. (1989) Recommendations for quantitation of the left ventricle by two-dimensional echocardiography. American Society of Echocardiography Committee on Standards, Subcommittee on Quantitation of Two-Dimensional Echocardiograms. J Am Soc Echocardiogr 2: 358–367.
24. Westermann D, Riad A, Lettau O, Roks A, Savvatis K, et al. (2008) Renin inhibition improves cardiac function and remodeling after myocardial infarction independent of blood pressure. Hypertension 52: 1068–1075.
25. Madrazo J, Kelly D (2008) The PPAR trio: regulators of myocardial energy metabolism in health and disease. J Mol Cell Cardiol 44: 968–975.
26. Duan SZ, Ivashchenko CY, Russell MW, Milstone DS, Mortensen RM (2005) Cardiomyocyte-Specific Knockout and Agonist of Peroxisome Proliferator-Activated Receptor-γ Both Induce Cardiac Hypertrophy in Mice. Circulation Research 97: 372–379.
27. Lister K, Autelitano D, Jenkins A, Hannan R, Sheppard K (2006) Cross talk between corticosteroids and alpha-adrenergic signalling augments cardiomyocyte hypertrophy: a possible role for SGK1. Cardiovasc Res 70: 555–565.
28. Brooks WW, Conrad CH (2009) Isoproterenol-induced myocardial injury and diastolic dysfunction in mice: structural and functional correlates. Comp Med 59: 339–343.
29. Li L, Fan D, Wang C, Wang J-Y, Cui X-B, et al. (2011) Angiotensin II increases periostin expression via Ras/p38 MAPK/CREB and ERK1/2/TGF-β1 pathways in cardiac fibroblasts. Cardiovascular Research 91: 80–89.
30. Dobaczewski M, Gonzalez-Quesada C, Frangogiannis NG (2010) The extracellular matrix as a modulator of the inflammatory and reparative response following myocardial infarction. Journal of Molecular and Cellular Cardiology 48: 504–511.
31. Gupta M (2007) Factors controlling cardiac myosin-isoform shift during hypertrophy and heart failure. J Mol Cell Cardiol 43: 388–403.
32. Solomon SD, Hee Shin S, Shah A, Skali H, Desai A, et al. (2011) Effect of the direct renin inhibitor aliskiren on left ventricular remodelling following myocardial infarction with systolic dysfunction. European Heart Journal 32: 1227–1234.
33. Yazawa H, Miyachi M, Furukawa M, Takahashi K, Takatsu M, et al. (2011) Angiotensin-Converting Enzyme Inhibition Promotes Coronary Angiogenesis in the Failing Heart of Dahl Salt-Sensitive Hypertensive Rats. Journal of Cardiac Failure 17: 1041–1050.

10

Cardiac Ankyrin Repeat Protein Attenuates Cardiac Hypertrophy by Inhibition of ERK1/2 and TGF-β Signaling Pathways

Yao Song[2◊], Jialin Xu[1◊], Yanfeng Li[1◊], Chunshi Jia[1], Xiaowei Ma[2], Lei Zhang[1], Xiaojie Xie[4], Yong Zhang[1], Xiang Gao[3]*, Youyi Zhang[2]*, Dahai Zhu[1]*

1 Department of Biochemistry and Molecular Biology, Institute of Basic Medical Sciences, Chinese Academy of Medical Sciences and Peking Union Medical College, Beijing, China, 2 Institute of Vascular Medicine, Peking University Third Hospital, Key Laboratory of Cardiovascular Molecular Biology and Regulatory peptides, Ministry of Health and Key Laboratory of Molecular Cardiovascular Science, Ministry of Education, Beijing, China, 3 National Resource Center for Mutant Mice Model Animal Research of Nanjing University, Pukou High-Tech District, Nanjing, China, 4 Department of Cardiology, Second Affiliated Hospital, Zhejiang University College of Medicine, Hangzhou, China

Abstract

Aims: It has been reported that cardiac ankyrin repeat protein is associated with heart development and diseases. This study is aimed to investigate the role of CARP in heart hypertrophy in vivo.

Methods and Results: We generated a cardiac-specific CARP-overexpressing transgenic mouse. Although such animals did not display any overt physiological abnormality, they developed less cardiac hypertrophy in response to pressure overload than did wildtype mice, as indicated by heart weight/body weight ratios, echocardiographic and histological analyses, and expression of hypertrophic markers. These mice also exhibited less cardiac hypertrophy after infusion of isoproterenol. To gain a molecular insight into how CARP attenuated heart hypertrophy, we examined expression of the mitogen-activated protein kinase cascade and found that the concentrations of phosphorylated ERK1/2 and MEK were markedly reduced in the hearts of transgenic mice subjected to pressure overload. In addition, the expressions of TGF-β and phosphorylated Smad3 were significantly downregulated in the hearts of CARP Tg mice in response to pressure overload. Furthermore, addition of human TGF-β1 could reverse the inhibitory effect of CARP on the hypertrophic response induced by phenylephrine in cardiomyocytes. It was also evidenced that the inhibitory effect of CARP on cardiac hypertrophy was not attributed to apoptosis.

Conclusion: CARP attenuates cardiac hypertrophy, in which the ERK and TGF-β pathways may be involved. Our findings highlight the significance of CARP as an anti-hypertrophic factor in therapy of cardiac hypertrophy.

Editor: Emilio Hirsch, University of Torino, Italy

Funding: This work was supported by the National Basic Research Program of China (http://www.973.gov.cn/English/Index.aspx) (grant nos. 2007CB946903, 2005CB522405, 2005CB522507, and 2011CB503903); the National Natural Science Foundation of China (http://www.nsfc.gov.cn/e_nsfc/desktop/zn/0101.htm) (grant nos. 30721063, 30971161 and 81030001); the Chinese National Programs for High Technology Research and Development (http://www.most.gov.cn/eng/programmes1/200610/t20061009_36225.htm) (grant no. 2007AA02Z109); and the Projects for International Cooperation and Exchanges NSFC (http://www.nsfc.gov.cn/e_nsfc/desktop/zn/0110.htm) (grant no. 30910103902). The funders had no role in study design, data collection and analysis, decision to publish, or preparation of the manuscript.

Competing Interests: The authors have declared that no competing interests exist.

* E-mail: dhzhu@pumc.edu.cn (DZ); zhangyy@bjmu.edu.cn (YZ); gaoxiang@nju.edu.cn (XG)

◊ These authors contributed equally to this work.

Introduction

Cardiac hypertrophy is an adaptive response of the myocardium to the increased workload that results from diverse cardiovascular diseases. Although this compensatory response to stress is considered to be an effective means to support increased cardiac output, prolonged hypertrophy ultimately leads to sudden death or progression to heart failure [1]. Pathological stress signals usually initiate cardiac hypertrophy through two classes of mechanisms: biomechanical/stretch-sensitive mechanisms and neurohumoral mechanisms [2]. Whichever mechanism serves as the initiating stimulus, the hypertrophic response is switched on at the level of

receptors or ion channels, which activate intracellular signaling cascades and transcriptional factors. The ultimate result is cardiomyocyte hypertrophy, fibroblast hyperplasia, and activation of the "fetal gene" program. An imbalance between the expression of pro- and anti-hypertrophic factors acting via a network of intracellular signaling pathways is responsible for development of cardiac hypertrophy [3]. However, previous research efforts have focused largely on signaling pathways that positively regulate cardiac hypertrophy. By comparison, negative regulators of cardiac hypertrophy have received much less attention. Accordingly, the therapeutic measures against cardiac hypertrophy developed to date principally target pro-hypertrophic pathways;

however, patient outcomes are far from ideal [4]. Against this backdrop, the development of new therapies aimed at enhancing the anti-hypertrophic effect is arguably a worthy undertaking.

CARP (cardiac ankyrin repeat protein), encoded by the *Ankrd1* (ankyrin repeat domain 1) gene, was originally identified in human dermal microvascular endothelial cells induced with interleukin (IL)-1A and tumor necrosis factor α (TNFα) [4], and was subsequently shown to be expressed predominantly in the heart. Developmental studies showed that *Ankrd1* transcripts are first detected at 8.5 days post-coitus in mouse embryos; thereafter, *Ankrd1* continues to be abundantly expressed in the embryonic heart but levels decrease in the adult heart. This pattern of expression suggested that CARP might function to negatively regulate transcription of cardiac genes in the fetal heart [5]. Additional studies have implicated CARP in myofibrillar assembly, stretch sensing, and communication between the sarcoplasm and the nucleus in the adult heart [6,7,8].

The most intriguing clue to the possible functional role of CARP comes from the observation that expression of the *Ankrd1* gene is rapidly induced in response to various hypertrophic stimuli, including pressure overload, denervation, stretch, and neurohumoral agonists (e.g., phenylephrine, endothelin, angiotensin II, and isoproterenol) [9]. Recent studies have also indicated that the *Ankrd1* gene is strongly upregulated in the hearts of both hypertrophic animal models [10,11,12] and those of heart-failure patients with dilated cardiomyopathy (DCM), ischemic cardiomyopathy (ICM), or arrhythmogenic right ventricular cardiomyopathy (ARVC) [13,14,15]. These lines of evidence point to an important role for the CARP protein in heart development generally, and in cardiac hypertrophy in particular. Interestingly, however, mice with complete germline ablation of the *Ankrd1* gene do not show any phenotypic change during development. It is therefore necessary to establish animal models with heart-specific *Ankrd1* deletion and/or overexpression of CARP to further investigate the *in vivo* function of CARP during heart development and cardiac hypertrophy.

In the present study, we generated cardiac-specific CARP-overexpressing transgenic (CARP Tg) mice and used these animals as a hypertrophic model to investigate the functional role of CARP in cardiac hypertrophy. Our results show that CARP has an important role in inhibiting cardiac hypertrophy induced by pressure overload and continuous isoproterenol infusion, and reveal an important regulatory role for transforming growth factor-β (TGF-β) signaling and the mitogen-activated protein kinase (MAPK) cascade, specifically the MEK/ERK1/2 (MAPK/ERK kinase/extracellular signal-regulated kinase) pathway, in mediating attenuation of cardiac hypertrophy and fibrosis by CARP.

Methods

All of the animal procedures were conducted in accordance with the Guide for the Care and Use of Laboratory Animals published by the US National Institutes of Health (NIH Publication No. 85-23, revised 1996) and were approved by the Institutional Animal Care and Use Committee of Chinese Academy of Medical Sciences & Peking Union Medical College.

Generation of Transgenic Mice

Transgenic mice were produced by microinjection of the α-MHC-CARP construct into fertilized mouse embryos (129 strain background). Four independent transgenic lines (B, D, E, and F) were established. The F-line transgenic mouse was backcrossed with C57/BL6J animals for more than five generations to create a >98.5% C57/BL6J background. Full details are provided in Supporting Information S1.

Animal Models

Pressure overload-induced cardiac hypertrophy was produced by transverse aortic constriction (TAC) surgery [16]. Male CARP Tg mice (9–11-weeks old) and wild-type (WT) littermates were anesthetized with ketamine/xylazine/atropine (100 mg/10 mg/1.2 mg per 1 kg IP). After the mice were confirmed in an anaesthetized state (e.g. no response to toe pinching), they were next ventilated by tracheal intubation using a rodent ventilator (Alcbio Corporation, Shanghai, China) with a tidal volume of 0.2 mL and a respiratory rate of 88 breaths/min. The chest was opened at the suprasternal fossa along the midsternal line, and the thymus glands were superiorly reflected. The transverse thoracic aorta between the innominate artery and the left common carotid artery was dissected, and a 6-0 silk suture was tied around the aorta against a 26-gauge needle. Both control groups underwent a sham operation involving thoracotomy and aortic dissection without constriction of the aorta. After 4 weeks, the mice were sacrificed by cervical dislocation after deep anesthesia with 2% isoflurane (Baxter Healthcare Corporation, New Providence, NJ, USA) and the ratios of heart weight to body weight (HW/BW) and tibia length (HW/TL) were determined.

The isoproterenol-induced cardiac hypertrophic model was established by infusing isoproterenol (Sigma, St Louis, Mo) in vivo using subcutaneously implanted micro-osmotic pumps (Alzet DURECT, Cupertino, CA; model 1002). In brief, 9–11-week-old male CARP Tg and WT mice were anesthetized with ketamine/xylazine/atropine (100 mg/10 mg/1.2 mg per 1 kg IP). After confirming an anaesthetized state of mice (e.g. no response to toe pinching), micro-osmotic pumps were implanted in the back of mice, and isoproterenol was delivered continuously at a rate of 30 mg/kg/day. The control mice received vehicle (100 μmol/L ascorbic acid). After 14 days, the mice were sacrificed by cervical dislocation after deep anesthesia with 2% isoflurane and the ratios of heart weight to body weight (HW/BW) and tibia length (HW/TL) were determined.

Cardiac hypertrophy and function were assessed by echocardiography before and after TAC surgery or isoproterenol infusion using a Vevo 770TM Imaging System (VisualSonics Inc., Toronto, Canada) equipped with a 30-MHz microprobe under anesthesia with 1.5% isoflurane allowing spontaneous breathing.

Histological Analysis

Histological analysis of tissues was performed according to standard protocols [17]. Full details are provided in Supporting Information S1.

Isolation and Culture of Rat Cardiomyocytes

Cardiomyocytes were isolated and cultured from 1–2-day-old neonatal Sprague-Dawley (SD) rats as described previously [18]. Briefly, a central thoracotomy was performed after the neonatal rats were deeply anaesthetized with 1.0% isoflurane. The hearts were quickly excised and immediately embedded in freezing hanks solution. Cardiomyocytes were dispersed by digestion with 0.1% (w/v) trypsin and 0.03% (w/v) collagenase at 37°C, then were collected after differential adhesion of non-cardiomyocytes and plated at a density of 150–200 cells/mm². Cultures were maintained in DMEM supplemented with 10% (v/v) fetal bovine serum; 100 μmol/L bromodeoxyuridine was included to prevent fibroblast proliferation.

Generation of Recombinant CARP-GFP Adenovirus

Full-length rat CARP cDNA with a C-terminal Myc tag was subcloned into the pAdTrack vector. The resulting plasmid was linearized by digestion with *Pme*I and was transformed into *Escherichia coli* BJ5183 cells together with the adenoviral backbone plasmid pAdEasy-1. Kanamycin-resistant recombinants were selected and recombination was confirmed by digestion with *Pac*I. The recombinant adenoviral plasmid was transfected into 293A cells to generate infectious CARP-GFP-expressing viral particles (Ad-CARP-GFP). Adenovirus was purified via standard CsCl ultracentrifugation and desalting procedures. Viral titers were determined by plaque assay.

Immunocytochemistry and Cell Size Measurements

Immunocytochemistry was performed with cardiomyocytes as described in Supporting Information S1.

Quantitative Real-time Reverse Transcription-polymerase Chain Reaction (RT-PCR)

Total RNA was extracted from ventricular tissue and cultured neonatal rat cardiomyocytes using TRIzol (Invitrogen, Carlsbad, CA). cDNA was synthesized from total RNA using AMV reverse transcriptase and oligo (dT) primers (Promega, Madison, WI), as instructed by the manufacturer. PCR-amplified target mRNAs were quantified using SYBR Green PCR Master Mix (Bio-Rad, Hercules, CA) and normalized to glyceraldehyde phosphate dehydrogenase (GAPDH) mRNA levels. The primer sequences for PCR were presented in Supporting Information S1.

Quantification of TGF-β1 Protein Production

The concentrations of TGF-β1 in heart homogenates and supernatants of cultured neonatal rat cardiomyocytes were measured using a specific ELISA kit (Shanghai ExCell Biology, Inc., Shanghai, China) employing the double-antibody sandwich method according to manufacturer's instruction. Full details are provided in Supporting Information S1.

Nuclear Staining and Laser Confocal Microscopy

Cardiomyocytes were fixed with 4% paraformaldehyde and permeabilized in 0.2% Triton X-100 for 30 min at 37°C. The cells were sequentially stained for 15 min with 0.1 µg/ml Hochest 33342. Nuclear structure was visualized on a Leica laser confocal microscope.

Western Blotting

Immunoblotting was performed with heart homogenates and cardiomyocytes as described in Supporting Information S1.

Statistical Analysis

Data are expressed as means ± SEMs. Differences between two groups were analyzed using unpaired Student's t-tests. Comparisons among different mice genotypes subjected to different treatments were made by two-way ANOVA. A *P*-value less than 0.05 was considered significant.

Results

Overexpression of CARP Inhibits Neurohumoral Agonist-induced Cardiomyocyte Hypertrophy *in vitro*

Because the *Ankrd1* gene is upregulated in the heart in response to various hypertrophic stimuli, such as phenylephrine, endothelin, or isoproterenol, it has been hypothesized that CARP might function as a pro- or anti-hypertrophic regulator. To test this

hypothesis, we first overexpressed CARP in isolated neonatal rat cardiomyocytes infected with a c-Myc-CARP-GFP-expressing recombinant adenovirus (Ad-CARP-GFP); Ad-GFP was used as a negative control. Adenoviral-mediated expression of CARP protein was confirmed by immunoblotting, using anti-CARP and anti-Myc antibodies, of cells infected with different doses of the recombinant adenovirus (25, 50, 100, and 200 MOI (Multiplicity of infection)) for 24 hours. As shown in Figure 1A, endogenous CARP protein was expressed in a dose-independent manner in Ad-GFP-infected cardiomyocytes, and no ectopically expressed CARP protein was detected in Ad-GFP-infected cardiomyocytes blotted with an anti-Myc antibody. Immunoblotting of samples from cardiomyocytes infected with Ad-CARP-GFP showed that both ectopic CARP (anti-Myc antibody) and total CARP protein (anti-CARP antibody) were expressed in an adenoviral-dose-dependent manner in these cells (Figure 1A).

To determine the effect of CARP on cardiac hypertrophy *in vitro*, we treated Ad-CARP-GFP- and Ad-GFP-infected cells, as well as non-infected cells (control), with phenylephrine (100 µM) for 24 hours to induce cardiac hypertrophy. As shown in Figure 1B and 1C, phenylephrine significantly increased the size of Ad-GFP-infected and non-infected cardiomyocytes. Importantly, we found that overexpression of CARP markedly inhibited phenylephrine-induced cardiomyocyte hypertrophy, as reflected by a decrease in myocyte area (Figure 1B and 1C) and reduced expression of the hypertrophic molecular markers α-actin, β-MHC, and ANF (Figure 1D and 1E). Together, these data indicate that over-expression of CARP in rat cardiomyocytes blocks phenylephrine-induced cardiac hypertrophy *in vitro*.

CARP Tg Mice are Less Susceptible to Pathological Cardiac Hypertrophy Induced by Pressure Overload and Neurohumoral Stimulation Compared with Wild Type Mice

The observation that CARP attenuates cardiomyocyte hyper-trophy *in vitro* prompted us to ask whether CARP might function in a similar manner *in vivo*. To investigate this possibility, we generated CARP Tg mice in which Myc-tagged CARP was selectively overexpressed in the heart under the control of the α-MHC promoter (Figure S1A). Four independent transgenic lines (B, D, E, and F) were obtained. All animals were born with the expected Mendelian ratios and were overtly normal. Transgenic mice from the F-line used in this study were characterized by PCR analysis of genomic DNA (Figure S1B) and by determination of *Ankrd1* mRNA levels (Figure S1C and S1D). To detect ectopically expressed CARP protein in transgenic mice, we analyzed total protein extracts from various tissues of 2-month-old CARP Tg mice by Western blotting using anti-Myc and anti-CARP antibodies. Figure S1E shows that ectopically expressed CARP was detected only in the hearts of CARP Tg mice. Furthermore, the level of CARP protein in the hearts of Tg mice was increased by more than 3-fold compared with that of WT mice (Figure S1F and S1G).

Because no overt physiological abnormalities were evident in CARP Tg mice under normal growth conditions, we next investigated CARP function in pathological cardiac hypertrophy. We first assessed the hypertrophic response of WT and CARP Tg mice to a stretch stimulus, performing pressure overload using TAC in CARP Tg mice and age/gender-matched WT littermates. Echocardiographic analyses were performed to evaluate cardiac structure and function. As shown in Figure 2A and Table S1, 4 weeks after TAC, left ventricular posterior wall thickness (LVPW;d) and the LV mass of WT mice had increased by

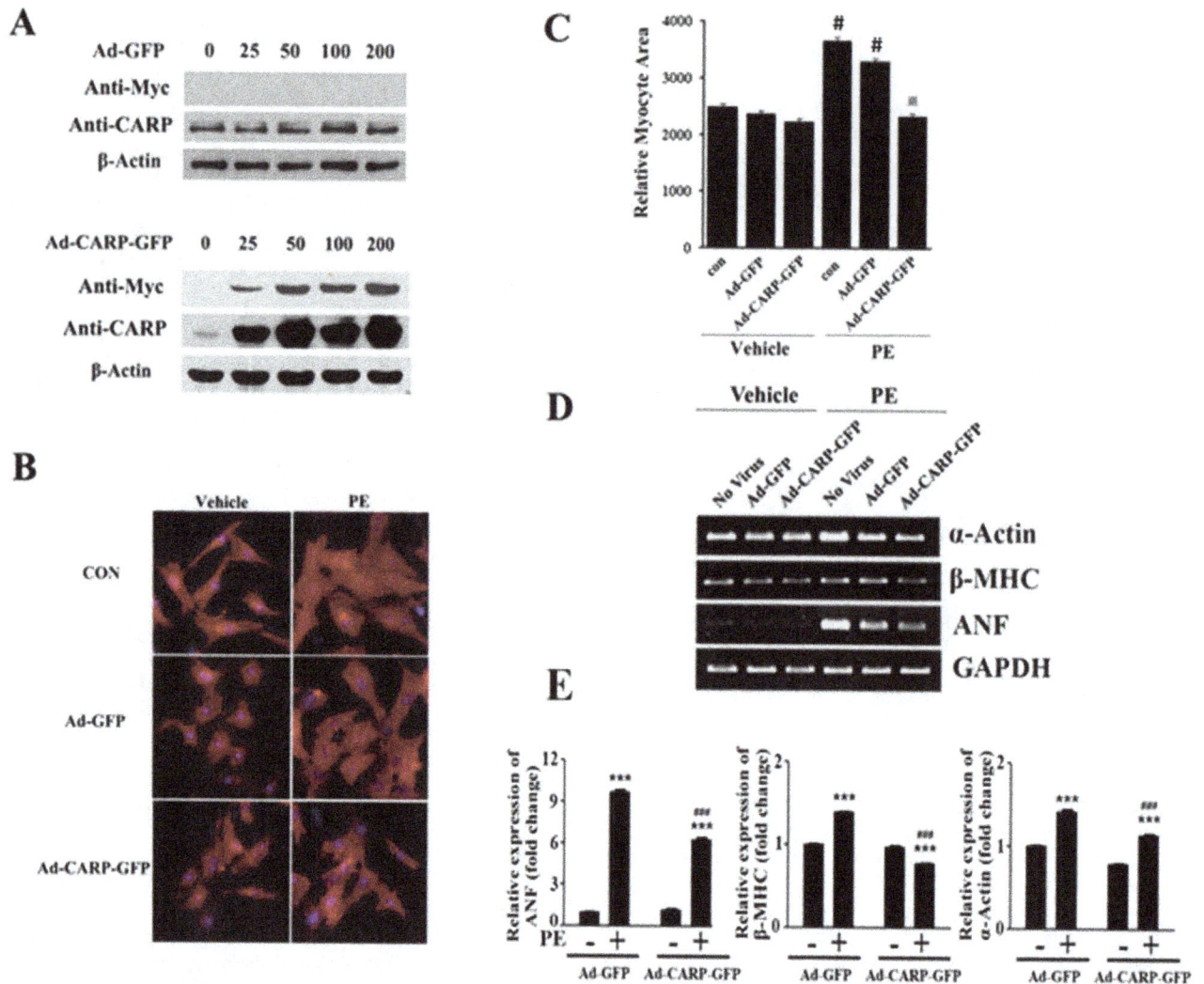

Figure 1. Overexpression of CARP inhibits phenylephrine-induced cardiomyocyte hypertrophy. (A) Primary neonatal rat cardiomyocytes were infected with adenoviruses expressing GFP or Myc-tagged CARP-GFP at the indicated MOIs. After 24 hours, CARP and Myc-tagged CARP levels were evaluated using Western blotting. (B) α-actin staining showed that adenoviral-mediated overexpression of CARP inhibited phenylephrine-induced cardiomyocyte hypertrophy. Cells were infected with Ad-GFP as a negative control. Nuclei were stained with DAPI. (C) Quantification of the cell surface areas shown in (B). 100–120 random cells were measured in each group. *$P<0.001$ relative to phenylephrine+Ad-GFP (PE+Ad-GFP), #$P<0.01$, compared with con+vehicle; (D) The effect of CARP overexpression on the levels of mRNA of α-actin, β-MHC, and ANF in cardiomyocytes exposed to phenylephrine or not. mRNA levels were measured via semi-quantitative RT-PCR; GAPDH was employed as an internal control; (E) Quantification of mRNA levels in (D). ***$P<0.001$, compared with Ad-GFP, ###$P<0.001$, compared with PE+Ad-GFP.

45.5% and 47.2%, respectively, compared with those of sham-operated mice; in contrast, these two parameters were only 25.8% and 33.8% higher in TAC/CARP Tg mice than in sham-operated/CARP Tg animals. These data suggest that over-expression of CARP in the heart reduces the hypertrophic response to TAC. However, no difference in cardiac function, measured as ejection fraction percentage (EF%) and fractional shortening percentage (FS%), was evident between CARP Tg and WT mice in response to TAC.

Mice were sacrificed 4 weeks after TAC and aspects of cardiac hypertrophy were examined. The levels of CARP in hearts from wild-type TAC, transgenic sham and transgenic TAC mice were 3.05 ± 0.20, 5.75 ± 1.10 and 8.60 ± 1.61 fold of that in hearts from wild-type sham mice, implying that TAC could increase CARP expression in hearts of both wild-type and transgenic mice, although showing no statistical difference (Figure S2). As shown in Figure 2B and 2C, significant increases in HW/BW and HW/TL

ratios were observed in both groups compared with sham-operated controls. Interestingly, the extent of cardiac hypertrophy in CARP Tg mice was significantly lower than that in WT animals. Examination of gross heart morphology and analysis of myocyte area on histological sections after 4 weeks of TAC also revealed that the heart size was smaller and the cellular hypertrophy less in CARP Tg mice compared with WT animals (Figure 2D, 2E, and 2F). Moreover, histological analysis of the extent of fibrosis using Picric acid-Sirius red (PSR) staining showed a substantial decrease in collagen deposition in the hearts of CARP Tg mice after TAC, compared with WT animals (Figure 2D and 2G).

We also found that the expression levels of mRNAs encoding the hypertrophic markers ANF, β-MHC, and α-actin were markedly decreased in CARP Tg mice after TAC compared with the levels seen in WT animals (Figure S3A and S3C). Meanwhile the expression levels of fibrosis markers, such as procollagen type

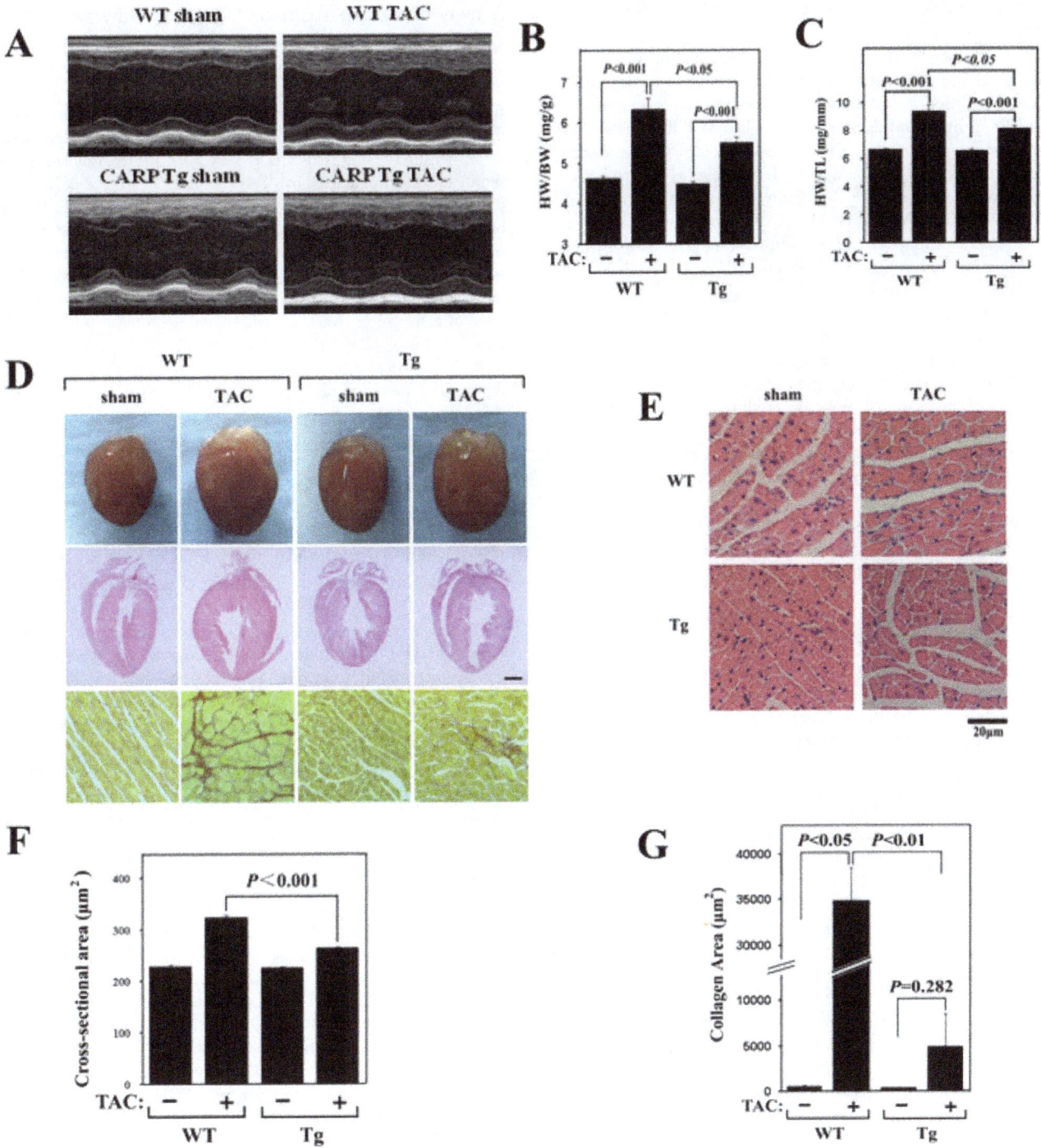

Figure 2. Pressure overload-induced cardiac hypertrophy is attenuated in CARP Tg mice. WT and CARP Tg mice were subjected to TAC or a sham operation. Cardiac hypertrophy and function were assessed by echocardiography. After 4 weeks, the mice were sacrificed for assessment of cardiac hypertrophy. (A) Representative examples of M-mode echocardiograms of hearts from WT and CARP Tg mice subjected to TAC or a sham operation. (B) The ratio of heart weight to body weight (HW/BW). (C) The ratio of heart weight to tibia length (HW/TL). (D) Staining of heart sections from WT and CARP Tg mice subjected to TAC or a sham operation. *Upper panel:* Gross heart morphology; *middle panel:* H&E-stained longitudinal sections; *lower panel:* PSR-stained sections. (E) H&E staining of sections from the left ventricular myocardium of WT and CARP Tg mice subjected to TAC or a sham operation. Scale bar = 20 μm. (F) Quantification of cross-sectional areas of the cardiomyocytes shown in (E). (G) Quantification of collagen areas in the myocytes shown in (D).

Iα2 (Col I), procollagen type III α1 (Col III), and connective tissue growth factor (CTGF), were upregulated in WT mice in response to TAC, but the effect was significantly blunted in TAC-treated CARP Tg mice (Figure S3D, S3E, and S3F). In contrast, the genes encoding myosin heavy polypeptide 6 (α-MHC) and sarco/endoplasmic reticulum Ca^{2+}-ATPase 2 (SERCA2) were downregulated in WT mice in response to TAC, but the expression levels were unchanged in TAC-treated CARP Tg animals (Figure S3G and S3H).

In addition to pressure overload stimulation, we also investigated the response of CARP Tg mice to a neurohumoral signal. We used isoproterenol to induce cardiac hypertrophy in CARP Tg mice and age/gender-matched WT littermates. After continuous infusion over 2 weeks, isoproterenol produced significant increases in LVPW;d in WT animals, as determined by echocardiography (Figure 3A, Table S2) and also increased the HW/BW and HW/TL ratios (Figure 3B and 3C), global heart size (Figure 3D), and myocyte area (Figure 3E and 3F). However, both LVPW;d and the ratios HW/BW and HW/TL were lower, and global heart size and myocyte area smaller, in CARP Tg mice than in WT animals after isoproterenol administration (Table S2 and Figure 3A–F). Furthermore, less collagen deposition was evident in the hearts of CARP Tg mice treated with isoproterenol than in the hearts of isoproterenol-treated WT animals (Figure 3D and 3G). The isoproterenol-induced increases in expression of ANF, β-MHC, and α-actin were also partially inhibited in CARP Tg mice (Figure 3H). These results indicate that overexpression of CARP markedly attenuates isoproterenol-induced cardiac hypertrophy.

Collectively, our findings provide the first experimental evidence that overexpression of CARP in the heart of the mouse attenuates cardiac hypertrophy.

CARP Overexpression Inhibits the MAPK/ERK Signaling Pathway both in vitro and in vivo

To investigate the potential mechanisms by which overexpression of CARP attenuates cardiac hypertrophy, we examined several signaling pathways often involved in development of cardiac hypertrophy. The phosphoinositol 3-kinase (PI3K)/Akt and ERK signaling pathways play important roles in pressure overload-induced cardiac hypertrophy. To determine whether these signaling pathways are involved in mediation of the CARP-inhibitory action in terms of cardiac hypertrophy, we used Western blot analysis to examine the phosphorylation status of MEK1/2, ERK1/2, p90RSK, Akt, and GSK3β (all are components of the two pathways mentioned above) in hearts from TAC-treated CARP Tg mice and WT mice. As shown in Figure 4A, the most prominent changes observed affected the ERK signaling pathway. We found that the levels of phosphorylated MEK1/2, ERK1/2, and p90RSK were significantly increased in WT mice following pressure overload. Importantly, the levels of phosphorylated MEK1/2, ERK1/2, and p90RSK proteins were strikingly reduced in the hearts of CARP Tg mice (Figure 4A). However, Akt and GSK3β phosphorylation status was unaffected (Figure 4A), suggesting that the Akt signaling pathway may not participate in CARP function. To further elucidate the functional role played by the MEK1/2 MAPK signaling pathway in the cardiac hypertrophy-attenuating function of CARP, we treated CARP-overexpressing cultured neonatal rat cardiomyocytes with phenylephrine and examined activation of the ERK signaling pathway. As demonstrated in our in vivo experiments, the levels of phosphorylated MEK1/2, ERK1/2, and p90RSK proteins were augmented by phenylephrine treatment in a time-dependent manner in mock-transfected cells. However, phosphorylation of MEK1/2, ERK1/2, and p90RSK after phenylephrine induction was blocked in CARP-overexpressing cells (Figure 4B and 4C). Together, our findings provide in vivo and in vitro experimental evidence suggesting that the ERK signaling pathway plays a critical role in mediating the partial inhibitory effect of CARP against cardiac hypertrophy.

Activity of the TGF-β/Smad3 Signaling Pathway in CARP Tg Mice is Decreased in Response to Pressure Overload

Because TGF-β has been implicated in cardiomyocyte growth, fibrosis, and re-expression of fetal genes, we investigated whether signal transduction via this pathway was relevant to CARP function. Expressions of TGF-β1, -β2, and -β3 at the mRNA level were measured using real-time RT-PCR. All three isoforms were significantly upregulated by TAC in the hearts of WT mice (Figure 5A). However, their induction in response to TAC was blocked in the hearts of CARP Tg animals. To provide further support for a role for TGF-β in mediation of CARP function, we measured the levels of TGF-β1 content in heart homogenates. We found that the content of TGF-β1 increased significantly in WT mice after pressure overload, whereas this increase was partially attenuated in CARP Tg mice (Figure 5B).

To further determine the functional role of the TGF-β signaling pathway in the inhibitory effect of CARP on cardiac hypertrophy, we measured TGF-β pathway activation by examining the phosphorylation level of Smad3. The level of phosphorylated Smad3 protein was increased in wild-type mice after TAC surgery (Figure 5C and 5D), but this increase was abrogated in CARP Tg mice (Figure 5C and 5D).

TGF-β1 Eliminates the Inhibitory Effect of CARP on Phenylephrine-induced Cardiomyocyte Hypertrophy

To investigate the role of TGF-β1 in mediating the effect of CARP on cardiac hypertrophy, we first examined the effect of CARP on TGF-β1 secretion from cardiomyocytes in response to a pro-hypertrophic factor, phenylephrine. As shown in Figure 6A, phenylephrine induced an approximately 1-fold increase in TGF-β1 release (compared with the baseline level) from cardiomyocytes (1.92±0.28 fold in the GFP/PE test vs 1 fold in the GFP control; $P<0.05$). However, overexpression of CARP resulted in a MOI-dependent inhibition of TGF-β1 release in response to phenylephrine; a 50% decrease was evident at an MOI of 50 compared with the level seen when an equivalent amount of control GFP-expressing virus was used for infection (0.97±0.11 fold in the CARP MOI 50/PE test vs 1.92±0.28 fold in the GFP MOI 50/PE control; $P<0.05$). Next, we investigated whether exogenous TGF-β1 could rescue the inhibitroy effects of CARP on the hypertrophic response of cardiomyocytes. Both phenylephrine and human TGF-β1 (hTGF-β1, R&D Systems) induced marked hypertrophy, as shown by expression of mRNAs encoding ANF and β-MHC (2.55±0.43- and 2.55±0.41-fold that of the GFP control, respectively, for ANF; $P<0.01$; 2.13±0.26- and 2.22±0.32-fold that of the GFP control, respectively, for β-MHC, $P<0.01$), whereas addition of hTGF-β1 plus phenylephrine did not further aggravate the hypertrophic response to phenylephrine (2.75±0.57- vs 2.55±0.43-fold for ANF and 2.14±0.35- vs 2.13±0.26-fold for β-MHC; Figure 6B). In contrast, neither phenylephrine nor hTGF-β1 induced significant hypertrophy in CARP-overexpressing cardiomyocytes (Figure 6B and 6C). However, addition of both hTGF-β1 and phenylephrine restored the hypertrophic response (2.59±0.10-fold of the GFP control for ANF and 1.91±0.08-fold of the GFP control for β-MHC) to a level similar to that in cardiomyocytes that were not transfected with CARP (2.75±0.57-fold of the GFP control level for ANF and 2.14±0.35-fold of the GFP control level for β-MHC; $P>0.05$, Figure 6B and 6C). Similarly, inhibition of phenylephrine-induced increase in cardiomyocyte size upon CARP overexpression (1.13±0.04-fold of GFP control) was also reversed to a great extent by addition of hTGF-β1(1.35±0.03-fold of GFP control; $P<0.05$, Figure 6D). Together, these results indicate that

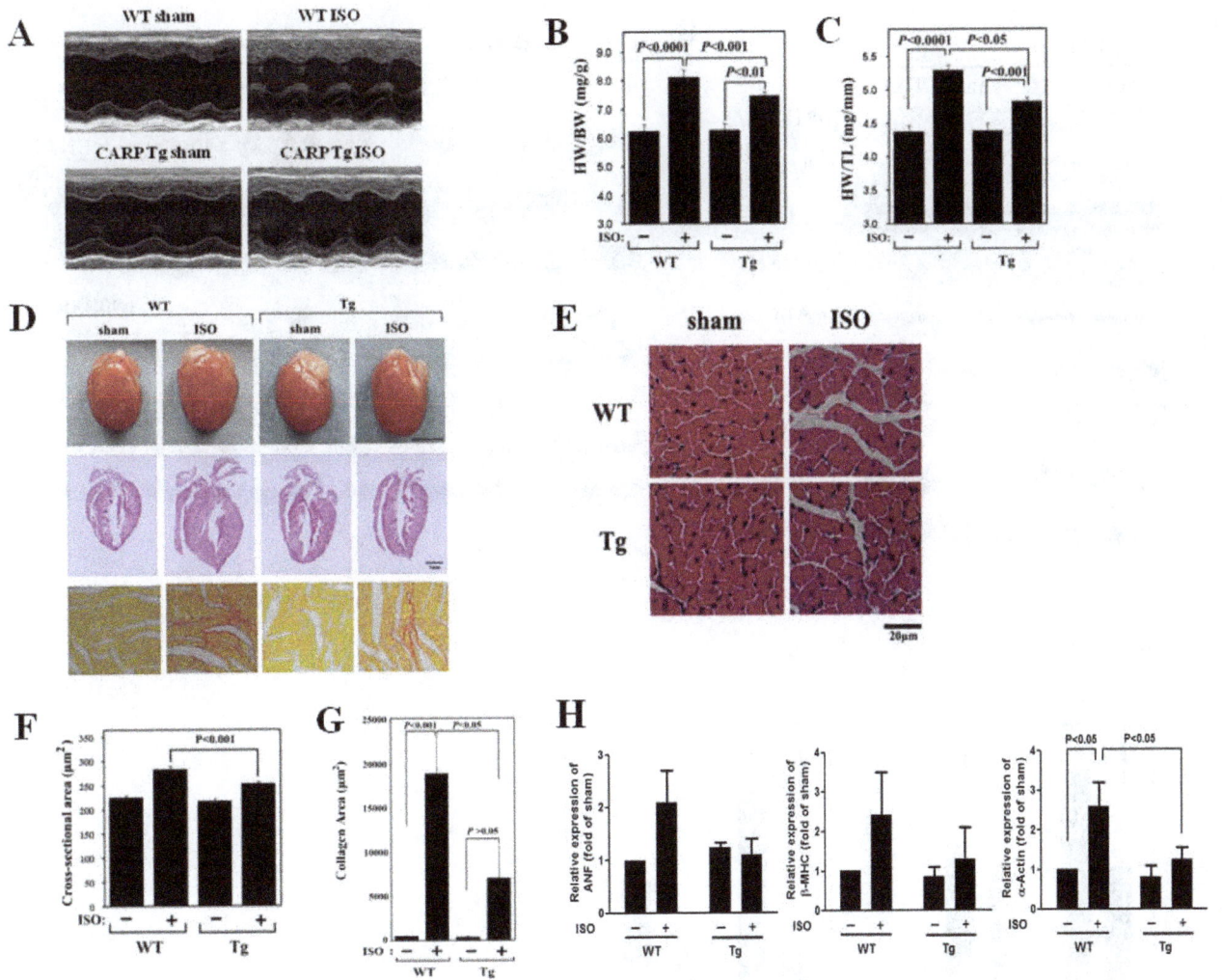

Figure 3. Isoproterenol-induced cardiac hypertrophy is attenuated in CARP Tg mice. WT and CARP Tg mice were continuously infused with vehicle (100 μmol/L ascorbic acid) or isoproterenol at a rate of 30 mg/kg/day using a subcutaneously implanted mini-osmotic pump. After 14 days, mice were sacrificed for assessment of cardiac hypertrophy. (A) Representative examples of M-mode echocardiograms of hearts from WT and CARP Tg mice infused with isoproterenol (ISO) or vehicle (sham). (B) The ratio of heart weight to body weight (HW/BW). (C) The ratio of heart weight to tibia length (HW/TL). (D) Staining of hearts from WT and CARP Tg mice infused with ISO or vehicle. *Upper panel:* Gross heart morphology; *middle panel:* H&E-stained longitudinal sections; *lower panel:* PSR-stained sections. (E) H&E staining of sections from the left ventricular myocardia of WT and CARP Tg mice infused with ISO or vehicle. Scale bar = 20 μm. (F) Quantification of cross-sectional areas in the cardiomyocytes shown in (E). (G) Quantification of collagen areas in the myocytes shown in (D). (H) Changes in the expression levels of mRNAs transcribed from the ANF, β-MHC, and α-actin genes after infusion of isoproterenol in WT and CARP Tg mice. mRNA expression levels were quantitated using real-time PCR.

the TGF-β/Smad3 signaling pathway, in concert with the ERK MAPK pathway, may play a role in regulating CARP-mediated attenuation of cardiac hypertrophy and fibrosis in response to pressure overload *in vivo*.

Apoptosis was not Involved in the Inhibitory Effect of CARP on Cardiac Hypertrophy

To exclude the possibility that the inhibitory effect of CARP on cardiac hypertrophy was due to apoptosis-dependent cell death, we investigated whether overexpression of CARP induced cardiomyocyte apoptosis. As shown in Figure S4A, overexpression of CARP did not cause nuclear condensation in the absence or presence of phenylephrine. Furthermore, compared with the myocytes infected with GFP alone, the levels of caspase-3 did not decrease and cleaved caspase-3 was not detected in myocytes overexpressing CARP (Figure S4B). Thus, it suggests that

apoptosis does not participate in the inhibitory effect of CARP on cardiac hypertrophy.

Discussion

Since its discovery in 1995, the *Ankrd1* gene transcript has attracted significant interest owing to its persistent upregulation in patients with cardiac hypertrophy and heart failure. However, the precise role played by the encoded CARP protein under these pathological conditions remains poorly understood. It has been proposed that inducible expression of CARP in the myocardium may indicate that the protein has a protective function, reflecting an adaptive response to various stresses [19]. To test this hypothesis, we generated cardiac-specific CARP Tg mice and investigated the functional role of CARP in cardiac hypertrophy induced by isoproterenol infusion and pressure overload. We found that overexpression of CARP markedly attenuates cardiac

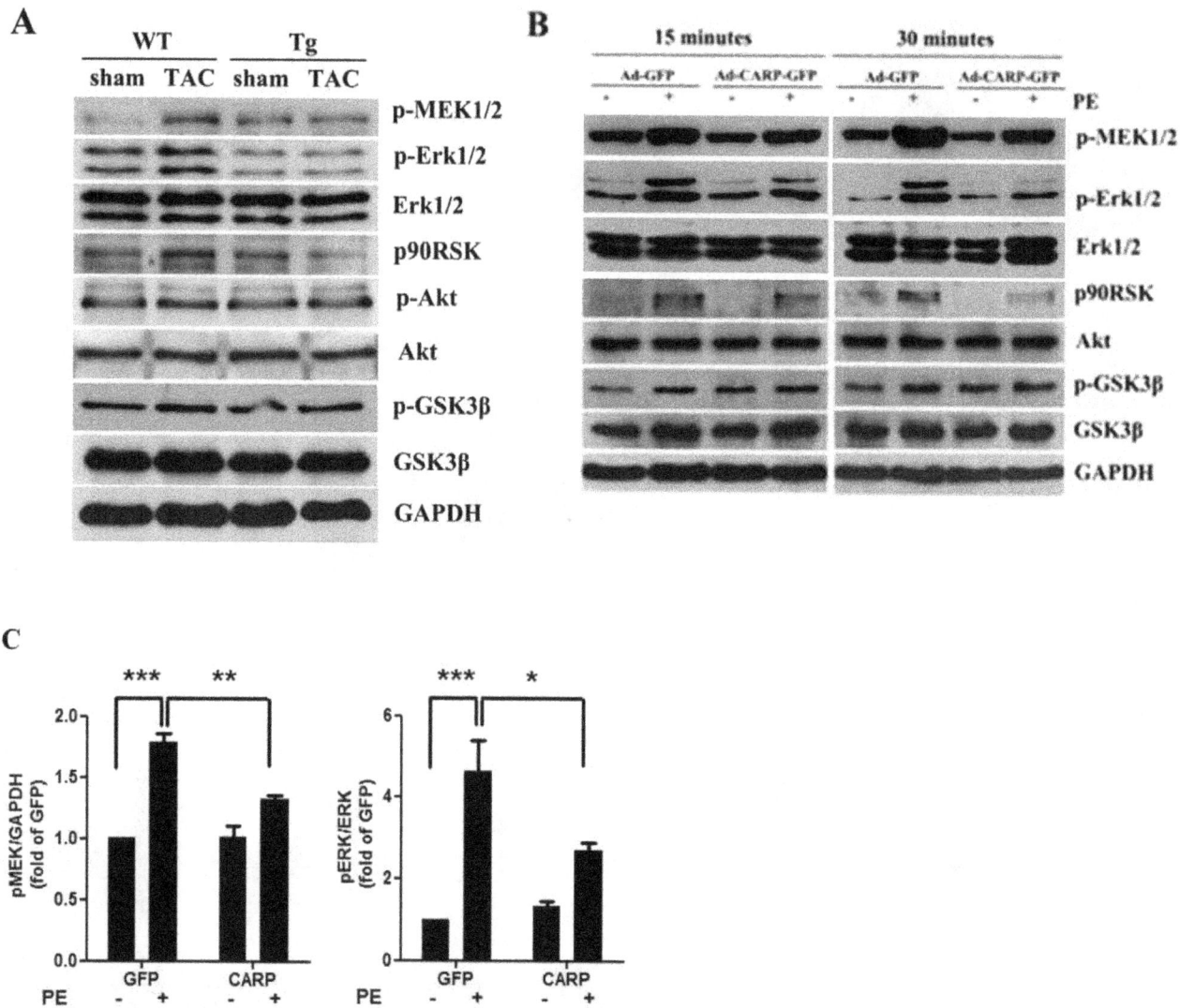

Figure 4. Overexpression of CARP inhibits the activation of MEK/ERK signaling by hypertrophic stimuli. (A) Western blotting of heart protein extracts to examine the levels of various phosphorylated and total kinases in WT and CARP Tg mice following TAC or a sham operation. A representative Western blot (from one of three independent experiments) is shown. (B) Western blotting of protein extracts to detect various phosphorylated and total kinase levels in parental and CARP-overexpressing cardiomyocytes subjected to phenylephrine treatment or not. A representative Western blot (from one of three independent experiments) is shown. (C) Quantification of the expression of the p-MEK1/2 and p-ERK1/2 proteins shown in (B) at 30 min after commencement of PE treatment.

hypertrophy and fibrosis induced by pressure overload *in vivo*. Furthermore, we provide experimental evidence showing that this action of CARP is mediated by inhibition of the ERK1/2 and TGF-β signaling pathways. Most importantly, our findings suggest that increased CARP level may be a potential mode of prevention and treatment of cardiac hypertrophy.

It has been reported that increased expression of the *Ankrd1* gene in the left ventricular myocardium is induced by various hypertrophic stimuli, both in animal models and in heart failure patients with dilated cardiomyopathy (DCM) or ischemic cardiomyopathy (ICM) [13,14]. Intriguingly, inducible expression of CARP also occurs in non-cardiomyocytes in response to stress. For example, the *Ankrd1* gene is upregulated in vascular endothelial cells during wound healing and promotes angiogenesis in granulation tissue [20]. Moreover, *Ankrd1* expression is strongly induced in regenerating rat skeletal muscles after damage by

a single injection of bupivacaine, peaking in level 3 days after injury and falling to undetectable levels after 28 days. In addition, high-level *Ankrd1* gene expression in DMD patients is restricted to regenerating myofibers, strongly suggesting that CARP could be involved in muscle satellite cell activation during regeneration in such patients [21]. Functional studies have shown that overexpression of CARP in rat embryonic H9C2 cardiomyoblasts protects against hypoxia-induced apoptosis [22]. Even more striking is the observed association between CARP expression and the sensitivity of ovarian cells to cisplatin reported by Scurr et al., who showed that *Ankrd1* expression was negatively correlated with cisplatin sensitivity in a panel of human cancer cell lines and was specifically and dramatically decreased in cisplatin-sensitive lines [23]. These data indicate that, although *Ankrd1* is predominantly expressed in cardiomyocytes during normal development, its expression can be induced in non-

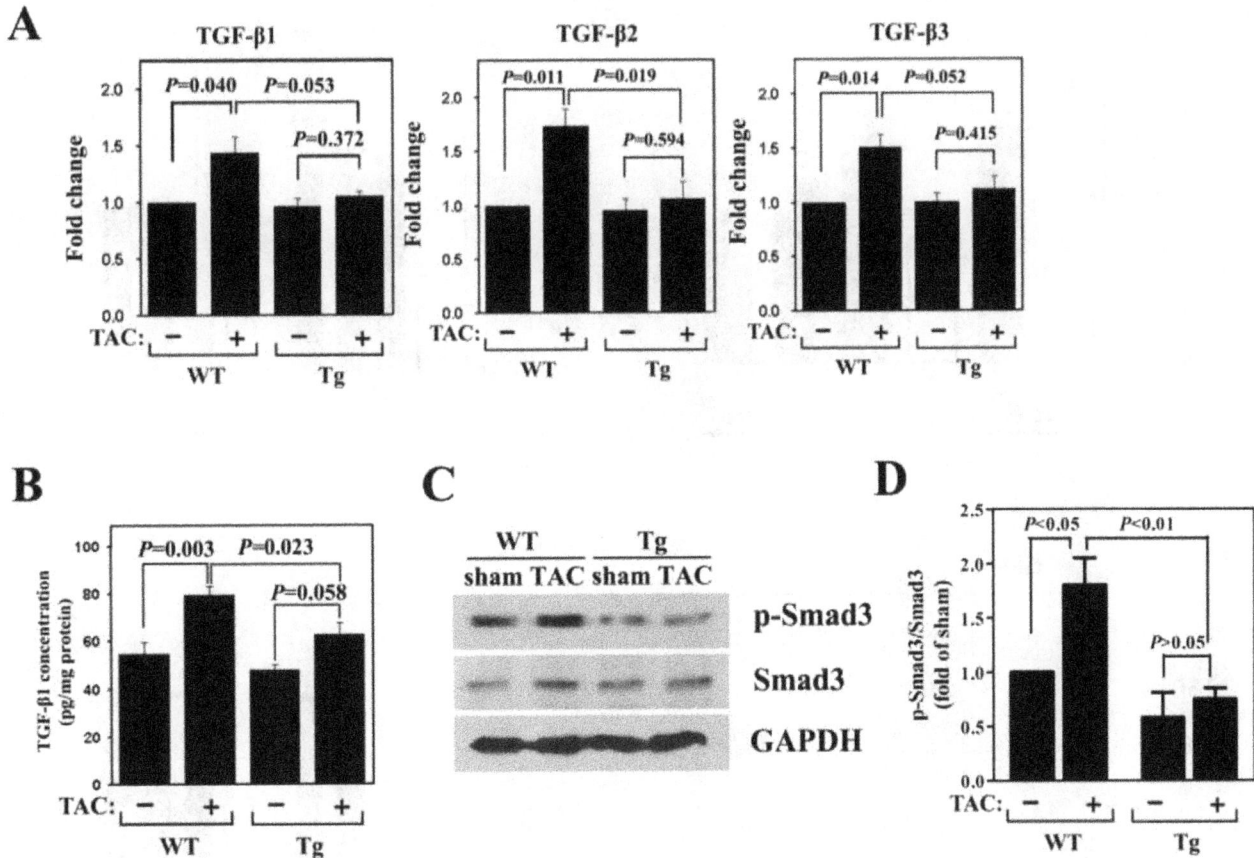

Figure 5. Upregulated TGF-β/Smad signaling is inhibited in CARP Tg mice following TAC. (A) Quantitative detection of TGF-β1, -β2, and -β3 mRNA expression by real-time PCR in hearts from WT and CARP Tg mice subjected to TAC or a sham operation. (B) ELISA measurements of TGF-β1 levels in heart homogenates from WT and CARP Tg mice subjected to TAC or a sham operation. (C) Western blotting to detect phosphorylated and total Smad3 protein in heart protein extracts from WT and CARP Tg mice subjected to TAC or a sham operation. (D) Quantification of the level of phosphorylated Smad 3 shown in (C).

cardiomyocytes in response to various stimuli. This stress-inducible feature of the *Ankrd1* gene, together with the evidence that CARP function is likely not restricted to cardiomyocytes, suggests that CARP is involved in a generalized response to various physiological or pathological stresses, which may be of profound cytoprotective significance. Collectively, these observations provide considerable evidence that the unique pattern of *Ankrd1* expression may reflect a general protective role of CARP in the adaptive responses of cells to stress and disease states.

In the present study, we applied 26-gauge instead of 27-gauge needle as a marker to ligate the aorta so as to exert relatively moderate pressure overload on the heart, which may simulate the course of chronic high blood pressure better. Similar to the previous work reported in our lab [16], the method did make a successful TAC model because: 1) Echocardiographic analysis showed that the blood flow velocity at the ligation site in the TAC mice markedly increased compared with that in sham-operated mice (2980.4±406.3 mm/s for WT-TAC and 3279.7±498.6 mm/s for Tg-TAC vs. 756.4±106.5 mm/s for WT-sham and 877.9±119.3 mm/s for Tg-sham, respectively, P<0.01, Figure S5); 2) Left ventricular hypertrophy was usually apparent at 3 weeks after TAC surgery as determined by echocardiogram (0.81±0.02 mm for WT-TAC vs. 0.65±0.02 mm for WT-sham as indicated by LVPW;d, data not shown), and became more severe at 4 weeks after TAC (Table S1);

3) Histological staining showed increased myocyte size and interstitial fibrosis; 4) Hypertrophic markers altered significantly, and etc. Since the aorta was moderately constricted, although cardiac hypertrophy happened soon after TAC surgery, the heart might gradually adapt to the stress and keep at the compensating state for quite a long period. This kind of model might better mimic the course of cardiac hypertrophy resulting from chronic high blood pressure, but could not progress into heart failure within a short time like some TAC surgeries which constriction is carried out against a 27-gauge needle or to a greater extend [24,25]. Although we could not observe if CARP protected against heart failure during a relatively short period, there were still some clues showing that CARP may play a protective role since overexpression of CARP decreased fibrosis deposition in heart and did not result in cardiomyocyte apoptosis. Besides, Cinquetti et al. found that CARP gene expression and mutation were evident in lymphoblastoid cell lines derived from both a translocation-bearing proband and an independent sporadic total anomalous pulmonary venous return (TAPVR) patient [26]. The study shed light on the functional role played by CARP in cardiomyopathies and suggested that *Ankrd1* gene therapy or modulation of CARP activity could be viable therapeutic strategies against different types of cardiomyopathies.

Several signaling pathways have been implicated in the regulation of cardiac hypertrophy; these include the Raf/MEK/

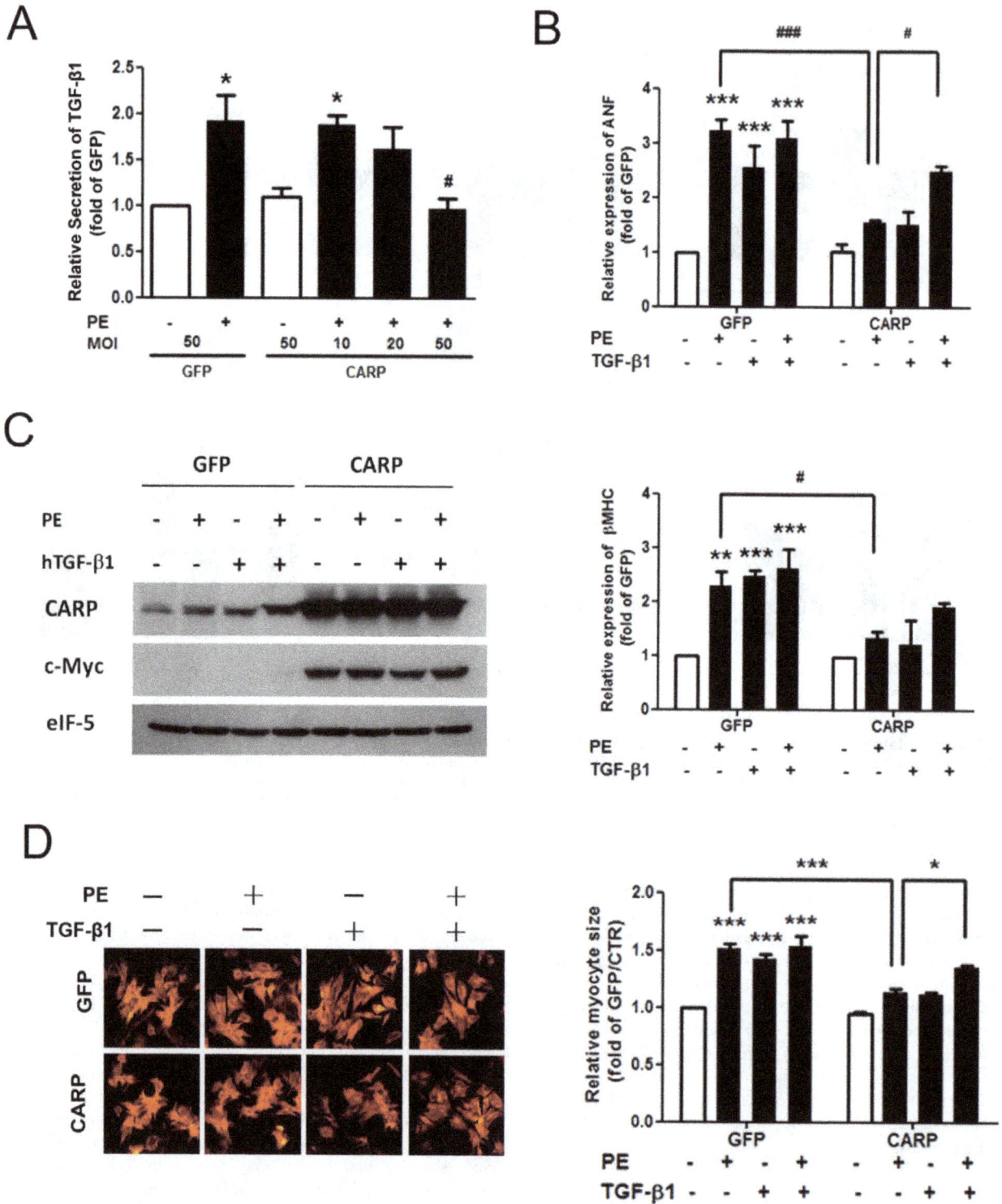

Figure 6. Addition of exogenous human TGF-β1 rescues the attenuation in cardiomyocyte hypertrophy evident upon CARP overexpression. (A) Overexpression of CARP inhibited phenylephrine-induced TGF-β1 secretion by cardiomyocytes. Cultured neonatal rat cardiomyocytes were infected with adenoviruses containing CARP/GFP or GFP alone and next exposed to 10 μM phenylephrine for 24 hours. The levels of TGF-β1 in culture supernatants were next determined using a double-antibody sandwich ELISA method and normalized to the concentrations in the corresponding cardiomyocytes. TGF-β1 secretion from cardiomyocytes infected with adenovirus/GFP alone was taken to be unity in each experiment. n = 4. *$P<0.05$, compared with the GFP control at an MOI of 50; #$P<0.05$, compared with the GFP control at an MOI of 50/PE. (B) Supplementation with exogenous TGF-β1 reversed the inhibitory effect of CARP on hypertrophic markers up-regulation in cardiomyocytes in response to phenylephrine. Cultured cardiomyocytes were infected with adenoviruses containing GFP alone or CARP/GFP/c-myc and next treated with phenylephrine, human TGF-β1, or phenylephrine plus human TGF-β1, for 24 hours. TRIzol was added and total RNA was extracted for determination of the levels of mRNA encoding ANF and β-MHC using real-time PCR. n = 3. **$P<0.01$, ***$P<0.001$, compared with GFP alone; #$P<0.05$, ###$P<0.001$. (C) Western blotting to explore expression of CARP and c-myc in the cardiomyocytes of (B) above. Data from one of four independent

experiments are shown. (D) The inhibitory effect of CARP overexpression on increase in cardiomyocyte size induced by phenylephrine was reversed by addition of hTFG-β1. Cultured cardiomyocytes infected with GFP or GFP/CARP adenoviruses were treated the same way as described in (B) and fixed in 4% (v/v) formaldehyde. Then F-actin was stained with Rhodamine phalloidin and myocyte size was assessed using a microscope equipped with a 200× objective and appropriate epifluorescence filters. 100 random cells were measured in each group and four independent experiments were performed. hTGF-β1, human TGF-β1; MOI, multiplicity of infection; PE, phenylephrine.

MAPK, PI3K/Akt, and JAK/STAT pathways [27]. It has been reported that three major MAPK pathways, ERK, SAPK/JNK (stress-activated/c-Jun N-terminal kinase), and p38 MAPK, are activated in the cardiac tissue of mice following TAC surgery [28]. ERK plays an essential role in mediating the cardiomyocyte hypertrophy induced by the hypertrophic agonists endothelin-1 and phenylephrine [29,30]. In the present study, we found that phosphorylation levels of MEK1/2, ERK1/2, and their downstream target, ribosomal S6 kinase (p90RSK), were remarkably increased after TAC in WT mice, but were unchanged in CARP Tg mice (Figure 6). In contrast, we observed no significant differences in p38, Stat3, or Akt phosphorylation levels between WT and CARP Tg mice subjected to TAC (data not shown). Thus, our data suggest that CARP alleviates cardiac hypertrophy, at least in part, via inhibition of the MEK1/2/ERK1/2 pathway. However, activation of the MEK1/2/ERK1/2 pathway appears to contribute only to cardiomyocyte hypertrophy and not to interstitial fibrosis.

Because TGF-β controls the expression of both ECM network components, such as the fibrillar collagens and fibronectin, and also protease inhibitors, including PAI-1 and TIMPs. TGF-β is an important regulator of extracellular matrix (ECM) deposition. These actions render TGF-β central to the development of tissue fibrosis. TGF-β1, the most important isoform in the cardiovascular system, has been reported to play a central role in the development of heart hypertrophy and heart failure. Transgenic mice overexpressing TGF-β1 display prominent cardiac hypertrophy caused by increases in both cardiomyocyte growth and intercellular fibrosis. We have shown that pressure overload-induced hypertrophy was partially inhibited in CARP Tg mice and, most importantly, that TGF-β1, TGF-β2, and TGF-β3 levels were decreased compared with those of WT animals. In addition, fibrotic marker expression levels were significantly decreased in CARP Tg mice after pressure overload, indicating that expression of the genes encoding collagen synthesis was blocked in the hearts of CARP transgenic mice in response to TAC. This observation is consistent with the results of PSR staining of ventricular heart tissue. Because we also found that TGF-β protein levels were downregulated in CARP Tg mice, it is reasonable to propose that the reduced expression and secretion of TGF-β in such animals, in response to TAC, may contribute to CARP functions in attenuating cardiomyocyte hypertrophy. Our experimental evidence supports this notion. Indeed, TGF-β1 secretion was significantly decreased in CARP-overexpressing cardiomyocytes, in a manner that appeared to be dependent on the MOI of the CARP-expressing viral vector. However, infection with adenovirus carrying GFP alone did not affect the TGF-β1 release level, suggesting that the decrease in TGF-β1 secretion is CARP-dependent. In addition, CARP overexpression inhibited cardiomyocyte hypertrophy in response to phenylephrine. Notably, addition of exogenous TGF-β1 (hTGF-β1) reversed this inhibitory effect of CARP, indicating that the TGF-β signaling pathway participates in the inhibitory action of CARP in terms of cardiac hypertrophy. It is worth mentioning that hTGF-β1 (16 ng/mL) also induced cardiomyocyte hypertrophy and that this effect was also inhibited when CARP was overexpressed. This may be due to that CARP functions as a negative regulator which can directly

inhibit quite a few pro-hypertrophic factors, including the downstream molecules of TGF-β1, so addition of hTGF-β1 alone could not reverse the inhibitory effect of CARP on cardiomyocyte hypertrophy. However, when hTGF-β1 and phenylephrine act together, some unknown synergistic mechanism may be triggered and thereby partly reversing the negative effect of CARP on hypertrophy.

Further support for the proposed deficiency in TGF-β function is provided by our finding that the levels of phosphorylated Smad3, a downstream target of TGF-β signaling, were significantly decreased in the hearts of CARP Tg mice. Smads play central roles in regulating ECM gene expression in response to TGF-β, and Smad3 mediates acute and chronic changes in gene expression that leads to inflammation and fibrosis. Smad3 also plays a role in mediating the effects of angiotensin II; chronic exposure to this protein promotes a profibrotic environment via multiple mechanisms, including increased expression of TGF-β1 and stimulation of Smad3-dependent gene expression.

Since apoptosis causes cell death and cell loss, which directly result in thinning of ventricular wall and heart failure without compensating hypertrophy, we asked whether CARP attenuated cardiac hypertrophy via activating apoptosis. However, our results showed that overexpression of CARP did not promote nuclear condensation and activation of caspase-3 pathway, which are regarded as the distinctive features of apoptosis at biochemical level [31]. The findings suggest that apoptosis is not involved in the inhibitory effect of CARP on cardiac hypertrophy.

It is well-known that analysis of genetically engineered mice has great advantages for our understanding of the in vivo function of a given gene and protein. In the present study we applied cardiac-specific transgenic mice as a model to investigate the function of CARP in cardiac hypertrophy. Cardiac-specific transgene can exclude the impacts of CARP overexpressed in other tissues or organs, and as a negative regulator, gain-of-function study (transgenic model) seems more suitable for investigation of CARP function. However, since the level of CARP in transgenic mice is much higher than normal level, some non-specific effects would inevitably occur.

In summary, our data provide the first evidence that overexpression of CARP decreases the activity of both the ERK1/2 and the TGF-β/Smads signaling pathways and subsequently attenuates cardiac hypertrophy and fibrosis in the hearts of CARP transgenic mice (Figure S6). Our findings thus provide compelling support for a role for CARP in inhibiting cardiac hypertrophy and fibrosis. More importantly, our results highlight the potential significance of CARP as an anti-hypertrophic factor with therapeutic potential against cardiac hypertrophy in humans.

Supporting Information

Figure S1 Establishment and identification of cardiac-specific CARP Tg mice. (A) Schematic diagram of the α-MHC-CARP plasmid. (B) Distinguishing CARP transgenic (Tg) mice from wild-type (WT) mice by PCR genotyping. (C) Expression of CARP in CARP Tg and WT mice as detected by semi-quantitative RT-PCR. GAPDH was used as an internal control. (D) Quantification of the CARP expression shown in (C). (E) Expression of CARP and CARP-Myc fusion proteins in the hearts of WT and CARP Tg mice as detected by Western blotting. β-tubulin was used as an internal control. (F) Quantification of the CARP expression shown in (E). (G) Tissue-specific expression of transgenic CARP in the heart, relative to other tissues (as indicated).

Figure S2 Relative levels of CARP in hearts from wild-type and CARP transgenic mice subjected to sham-operation or TAC. Heart tissue lysates were separated with electrophoresis and the relative levels of CARP and c-myc were detected by Western blotting. Quantification of CARP expression was also shown here. The data were representative of 2 separate experiments (4 samples for each group, i.e. n = 4).

Figure S3 Molecular markers of cardiac hypertrophy are inversely regulated in CARP Tg mice in response to pressure-overload. Expression of mRNAs encoding molecular markers in the hearts of WT and CARP Tg mice subjected to TAC or a sham operation were detected using real-time PCR. Col I, procollagen type Iα2; Col III, procollagen type III α1; Myh6, α-MHC.

Figure S4 Overexpression of CARP did not induce apoptosis of cardiomyocytes. Cardiomyocytes infected with indicated adenovirus constructs were incubated for 48 hours in serum-free medium and treated with or without phenylephrine for 24 hours then: (A) The cells were fixed and stained for nuclear chromatin with Hochest 33342. Fluorescent confocal micrographs were obtained using 2 different filters to visualize GFP or GFP-CARP expression (top), nucleus (medium) and overlapped image (bottom) without changing the viewing field. Note that neither nuclear chromatin nor karyorrhexis occurred in CARP-over-expressed myocytes treated with or without phenylephrine. Scale bar = 50 μm, from 100 infected cells for each of the treatment condition. (B) Cardiomyocytes were collected and the levels of caspase-3 were assessed by Western blotting. Neither decrease in caspase-3 expression nor cleaved caspase-3 was detected in CARP-overexpressed cells. Data are representative of 3 separate experiments.

Figure S5 Representative examples of Doppler echo-cardiography detecting the aortic blood flow at the ligation site of TAC surgery. The wild type and CARP Tg mice were subjected to TAC or sham-operation. Four weeks later, the mice were assessed by echocardiography under anesthesia.

The Doppler images showed velocity of aortic blood flow at ligation site were much higher in the mice subjected to TAC than that in sham-operated mice.

Figure S6 A Schematic Model for CARP Function in Protecting Cardiac Hypertrophy and Fibrosis.

Table S1 Echocardiographic analysis of LV remodeling in response to TAC in CARP Tg mice and WT littermates. All values are means ± SEMs. EF, ejection fraction; FS, fractional shortening; HR, heart rate; LVID;d, end-diastolic left ventricular internal dimension; LVID;s, end-systolic left ventricular internal dimension; LV mass, left ventricular mass, which equals to $1.053*[(LVID;d+LVPW;d+LVAW;d)^3-LVID;d^3]*0.8$; LVPW;d, end-diastolic left ventricular posterior wall; LVPW;s, end-systolic left ventricular posterior wall; LVAW;d, end-diastolic left ventricular anterior wall; LVAW;s, end-systolic left ventricular anterior wall;. $^{**}P<0.01$, $^{***}P<0.001$, compared to sham-operated mice; $^{\#}P<0.05$, $^{\#\#\#}P<0.001$, compared to WT mice subjected to TAC.

Table S2 Echocardiographic analysis of LV remodeling in response to isoproterenol infusion in CARP Tg mice and WT littermates. All values shown are means ± SEMs. EF, ejection fraction; FS, fractional shortening; HR, heart rate; ISO, isoproterenol; LVID;d, end-diastolic left ventricular internal dimension; LVID;s, end-systolic left ventricular internal dimension; LV mass, left ventricular mass, which equals to $1.053*[(LVID;d+LVPW;d+LVAW;d)^3-LVID;d^3]*0.8$; LVPW;d, end-diastolic left ventricular posterior wall; LVPW;s, end-systolic left ventricular posterior wall; LVAW;d, end-diastolic left ventricular anterior wall; LVAW;s, end-systolic left ventricular anterior wall. $^{**}P<0.01$, $^{***}P<0.001$, compared to vehicle-infused mice; $^{\#\#}P<0.01$, $^{\#\#\#}P<0.001$, compared to WT mice treated with ISO.

Author Contributions

Conceived and designed the experiments: DZ Youyi Zhang. Performed the experiments: YS JX YL. Analyzed the data: CJ XM LZ. Contributed reagents/materials/analysis tools: XX Yong Zhang XG. Wrote the paper: YS JX.

References

1. Frey N, Olson EN (2003) Cardiac hypertrophy: The good, the bad, and the ugly. Annu Rev Physiol 65: 45–79.
2. Heineke J, Molkentin JD (2006) Regulation of cardiac hypertrophy by intracellular signalling pathways. Nat Rev Mol Cell Biol 7: 589–600.
3. Hardt SE, Sadoshima J (2004) Negative regulators of cardiac hypertrophy. Cardiovasc Res 63: 500–509.
4. Dahlof B, Pennert K, Hansson L (1992) Reversal of left ventricular hypertrophy in hypertensive patients. A metaanalysis of 109 treatment studies. Am J Hypertens 5: 95–110.
5. Jeyaseelan R, Poizat C, Baker RK, Abdishoo S, Isterabadi LB, et al. (1997) A novel cardiac-restricted target for doxorubicin. Carp, a nuclear modulator of gene expression in cardiac progenitor cells and cardiomyocytes. J Biol Chem 272: 22800–22808.
6. Granzier HL, Labeit S (2004) The giant protein titin: A major player in myocardial mechanics, signaling, and disease. Circ Res 94: 284–295.
7. Miller MK, Granzier H, Ehler E, Gregorio CC (2004) The sensitive giant: The role of titin-based stretch sensing complexes in the heart. Trends Cell Biol 14: 119–126.
8. Purevjav E, Arimura T, Augustin S, Huby AC, Takagi K, et al. (2012) Molecular basis for clinical heterogeneity in inherited cardiomyopathies due to myopalladin mutations. Hum Mol Genet 21: 2039–2053.
9. Mikhailov AT, Torrado M (2008) The enigmatic role of the ankyrin repeat domain 1 gene in heart development and disease. Int J Dev Biol 52: 811–821.
10. Torrado M, Lopez E, Centeno A, Castro-Beiras A, Mikhailov AT (2004) Left-right asymmetric ventricular expression of carp in the piglet heart: Regional response to experimental heart failure. Eur J Heart Fail 6: 161–172.
11. Arber S, Hunter JJ, Ross J Jr., Hongo M, Sansig G, et al. (1997) MLP-deficient mice exhibit a disruption of cardiac cytoarchitectural organization, dilated cardiomyopathy, and heart failure. Cell 88: 393–403.
12. Aihara Y, Kurabayashi M, Arai M, Kedes L, Nagai R (1999) Molecular cloning of rabbit carp cdna and its regulated expression in adriamycin-cardiomyopathy. Biochim Biophys Acta 1447: 318–324.
13. Zolk O, Frohme M, Maurer A, Kluxen FW, Hentsch B, et al. (2002) Cardiac ankyrin repeat protein, a negative regulator of cardiac gene expression, is augmented in human heart failure. Biochim Biophys Res Commun 293: 1377–1382.

14. Nagueh SF, Shah G, Wu Y, Torre-Amione G, King NM, et al. (2004) Altered titin expression, myocardial stiffness, and left ventricular function in patients with dilated cardiomyopathy. Circulation 110: 155–162.

15. Wei YJ, Cui CJ, Huang YX, Zhang XL, Zhang H, et al. (2009) Upregulated expression of cardiac ankyrin repeat protein in human failing hearts due to arrhythmogenic right ventricular cardiomyopathy. Eur J Heart Fail 11: 559–566.

16. Xiao H, Ma X, Feng W, Fu Y, Lu Z, et al. (2010) Metformin attenuates cardiac fibrosis by inhibiting the TGFβ1–Smad3 signalling pathway. Cardiovasc Res 87: 504–513.

17. Lim HW, De Windt LJ, Steinberg L, Taigen T, Witt SA, et al. (2000) Calcineurin expression, activation, and function in cardiac pressure-overload hypertrophy. Circulation 101: 2431–2437.

18. Moulik M, Vatta M, Witt SH, Arola AM, Murphy RT, et al. (2009) Ankrd1, the gene encoding cardiac ankyrin repeat protein, is a novel dilated cardiomyopathy gene. J Am Coll Cardiol 54: 325–333.

19. Takeda S, Hisatome I (2001) Overexpression of CARP, a cell type-restricted ankyrin repeat protein, inhibits cardiac hypertrophy. J Yonago Medical Association 52: 144–152.

20. Shi Y, Reitmaier B, Regenbogen J, Slowey RM, Opalenik SR, et al. (2005) Carp, a cardiac ankyrin repeat protein, is up-regulated during wound healing and induces angiogenesis in experimental granulation tissue. Am J Pathol 166: 303–312.

21. Nakada C, Tsukamoto Y, Oka A, Nonaka I, Takeda S, et al. (2003) Cardiac-restricted ankyrin-repeated protein is differentially induced in duchenne and congenital muscular dystrophy. Lab Invest 83: 711–719.

22. Han XJ, Chae JK, Lee MJ, You KR, Lee BH, et al. (2005) Involvement of gadd153 and cardiac ankyrin repeat protein in hypoxia-induced apoptosis of h9c2 cells. J Biol Chem 280: 23122–23129.

23. Scurr LL, Guminski AD, Chiew YE, Balleine RL, Sharma R, et al. (2008) Ankyrin repeat domain 1, ankrd1, a novel determinant of cisplatin sensitivity expressed in ovarian cancer. Clin Cancer Res 14: 6924–6932.

24. Barrick CJ, Rojas M, Schoonhoven R, Smyth SS, Threadgill DW (2007) Cardiac response to pressure overload in 129S1/SvImJ and C57BL/6J mice: temporal- and background-dependent development of concentric left ventricular hypertrophy. Am J Physiol Heart Circ Physiol 292: H2119–H2130.

25. Xu Q, Lekgabe ED, Gao XM, Ming Z, Tregear GW, et al. (2008) Endogenous relaxin does not affect chronic pressure overload-induced cardiac hypertrophy and fibrosis. Endocronology 149: 476–482.

26. Cinquetti R, Badi I, Campione M, Bortoletto E, Chiesa G, et al. (2008) Transcriptional deregulation and a missense mutation define ankrd1 as a candidate gene for total anomalous pulmonary venous return. Hum Mutat 29: 468–474.

27. Rohini A, Agrawal N, Koyani CN, Singh R (2010) Molecular targets and regulators of cardiac hypertrophy. Pharmacol Res 61: 269–280.

28. Esposito G, Prasad SV, Rapacciuolo A, Mao L, Koch WJ, et al. (2001) Cardiac overexpression of a G(q) inhibitor blocks induction of extracellular signal-regulated kinase and c-jun nh(2)-terminal kinase activity in in vivo pressure overload. Circulation 103: 1453–1458.

29. Yue TL, Gu JL, Wang C, Reith AD, Lee JC, et al. (2000) Extracellular signal-regulated kinase plays an essential role in hypertrophic agonists, endothelin-1 and phenylephrine-induced cardiomyocyte hypertrophy. J Biol Chem 275: 37895–37901.

30. Bueno OF, De Windt LJ, Tymitz KM, Witt SA, Kimball TR, et al. (2000) The mek1-erk1/2 signaling pathway promotes compensated cardiac hypertrophy in transgenic mice. EMBO J 19: 6341–6350.

31. Kotamraju S, Konorev EA, Joseph J, Kalyanaraman B (2000) Doxorubicin-induced apoptosis in endothelial cells and cardiomyocytes is ameliorated by nitrone spin traps and Ebselen. J Biol Chem 275: 33585–33592.

11

Rac-Induced Left Ventricular Dilation in Thyroxin-Treated ZmRacD Transgenic Mice: Role of Cardiomyocyte Apoptosis and Myocardial Fibrosis

Mohammad T. Elnakish[1,2]**, Mohamed D. H. Hassona**[1]**, Mazin A. Alhaj**[1]**, Leni Moldovan**[3]**,
Paul M. L. Janssen[2]**, Mahmood Khan**[4]**, Hamdy H. Hassanain**[1]*

1 Department of Anesthesiology, and Dorothy M. Davis Heart and Lung Research Institute, The Ohio State University, Columbus, Ohio, United States of America,
2 Department of Physiology and Cell Biology, and Dorothy M. Davis Heart and Lung Research Institute, The Ohio State University, Columbus, Ohio, United States of America, 3 Department of Pulmonary, Allergy, Critical Care and Sleep Medicine, and Dorothy M. Davis Heart and Lung Research Institute, The Ohio State University, Columbus, Ohio, United States of America, 4 Department of Internal Medicine, and Dorothy M. Davis Heart and Lung Research Institute, The Ohio State University, Columbus, Ohio, United States of America

Abstract

The pathways inducing the critical transition from compensated hypertrophy to cardiac dilation and failure remain poorly understood. The goal of our study is to determine the role of Rac-induced signaling in this transition process. Our previous results showed that Thyroxin (T4) treatment resulted in increased myocardial Rac expression in wild-type mice and a higher level of expression in Zea maize RacD (ZmRacD) transgenic mice. Our current results showed that T4 treatment induced physiologic cardiac hypertrophy in wild-type mice, as demonstrated by echocardiography and histopathology analyses. This was associated with significant increases in myocardial Rac-GTP, superoxide and ERK1/2 activities. Conversely, echocardiography and histopathology analyses showed that T4 treatment induced dilated cardiomyopathy along with compensatory cardiac hypertrophy in ZmRacD mice. These were linked with further increases in myocardial Rac-GTP, superoxide and ERK1/2 activities. Additionally, there were significant increases in caspase-8 expression and caspase-3 activity. However, there was a significant decrease in p38-MAPK activity. Interestingly, inhibition of myocardial Rac-GTP activity and superoxide generation with pravastatin and carvedilol, respectively, attenuated all functional, structural, and molecular changes associated with the T4-induced cardiomyopathy in ZmRacD mice except the compensatory cardiac hypertrophy. Taken together, T4-induced ZmRacD is a novel mouse model of dilated cardiomyopathy that shares many characteristics with the human disease phenotype. To our knowledge, this is the first study to show graded Rac-mediated $O_2 \cdot^-$ results in cardiac phenotype shift *in-vivo*. Moreover, Rac-mediated $O_2 \cdot^-$ generation, cardiomyocyte apoptosis, and myocardial fibrosis seem to play a pivotal role in the transition from cardiac hypertrophy to cardiac dilation and failure. Targeting Rac signaling could represent valuable therapeutic strategy not only in saving the failing myocardium but also to prevent this transition process.

Editor: Tianqing Peng, University of Western Ontario, Canada

Funding: This work was supported by Startup fund, Department of Anesthesiology, The Ohio State University. Mohammad T. Elnakish was supported by a scholarship from The Egyptian Government. The funders had no role in study design, data collection and analysis, decision to publish, or preparation of the manuscript.

Competing Interests: The authors have declared that no competing interests exist.

* E-mail: dr.hamdyhassanain@gmail.com

Introduction

Cardiovascular diseases remain the main cause of death in the Western world, with heart failure representing the highest increasing subclass over the past decade [1]. Heart failure is classically induced by several common disease stimuli, such as hypertension, myocardial infarction or ischemic coronary artery diseases [2,3]. Most of these stimuli initially provoke a stage of cardiac hypertrophy [4]. Hypertrophy can be a compensatory response to enhance contractility and preserve cardiac output exclusive of undesirable pathology. Nevertheless, persistent stress can progress this compensatory process into a decompensated state with reflective alterations in gene expression profile, contractile dysfunction, and extracellular remodeling [5,6]. Pathological signs in end-stage heart failure share various common features apart from the causal etiologies, such as ventricular wall thinning, chamber dilation, cardiomyocyte loss, and severely increased interstitial fibrosis [7], signifying that intracellular signaling pathways triggered by different stressors may congregate to a number of common targets [8]. As highly conserved signaling pathway, the Rho/Rac signaling may be a common mediator in these pathological remodeling processes.

Previous studies using isolated cardiomyocytes from transgenic mice over-expressing Rac1 in the myocardium showed the importance of Rac1 in the development of cardiac hypertrophy [9]. Also, over-expression of a constitutively active form of human Rac1 in the hearts of transgenic mice resulted in cardiac hypertrophy and cardiac dilation [10]. Additionally, It has been reported that in human heart failure, increased NADPH oxidase–dependent ROS production is coupled with increased membrane expression and activity of Rac1 [11]. More recently, we have shown for the first time the conservation of Rho/Rac proteins in both plant and animal kingdoms *in-vivo*. Furthermore, we showed that over-expression of a constitutively active cardiac-specific form of ZmRacD gene in the transgenic mice resulted in cardiac hypertrophy as well as a moderate decrease in systolic function in older mice. Besides, the activation of ZmRacD expression with T4 for two weeks led to cardiac dilation and severe systolic dysfunction in adult transgenic mice. However, the same T4 treatment in wild-type mice resulted in a lower increase in myocardial expression of endogenous Rac with preserved cardiac function and left ventricular (LV) internal diameters [12]. Moreover, our current data shows that this preserved cardiac function in wild-type mice after T4 treatment is linked to physiologic cardiac hypertrophy.

While physiological versus pathological hypertrophy can be obviously distinguished by numerous qualitative and quantitative parameters, the basic mechanisms and their interrelationship remain divisive. Most notably, the signaling mechanisms inducing the critical transition from compensated hypertrophy to decompensated heart failure remain poorly understood [6,13]. In the current study we hypothesize that recognizing the functional, structural, and molecular differences between these two distinct phenotypes; the Rac- induced physiologic cardiac hypertrophy in wild-type mice and pathologic cardiac dilation in ZmRacD transgenic mice after T4 treatment, will provide better understanding of the molecular mechanisms behind these diseases. This will allow for better treatment options in the future.

Methods

Animals

Mice were bred and maintained at the W.M. Keck Genetic Research Facility of The Ohio State University (OSU), and all experimental procedures and protocols used in this study were approved by the Animal Care and Use Committee of OSU, conforming with the guide for care and use of laboratory animals published by U.S. National Institutes of Health (NIH publication No. 85-23, revised 1996). 6-to-8-months-old sex-matched heterozygous ZmRacD transgenic mice and nontransgenic wild-type littermates were used in this study. Unless otherwise stated 6 to 8 mice per genotype were used for each experiment.

Thyroxin (T4) and Drug Treatments

T4 was prepared as described by Pierres and Gaugain-Hamidi [14] with slight modification to increase both the solubility and stability of T4 preparation. Briefly, each 100 ml of the preparation contained all of the following: (Sodium-L-thyroxin: 2 mg, NaHCO$_3$: 0.336 g, hydroxypropyl-β-cyclodextrin: 2 g, EDTA: 0.1 g, ammonium chloride: 0.5 g, ethanol: 15 ml, all obtained from Sigma), *p*H was adjusted to 8.5, then completed to 100 ml with double distilled water and stored at 4 C°.

Animals were divided into 6 groups based on genetic background and treatment (n = 8/group) as follows: wild-type; wild-type + T4; ZmRacD; ZmRacD + T4; ZmRacD + carvedilol + T4; ZmRacD + pravastatin + T4. The study duration was extended to 3 weeks instead of 2 weeks [12] based on previous studies demonstrating that the largest part (70–80%) of the myocardial remodeling process in rodent e.g. rat occurs within the first 3 weeks [15]. Basal echocardiography parameters were determined before starting T4 treatment and on a weekly basis thereafter, till the experiment was terminated. T4 (200 µg/Kg) was injected intraperitoneally as previously described [12].

Carvedilol (2 mg/Kg) or pravastatin (10 mg/Kg) were administered by intraperitoneal injection 1 hour before T4 administration. Carvedilol was prepared as reported in [16] with some modifications. Briefly, carvedilol from Sigma was dissolved in a minimal amount of DMSO, and then diluted with 5% dextrose solution containing 1–2 drops of glacial acetic acid (final DMSO concentration ≤0.1%). The dose of carvedilol used in this study was based on previous studies that showed its effectiveness in a rat model of cardiac dilation and it is roughly equivalent to the carvedilol dose in human [17]. Pravastatin was prepared and injected as previously described [12]. At the end of the treatment period animals underwent echocardiography. Directly after echocardiography, animals were sacrificed, and hearts were excised and processed for further experiments.

Echocardiography

In- vivo cardiac dimension and contractile function in both wild-type and transgenic mice were evaluated using a high-frequency ultrasound imaging system (VEVO 2100, Visual Sonics, Toronto, ON, Canada). Experimental mice were initially anesthetized with isoflurane at a concentration of 2% and thereafter maintained at 1% isoflurane using nasal prongs during the whole procedure. The measurements were taken from the parasternal short-axis view in M-mode to view the LV movement during diastole and systole corresponding to the electrocardiogram. All data and imaging were analyzed by the Visual Sonics Cardiac Measurements Package.

Myocardial Rac-GTP Activity

Rac-GTP activity was detected using a new commercially available antibody that has been reported to be specific for the active GTP-bound state of Rac1 (Neweast Biosciences, cat. #: 26903). This antibody has been recently characterized as a probe to examine Rac1 activation status in formalin-fixed paraffin embedded (FFPE) samples [18]. Immunohistochemical staining of Rac1-GTP was performed on 4-µm sections from FFPE midventricles. Antigen retrieval was performed by a heat method in which the specimens were placed in Dako's target retrieval solution, pH 6.1 (Dako code S1699) for 25 minutes at 95°C using a steamer and cooled for 15 minutes in solution. Slides were then placed on a Dako Autostainer, immunostaining system. To minimize nonspecific staining, the Animal Research Kit from Dako (code K3955) was used according to the package insert. Primary antibody was diluted 1:150. Slides were initially blocked for endogenous biotin, and then the biotinylated primary antibody was added for 1 hour, followed by the labeled streptavidin for 30 minutes. Finally, the slides were developed with diaminobenzidine (DAB) chromogen for 10 minutes, lightly counterstained in Richard Allen hematoxylin, dehydrated through graded ethanol solutions and coverslipped. 3 to 5-images per heart were acquired with a 20× objective for morphometric evaluation of the brownstained Rac-GTP using MetaMorph image analysis software 7.1.2.0 (Molecular Devices, CA).

Myocardial Superoxide (O$_2$·$^-$) Production

In-situ production of myocardial O$_2$·$^-$ was assessed by the fluorescent dye, dihydroethidium (DHE) as described previously [12]. Briefly, hearts from both wild-type and transgenic mice were placed immediately in ice-cold PBS, washed and then embedded in OCT for cryosectioning. Frozen sections (6-µm) from the hearts were incubated with DHE (10 µM; Sigma-Aldrich) for 30 min at 37°C in a dark chamber. After rinsing with PBS, sections were mounted in aqueous medium (Gel Mount, Sigma) and 3 to 5-images per heart were acquired with a 40× objective using a fluorescence microscope (Nikon TE 300, Tokyo, Japan). The red fluorescence intensity was determined using the MetaMorph image analysis software 7.1.2.0.

Cardiomyocyte Length and Cross Sectional Area

4-μm FFPE mid-ventricles sections were lightly stained with Masson's trichrome. 3 to 5-images per heart were acquired with a 40× objective with a Nikon Eclipse TS-100F inverted microscope equipped with a Lumenera Infinity 1-2C camera (Nikon Instruments Inc., Melville, NY). The length and cross sectional area of cardiomyocytes were measured using the MetaMorph image analysis software 7.1.2.0 as previously described [12]. An average of 50–150 cells/group have been evaluated for cardiomyocyte length and 200–500 cells/group have been evaluated for cardiomyocyte cross sectional area.

Myocardial Fibrosis

Standard Masson's trichrome staining was performed on 6-μm sections from FFPE mid-ventricles. 3 to 5-images per heart were acquired with a 40× objective for morphometric evaluation using MetaMorph image analysis software 7.1.2.0 and collagen deposition areas in both ventricles were calculated from different animals.

Western Blot Analysis

Western blots were performed to determine the relative cardiac expression of the extracellular signal-regulated kinase (ERK1/2), p-ERK1/2, jun NH2-terminal kinase (JNK), p-JNK, p38 MAPK, p-p38 MAPK, caspase-8, cleaved caspase-3 and tumor necrosis factor-α (TNF-α) in both wild-type and transgenic mice as described in our previous reports [19]. Membranes were incubated with specific antibody for p-ERK1/2 and p38 MAPK (1:1000; Cell Signaling), ERK1/2, JNK and p-JNK (1:500; Santa Cruz), p-p38 MAPK (1:500; Cell Signaling), or caspase-8, cleaved caspase-3 and TNF-α (1:250; Cell Signaling). Secondary antibodies were goat anti-rabbit and anti-mouse IgG-HRP (1:2000; Santa Cruz). Antibody signals were detected by an enhanced chemiluminescence kit (Pierce, USA), and GAPDH (1:3000; Cell Signaling) was used as an internal control for equal protein loading. All Western blot results are expressed as the ratio of respective proteins to GAPDH.

Myocardial Cell Apoptosis

To detect fragmented DNA, in-situ terminal deoxynucleotidyl transferase-mediated nick-end labeling (TUNEL) assay was performed as specified in the in-situ apoptosis detection kit instructions (Roche, cat. # 11 684 817 910) using 4-μm FFPE mid-ventricles sections. The slides were developed with a DAB chromogen for 10 minutes. Slides were then lightly counterstained in Richard Allen hematoxylin, dehydrated through graded ethanol solutions and coverslipped. 3 to 5-images per heart were acquired with a 40× objective for morphometric evaluation of the brown-stained apoptotic nuclei using MetaMorph image analysis software 7.1.2.0. Data are expressed as the percentage of apoptotic nuclei relative to normal nuclei.

Data Analysis

Data were analyzed by ANOVA followed by Tukey-Kramer Multiple Comparisons post-hoc test, and are presented as means ± SEM. A two-tailed value of $P < 0.05$ was considered statistically significant.

Results

T4-Stimulated Rac Expression is Associated with Increased Myocardial Rac-GTP Activity and Superoxide ($O_2 \cdot {}^-$) Production

Our current data confirmed our previous finding [12] and showed significant increases in myocardial Rac expression in transgenic (0.63 ± 0.03; $p < 0.05$) compared to wild-type (0.38 ± 0.04) mice at basal conditions. In addition, T4 supplementation resulted in increased myocardial Rac expression in wild-type (0.66 ± 0.04; $p < 0.01$) compared to untreated adult wild-type mice, and resulted in further increase in myocardial Rac expression in transgenic mice (1.20 ± 0.03; $p < 0.001$) compared to all other groups. Pre-treatment of T4-supplemented mice with carvedilol, a mixed α, β-blocker with antioxidant activity [17], or pravastatin, an antihyperlipidemic with Rac-GTPase inhibiting activity [12] did not significantly (1.1 ± 0.03 and 1.3 ± 0.07, respectively) affect T4-induced myocardial Rac expression in ZmRacD mice (Figure 1A).

Interestingly, our current results demonstrate that T4-induced myocardial Rac expression is associated with corresponding increases in both Rac-GTP activity and $O_2 \cdot {}^-$ production in the mouse hearts. Immunostaining of Rac-GTP and DHE staining of $O_2 \cdot {}^-$ showed significant increases in myocardial Rac-GTP activity and $O2 \cdot {}^-$ levels in transgenic mice (7.10 ± 0.40 and 2.50 ± 0.10; $p < 0.001$) compared to adult wild-type mice (0.70 ± 0.10 and 0.90 ± 0.10), respectively, at basal conditions. Similarly, T4-stimulated Rac expression in wild-type mice was associated with significant increases in myocardial Rac-GTP activity and $O2 \cdot {}^-$ levels (5.61 ± 0.15; $p < 0.05$ and 2.60 ± 0.15; $p < 0.001$), respectively, compared to untreated wild-type mice. Furthermore, T4-stimulated myocardial Rac expression in transgenic mice was associated with highly significant increases in myocardial Rac-GTP activity and $O2 \cdot {}^-$ levels (14.10 ± 2.24 and 3.70 ± 0.15; $p < 0.001$), respectively, compared to all other groups (Figure 1B, C, D, E). On the other hand, our data show that pravastatin (6.40 ± 0.60; $p < 0.001$) but not carvedilol (11.40 ± 0.50) significantly reduced T4-induced myocardial Rac-GTP activity to levels that were not significant from untreated transgenic and T4-treated wild-type mice , while still significantly higher compared to untreated wild-type mice ($p < 0.01$) (Figure 1B, C). Conversely, both carvedilol (1.70 ± 0.17; $p < 0.001$) and pravastatin (1.82 ± 0.21; $p < 0.001$) significantly reduced T4-induced myocardial $O2 \cdot {}^-$ to levels that were significantly lower from those of untreated transgenic ($p < 0.01$ and 0.05, respectively) and T4-treated wild-type mice ($p < 0.01$), while still significantly higher compared to untreated wild-type mice ($p < 0.01$) (Figure 1D, E).

T4-Stimulated Myocardial Rac Expression and Activity Led to Physiologic Cardiac Hypertrophy in Wild-Type Mice and Dilated Cardiomyopathy in Transgenic Mice

Heart weight (HW) and body weight (BW) data are shown in (Table 1). Initially, BW did not significantly change among groups. However, T4-treated wild-type mice demonstrated significant increases in both HW ($p < 0.001$) and HW/BW ratios ($p < 0.001$) compared to untreated wild-type and transgenic mice. Similarly, T4-treated transgenic mice showed significant increases in both HW ($p < 0.001$) and HW/BW ratios ($p < 0.01$) compared to untreated wild-type and transgenic mice. Nonetheless, carvedilol and pravastatin did not significantly affect both HW and HW/BW ratios of T4-treated transgenic mice (Table 1).

Using echocardiography, cardiac dimensions and function were evaluated in wild-type and transgenic mice under basal conditions,

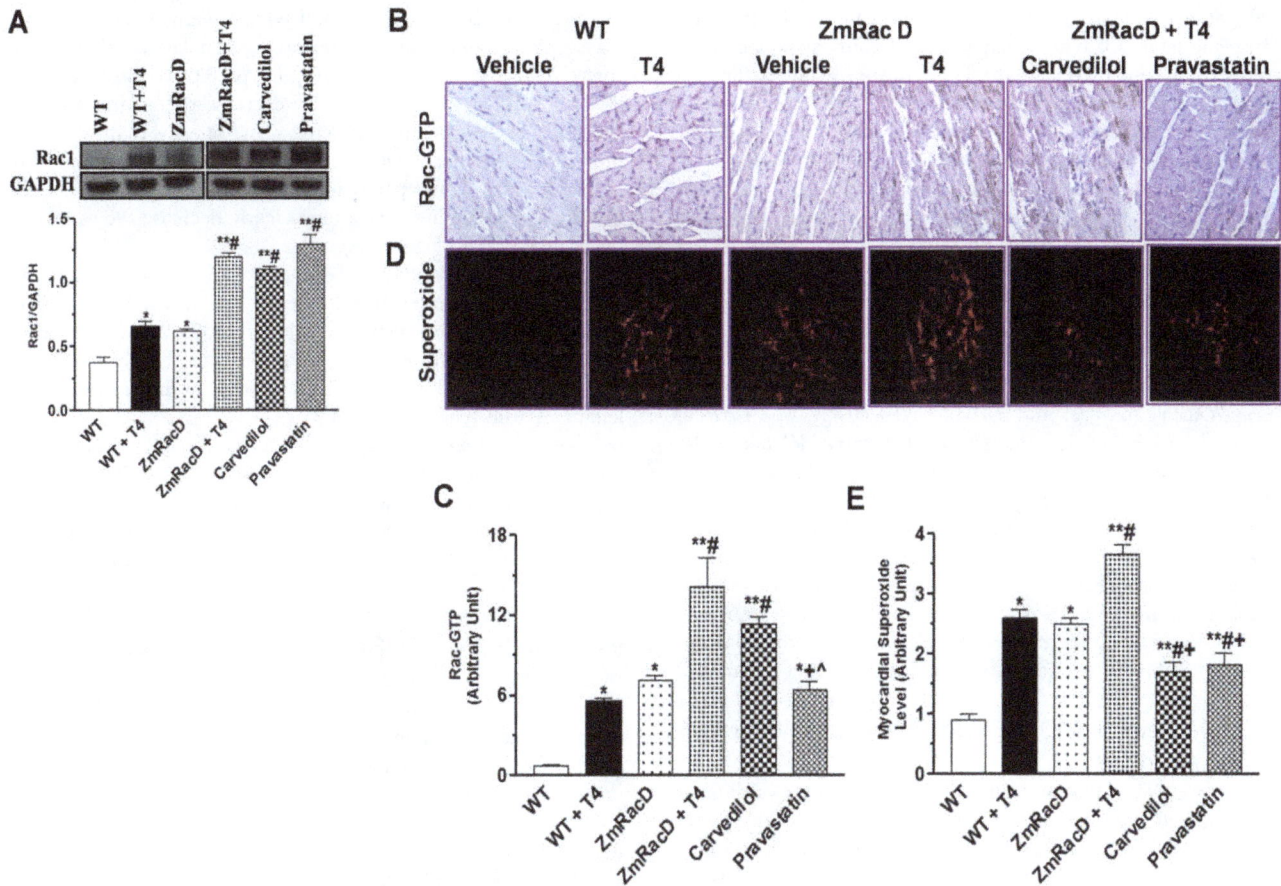

Figure 1. T4-Stimulated Rac Expression is Associated with Increased Myocardial Rac-GTP Activity and Superoxide (O2·⁻) Production. Western blot analyses of myocardial Rac1 (**A**) Representative images of Rac-GTP immunostaining in FFPE mid-ventricle sections, with bar graph for the mean intensity of the brown colored active Rac-GTP in arbitrary units (**B & C**). Representative images of myocardial $O_2^{\cdot-}$ generation with DHE in frozen sections of mice hearts, with bar graphs for mean fluorescence intensity in arbitrary units (**D & E**). * is significant change compared to untreated WT mice, ** is significant change compared to T4-treated and untreated WT mice, # is significant change compared to untreated transgenic mice, + is significant change compared to T4-treated transgenic mice, and ^ is significant change compared to T4-supplemented transgenic mice that pre-treated with carvedilol (n = 8/group).

as well as after T4 stimulation (Table 2). Our current results show no significant differences in cardiac dimensions and function between adult transgenic and wild-type mice at basal conditions. Likewise, T4-treated wild-type mice demonstrated non-significant changes in cardiac dimensions and function compared to untreated wild-type mice. However, these mice showed significant increases in both LV mass (p<0.001) and LV mass/BW ratio (p<0.05) compared to untreated wild-type and transgenic mice. In contrast, T4-treated transgenic mice experienced remarkable

cardiac dysfunction, as shown by decreased LV ejection fraction (EF) (p<0.001) and fractional shortening (FS) (p<0.001) and exhibited enlarged left chambers, as shown by increased systolic (p<0.001) and diastolic (p<0.001) internal diameters, compared to all other groups. Furthermore, these T4-treated mice demonstrated significantly smaller posterior wall thickness during diastole compared to untreated and T4-treated wild-type (p<0.01) and untreated transgenic (p<0.001) mice. Moreover, there were significant increases in both LV mass (p<0.001) and LV mass/

Table 1. Body Weight and Heart Weight Data.

	WT		ZmRacD		ZmRacD + T4	
	Vehicle	T4	Vehicle	T4	Carvedilol	Pravastatin
BW (g)	29±0.95	33±0.74	34±1	35±2.5	28±1.4	29±2.01
HW (mg)	116±5.22	178±2.7*#	127±5.2	188±5.2*#	163±13.20*#	168±5.8*#
HW/BW (mg/g)	3.74±0.33	5.43±0.16*#	4.01±0.08	5.20±0.10*#	4.90±0.26*#	5.30±0.12*#

*is significant change compared to untreated WT mice, and,
#is significant change compared to untreated transgenic mice, (n = 8/group).

BW ratio (p<0.001) compared to untreated wild-type and transgenic mice. Of note, extending the treatment period of T4 to 3 weeks in this current study slightly increased the pathogenic effect of T4 on the transgenic mice; however, this did not reach significance compared to the 2 weeks T4 treatment used in our previous report [12] (Figure S1).

Echocardiography analysis demonstrated that both carvedilol and pravastatin significantly improved the cardiac functions of the T4-treated transgenic mice as indicated by increased EF (p<0.001) and FS (p<0.001). In addition, carvedilol and pravastatin significantly reduced the LV chamber dilation in T4-treated transgenic mice as evident by decreased systolic (p<0.05) and diastolic (p<0.001) internal diameters. Furthermore, carvedilol and pravastatin significantly increased posterior wall thickness during diastole (p<0.01 and p<0.05), respectively, in T4-treated transgenic mice. On the contrary, neither carvedilol nor pravastatin significantly affected LV mass or LV mass/BW ratios in T4-treated transgenic mice (Table 2).

It is worth mentioning that our recent experiments with propranolol, a β-blocker lacking the antioxidant activity [20], showed inferior efficacy compared to carvedilol. Propranolol was unable to improve the cardiac functions of T4-treated transgenic mice; however, it significantly decreased the LV internal diameter to a remarkably lower extent compared to carvedilol (Figure S2).

Structural Remodeling of Cardiac Myocytes in the Hearts of T4-Treated Mice

Both transversal and longitudinal sections through cardiomyocytes stained with Masson's trichrome were obtained and analyzed. For the transversal sections we measured the cross sectional area of the cardiomyocytes. Our results show no statistical difference between wild-type mice ($297 \pm 9 \ \mu m^2$) and transgenic mice ($320 \pm 5 \ \mu m^2$) under basal conditions. However, a statistically significant increase was observed in T4-treated wild-type mice ($385 \pm 8 \ \mu m^2$) compared to untreated wild-type and transgenic mice (p<0.01). In striking contrast to all groups, T4-treated transgenic mice exhibited a dramatically significant increase in the cross sectional area ($702 \pm 14 \ \mu m^2$; p<0.001)

(Figure 2A, B). In addition, we noticed that many of the T4-treated transgenic cardiomyocytes appeared vacuolated (Figure 2A). Interestingly, carvedilol ($518 \pm 20 \ \mu m^2$; p<0.001) and pravastatin ($498 \pm 10 \ \mu m^2$; p<0.001) markedly decrease the enlarged cardiomyocytes of T4-treated transgenic mice. However, they did not normalize the cardiomyocyte size and it was still significantly higher (p<0.001) compared to all other groups (Figure 2A, B). Besides, carvedilol and pravastatin clearly decrease the cardiomyocyte vacuolation (Figure 2A).

Cardiomyocyte lengths were measured in those sections with clearly delineated intercalated discs at both ends. We found no significant differences between wild-type ($37 \pm 2 \ \mu m$) and transgenic ($38 \pm 1 \ \mu m$) mice under basal conditions. In contrast, T4 stimulation resulted in a significant increase in the cardiomyocyte length of wild-type mice ($50 \pm 3 \ \mu m$; p<0.001) compared to all other groups. Unexpectedly, T4-treated transgenic mice showed no significant difference in the cardiomyocyte length ($38 \pm 1 \ \mu m$) compared to untreated wild-type and transgenic mice. Likewise, carvedilol ($35 \pm 1 \ \mu m$) and pravastatin ($36 \pm 2 \ \mu m$) did not significantly change the lengths of T4-treated transgenic mice (Figure 2C, D).

Increased Myocardial Fibrosis in Dilated Cardiomyopathy of T4-Treated Transgenic mice

As evident by Masson's trichrome staining our results showed no apparent fibrosis in wild-type mice under basal conditions (4.40 ± 0.50). Also, the total collagen content in the hearts of untreated transgenic (6.50 ± 0.95) and T4-treated wild-type (7.00 ± 0.53) mice did not significantly changed compared to untreated wild-type mice. Conversely, Masson's trichrome staining clearly demonstrated significantly higher levels of cardiac fibrosis in the ventricles of T4-treated transgenic mice with extremely significant higher total collagen content (16.40 ± 1.20; p<0.001) compared to all other groups (Figure 3A, B). In contrast, carvedilol (6.90 ± 0.60; p<0.001) and pravastatin (5.10 ± 0.40; p<0.001) significantly attenuated the cardiac fibrosis and decreased the total collagen content in the hearts of T4-treated transgenic mice

Table 2. Ech Table 2. Echocardiography Analysis.

	WT		ZmRacD		ZmRacD + T4	
	Vehicle	T4	Vehicle	T4	Carvedilol	Pravastatin
% LVEF	69±3.6	74±3.3	71±2.4	35±1.6**#	65±2.33+	64±6.43+
% LVFS	42±2.4	42±2.9	39±1.5	16±1.23**#	34±1.87+	35±4.73+
IVS,s (mm)	1.3±0.12	1.4±0.05	1.43±0.04	1.24±0.07	1.5±0.04	1.38±0.09
IVS,d (mm)	0.8±0.08	0.98±0.08	1.04±0.04	0.92±0.09	1.01±0.05	1.05±0.09
LVID,s (mm)	2.6±.09	3±0.16	2.7±0.11	3.8±0.12**#	2.95±0.27+	2.98±0.19+
LVID,d (mm)	3.7±0.11	4.1±0.06	3.94±0.02	4.9±0.13**#	3.96±0.21+	3.96±0.16+
LVPW,s (mm)	1.3±0.1	1.5±0.1	1.43±0.09	1.18±0.07	1.43±0.07	1.15±0.09
LVPW,d (mm)	1.08±0.1	1.1±0.03	1.12±0.04	0.74±0.04**#	1.05±0.06+	1.00±0.05+
LV mass (mg)	100±4.1	143±6.1*#	103±2.8	160±2.03*#	135±7.03*#	142±9.82*#
LV mass/Body Weight (mg/g)	2.62±0.12	4.2±0.2*#	2.63±0.12	5.2±0.5*#	4.60±0.34*#	4.72±0.44*#

IVS, interventricular septum; LVID, left ventricular internal diameter; LVPW, left ventricular posterior wall; s, systole; d; diastole; BW, body weight; EF, ejection fraction; FS, fractional shortening.
*is significant change compared to untreated WT mice,
**is significant change compared to T4-treated and untreated WT mice,
#is significant change compared to untreated transgenic mice, and.
+is significant change compared to T4-treated transgenic mice (n = 8/group).

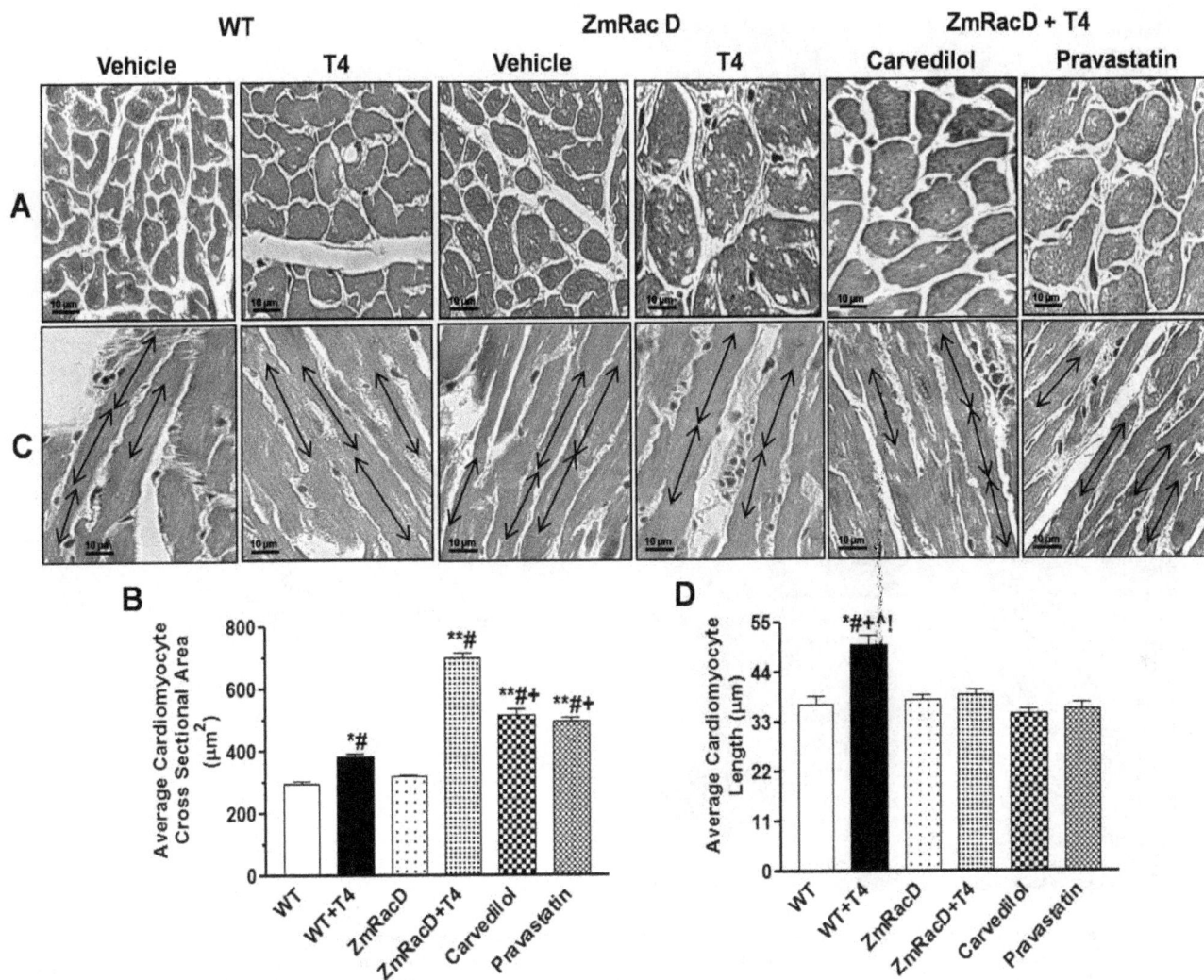

Figure 2. Structural Remodeling of Cardiac Myocytes in the Hearts of T4-Treated Mice. Masson's trichrome staining images with representative bar graphs for average cardiac myocytes cross sectional areas (**A & B**). Masson's trichrome staining images with representative bar graphs for average cardiac myocytes lengths (**C & D**); Magnifications are the same for all panels (size bar, 10 μm). * is significant change compared to untreated WT mice, ** is significant change compared to T4-treated and untreated WT mice, # is significant change compared to untreated transgenic mice, + is significant change compared to T4-treated transgenic mice, ∧, ! are significant change compared to T4-supplemented transgenic mice that pre-treated with carvedilol and pravastatin, respectively, (n = 8/group).

to levels that were not significant from those of all other groups (Figure 3A, B).

Differential Activation of MAPK in the Cardiac Remodeling of T4-treated Mice

Unregulated Ras/MAPK signaling can result in both cardiac hypertrophy and pathological remodeling in the heart [8]. Therefore, we sought to assess the activation of three key kinases in the MAPK cascade; ERK1/2, JNK, and p38-MAPK in the hearts of both wild-type and transgenic mice under basal conditions, and after T4 stimulation. Our results showed no significant difference in ERK1/2 activation between wild-type (0.60 ± 0.04) and transgenic mice (0.62 ± 0.04) under basal conditions. In contrast, T4 supplementation resulted in a moderate but significant increase in ERK1/2 activation in wild-type mice $(0.92\pm0.03; p<0.01)$ compared to untreated wild-type and transgenic mice. Interestingly, T4-treated transgenic mice exhibited a highly significant increase in ERK1/2 activation

$(1.31\pm0.07; p<0.001)$ compared to all other groups (Figure 4A). Conversely, carvedilol $(0.70\pm0.03; p<0.001)$ and pravastatin $(0.78\pm0.01; p<0.001)$ significantly decreased the activation of ERK in the hearts of T4-treated transgenic mice to levels that were not significantly different from those of untreated wild-type and transgenic mice. Additionally, ERK activity in the hearts of T4-supplemented transgenic mice that pre-treated with carvedilol but not pravastatin showed slight but significant $(p<0.05)$ decrease compared to T4-treated wild-type mice (Figure 4A).

On the other hand, we found no significant difference in the JNK activation in the hearts of both wild-type and transgenic mice under basal conditions $(0.71\pm0.03$ and $0.85\pm0.04)$, or after T4 stimulation $(0.91\pm0.07$ and $0.77\pm0.07)$, respectively. Similarly, there were no significant changes in JNK activation in the hearts of T4-supplemented transgenic mice that pre-treated with carvedilol (0.76 ± 0.07) or pravastatin (0.82 ± 0.11) (Figure 4B).

Furthermore, p38-MAPK activation was not significantly different between wild-type (1.80 ± 0.30) and transgenic mice

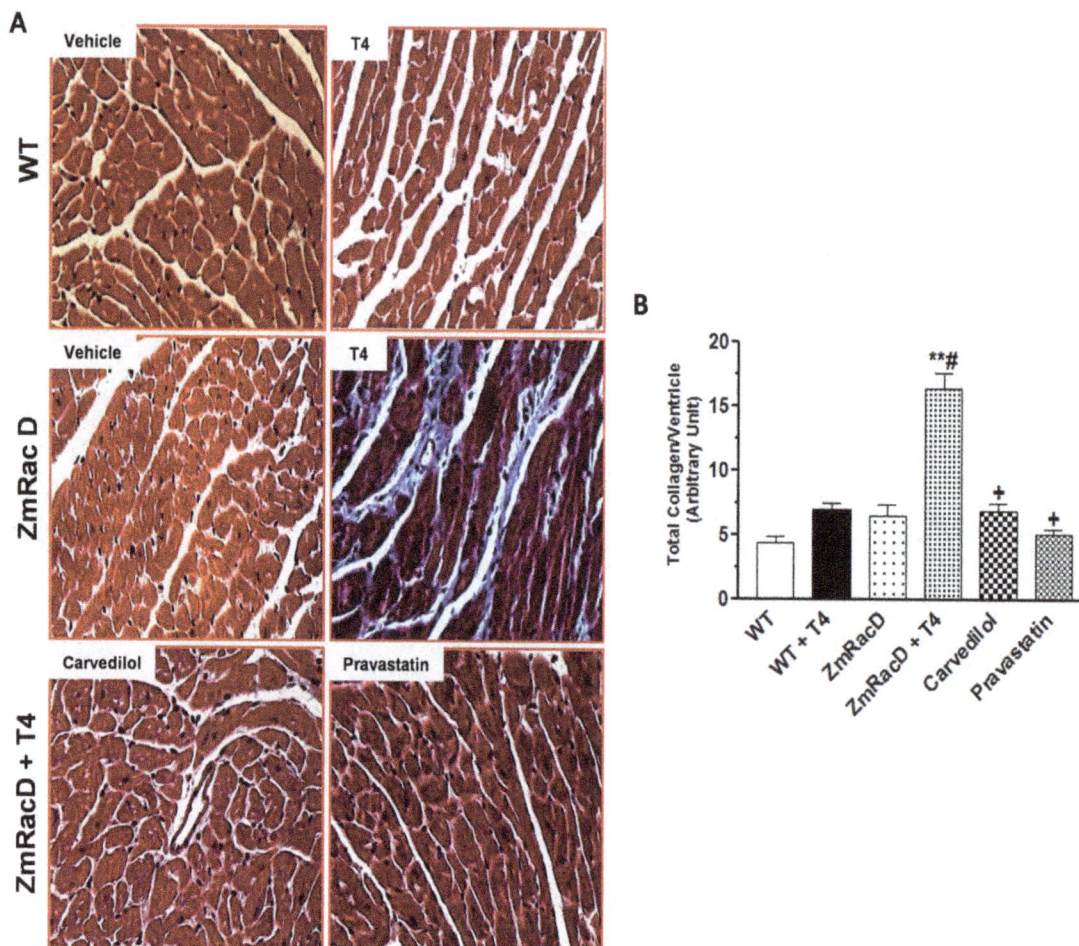

Figure 3. Increased Myocardial Fibrosis in Dilated Cardiomyopathy of T4-Treated Transgenic mice. Masson's trichrome staining shows distinct interstitial fibrosis in the hearts of T4-treated transgenic hearts (**A**); Magnifications are the same for all panels. Representative bar graph showing quantitative results on total collagen deposition in mice hearts (**B**). * is significant change compared to untreated WT mice, ** is significant change compared to T4-treated and untreated WT mice, # is significant change compared to untreated transgenic mice, and + is significant change compared to T4-treated transgenic mice (n = 8/group).

(1.92±0.23) under basal conditions. Similarly, T4-treated wild-type mice showed no significant difference in the activation of this kinase (1.82±0.07) compared to untreated wild-type and transgenic mice. In contrast, T4 treatment resulted in a significant decrease in p38-MAPK activation in the hearts of transgenic mice (0.84±0.03) compared to untreated wild-type (p<0.05), transgenic (p<0.01) and T4-treated wild-type (p<0.01) mice. In contrast, carvedilol (1.78±0.03; p<0.05) and pravastatin (1.73±0.06; p<0.05) significantly increased the activation of p38-MAPK in the hearts of T4-treated transgenic mice to levels that were not significant from those of all other groups (Figure 4C).

Dilated Cardiomyopathy of T4-Treated Transgenic Mice is Associated with increased Expression of Caspase-8 and Activation of Caspase-3 along with Enhanced Myocardial Apoptosis and TNF-α expression

Recently, initiator caspase-8 and activating caspase-3 have been reported to play a role in pathological cardiac hypertrophy, cardiac dilation and failure [21,22]. Therefore, we sought to assess the role of these two key caspases in the cardiac hypertrophy and cardiac dilation developed in wild-type and transgenic mice, respectively, after T4 treatment. Our results showed no significant

difference in caspase-8 levels between wild-type (0.20±0.01) and transgenic mice (0.22±0.02) under basal conditions. Similarly, T4-treated wild-type mice showed no significant difference in the expression of this caspase (0.28±0.04) compared to untreated wild-type and transgenic mice. However, T4 treatment resulted in a significant increase in caspase-8 expression in the hearts of the transgenic mice (0.57±0.04; p<0.001) compared to all other groups. In contrast, carvedilol (0.20±0.03; p<0.001) and pravastatin (0.30±0.05; p<0.001) significantly decreased caspase-8 expression in the hearts of T4-treated transgenic mice to levels that were not significant from those of all other groups (Figure 5A, B).

Likewise, there was no significant difference in activated caspase-3 between wild-type (0.20±0.03) and transgenic mice (0.18±0.02) under basal conditions. Also, T4-treated wild-type mice showed no significant difference in the expression of this caspase (0.26±0.03) compared to untreated wild-type and transgenic mice. Nevertheless, T4 treatment resulted in a highly significant increase in cleaved caspase-3 in transgenic mice (0.60±0.11) compared to untreated wild-type (p<0.001), transgenic (p<0.001) and T4-treated wild-type (p<0.01) mice. Conversely, carvedilol (0.20±0.02; p<0.001) and pravastatin (0.28±0.03; p<0.01) significantly decreased caspase-3 activity in

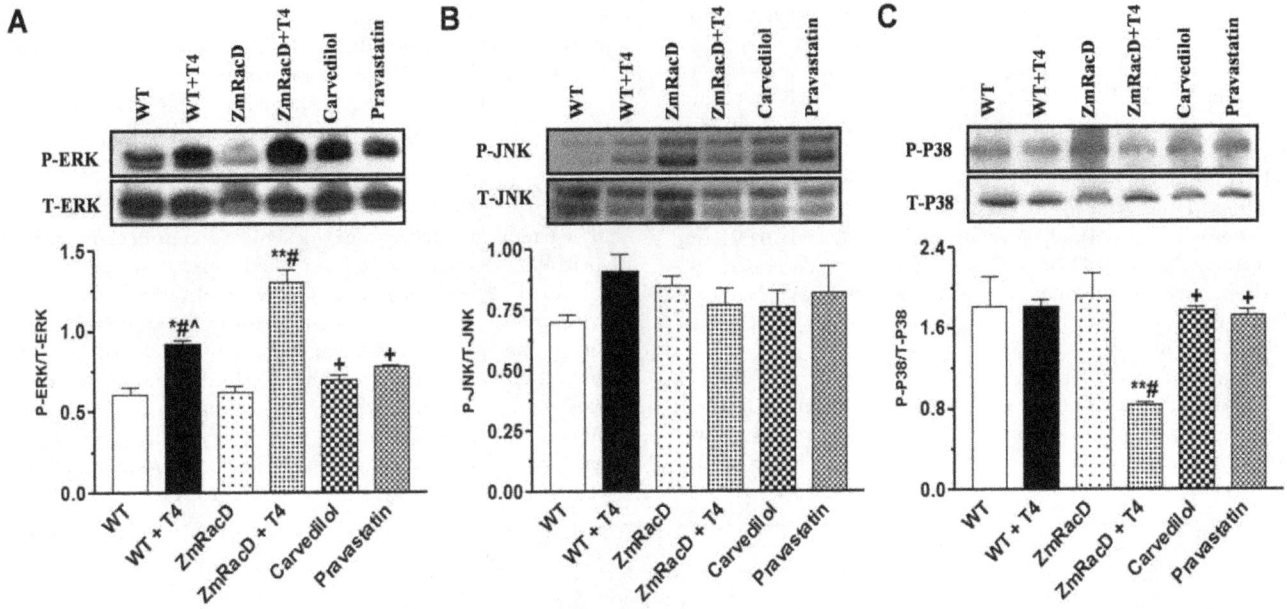

Figure 4. Differential Activation of MAPK in the Cardiac Remodeling of T4-treated Mice. Western blot analyses of total and phospho-ERK1/2 (**A**), total and phospho-JNK (**B**), and total and phospho-p38 (**C**) in the mice hearts. * is significant change compared to untreated WT mice, ** is significant change compared to T4-treated and untreated WT mice, # is significant change compared to untreated transgenic mice, + is significant change compared to T4-treated transgenic mice, ^ is significant change compared to T4-supplemented transgenic mice that pre-treated with carvedilol (n = 8/group).

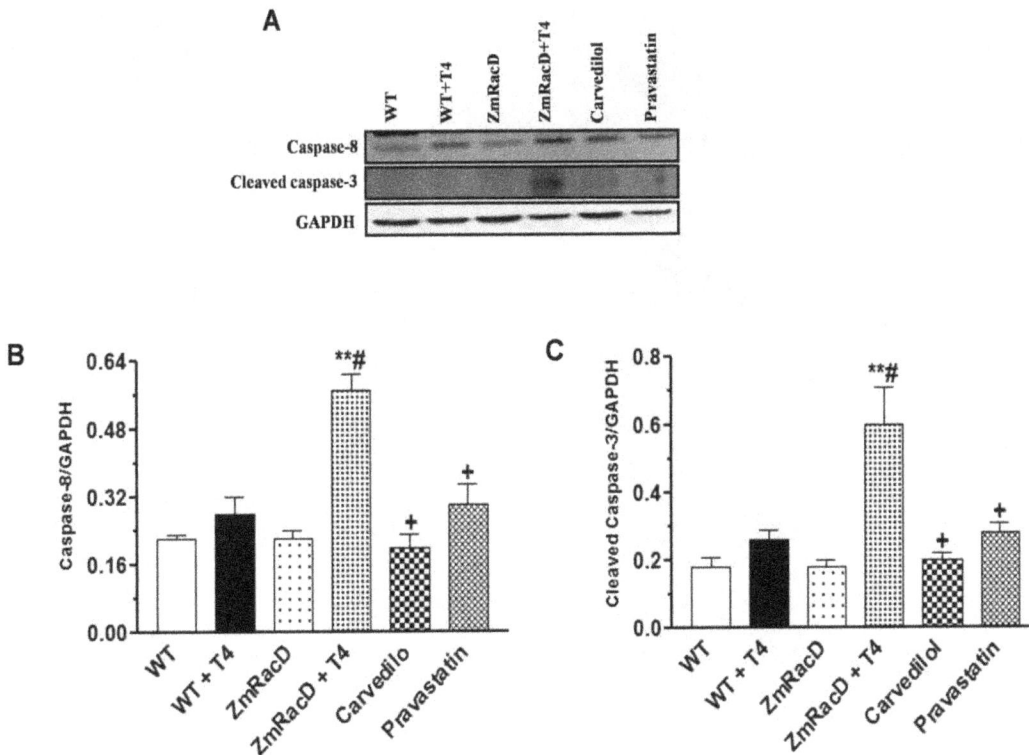

Figure 5. Dilated Cardiomyopathy of T4-Treated Transgenic Mice is Associated with Increased Expression of Caspase-8 and Activation of Caspase-3. Representative images for western blot analysis (**A**) with bar graphs for caspase-8 expression (**B**) and cleaved caspase-3 (**C**) in the mice hearts. * is significant change compared to untreated WT mice, ** is significant change compared to T4-treated and untreated WT mice, # is significant change compared to untreated transgenic mice, and + is significant change compared to T4-treated transgenic mice (n = 8/group).

the hearts of T4-treated transgenic mice to levels that were not significant from those of all other groups (Figure 5A, C).

To confirm the presence of cardiomyocyte apoptosis we performed TUNEL assays. Our results show that TUNEL-positive nuclei were absent in the hearts of untreated wild-type, untreated transgenic and T4-treated wild-type mice, whereas the number of TUNEL-positive nuclei was markedly increased in the hearts of T4-treated transgenic mice ($30\pm3.60\%$; $p<0.001$) compared to all other groups. Then again, carvedilol ($0.78\pm0.68\%$; $p<0.001$) and pravastatin ($0.77\pm0.41\%$; $p<0.001$) significantly decreased TU-NEL-positive nuclei in the hearts of T4-treated transgenic mice to levels that were not significant from that of all other groups (Figure 6A, B).

Since ROS can induce cardiomyocyte apoptosis partly through TNF-α [23], we assessed the level of this cytokine in the hearts of T4-treated and untreated transgenic mice. Our results showed significant increases in TNF-α expression in the hearts of T4-

treated transgenic mice (1.43 ± 0.16; $p<0.001$) compared to untreated transgenic mice (0.40 ± 0.04). In contrast, both carvedilol (0.52 ± 0.05; $p<0.01$) and pravastatin (0.66 ± 0.05; $p<0.01$) significantly attenuated this increase to levels that were not significant from that of untreated transgenic mice (Figure 6C).

Discussion

The pathways inducing the critical transition from compensated hypertrophy to cardiac dilation and failure remain poorly understood. In the present study, we took advantage of two cardiac models; a model of physiologic cardiac hypertrophy and another one of cardiac dilation, that were developed after T4 administration to wild-type and ZmRacD transgenic mice, respectively. This allowed us to investigate the functional, structural and molecular changes associated with these distinct phenotypes. These cardiac models will help us to understand the

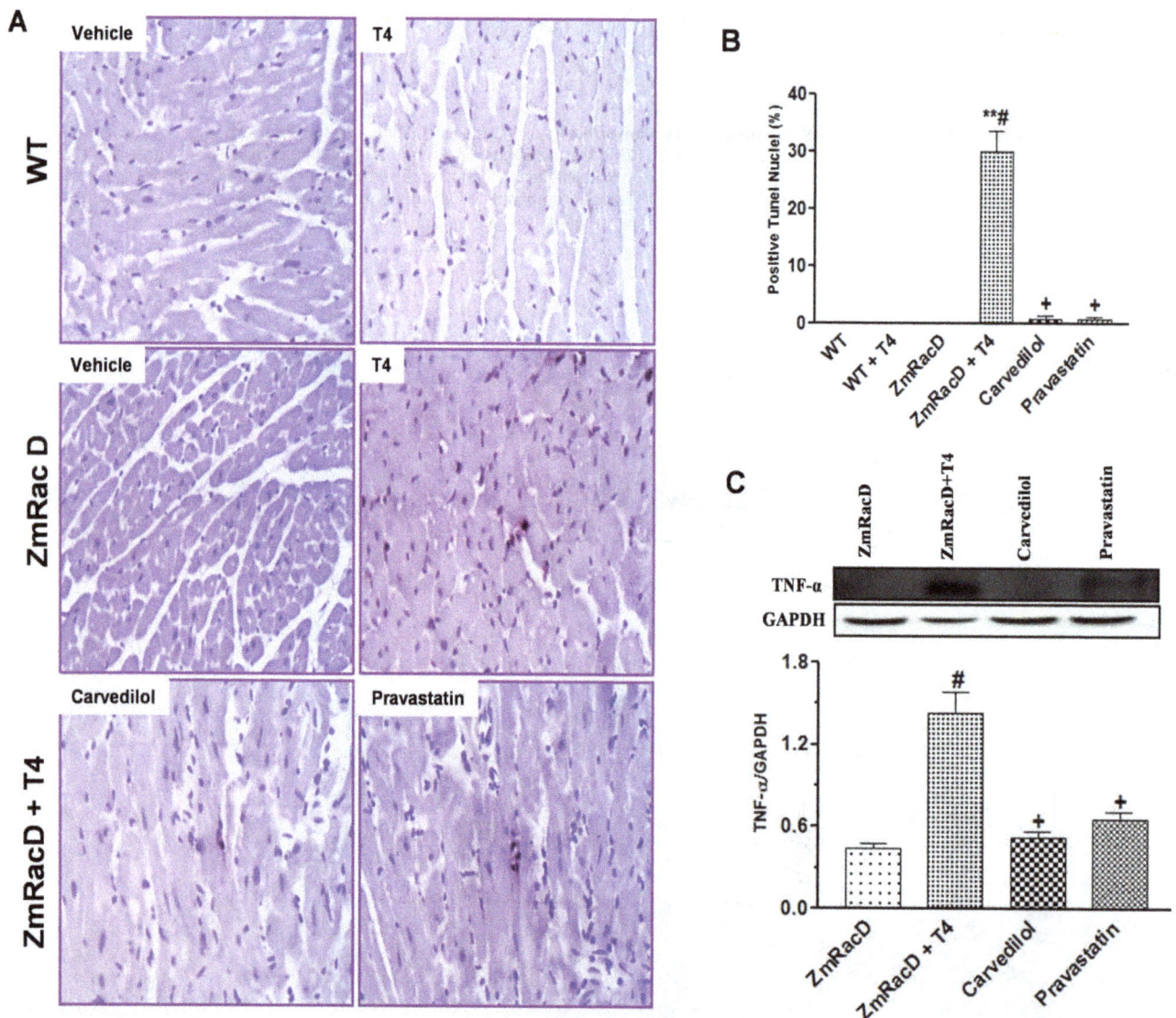

Figure 6. Dilated Cardiomyopathy of T4-Treated Transgenic Mice is Associated with Increased Cardiomyocyte Apoptosis and TNF-α expression. Representative images of in situ terminal deoxynucleotidyl transferase-mediated nick-end labeling (TUNEL) staining in FFPE mid-ventricle sections, with bar graph for the mean % of the brown colored apoptotic nuclei (**A & B**). Western blot analysis of TNF-α in transgenic mice hearts (**C**). * is significant change compared to untreated WT mice, ** is significant change compared to T4-treated and untreated WT mice, # is significant change compared to untreated transgenic mice, and + is significant change compared to T4-treated transgenic mice (n = 8/group).

role of Rac-induced signaling in the development and progression of cardiac remodeling, and to identify the mechanism(s) involved in the transition from cardiac hypertrophy into dilation and failure.

Recently, we have shown the conservation of Rho/Rac proteins in both plant and animal kingdoms *in-vivo* [12]. We showed that over-expression of a constitutively active form of ZmRacD specifically in the hearts of the transgenic mice resulted in cardiac hypertrophy and moderate decrease in systolic function in older mice. Additionally, we showed the increased myocardial Rac expression after T4 treatment in wild-type mice for 2 weeks. Confirming reported data [10], the same T4 treatment of ZmRacD mice up-regulated the α-MHC promoter and led to a higher expression level of ZmRacD transgene [12]. Besides, we illustrated that T4 treatment did not alter the cardiac function and LV internal dimensions in wild-type mice. However, it resulted in cardiac dilation and severe systolic dysfunction in adult transgenic mice within 2 weeks as evident by echocardiography analysis [12]. Notably, in this current report the study duration was extended to 3 weeks instead of 2 weeks [12] based on previous studies demonstrating that the largest part (70–80%) of the myocardial remodeling process in rodent e.g. rat occurs within the first 3 weeks [15]. Although this extended treatment resulted in further decrease in cardiac function and worsened the LV remodeling in the transgenic mice, these changes were not significantly different compared to the 2 weeks treatment used in our previous report [12]. Similar to this finding Kuzman et al. [24] showed that T4 treatment (500 µg/Kg) for 2 weeks resulted in cardiac hypertrophy in wild-type mice, and the same cardiac growth was maintained after extending the treatment period for 4 weeks.

It is becoming progressively clear that Rac, Rac-GTP activity, and Rac-mediated production of $O_2 \cdot^-$ play a key role in cardiac remodeling and heart failure [9–12]. In agreement with these studies, our current results showed marked increases in Rac expression, Rac-GTP activity and $O_2 \cdot^-$ generation in the hearts of T4-treated wild-type mice with higher increases in the hearts of the transgenic mice. Interestingly, these graded increases in Rac-GTP activity and $O_2 \cdot^-$ levels were associated with a graded phenotype shift in the heart, from growth and hypertrophy at a low level of Rac-mediated $O_2 \cdot^-$ in wild-type mice, to apoptosis and dilation at the higher level of Rac-mediated $O_2 \cdot^-$ in transgenic mice. This key finding is in line with previous reports showing that graded rises in the level of myocyte oxidative stress *in-vitro* either directly [25], or indirectly via stretch amplitude [26], provoke a graded shift in cardiac myocyte phenotype, from hypertrophy at low levels of oxidative stress, to apoptosis at higher levels.

In T4-treated wild-type mice, activated Rac/ROS signaling resulted in cardiac hypertrophy as evidenced by increased HW/BW and LV mass/BW ratios. This finding was confirmed by histopathology analysis that showed parallel increases in cardiomyocyte lengths and cross sectional areas. Interstitial fibrosis was absent and cardiac function was normal in these mice signifying a state of typical physiologic cardiac hypertrophy as described by Heineke and Molkentin [1]. In agreement with our finding, previous reports showed the development of physiologic cardiac hypertrophy in rodents after T4 treatment and the involvement of redox signaling in the T4-induced cardiac hypertrophy [27–29]. In contrast to our results, Kuzman et al. [29], showed that T4-induced physiologic cardiac hypertrophy in rats was associated with improved cardiac function. This exaggerated response may be due to the higher T4 dose (1 mg/kg) that has been used in this study [29]. However, this latter study as well as our data are in

agreement that in hypertrophic cardiomyopathy systolic function is typically normal or enhanced [30].

On the other hand, activated Rac/ROS signaling in the hearts of T4-treated transgenic mice resulted in enlarged LV chambers and severe systolic dysfunction, as evident by increased systolic and diastolic LV internal diameters and decreased LV EF and FS. Furthermore, there was a remarkable decrease in LV posterior wall thickness during diastole. These echocardiogrphic changes are consistent with a typical state of dilated cardiomyopathy [30]. The anatomic origin of cardiac dilation has been proposed to be due to: 1) a slight lengthening of cardiac myocyte, 2) slippage of the cardiac myocytes with subsequent thinning of ventricular wall, and 3) cardiac myocytes loss with subsequent replacement by scar tissue. Additionally, myocardial fibrosis seems to be a main component of dilated cardiomyopathy [31]. Although the increase in myocyte length with increased length/width ratio, are the most commonly observed anatomic changes in dilated cardiomyopathy, other studies showed that cardiac dilation was associated with decreased cardiac myocyte length and unaltered cross sectional area [32] or unchanged cardiac myocyte length and cross sectional area [33]. In the two latter studies [32,33], the incidence of cardiac dilation was attributed to the slippage of cardiac myocytes with subsequent thinning of ventricular wall. At variance with these studies, cardiac dilation in T4-treated ZmRacD mice was coupled with insignificant change in cardiomyocyte length but highly significant increase in cross sectional area. So, the question remains to be answered: what is the cause of dilated cardiomyopathy in T4-treated ZmRacD mice? While, slippage of cardiac myocytes cannot be excluded, we anticipate that cardiac dilation in T4-treated ZmRacD mice mainly occurred due to cardiac myocyte loss and increased myocardial fibrosis. In support of this hypothesis, our results demonstrated extremely significant increases in the total myocardial collagen content and fibrosis in the T4-treated ZmRacD mice. Furthermore, the level of cleaved caspase-3 was increased in the hearts of these mice, suggesting that caspase-3 is activated. This would then imply that cardiac myocyte apoptosis is enhanced in the hearts of these mice. Moreover, the incidence of oncotic cell death cannot be debarred, since some myocytes in the dilated hearts displayed formation of vacuoles corresponded to severe loss of sarcomere (myolysis) with accumulation of abundant mitochondria and mild increase in infiltration of inflammatory cells [32,34,35]. We consistently observed a marked increase in the number of TUNEL-positive cells in the hearts of T4-treated ZmRacD mice. Whether the TUNEL-positive cells in the hearts of T4-treated ZmRacD mice stand for apoptosis or oncosis remains to be revealed. In agreement with our findings, increased apoptosis, oncosis and interstitial fibrosis have been previously reported in transgenic mice and human patients with cardiac dilation [32,34,35].

In harmony with the concept that dilated cardiomyopathy is a hypertrophic myopathy in which myocyte growth seems unable to regularize the rise in mural stress formed by the interaction of hemodynamic factors and ventricular anatomical properties [31]; cardiac dilation in T4-treated ZmRacD mice was associated with significant amount of myocyte cellular hypertrophy which resulted in increased cardiac muscle mass as indicated by increased HW/BW and LV mass/BW ratios. Compensatory hypertrophy associated with cardiac dilation was proposed to normalize wall stress, preserve systolic force generation, and compensate for loss of cardiac mass caused by apoptosis [32,36]. Furthermore, a greater hypertrophic response may partially explain why particular hearts did not exhibit early failure, as proposed by the inspection that the compensated phase of ventricular remodeling leans to be of a longer duration in hearts with greater LV weights [37].

Therefore, we suggest that cardiac hypertrophy associated with the cardiac dilation in the T4-treated ZmRacD mice could explain the survival of these mice. In agreement with our results, cardiac hypertrophy has been reported to be associated with dilated cardiomyopathy in both mice [10] and humans [31].

Another question needs to be answered: what is the mechanism of the profound systolic dysfunction occurred in T4-induced cardiac dilation in ZmRacD mice? Previous reports showed that tissue injury with myocyte cell death and collagen accumulation is followed by a progressive decline of cardiac pump function in aging and in numerous cardiovascular disorders [31]. In addition, it has been reported that TNF-α is a well established mediator to impair cardiac function and it is implicated in different cardiac pathologies [38–40]. TNF-α can impair heart function either directly through its negative inotropic effect [38] or indirectly through inducing apoptosis [39] or activating cardiac caspases e.g. caspase-8 and caspase-3 without significant cell death [40]. Activation of caspases may initiate the progressive cleavage of myocardial contractile proteins, or it may activate other proteolytic enzymes e.g. matrix metalloproteinase that can degrade myocardial extracellular protein with subsequent decline in LV systolic function [40]. In line with these studies our current results presented that increased TNF-α, cardiac caspases, myocyte apoptosis and myocardial fibrosis are key players in the development of LV systolic dysfunction in T4-induced cardiac dilation in ZmRacD mice.

Among the most conserved signal transduction systems in the heart is the MAPK cascade. It involves consecutively acting protein kinases leading to the activation of three terminal MAPKs; ERK, JNK, and p38 kinase. Once activated, these kinases phosphorylate a wide range of intracellular targets that include various transcription factors leading to reprogramming of gene expression. Unregulated MAPK signaling can result in both cardiac hypertrophy and pathological remodeling in the heart [8]. Here we show that T4-induced cardiac hypertrophy in wild-type mice was coupled with increased activation of ERK1/2; however, there was no significant change in the activities of both JNK and p38-MAPK. Similarly, Kuzman et al. [29], showed that T4-induced cardiac hypertrophy in rats was associated with unchanged JNK and p38-MAPK activities. Yet, these rats also exhibited no significant change in the ERK1/2 activity either [29], while Araujo et al. [41], showed that T4-induced cardiac hypertrophy in rats was associated with increased ERK1/2 but not increased JNK activity. Low levels of oxidative stress were also found to be involved in cardiac myocyte hypertrophy, with increased ERK1/2 but not JNK activity in-vitro [26].

To date, reported results on MAPKs activity in failing myocardium are inconsistent. Various reports showed either increased ERK1/2, JNKs and p38-MAPK activities, increased JNK and p38-MAPK activities, but not ERK1/2 activity, or decreased p38-MAPK activity [42]. Our current data showed that T4-induced dilated cardiomyopathy in ZmRacD mice was associated with increased ERK1/2 activity and down-regulation of p38-MAPK activity; however, there was no significant change in JNK activity. Compatible with our findings increased ERK1/2 and decreased p38-MAPK activities have been previously reported in failing myocardium both in animals [43,44] and humans [42,45,46]. JNK activity has been shown to be either up-regulated [43] or down-regulated [42,44] in failing myocardium, while our results showed unchanged JNK activity in dilated hearts of ZmRacD mice.

It is worth noting that ERK1/2 activity is significantly higher, however, p38-MAPK activity is significantly lower in T4-induced cardiac dilation in ZmRacD mice compared to their correspond-

ing activities in T4-induced cardiac hypertrophy in wild-type mice. This may indicate an important role for both kinases in the transition from physiologic cardiac hypertrophy to cardiac dilation and failure. Yet, this remains to be determined.

Apoptosis has been coupled with numerous forms of heart failure, e.g. myocarditis, ischemia/reperfusion injury, and congestive heart failure. Two major apoptotic pathways have been reported, and both congregate on the activation of caspases [40]. Caspase-8 is one of the most upstream caspases involved in cardiac myocyte death. Transgenic mice that express a conditionally cardiac-specific active caspase-8 exhibited a lethal dilated cardiomyopathy [22]. In addition, caspase-3 is a downstream effecter of caspase-8 in apoptotic cell death [47]. Increased caspase-3 was evident in pathological LV hypertrophy with LV dysfunction and LV dilation, but not in physiological hypertrophy [21,32,36]. Additionally, increased Rac/ROS activity resulted in LV remodeling and increased caspase-3 expression [48]. Consistent with these findings we show here increased caspase-8 expression and caspase-3 activity in T4-induced cardiac dilation in ZmRacD mice, whereas there were no significant differences in both caspases in T4-induced physiologic cardiac hypertrophy in wild-type mice.

It has been demonstrated that ROS can induce cardiomyocyte apoptosis partially through TNF-α [23]. The TNF-α mediated pathway has been shown to be responsible for myocardial caspase-3 and -8 activation [40]. On the other hand, it has been reported that p38-MAPK may protect cardiac myocyte from apoptosis and p38 knockout mice exhibit increased apoptosis and caspase-3 activity compared to control [33]. Furthermore, it has been recently shown that activation of ERK1/2 contributes to cell death in some cell types and organs and it may act upstream to TNF-α, caspase-8 or caspase-3 in the apoptotic pathway [47]. In the present study one or more of these effectors (i.e. increased TNF-α and ERK1/2, or decreased p38-MAPK) may be involved in the ROS-induced apoptosis in our model. However, the exact mechanism remains to be elucidated.

To confirm the role of Rac and Rac-mediated $O_2 \cdot^-$ generation in the developed cardiac phenotypes in our model, T4-treated transgenic mice were pre-treated with either carvedilol or pravastatin. Carvedilol is a non-selective vasodilating β-blocker working on β_1-, β_2-, and α_1-adrenoceptors. Additionally, Carvedilol and its metabolites are potent antioxidants [17,20] due to their abilities to 1) scavenge $O2 \cdot^-$, 2) inhibit $O2 \cdot^-$ production, 3) attenuate lipid peroxidation, and 4) spare the consumption of endogenous antioxidants [20,49]. Recently, inhibition of $O2 \cdot^-$ production by carvedilol has been also accredited to its ability to decrease NADPH oxidase subunits (P^{47phox} and P^{67phox}) in the heart [50]. On the other hand, pravastatin is an antihyperlipidemic agent that inhibits Rac-GTPase and NADPH oxidase activities both in animal [12,51] and human [11] hearts, decreases myocardial $O_2 \cdot^-$ levels [52] and stimulates the endogenous antioxidant mechanism in the heart [51]. In our experiments, carvedilol significantly decreased $O_2 \cdot^-$ but not Rac-GTPase activity in dilated transgenic mice hearts, while; pravastatin inhibited both. Both treatments attenuated all downstream signaling: ERK1/2 activity, TNF-α expression, caspase-8 expression and caspase-3 activity. Conversely, they increased p38-MAPK activity. This led to marked decrease in cardiac myocyte size and ablation of myocardial fibrosis and apoptosis, with subsequent normalization of systolic and diastolic LV dimensions and preservation of heart functions. Thus, we confirm previous studies that showed the effectiveness of carvedilol [17,49,53–55] and pravastatin [11,51,52,56] in decreasing oxidative response,

TNF-α expression, fibrosis, apoptosis and attenuating cardiac dilation and failure both in animals and humans.

β-blockers are useful antioxidative therapy in patients with heart failure. They exert their antioxidatant effects either via blocking β-adrenoreceptors with subsequent inhibition of catecholamine-induced oxidative stress or via direct antioxidant properties of some β-blockers such as carvedilol [57]. To confirm that the antioxidant activity but not the β-blocking activity of carvedilol is the main contributor in these improvements observed in our model, propranolol, a β-blocker lacking the antioxidant activity, at higher dose (10 mg/kg) failed to improve the LV function of the dilated transgenic hearts, and it only resulted in significantly less improvements in LV dimensions of these hearts compared to carvedilol at the low dose (2 mg/kg) used in this current study. This is consistent with previous studies [20].

Another important effect of carvedilol [17,54,55] and prava-statin [56,58] is the decrease in cardiomyocyte size, HW and LV mass. In contrast, in a rat model of cardiac dilation with compensatory hypertrophy, pravastatin significantly decreased Rac and NADPH oxidase activity leading to inhibition of cardiac dilation, but not LV mass or cardiomyocyte size [51]. Consistent with this latter study [51], our current results showed that carvedilol and pravastatin were unable to significantly decrease HW or LV mass; however both drugs significantly decreased the cardiomyocyte size. This clearly indicates the involvement of Rac-mediated $O_2 \cdot^-$ in the development of cardiac hypertrophy in our model. The inability of carvedilol and pravastatin to normalize the HW and LV mass could indicate the involvement of other signaling pathways besides Rac signaling in the development of T4-induced cardiac hypertrophy in these mice such as PI3K, PKB/Akt, or the rennin-angiotensin system [59].

Taken together, our data demonstrate that T4-induced ZmRacD is a novel mouse model of dilated cardiomyopathy that shares many characteristics with the human disease phenotype. To our knowledge, this is the first study to show graded Rac-mediated $O_2 \cdot^-$ results in cardiac phenotype shift *in-vivo*. Moreover, Rac-mediated $O_2 \cdot^-$ generation, cardiomyocyte apoptosis and myocardial fibrosis seem to play a pivotal role in the transition from cardiac hypertrophy to cardiac dilation and failure. Targeting Rac signaling could represent valuable therapeutic strategy not only in saving the failing myocardium but also to prevent this transition process.

A limitation of the present study is that cardiomyocyte length is generally in the range of 78–127 μm as revealed from isolated cardiomyocytes [60]. However, in this current study cardiomyocyte lengths were obtained from stained cardiac tissue. Smaller cardiomyocyte lengths reported here (35–50 μm), may be partially due to the effect of tissue processing and sectioning. Even though, our data are consistent with other studies [61], that reported the same cardiac cell length (about 35 μm) in wild-type mice of approximate age (5–7 months) to our mice (6–8 months).

Supporting Information

Figure S1 Effect of Thyroxine (T4) treatment on the hearts of ZmRacD Mice. M-mode echocardiography images of the left ventricle (LV) of ZmRacD mice at basal condition (**A**), and after T4-treatment for 1 week (**B**), 2 weeks (**C**) and 3 weeks (**D**). Representative bar graphs for LV ejection fraction (EF) (**E**), fractional shortening (FS) (**F**), internal diameter during systole (LVID, s) (**G**), and internal diameter during diastole (LVID, d) (**H**). * is significant change compared to basal conditions and # is significant change compared to 1 week T4 treatment.

Figure S2 Comparative Effects of Carvedilol and Pro-pranolol on the Left Ventricle (LV) Function and Internal Diameters of T4-treated ZmRacD Mice. Representative bar graphs for LV ejection fraction (EF) (**A**), fractional shortening (FS) (**B**), internal diameter during systole (LVID, s) (**C**), and internal diameter during diastole (LVID, d) (**D**). # is significant change compared to untreated ZmRacD mice,+ is significant change compared to T4-treated ZmRacD mice and ^ is significant change compared to T4-supplemented transgenic mice that pre-treated with carvedilol.

Author Contributions

Performed the experiments: MTE MDHH MAA LM MK. Analyzed the data: MTE MDHH MAA LM MK. Wrote the paper: MTE HHH. Interpreted results of experiments: MTE MDHH MAA LM PMLJ MK HHH. Prepared figures: MTE LM MK. Edited and revised the manuscript: MTE MDHH MAA LM PMLJ MK. Approved the final version of manuscript: MTE MDHH MAA LM PMLJ MK HHH.

References

1. Heineke J, Molkentin JD (2006) Regulation of cardiac hypertrophy by intracellular signalling pathways. Nat Rev Mol Cell Biol 7:589–600.
2. Klein L, O'Connor CM, Gattis WA, Zampino M, de Luca L, et al. (2003) Pharmacologic therapy for patients with chronic heart failure and reduced systolic function: review of trials and practical considerations. Am J Cardiol 91: 18F–40F.
3. Lips DJ, deWindt LJ, van Kraaij DJ, Doevendans PA (2003) Molecular determinants of myocardial hypertrophy and failure: alternative pathways for beneficial and maladaptive hypertrophy. Eur Heart J 24: 883–896.
4. Berenji K, Drazner MH, Rothermel BA, Hill JA (2005) Does load-induced ventricular hypertrophy progress to systolic heart failure? Am J Physiol Heart Circ Physiol 289: H8–H16.
5. Diwan A, Dorn GW II (2007) Decompensation of cardiac hypertrophy: cellular mechanisms and novel therapeutic targets. Physiology 22: 56–64.
6. Selvetella G, Hirsch E, Notte A, Tarone G, Lembo G (2004) Adaptive and maladaptive hypertrophic pathways: points of convergence and divergence. Cardiovasc Res 63: 373–380.
7. Dorn GW (2009) Novel pharmacotherapies to abrogate postinfarction ventricular remodeling. Nat Rev Cardiol 6: 283–291.
8. Rose BA, Force T, Wang Y (2010) Mitogen-activated protein kinase signaling in the heart: angels versus demons in a heart-breaking tale. Physiol Rev 90:1507–1546.
9. Lezoualc'h F, Metrich M, Hmitou I, Duquesnes N, Morel E (2008) Small GTP-binding proteins and their regulators in cardiac hypertrophy. J Mol Cell Cardiol 44:623–632.

10. Sussman MA, Welch S, Walker A, Klevitsky R, Hewett TE, et al. (2000) Altered focal adhesion regulation correlates with cardiomyopathy in mice expressing constitutively active rac1. J Clin Invest 105:875–886.
11. Maack C, Kartes T, Kilter H, Schäfers HJ, Nickenig G, et al. (2003) Oxygen free radical release in human failing myocardium is associated with increased activity of rac1-GTPase and represents a target for statin treatment. Circulation 108:1567–1574.
12. Elnakish MT, Awad MM, Hassona MD, Alhaj MA, Kulkarni A, et al. (2011) Cardiac Remodeling Caused by Transgenic Over-expression of a Corn Rac Gene. Am J Physiol Heart Circ Physiol 301:H868–H880.
13. Frey N, Olson EN (2003) Cardiac hypertrophy: the good, the bad, and the ugly. Annu Rev Physiol 65: 45–79.
14. Pierres C, Gaugain-Hamidi A (2009) Concentrated Liquid Thyroid Hormone Composition. Patentdocs website. Available: http://www.faqs.org/patents/app/20090270507#ixzz1R067AyTq. Accessed: 2012 August 3.
15. Pfeffer MA, Braunwald E (1990) Ventricular remodeling after myocardial infarction. Circulation 81:1161–1172.
16. Schaefer WH, Politowski J, Hwang B, Dixon F Jr, Goalwin A, et al. (1998) Metabolism of carvedilol in dogs, rats, and mice. Drug Metab Dispos 26:958–969.
17. Watanabe K, Ohta Y, Nakazawa M, Higuchi H, Hasegawa G, et al. (2000) Low dose carvedilol inhibits progression of heart failure in rats with dilated cardiomyopathy. Br J Pharmacol 130:1489–1495.

18. Samuel MS, Lourenço FC, Olson MF (2011) K-Ras mediated murine epidermal tumorigenesis is dependent upon and associated with elevated Rac1 activity. PLoS One 6:e17143.

19. Hassona MD, Elnakish MT, Abouelnaga ZA, Alhaj M, Wani AA, et al. (2011) The Effect of Selective Antihypertensive Drugs on the Vascular Remodeling-associated Hypertension: Insights from a Profilin1 Transgenic Mouse Model. J Cardiovasc Pharmacol 57:550–558.

20. Feuerstein GZ, Ruffolo RR Jr (1996) Carvedilol, a novel vasodilating beta-blocker with the potential for cardiovascular organ protection. Eur Heart J 17:24–29.

21. Balakumar P, Singh M (2006) The possible role of caspase-3 in pathological and physiological cardiac hypertrophy in rats. Basic Clin Pharmacol Toxicol 99:418–424.

22. Wencker D, Chandra M, Nguyen K, Miao W, Garantziotis S, et al. (2003) A mechanistic role for cardiac myocyte apoptosis in heart failure. J Clin Invest 111:1497–1504.

23. Aikawa R, Nitta-Komatsubara Y, Kudoh S, Takano H, Nagai T, et al. (2002) Reactive oxygen species induce cardiomyocyte apoptosis partly through TNF-alpha. Cytokine 18:179–183.

24. Kuzman JA, O'Connell TD, Gerdes AM (2007) Rapamycin prevents thyroid hormone-induced cardiac hypertrophy. Endocrinology 148:3477–3484.

25. Siwik DA, Tzortzis JD, Pimental DR, Chang DL, Pagano PJ, et al. (1999) Inhibition of copper-zinc superoxide dismutase induces cell growth, hypertrophic phenotype, and apoptosis in neonatal rat cardiac myocytes in vitro. Circ Res 85:147–153.

26. Pimentel DR, Amin JK, Xiao L, Miller T, Viereck J, et al. (2001) Reactive oxygen species mediate amplitude-dependent hypertrophic and apoptotic responses to mechanical stretch in cardiac myocytes. Circ Res 89:453–460.

27. Araujo AS, Schenkel P, Enzveiler AT, Fernandes TR, Partata WA, et al. (2008) The role of redox signaling in cardiac hypertrophy induced by experimental hyperthyroidism. J Mol Endocrinol 41:423–430.

28. Florini JR, Saito Y, Manowitz EJ (1973) Effect of age on thyroxin-induced cardiac hypertrophy in mice. J Gerontol 28:293–297.

29. Kuzman JA, Vogelsang KA, Thomas TA, Gerdes AM (2005) L-Thyroxine activates Akt signaling in the heart. J Mol Cell Cardiol 39: 251–258.

30. Freeman K, Colon-Rivera C, Olsson MC, Moore RL, Weinberger HD, et al. (2001) Progression from hypertrophic to dilated cardiomyopathy in mice that express a mutant myosin transgene. Am J Physiol Heart Circ Physiol 280:151–159.

31. Beltrami CA, Finato N, Rocco M, Feruglio GA, Puricelli C, et al. (1995) The cellular basis of dilated cardiomyopathy in humans. J Mol Cell Cardiol 27:291–305.

32. Yamamoto S, Yang G, Zablocki D, Liu J, Hong C, et al. (2003) Activation of Mst1 causes dilated cardiomyopathy by stimulating apoptosis without compensatory ventricular myocyte hypertrophy. J Clin Invest 111:1463–1474.

33. Nishida K, Yamaguchi O, Hirotani S, Hikoso S, Higuchi Y (2004) P38 alpha mitogen-activated protein kinase plays a critical role in cardiomyocyte survival but not in cardiac hypertrophic growth in response to pressure overload. Mol Cell Biol 24:10611–10620.

34. Fentzke RC, Korcarz CE, Lang RM, Lin H, Leiden JM (1998) Dilated cardiomyopathy in transgenic mice expressing a dominant-negative CREB transcription factor in the heart. J Clin Invest 101:2415–2426.

35. Corradi D, Tchana B, Miller D, Manotti L, Maestri R, et al. (2009) Dilated form of endocardial fibroelastosis as a result of deficiency in respiratory-chain complexes I and IV. Circulation 120:e38–40.

36. Philipp S, Pagel I, Höhnel K, Lutz J, Buttgereit J, et al. (2004) Regulation of caspase-3 and Fas in pressure overload-induced left ventricular dysfunction. Eur J Heart Fail 6:845–851.

37. Brower GL, Janicki JS (2001) Contribution of ventricular remodeling to pathogenesis of heart failure in rats. Am J Physiol Heart Circ Physiol 280:H674–H683.

38. Yokoyama T, Vaca L, Rossen RD, Durante W, Hazarika P, et al. (1993) Cellular basis for the negative inotropic effects of tumor necrosis factor-alpha in the adult mammalian heart. J Clin Invest 92:2303–2312.

39. Lu X, Hamilton JA, Shen J, Pang T, Jones DL, et al. (2006) Role of tumor necrosis factor-alpha in myocardial dysfunction and apoptosis during hindlimb ischemia and reperfusion. Crit Care Med 34:484–491.

40. Carlson DL, Willis MS, White DJ, Horton JW, Giroir BP (2005) Tumor necrosis factor-alpha-induced caspase activation mediates endotoxin-related cardiac dysfunction. Crit Care Med 33:1021–1028.

41. Araujo AS, Fernandes T, Ribeiro MF, Khaper N, Belló-Klein A (2010) Redox regulation of myocardial ERK 1/2 phosphorylation in experimental hyperthyroidism: role of thioredoxin-peroxiredoxin system. J Cardiovasc Pharmacol 56:513–517.

42. Communal C, Colucci WS, Remondino A, Sawyer DB, Port JD, et al. (2002) Reciprocal modulation of mitogen-activated protein kinases and mitogen-activated protein kinase phosphatase 1 and 2 in failing human myocardium. J Card Fail 8:86–92.

43. Muchir A, Pavlidis P, Decostre V, Herron AJ, Arimura T, et al. (2007) Activation of MAPK pathways links LMNA mutations to cardiomyopathy in Emery-Dreifuss muscular dystrophy. J Clin Invest 117:1282–1293.

44. Tenhunen O, Soini Y, Ilves M, Rysä J, Tuukkanen J, et al. (2006) p38 Kinase rescues failing myocardium after myocardial infarction: evidence for angiogenic and anti-apoptotic mechanisms. FASEB J 20:E1276–E1286.

45. Dong Y, Gao D, Chen L, Lin R, Conte JV, et al. (2006) Increased ERK activation and decreased MKP-1 expression in human myocardium with congestive heart failure. J Cardiothorac Ren Res 1: 123–130.

46. Lemke LE, Bloem LJ, Fouts R, Esterman M, Sandusky G, et al. (2001) Decreased p38 MAPK activity in end-stage failing human myocardium: p38 MAPK alpha is the predominant isoform expressed in human heart. J Mol Cell Cardiol 33:1527–1540.

47. Zhuang S, Schnellmann RG (2006). A death-promoting role for extracellular signal-regulated kinase. J Pharmacol Exp Ther 319:991–997.

48. Worou ME, Belmokhtar K, Bonnet P, Vourc'h P, Machet MC, et al. (2011) Hemin decreases cardiac oxidative stress and fibrosis in a rat model of systemic hypertension via PI3K/Akt signalling. Cardiovasc Res 91:320–329.

49. Yaoita H, Sakabe A, Maehara K, Maruyama Y (2002) Different effects of carvedilol, metoprolol, and propranolol on left ventricular remodeling after coronary stenosis or after permanent coronary occlusion in rats. Circulation 105:975–980.

50. Arozal W, Watanabe K, Veeraveedu PT, Ma M, Thandavarayan RA, et al. (2010) Protective effect of carvedilol on daunorubicin-induced cardiotoxicity and nephrotoxicity in rats. Toxicology 274: 18–26.

51. Ichihara S, Noda A, Nagata K, Obata K, Xu J, et al. (2006) Pravastatin increases survival and suppresses an increase in myocardial matrix metalloproteinase activity in a rat model of heart failure. Cardiovasc Res 69:726–735.

52. Cheng CF, Juan SH, Chen JJ, Chao YC, Chen HH, et al. (2008) Pravastatin attenuates carboplatin-induced cardiotoxicity via inhibition of oxidative stress associated apoptosis. Apoptosis 13:883–894.

53. Chua S, Sheu JJ, Chang LT, Lee FY, Wu CJ, et al. (2008) Comparison of losartan and carvedilol on attenuating inflammatory and oxidative response and preserving energytranscription factors and left ventricular function in dilated cardiomyopathy rats. Int. Heart J 49: 605–619.

54. Li B, Liao YH, Cheng X, Ge H, Guo H, et al. (2006) Effects of carvedilol on cardiac cytokines expression and remodeling in rat with acute myocardial infarction. Int J Cardiol 111:247–255.

55. Palazzuoli A, Bruni F, Puccetti L, Pastorelli M, Angori P, et al. (2002) Effects of carvedilol on left ventricular remodeling and systolic function in elderly patients with heart failure. Eur J Heart Fail 4:765–770.

56. Zhao H, Liao Y, Minamino T, Asano Y, Asakura M, et al. (2008) Inhibition of cardiac remodeling by pravastatin is associated with amelioration of endoplasmic reticulum stress. Hypertens Res 31:1977–1987.

57. Nakamura K, Murakami M, Miura D, Yunoki K, Enko K, et al. (2011) Beta-Blockers and Oxidative Stress in Patients with Heart Failure. Pharmaceuticals 4:1088–1100.

58. Xu Z, Okamoto H, Akino M, Onozuka H, Matsui Y, et al. (2008) Pravastatin attenuates left ventricular remodeling and diastolic dysfunction in angiotensin II-induced hypertensive mice. J Cardiovasc Pharmacol 51:62–70.

59. Ojamaa K (2010) Signaling mechanisms in thyroid hormone-induced cardiac hypertrophy. Vascul Pharmacol 52:113–119.

60. Korecky B, Rakusan K (1978) Normal and hypertrophic growth of the rat heart: changes in cell dimensions and number. Am J Physiol 234:H123–H128.

61. Helms SA, Azhar G, Zuo C, Theus SA, Bartke A, et al. (2010) Smaller cardiac cell size and reduced extra-cellular collagen might be beneficial for hearts of Ames dwarf mice. Int J Biol Sci 6:475–490.

12

Src is Required for Mechanical Stretch-Induced Cardiomyocyte Hypertrophy through Angiotensin II Type 1 Receptor-Dependent β-Arrestin2 Pathways

Shijun Wang[1,2,9], Hui Gong[1,2,9], Guoliang Jiang[2,9], Yong Ye[2,9], Jian Wu[2], Jieyun You[2], Guoping Zhang[2], Aijun Sun[1,2], Issei Komuro[3], Junbo Ge[1,2], Yunzeng Zou[1,2]*

1 Shanghai Institute of Cardiovascular Diseases, Zhongshan Hospital, Fudan University, Shanghai, China, **2** Institutes of Biomedical Science, Fudan University, Shanghai, China, **3** Department of Cardiovascular Medicine, the University of Tokyo Graduate School of Medicine, Tokyo, Japan

Abstract

Angiotensin II (AngII) type 1 receptor (AT1-R) can be activated by mechanical stress (MS) without the involvement of AngII during the development of cardiomyocyte hypertrophy, in which G protein-independent pathways are critically involved. Although β-arrestin2-biased signaling has been speculated, little is known about how AT1-R/β-arrestin2 leads to ERK1/2 activation. Here, we present a novel mechanism by which Src kinase mediates AT1-R/β-arrestin2-dependent ERK1/2 phosphorylation in response to MS. Differing from stimulation by AngII, MS-triggered ERK1/2 phosphorylation is neither suppressed by overexpression of RGS4 (the negative regulator of the G-protein coupling signal) nor by inhibition of $G\alpha q$ downstream protein kinase C (PKC) with GF109203X. The release of inositol 1,4,5-triphosphate (IP_3) is increased by AngII but not by MS. These results collectively suggest that MS-induced ERK1/2 activation through AT1-R might be independent of G-protein coupling. Moreover, either knockdown of β-arrestin2 or overexpression of a dominant negative mutant of β-arrestin2 prevents MS-induced activation of ERK1/2. We further identifies a relationship between Src, a non-receptor tyrosine kinase and β-arrestin2 using analyses of co-immunoprecipitation and immunofluorescence after MS stimulation. Furthermore, MS-, but not AngII-induced ERK1/2 phosphorylation is attenuated by Src inhibition, which also significantly improves pressure overload-induced cardiac hypertrophy and dysfunction in mice lacking AngII. Finally, MS-induced Src activation and hypertrophic response are abolished by candesartan but not by valsartan whereas AngII-induced responses can be abrogated by both blockers. Our results suggest that Src plays a critical role in MS-induced cardiomyocyte hypertrophy through β-arrestin2-associated angiotensin II type 1 receptor signaling.

Editor: Tianqing Peng, University of Western Ontario, Canada

Funding: This work was supported by the National Natural Science Fund of China (81220108003; 81000041); China Doctoral Foundation (20110071110051) and Technology Commission of Shanghai Municipality (11JC1402400). The funders had no role in study design, data collection and analysis, decision to publish, or preparation of the manuscript.

Competing Interests: The authors have declared that no competing interests exist.

* E-mail: zou.yunzeng@zs-hospital.sh.cn

⑨ These authors contributed equally to this work.

Introduction

Angiotensin II type 1 (AT1) receptor, belonging to the G-protein-coupled receptor family (GPCRs), shares a common structure of 7-transmembrane receptor (7TMRs), and mediates the signal response of Angiotensin II (AngII), thereby regulates blood pressure, cardiac hypertrophy and heart failure [1,2]. Recent studies demonstrate that AT1-R acts as a stress-sensitive switcher which can be triggered by mechanical stress without the ligand binding [3–5]. We have previously showed that some kinds of angiotensin II receptor blockers (ARBs), such as candesartan and olmesartan, inhibit pressure overload-induced cardiac hypertrophy in angiotensinogen knockout (AGT KO) mice, while others like valsartan, exert the inhibitory effect in the presence of AngII [6]. However, the detailed molecular mechanisms of how mechanical stress-induced AT1-R activation and its inhibition are regulated by ARBs still remain elucidative.

A growing body of evidences indicated that biased agonism might selectively induce the conformational switch of GPCRs, which preferentially activated or inhibited a subset of downstream signaling [7,8]. We thus assumed there might be an unique pathway involved in mechanical stress (MS)-induced AT1-R activation and signal transduction, which was different from that induced by AngII, and resulted in the divergent effects of various ARBs. Rakesh K. previously reported that β-arrestin2 dependent pathway rather than G-protein coupling played a pivotal role in MS-induced AT1-R signaling [7]. However, little was known regarding to the downstream pathway subsequent to β-arrestin2-mediated AT1-R and ERK1/2 activation by mechanical stress. It was believed that AngII stimulated G-protein-dependent ERK1/2 activation through binding to AT1-R, but overexpression of AT1-R mutant lacking $G\alpha q/G\alpha i$ coupling also induced ERK1/2 phosphorylation and developed severe myocardial hypertrophy both in vitro and in vivo [9,10]. We previously reported that G protein-independent calcineurin was critically involved in mechanical stretch induced myocardial hypertrophy [11], and candesartan could attenuate the hypertrophic response through regulating the tyrosine kinases cascade [3]. Therefore, we hypothesized that Src family kinase, the non-receptor tyrosine kinase, might mediate G protein-independent AT1-R signaling and cardiac hypertrophy induced by MS.

Src is a stress-sensitive kinase which plays an important role in the pathophysiological mechanisms for pressure overload-induced myocardial hypertrophy and pulmonary arterial hypertension, Src inhibition can effectively reverse the hypertensive response and hypertrophic signaling [12,13]. MS-mediated autophosphorylation of Src is highly associated with ERK1/2 activation [14]. Recent study revealed the expression and distribution of Src in the nucleus of cardiomyocytes with hypertrophy [15], and β-arrestin2 enhanced nuclear localization of ERK1/2 via GPCRs activation [16]. Mutant AT1 receptor lacking the docking site impaired Src-dependent nuclear translocation of ERK1/2 [10]. These findings prompted us to assume that Src kinase might be involved in β-arrestin2-meidated ERK1/2 activation and cardiac hypertrophy subsequent to AT1-R activation by MS. In the present study, we focused on the changes of AT1-R downstream signals, especially the role of Src kinase, in regulating β-arrestin2-dependent and AT1-R-induced signal transduction after MS.

Materials and Methods

Reagents

Anti-ERK1/2 (#9102), anti-phospho-ERK1/2 at Thr^{202}/Tyr^{204} (#9101) and anti-phospho-Src at Tyr^{416} (#2101) were purchased from Cell-signaling Technology; anti-Angiotensin II type 1 receptor (ab9391) were purchased from Abcam, plc; anti-FLAG-probe (#F7425), GF109203X (#G2911) were purchased from Sigma-Aldrich; anti-HA-probe (sc-805), anti-β-arrestin2 (sc-13140) were purchased from Santa Cruz Biotechnology; and SU6656 (#572635) was purchased from Calbiochem, Merck KGaA. Mechanic stretch-model culture plates were provided as kind gifts from Chiba University Graduate School of Medicine.

Plasmids Constructs

HA-tagged ERK2, FLAG-tagged β-arrestin1 and 2 were kindly provided by professor Issei Komuro (Tokyo University, Japan). Wild-type FLAG-tagged β-arrestin2 in vector pcDNA3 was used as the template. PCR based site-directed mutagenesis approach was performed to make a valine(54)-to-aspartic substitution in the wild-type β-arrestin2 using Pfu polymerase (Takara), the mutagenic primers were as follows: 5'-GACCGGAAAGACTTTGT-GACC-3' (forward) and 5'-GGTCACAAAGTCTTTCCGGTC-3' (reverse). The mutant β-arrestin2-V54D was amplified and then cloned into plasmid pcDNA3. The SRC gene was amplified by PCR using primers 5'-CGGGATCCACTAGTAACGGCCGC-CAG-3' (forward) with a BamHI restriction site and 5'-CGCTCGAGCGAGGTTCTCTCCAGGCTG-3' with a XhoI restriction site, and subcloned into the pcDNA3 plasmid containing a HA tag-encoding sequence.

Cell Culture and transfection

In vitro cardiacmyocytes were cultured as previously reported [34]. In brief, neonatal (one-day-old) rats were sacrificed under ether anesthesia, and then ventricular tissues were surgically isolated from the anesthetized rats, all operations were made to minimize suffering. The isolated tissues were minced and placed in culture medium containing the buffers of 5.4 mmol/L KCl, 0.44 mmol/L NaH_2PO_4, 137 mmol/L NaCl, 4.2 mmol/L $NaHCO_3$ and 5 mmol/L glucose at pH 7.4. Cells were then

dissociated at 37°C by a combination of mechanical agitation and enzymatic digestion with 0.1 mg/mL DNase II (Sigma) and 0.125% pancreatin trypsin (Calbiochem). Cells were pre-plated for 2 h in 100 mm dishes with Dulbecco's modified Eagle's medium (DMEM) with 10% defined bovine calf serum (FBS, HyClone), penicillin (100 units/mL) and streptomycin (100 mg/mL) (Sigma), then the unattached cardiomyocytes were collected and plated at a field density of 1×10^5 cells/cm^2 on silicone rubber culture dishes. Stretching of cardiacmyocytes by 10% was conducted as described previously [3]. HEK-293-AT1 cells lines were kindly provided by professor Issei Komuro (Tokyo University, Japan), and were cultured in Dulbecco's modified Eagles medium (DMEM) with 10% FBS and 1% penicillinystreptomycin as described previously [3]. Transient transfection of AT1 plasmids into cells were performed by using Gene Transfection System (Invitrogen) according to the manufacturer's instructions. The stable selection of transfection cells were achieved by adding Aminoglycoside G418 (200 ug/mL) to cells 3 day after transfection. All cell cultures were transferred to serum-free media 24 h before experiment.

Experimental Animal Model

Angiotensinogen gene knockout (AGT KO) mice were provided as kind gifts from professor Issei Komuro. Aged 8~10 weeks of AGT KO mice were used in the present study and wide-type (WT) C57BL/6 mice were used as control littermates. All the procedures involving animals were carried out in accordance with the recommendations of the guidelines for the Care and Use of Laboratory Animals from China Council on Animal Care. The experiment was approved by the Experimental Animal Ethics Committee, Fudan University Shanghai Medical College with the permit number of 20110307-092. Pressure overload model was established by transverse aorta constriction (TAC) for 2 weeks as previously described [6,11]. To ameliorate suffering, the mice were anesthetized by intraperitoneal injection of a combination of ketamine (100 mg/kg) with xylazine (5 mg/kg), and respiration was artificially controlled with a tidal volume of 0.2 ml and a respiratory rate of 110 breaths/min. The transverse aorta was constricted with the 7-0 nylon strings by ligating the aorta together with a blunted 27-gauge needle to yield a narrowing of 0.4 mm in diameter, and the needle was pulled out later. SU6656 (1 mg/kg/day) was continuously administered by Alzet osmotic mini pumps (DURECT, Cupertino, California) and was implanted subcutaneously into the back of mice right after anesthetized with 2% inhaled isoflurane from 3 days before TAC to 2 weeks after TAC. At 2 weeks after TAC, all mice were anesthetized by inhaled anesthetic isoflurane for cardiac echocardiography and hemodynamics analysis, and then mice were quickly sacrificed before they woke up. The hearts were excised for further examination, and the bodies were recorded, collected and centralized processing.

ERK2 kinase activity Assay

HA-tagged ERK2 plasmid was transient transfected into cardiomyocytes 24 h after plating the cells on stretch-model culture plates. ERK2 kinase activity was determined as we described previously [17]. In brief, RGS4 plasmid DNA (7.5 μg) was co-transfected into each dish of HEK-293-AT1 cells with or without HA tagged-ERK2 (2.5 μg), then the transfected cells were lysed, and the lysates were incubated with anti-HA antibody for 1 h at 4°C. Then, the immunocomplex was precipitated using A/G Plus-agarose beads, washed, resuspended in 25 ml kinase buffer with 2 m Ci of [γ-^{32}P] ATP, and incubated with 25 mg of MBP as the substrate at 25°C for 10 min. After incubation, the reaction was terminated by adding Laemmli sample buffer (0.002% bromphenol blue, 0.01M sodium phosphate buffer, pH 7.0, 10%

glycerol, 0.4%SDS, and 1% 2-mercaptoethanol) to the samples, and the samples were boiled for 5 min. The supernatants were subjected to SDS-polyacrylamide gel electrophoresis, and the gel was washed with 7% acetic acid for 30 min and with 3% glycerol for 30 min, dried, and then subjected to autoradiography.

RT-PCR analysis

Total RNA were extracted from cardiomyocytes using Trizol (Invitrogen) after mechanical stretch for 10 min. The cDNA was synthesized and optimized using a cDNA reverse transcription Kit (Takara), and the PCR primers used as follows:β-arrestin1, the sense primer:5′-CTGGATGTCTTGGGTCTGA-3′ and anti-sense primer: 3′-CGGATGGGGAAGTGGAAAC-5′; β-arrestin2, the sense primer: 5′-CCCTATGCTCAGAAACGAA-3′ and the anti-sense primer: 3′-TAGACAAGTAGCGGTGGAT-5′. The amplification of target genes were carried out on MJ Mini™ Gradient Thermal Cycler with a program of 95°C for 3 min followed by 35 cycles of 95°C for 30 s, 54°C for 30 s and 72°C for 30 s, and by a single incubation at 72°C for 5 min. PCR products were separated by electrophoresis on 1.2% agarose gels.

Western blotting (WB) Analysis

Cardiomyocytes were digested and separated to mini tubes. After incubating with cell lysates for 30 min on ice, cells supernatant was obtained by centrifugating for 30 min.Total protein extracts were size-fractionated by SDS-PAGE and were transferred to PVDF membranes. The membranes were blocked with 5% FBS in TBS-T buffer (20 umol/L Tris pH 7.4, 150 mmol/L NaCl and 0.05% Tween 20) for 2 h, then were incubated with antibody at 4°C overnight. After washing them for 3 times, the second antibody was adding, finally the membranes were treated with supersignal West Pico Chemiluminescent Substrate (Thermo), and the immunoreactive bands were detected by chemiluminescence system (Bio-Rad).

Immunoprecipitation (IP) and WB analysis

Cultured cells were transfected with various plasmids as indicated. After transfection for 24 h, cells were harvested by lysis buffer (10 mmol/L Tris-HCl, pH 7.4, 150 mmol/L NaCl, 1 mmol/L EDTA, 1% Triton X-100, 2.5 mmol/L sodium pyrophosphate, 25 mmol/L β-glycerol phosphate, 10 mmol/L NaF, 10 μg/mL aprotinin, 10 μg/mL leupeptin, 1 mmol/L PMSF). Cell extracts were sonicated and then centrifuged at 15000 g for 30 min at 4°C. Supernatants were subjected to immunoprecipitaion with indicated antibodies and co-incubated with protein A/G Plus-agarose beads (Santa Cruz Biotechnology) at 4°C for 3 h. Then the beads were spun down at 800 g for 2 min, washed with 700 μL lysis buffer for 3 times. The beads were eluted with SDS/PAGE loading buffer after extensive washed with 0.1 mol/L Tris-buffered saline. Finally the immunoprecipitates and total cell lysates were subjected to SDS/PAGE and determined by Western blotting with indicated antibodies.

Immunocytochemistry Analysis

In vitro cultured cardiomyocytes were seeded in photic-bottomed stretch plate, and were transfected with β-arrestin2-GFP-WT or β-arrestin2-GFP-V54D mutant. Cells were stretched for 10 min, and washed with 1×PBS and fixed in 4% formaldehyde for 15 minutes at room temperature. After permeabililized with 0.1% triton X-100 for 10 minutes at room temperature, cells were blocked in 5% BSA for 1.5 hours. Immunostaining was performed by using anti-phospho-Src antibody overnight at 4°C. Oil immersion lens in a multitrack

mode using a dual excitation (Alexa Fluor488 and Alexa Fluor555) filter sets. All Cells were counterstained with DAPI staining. Immunostaining was visualized by using laser scanning microscope (Leica Microsystems, Bensheim, Germany).

Detection of Inositol Phosphates

Determination of IP_3 was according to the methods as described previously [16]. In brief, cells were replated into 24-well plates at 1.5×10^5 cells per well and labeled for 24 h at 37°C with myo-[^{3}H] inositol (1.0 μCi/mL). After terminated labeling by aspirating the medium, cells were rinsing twice and the pellet was resuspended and harvested with phosphate-buffered saline (0.02% EDTA). Cells were transferred to culture template for re-adherence, and after subjecting to mechanical stretch or incubated with AngII (10^{-7} mol/L), cell lysates were prepared in 0.4M perchloric acid and neutralized in 0.72M KOH and 0.6M $KHCO_3$ in the presence of 5 mM LiCl. The lysates were then applied to Dowex columns (AG1-X8; Bio-Rad), washed, and eluted. The eluates were counted in a liquid scintillation counter. IP_3 releasing was estimated by determining the ratio of inositol phosphate radioactivity to the sum of total inositol phosphate.

Echocardiography Analyses and Hemodynamic Measurements

Transthoracic echocardiography was performed by animal specific instrument (Visual Sonics® Vevo770®, VisualSonics Inc. Canada). Mice were anesthetized and M-mode images of the left ventricle were record when mice partially recovered from anesthesia. The anterior and posterior wall thickness of left ventricular (LVAWD, LVPWD) at end-diastole and papillary muscle level was measured by two-dimensional short-axis views of the left ventricle and M-mode tracings. Left ventricle ejection fraction (LVEF) was obtained using Simpson approach. Left ventricular hemodynamics was also evaluated at 2 weeks after TAC. Briefly, a micronanometer catheter (Millar 1.4F, SPR 835, Millar Instruments, Houston, TX, USA) was inserted through the right common carotid artery into the aorta and carefully introduced into left ventricular. Left ventricular end systolic pressure (LVSBP) was measured as previously described [6].

Statistical Analysis

All data were expressed as means ± s.e.m. The between-group comparisons of means were done by one-way ANOVA followed by Tukey-Kramer test. *P* values smaller than 0.05 were considered statistical significance.

Results

RGS4 failed to inhibit mechanical stretch-induced ERK1/2 phosphorylation

Increasing evidence implicated that AT1-R could function through a heterotrimeric G-protein coupling or a G-protein-independent mode [18–20]. AngII, as the receptor agonist, activated AT1-R via a traditional GTP analog sensitive pathway. Ligand binding to G-protein-coupled receptors (GPCRs) induced GTP binding to the Gα subunit and dissociation from the βγ subunits. Here, we tested the possibility of Gα subunit activation during the process of mechanical stretch-induced AT1-R activation. It was reported that RGS4 negatively regulated Gαq signaling though promoting the hydrolysis of GTP [19,20]. Thus, the effect of Gαq coupling was attenuated by overexpressing RGS4 in cardiomyocytes. As shown in Figure 1A, Gαq-dependent phosphorylation of ERK1/2 was significantly reduced in AngII

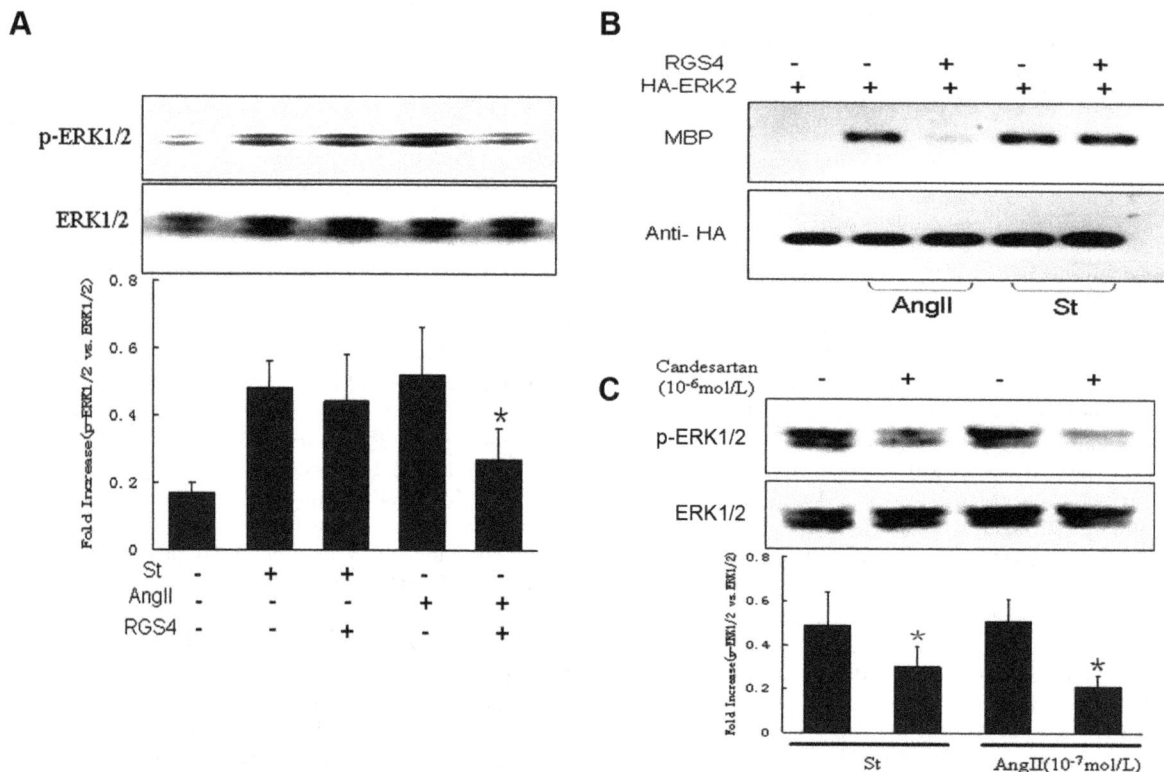

Figure 1. Mechanical stretch induced ERK1/2 signaling via activation of AT1-R, but not affected by G protein inhibition. (A) In vitro cultured cardiomyocytes were transfected with or without RGS4 plasmid, and then stimulated by stretch or AngII (10^{-7} mol/L) for 10 min, total proteins were collected and the expressions of phosphorylated ERK1/2 and total ERK1/2 were determined by Western blotting. **(B)** HA-tagged ERK2 was co-transfected with RGS4 plasmid into HEK-293 AT1 expressed cells for 24 h, ERK2 activity (indicated by MBP expression) was detected in cells induced by stretch or AngII, respectively. **(C)** Cardiomyocytes were pretreated with candesartan (10^{-6} mol/L) and then induced by stretch or AngII for 10 min, the expressions of phosphorylated ERK1/2 and total ERK1/2 were determined. * $P < 0.05$ vs. stretch-induced group (n = 3 separated experiments).

(10^{-7} mol/L)-induced cardiomyocytes after overexpressing RGS4. In contrast, RGS4 induced suppression of ERK1/2 was largely prevented by mechanical stretch.

To confirm the role of AT1-R in mechanical stretch evoked signal transduction, we then co-transfected HA-tagged ERK2 with RGS4 in HEK-293-AT1 expressed cells. After transient transfection for 24 h, the cells were stimulated by AngII (10^{-7} mol/L) and mechanical stretch, respectively. Immunoblotting analyses showed that ERK2 phosphorylation (indicated by MBP activity) was markedly attenuated in RGS4 overexpressed cells followed by AngII induction but not by mechanical stretch (Fig. 1B). Of note, both stretch-induced and AngII-stimulated ERK1/2 activation were inhibited by candesartan (10^{-6} mol/L) (Fig. 1C), indicating a critical role of AT1-R in regulating ERK1/2 phosphorylation during mechanical stretch.

Mechanical stretch-induced ERK1/2 phosphorylation did not depend on Gα coupling pathway

Previous in vivo studies showed that mechanical stretch-induced ERK1/2 activation was significantly attenuated in hearts from β-arrestins KO mice [7,18]. To explore whether mechanical stretch induced ERK1/2 response via β-arrestin-dependent pathway or Gα-dependent signaling, we first determined the release of inositol 1,4,5-triphosphate (IP_3) in stretch-induced cardiomyocytes, since CAMP-dependent IP_3 bioactivity was the major event of GPCRs

activation through Gα protein coupling. As shown in Figure. 2A, IP_3 release was significantly attenuated in stretching-induced cardiomyocytes compared with that in AngII (10^{-7} mol/L)-induced cardiomyocytes. Both AngII and mechanical stretch mediated IP_3 release were blocked by candesartan (10^{-6} mol/L), suggesting that AT1 receptor was essential for Gα protein coupling. In addition, inhibition of PKC with GF109203X, a specific PKC inhibitor, effectively attenuated AngII (10^{-7}M) induced ERK1/2 phosphorylation, but the phosphorylation level of ERK1/2 stimulated by stretching was not affected (Fig. 2B). These data suggested that mechanical stretch mediated ERK1/2 signal might not through activating the "classical" G-protein-dependent pathway.

Next, we examined the role of β-arrestin in ERK1/2 activation induced by mechanical stretch. Results showed that both the mRNA and protein levels of β-arrestin1/2 remained unchanged in response to mechanical stretch (Fig. 2C). However, knocking down endogenous β-arrestin1/2 caused a significant decrease in the phosphorylation level of ERK1/2 in response to mechanical stretch (Fig. 2D). We further found that a robust increase of phosphorylated ERK1/2 at 10 min after stretching, which was induced by β-arrestin2 but not by β-arrestin1 in β-arrestin1 or 2 single transfected HEK-293-AT1 cells after knocking down the endogenous β-arrestin1/2 with specific siRNA (Fig. 2E).

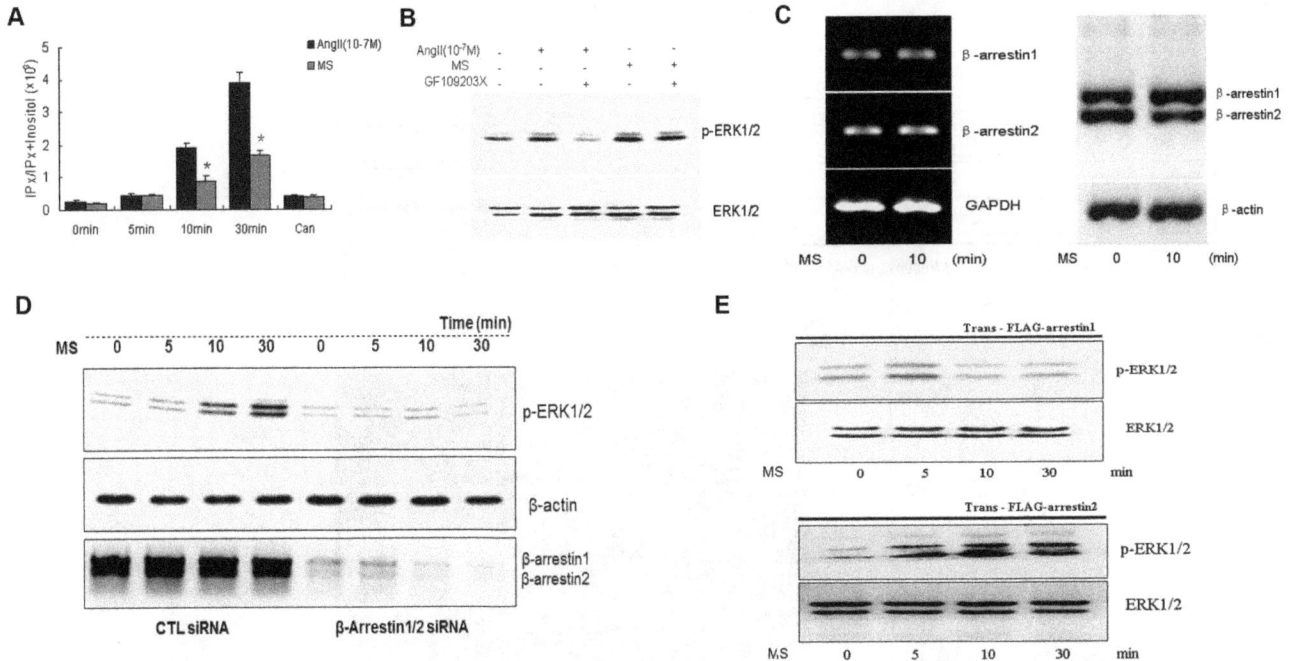

Figure 2. Mechanical stretch preferentially activated a heterotrimeric G protein-independent AT1 signaling pathway. (A) In vitro cultured cardiomyocytes were seeded on 24 well plates (1.5×10^5 cells) and labeled by myo-[^{3}H] inositol (1.0 μCi/mL) at 37°C for 24 h. Inositol phosphates (IPx) release was determined at the different indicated time points triggered by AngII (10^{-7} mol/L) or stretch respectively, and including the treatment of candesartan. **(B)** The effect of GF109203X on ERK1/2 phosphorylation stimulated by stretch or AngII (10^{-7} mol/L). **(C)** The endogenous mRNA and protein levels of β-arrestin1 and β-arrestin2 in cardiomyocytes were determined before and after stretch for 10 min. **(D)** Time-dependent ERK1/2 phosphorylation was determined after treatment with β-arrestin1/2 siRNA or scrambled siRNA. **(E)** Mechanical stretch-induced expression of phosphorylated ERK1/2 was determined in a single plasmid (β-arrestin1 or β-arrestin2) transfected HEK-293-AT1 cells after knock-down of endogenous β-arrestin1/2. * $P<0.05$ vs. AngII-induced group (n = 3 separated experiments).

β-arrestin2 regulated ERK1/2 phosphorylation through interacting with the tyrosine kinase Src during mechanical stretch

Above data indicated that β-arrestin2 was critically involved in mechanical stretch-induced ERK1/2 phosphorylation, however, both mRNA and protein levels of β-arrestin2 were not affected by stretching, but the phosphorylation level of Src was suppressed by knocking down of β-arrestin2 (Fig. 3A). Therefore, we assumed that β-arrestin2 might be the scaffold protein that mediated AT1-R-dependent tyrosine kinase phosphorylation. In the Co-IP analysis, we revealed that Src was immunoprecipitated by anti-AT1-R antibody in a time dependent manner (Fig. 3B), suggesting that Src was recruited to the cell membrane and interact with AT1-R during stretching. Our previous observation indicated that one kind of Src family tyrosine kinase was critically involved in mechanical stretch-evoked AT1-R signaling [3], but a direct interaction between Src and β-arrestin2 had not been demonstrated in the model of mechanical stretch. Hence, we co-transfected FLAG-tagged β-arrestin2 and HA-tagged Src into HEK-293-AT1 cells. Afterwards, co-immunoprecipitation assays were conducted in stretched or unstretched HEK-293-AT1 cells. The proteins were collected after stretching for 10 min, and followed by immunoprecipitation of β-arrestin2 with anti-FLAG antibody. We probed the immunoprecipitated sample by Western blotting using anti-HA antibody. The results showed that β-arrestin2 interacted with Src only in stretched cells (Fig. 3C), suggesting that AT1-R mediated recruitment of β-arrestin2 might be important for Src binding and activation. But Src kinase was markedly reduced in sample from cells transfected with dominant negative β-arrestin2-V54D (Fig. 3C). Previous studies reported that β-arrestin, which functioned as a scaffold protein, could recognize and interact with the catalytic domain of Src, by which regulated its kinase activity. Therefore, the attenuated interaction between Src and β-arrestin2-V54D might be due to the lack of binding site for SH2 domain kinase docking [25]. Cell immunofluorescence further confirmed that Src kinase was phosphorylated and recruited to membrane by accumulated β-arrestin2 after mechanical stretch, but this effect was abolished by mutating the Src binding site in β-arrestin2-V54D transfected cardiomyocytes (Fig. 3D). Taken together, these data suggested that mechanical stretch-induced translocation of β-arrestin2 was essential for Src docking and signal transduction. To further investigate the effect of β-arrestin2/Src interaction after stretching on cardiomyocyte hypertrophy, we examined stretch-induced ERK1/2 phosphorylation in both β-arrestin2 and β-arrestin2-V54D transfected cardiomyocytes. The results showed that ERK1/2 phosphorylation was significantly attenuated in cells transfected with β-arrestin2-V54D compared with that in β-arrestin2 transfected cells (Fig. 3E). In addition, mechanical stretch-induced ERK1/2 activation was also inhibited by pretreating cardiomyocytes with SU6656 (10 μmol/L), a selective Src family kinase inhibitor. Of note, the inhibitory effect of SU6656 on ERK1/2 phosphorylation was not observed in cardiomyocytes stimulated by AngII (10^{-7} mol/L) (Fig. 3F). Collectively, these data confirmed that β-arrestin2/Src interaction was uniquely involved in mechanical stretch-mediated ERK1/2 activation.

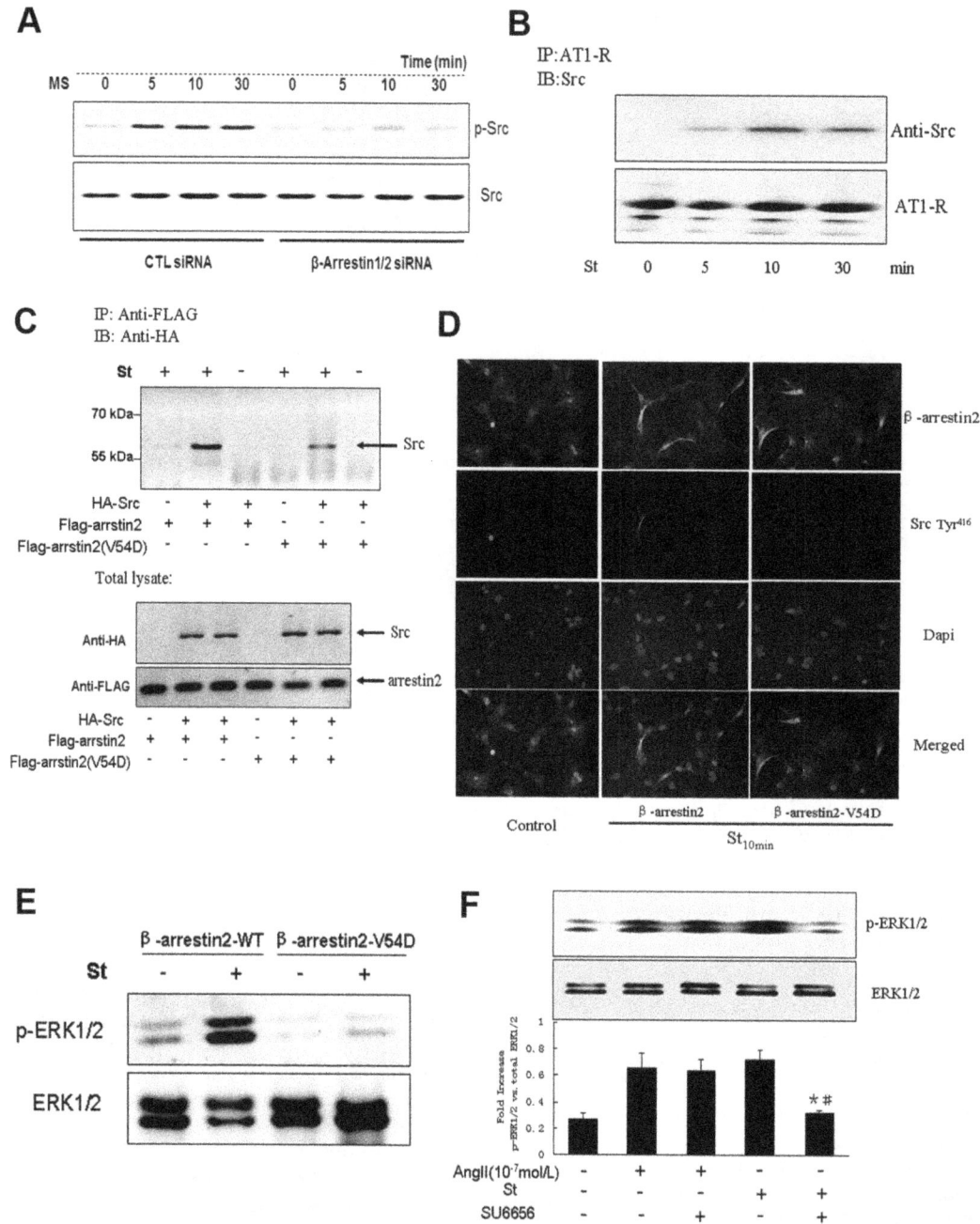

Figure 3. Src/β-arrestin2 signal complex was required for mechanical stretch-mediated AT1-R signaling. (**A**) Western blotting analyses of time-dependent Src phosphorylation after treatment with β-arrestin1/2 siRNA or scrambled siRNA. (**B**) Coimmunoprecipitation analyses of Src and AT1-R in lysates of stretched cardiomyocytes in a time-dependent manner. (**C**) HA-tagged Src and FLAG-tagged β-arrestin2 (or dominant negative β-arrestin2-V54D) were transient transfected into HEK-293-AT1 cells, whole cell extracts were immunoprecipitated with anti-FLAG monoclonal antibody, and the proteins in the immunoprecipitates and in the total lysates were probed by Western blotting using an anti-HA antibody. (**D**) The intercellular location of Src kinase in GFP-tagged β-arrestin2 WT and dominant negative GFP-tagged β-arrestin2-V54D transfected HEK-293-AT1 cells was visualized by immunofluorescence after stretching cells for 10 min. (**E**) The effect of β-arrestin2 WT or β-arrestin2-V54D transfection on mechanical stretch-induced ERK1/2 phosphorylation. (**F**) The effect of SU6656 (5 mmol/L) on ERK1/2 phosphorylation in cardiomyocytes stimulated by mechanical stretch or AngII (10^{-7} mol/L). * $P<0.05$ vs. both AngII and SU6656 treated groups; # $P<0.05$ vs. stretched groups (n = 3 separated experiments).

Src inhibition attenuated pressure overload-induced myocardial hypertrophy

We then investigated the in vivo consequence of the inhibition of β-arrestin2/Src signaling on pressure overload-induced myocardial hypertrophy in AGT KO mice. At 2 weeks after TAC,

echocardiography assessment showed a significant increase of left ventricular anterior wall at end-diastolic (LVAWd) and posterior wall at end-diastolic (LVPWd) thickerness in both C57BL/6 mice and AGT KO mice, accompanied by higher left ventricular ejection fraction (LVEF) and left ventricular end-systolic pressure (LVESP). However, Efficacy of attenuating myocardial hypertrophy by pretreatment with SU6656 was more pronounced in AGT KO mice than in C57BL/6 mice (Fig. 4A). Cardiac reprogramming of specific genes expressions were activated during pressure overload, we therefore determined the immediate-early response genes and fetal genes in the heart after TAC. Pressure overload enhanced the transcriptional levels of ANP, BNP and α-skeleton in AGT KO mice and C57BL/6 littermates, but expression of these re-enhanced genes was significantly lower in AGT KO mice than in C57BL/6 mice after SU6656 treatment, except for sarcoplasmic reticulum Ca^{2+}-ATPase (SERCA) (Fig. 4B).

Effects of different ARBs on AngII and TAC-induced cardiac hypertrophic response in AGT KO mice

We further compared the effects of candesartan and valsartan on myocardial hypertrophic response induced by TAC and AngII stimulation in AGT KO mice. Results showed that both candesartan and valsartan exerted inhibitory impacts on AngII-induced cardiac hypertrophy, but only candesartan effectively reversed TAC-induced hypertrophic response (Fig. 5A–B). Furthermore, Src was weakly upregulated by AngII but robustly enhanced by TAC for 2 weeks, and AngII-induced upregulation of

Src was inhibited by both candesartan and valsartan, while TAC-induced Src activation was inhibited only by candesartan (Fig. 5C).

Discussion

Cardiac hypertrophy is one of the independent risk factors responsible for myocardial injury and remodeling, and such compensatory response may transit to heart failure. Plenty of previous studies have demonstrated that AT1-R is one of the most important receptors mediating cardiac hypertrophic response through multiple signaling pathways [2,3,21,22]. However, the diversity of AT1-R-mediated signaling in response to hypertrophic stimuli in the heart is still not fully understood. We have previously revealed that mechanical stretch can activate AT1-R without the involvement of AngII [3]. In this study, we further confirm a critical role of Src in regulating AT1-R-mediated intercellular signaling transduction stimulated by mechanical stretch.

Immerging evidences indicated that activation model of GPCRs might undergo different phases due to different stimuli. It was generally believed the first phase of AT1-R activation was G-protein coupling dependent, and this process was hypersensitive to ligand binding. G-protein signaling subtype 4 (RGS4), an

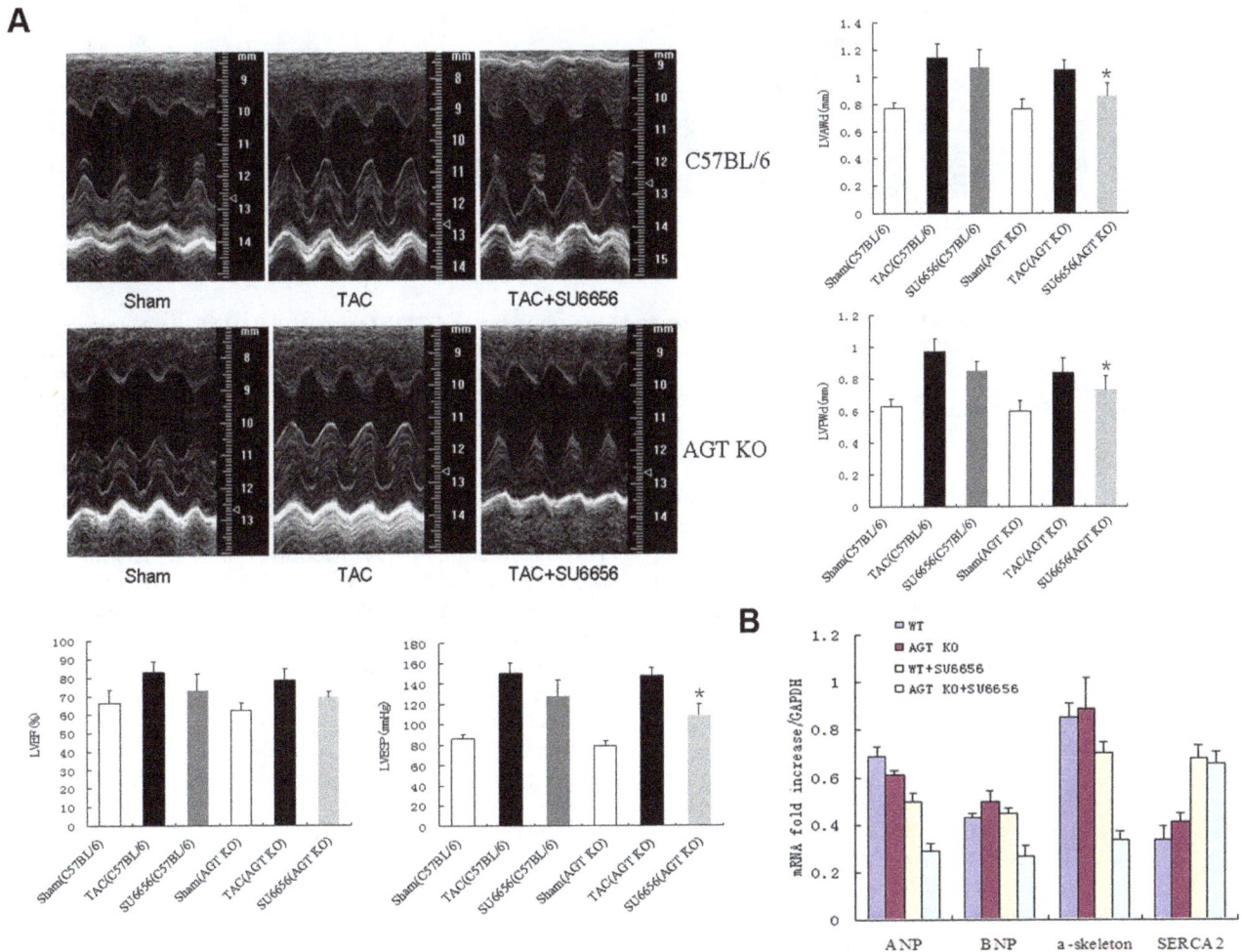

Figure 4. In vivo analyses of the cardiac function by echocardiography and hemodynamic measurements. Both AGT KO mice and the C57BL/6 WT littermates were pretreated with or without Src kinase inhibitor (SU6656), followed by TAC for 2 weeks. (**A**) Quantifications of LVAWd, LVPWd, LVEF and LVESP by representative M-mode tracing and hemodynamic recording from five mice. (**B**) Quantifications of cardiac immediate-early response genes in C57BL/6 mice and AGT KO mice with or without pretreatment of SU6656 (n = 5 separated experiments). * P<0.05 vs. saline-treated TAC-operated AGT KO mice.

A

Control   AngII   AngII+Val   AngII+Can

Sham   TAC   TAC+Val   TAC+ Can

B

C

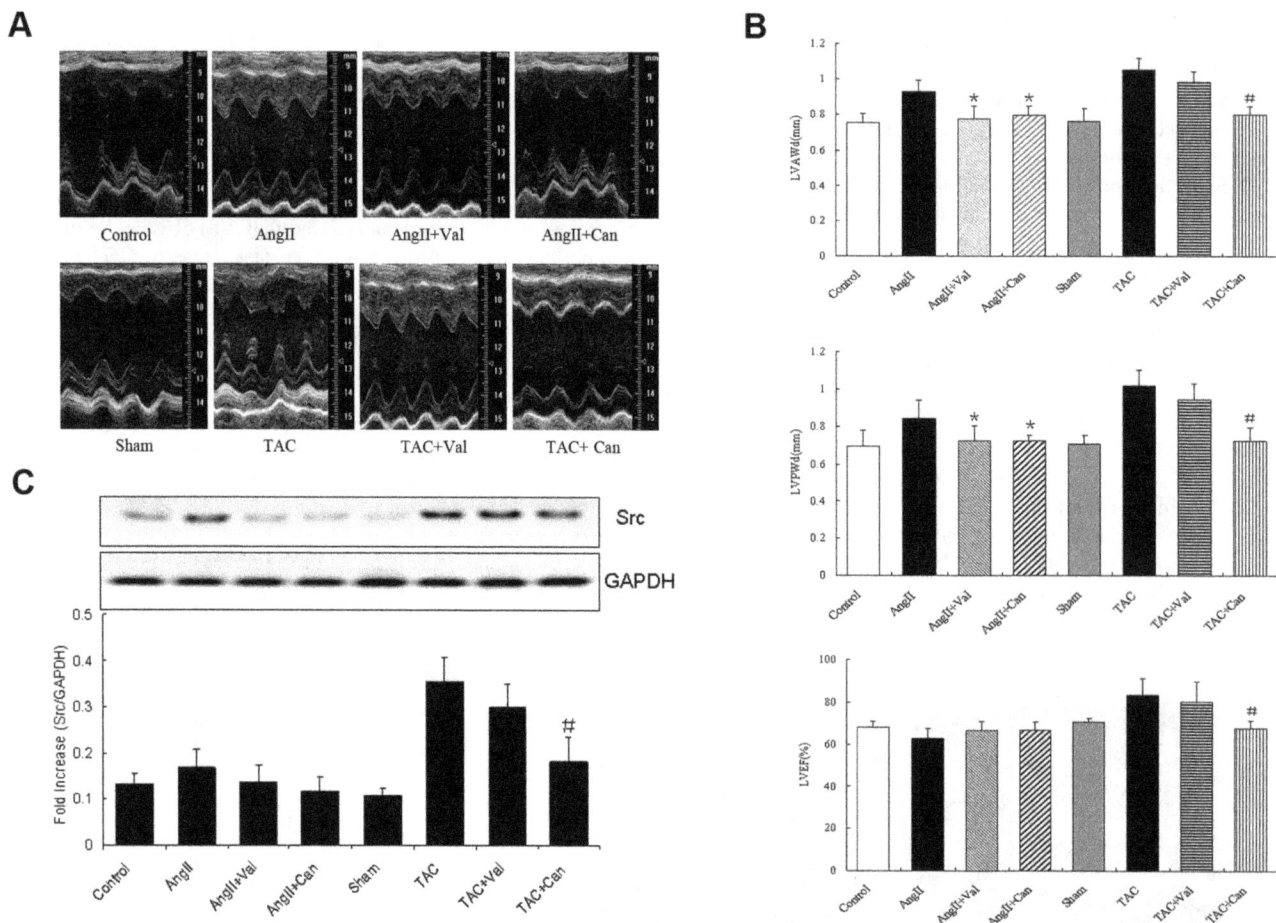

Figure 5. The effects of different ARBs on the cardiac function and Src expression in AGT KO mice. AGT KO mice were induced by AngII or TAC for 2 weeks with or without the pretreatment of valsartan or candesartan. (**A**) Representative M-mode tracings of AGT KO hearts stimulated by AngII (10^{-5} mol/L, top line) or by TAC for 2 weeks (bottom line). (**B**) Representative recording of LVAWd, LVPWd and LVEF in AGT KO mice from each group. (**C**) The expression of Src in myocardium of AGT KO mice from each group was determined. Data were presented as mean ± s.e.m. from five to eight mice. * $P<0.05$ vs. AngII-treated AGT KO mice; # $P<0.05$ vs. TAC-treated AGT KO mice.

inhibitory regulator of GPCR signaling through accelerating GTPase activity, was mainly expressed on cardiomyocytes [23,24]. In this study, intervention of G-protein coupling by overexpressing RGS4 in cardiomyocytes effectively blocked AngII-stimulated ERK1/2 phosphorylation, the indicator of hypertrophic response, but this effect was almost invisible in mechanical stretched cardiomyocytes. These resgults suggested that stretch-mediated AT1-R activation in the absence of the ligand binding might be sensitive to a second phase of G-protein signaling transduction which was independent of G-protein coupling.

Previous studies illustrated that PKC and IP_3, two important molecules were required for AngII-mediated modulation of myofilament calcium sensitivity and cardiac excitation-contraction coupling [17,25]. However, IP_3 was not fully activated in cardiomyocytes by short time effect of mechanical stretch. Interestingly, MS-induced ERK1/2 phosphorylation was not, suppressed by blocking PKC, suggesting a G-protein coupling independent signaling pathway was involved in stretching-induced cardiac hypertrophy. Of note, SU6656, a Src kinase inhibitor, effectively suppressed stretching-induced ERK1/2 activation, indicating a crucial role of Src but not PKC was required for mechanical stretch-mediated AT1 activation and intracellular signaling.

Rakesh K. previously reported that mechanical stretch evoked an abundant increase of ERK1/2 phosphorylation in hearts from WT mice, but not from AT1-R KO or arrestin2 KO mice [7]. It was believed that distinct conformational states of AT1-R might selectively stimulate signaling via G-protein dependent or independent pathway, while β-arrestin–biased agonism might serve as the central mechanism for mechanical stretch-mediated GPCR signaling, In line with this finding, our data suggested that β-arrestin2 not β-arrestin1 was required for stretch-induced ERK1/2 phosphorylation. However, both mRNA and protein levels of β-arrestin2 remained unchanged after mechanical stretch. Instead, stretch triggered β-arrestin2 translocation to the membrane of cardiomyocyte. Previous reports indicated the divergent roles of β-arrestin1 and β-arrestin2 in regulating intercellular signal via translocation to nucleus and cell surface [16,18,26,27]. In this study, we revealed that β-arrestin2 was highly expressed on cell membrane suggesting that mechanical stretch promoted the membrane recruitment of β-arrestin2 and binding with AT1-R. Plenty of studies demonstrated that GPCRs-mediated β-arrestin2 recruitment was essential not only for receptor internalization, but also for signal transduction [18,26]. It was also proved that tyrosine kinases-dependent signal cascade was crucial for GPCRs mediated ERK1/2 phosphorylation through transactivating

EGFR [7,27,28]. However, the underlying mechanism was not yet fully clear. Our data demonstrated that AT1-R-mediated accumulation of Src kinase in response to mechanical stretch was β-arrestin2 dependent, dominant negative β-arrestin2 greatly attenuated Src docking and accumulation after stretching. Recruitment of Src to activated GPCRs had multiple functions, such as MAP kinase activation, receptor internalization, and granule release [29,30]. In our study, Src activation was essential for β-arrestin2-mediated ERK1/2 phosphorylation. Transfection with mutant β-arrestin2 V54D or inhibition of Src by SU6656 in cardiomyocytes effectively suppressed MS-induced ERK1/2 activation. Src-dependent Ras-ERK1/2 pathway was also reported in the activation of AT1a-i2m receptor, which lacking the binding site for G-protein [9,10]. Therefore, we proposed that β-arrestin2-mediated Src activation might play an important role in G-protein-independent AT1-R activation and subsequent hypertrophic response.

The activation of cellular oncogenes such as c-myc and c-Src were critically involved in the reprogram progress of gene expression during pressure overload-induced myocardial hypertrophy [31]. Here, we also found enhanced that cardiac reprogramming genes were enhanced in the pressure overload model of AGT KO mice, which indicated that AngII binding signal was not essential for regulation of fetal genes reprogramming and hypertrophy induced by mechanical stretch. Instead, inhibition of Src effectively suppressed the transcripts of ANP, BNP and α-skeleton, reversed the ventricular remodeling and hypertrophic response. In this study, we also found that mechanical stress-induced ERK1/2 response could only be suppressed by candesartan, one kind of inverse agonism, but not by valsartan.. Of note, candesartan inhibited the AT1-R activation through binding two domains of Gln257 in TM6 and Thr287 in TM7, both located at the carboxyl of the receptor, thereby stabilized AT1-R in the inactive state [4,32]. Previous studies suggested that the carboxyl-terminal residues of AT1-R were required for G-protein independent signal transduction and transactivation of EGFR [28,33]. Mutation of the conserved YIPP motif in the C terminus of AT1-R, resulted in diminished EGFR transactivation and cardiac hypertrophy in Tg-Y319F mice [33]. Because β-arrestin2-dependent Src recruitment was critically involved in GPCRs-mediated EGFR transactivation, the data presented here further supported the notion that the special effect of candesartan on mechanical stretch-induced ERK1/2 phosphorylation was achieved via inhibition of G-protein independent but β-arrestin2 dependent Src recruitment.

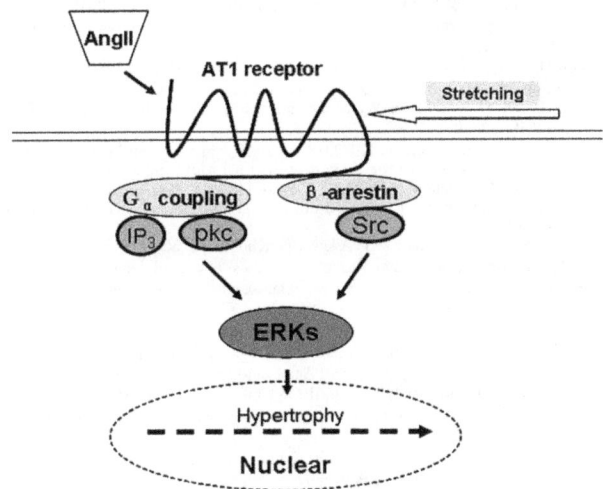

Figure 6. Schema for the mechanism of cardiac hypertrophy via AT1-R-dependent signaling pathway induced by AngII or mediated by mechanical stretch, respectively.

In summary, our study presented the divergent mechanisms for mechanical stretch- and AngII-mediated β-arrestin2-dependent and G-protein coupling-dependent signaling pathway in cardiac hypertrophy. Mechanical stretch-induced conformational switch of AT1-R might be different from that stimulated by AngII, thus resulted in different signal transduction (Fig. 6). The uncovering of β-arrestin2/Src-mediated ERK1/2 phosphorylation in response to mechanical stretch might be crucial for the establishment of pressure overload-induced cardiac hypertrophy, and clarification of this novel mechanism might be helpful for the development of more potent inverse agonist for AT1-R.

Acknowledgments

We thanked Professor Weidong Zhu (Department of Cardiology, Shanghai East hospital, Tongji University) for helpful discussion and technical assistance.

Author Contributions

Conceived and designed the experiments: YZ SW HG. Performed the experiments: SW GJ YY JW. Analyzed the data: SW JY. Contributed reagents/materials/analysis tools: GZ IK JG. Wrote the paper: SW YZ. Helped to complete the response work and gave suggestions for study: AS.

References

1. Murphy TJ, Alexander RW, Griendling KK, Runge MS, Bernstein KE (1991) Isolation of a cDNA encoding the vascular type-1 angiotensin II receptor. Nature 351: 233–236.

2. Lorell BH (1999) Role of angiotensin AT1, and AT2 receptors in cardiac hypertrophy and disease. Am J Cardiol 83: 48H–52H.

3. Zou Y, Akazawa H, Qin Y, Sano M, Takano H, et al. (2004) Mechanical stress activates angiotensin II type 1 receptor without the involvement of angiotensin II. Nat Cell Biol 6: 499–506.

4. Yasuda N, Akazawa H, Qin Y, Zou Y, Komuro I (2008) A novel mechanism of mechanical stress-induced angiotensin II type 1-receptor activation without the involvement of angiotensin II. Naunyn Schmiedebergs Arch Pharmacol 377: 393–399.

5. Akazawa H, Yasuda N, Komuro I (2009) Mechanisms and functions of agonist-independent activation in the angiotensin II type 1 receptor. Mol Cell Endocrinol 302: 140–147.

6. Li L, Zhou N, Gong H, Wu J, Lin L, et al. (2010) Comparison of angiotensin II type 1-receptor blockers to regress pressure overload-induced cardiac hypertrophy in mice. Hypertens Res 33: 1289–1297.

7. Rakesh K, Yoo B, Kim IM, Salazar N, Kim KS, et al. (2010) beta-Arrestin-biased agonism of the angiotensin receptor induced by mechanical stress. Sci Signal 3: ra46.

8. Godin CM, Ferguson SS (2012) Biased agonism of the angiotensin II type 1 receptor. Mini Rev Med Chem 12: 812–816.

9. Zhai P, Yamamoto M, Galeotti J, Liu J, Masurekar M, et al. (2005) Cardiac-specific overexpression of AT1 receptor mutant lacking G alpha q/G alpha i coupling causes hypertrophy and bradycardia in transgenic mice. J Clin Invest 115: 3045–3056.

10. Seta K, Nanamori M, Modrall JG, Neubig RR, Sadoshima J (2002) AT1 receptor mutant lacking heterotrimeric G protein coupling activates the Src-Ras-ERK pathway without nuclear translocation of ERKs. J Biol Chem 277: 9268–9277.

11. Zhou N, Li L, Wu J, Gong H, Niu Y, et al. (2010) Mechanical stress-evoked but angiotensin II-independent activation of angiotensin II type 1 receptor induces cardiac hypertrophy through calcineurin pathway. Biochem Biophys Res Commun 397: 263–269.

12. Pullamsetti SS, Berghausen EM, Dabral S, Tretyn A, Butrous E, et al. (2012) Role of Src tyrosine kinases in experimental pulmonary hypertension. Arterioscler Thromb Vasc Biol 32: 1354–1365.

13. Reineke EL, York B, Stashi E, Chen X, Tsimelzon A, et al. (2012) SRC-2 coactivator deficiency decreases functional reserve in response to pressure overload of mouse heart. PLoS One 7: e53395.

14. Boutahar N, Guignandon A, Vico L, Lafage-Proust MH (2004) Mechanical strain on osteoblasts activates autophosphorylation of focal adhesion kinase and proline-rich tyrosine kinase 2 tyrosine sites involved in ERK activation. J Biol Chem 279: 30588–30599.

15. Chen P, Li F, Xu Z, Li Z, Yi XP (2013) Expression and distribution of Src in the nucleus of myocytes in cardiac hypertrophy. Int J Mol Med 32: 165–173.

16. Kobayashi H, Narita Y, Nishida M, Kurose H (2005) Beta-arrestin2 enhances beta2-adrenergic receptor-mediated nuclear translocation of ERK. Cell Signal 17: 1248–1253.

17. Zou Y, Komuro I, Yamazaki T, Aikawa R, Kudoh S, et al. (1996) Protein kinase C, but not tyrosine kinases or Ras, plays a critical role in angiotensin II-induced activation of Raf-1 kinase and extracellular signal-regulated protein kinases in cardiac myocytes. J Biol Chem 271: 33592–33597.

18. Rajagopal K, Whalen EJ, Violin JD, Stiber JA, Rosenberg PB, et al. (2006) Beta-arrestin2-mediated inotropic effects of the angiotensin II type 1A receptor in isolated cardiac myocytes. Proc Natl Acad Sci U S A 103: 16284–16289.

19. Yan Y, Chi PP, Bourne HR (1997) RGS4 inhibits Gq-mediated activation of mitogen-activated protein kinase and phosphoinositide synthesis. J Biol Chem 272: 11924–11927.

20. Mukhopadhyay S, Ross EM (1999) Rapid GTP binding and hydrolysis by G(q) promoted by receptor and GTPase-activating proteins. Proc Natl Acad Sci U S A 96: 9539–9544.

21. Dostal DE, Baker KM (1992) Angiotensin II stimulation of left ventricular hypertrophy in adult rat heart. Mediation by the AT1 receptor. Am J Hypertens 5:276–280.

22. Sadoshima J, Izumo S (1993) Molecular characterization of angiotensin II–induced hypertrophy of cardiac myocytes and hyperplasia of cardiac fibroblasts. Critical role of the AT1 receptor subtype. Circ Res 73:413–423.

23. Tamirisa P, Blumer KJ, Muslin AJ (1999) RGS4 inhibits G-protein signaling in cardiomyocytes. Circulation 99: 441–447.

24. Tokudome T, Kishimoto I, Horio T, Arai Y, Schwenke DO, et al. (2008) Regulator of G-protein signaling subtype 4 mediates antihypertrophic effect of locally secreted natriuretic peptides in the heart. Circulation 117: 2329–2339.

25. Purdy KE, Arendshorst WJ (2001) Iloprost inhibits inositol-1,4,5-trisphosphate-mediated calcium mobilization stimulated by angiotensin II in cultured preglomerular vascular smooth muscle cells. J Am Soc Nephrol 12: 19–28.

26. Shenoy SK, Drake MT, Nelson CD, Houtz DA, Xiao K, et al. (2006) beta-arrestin-dependent, G protein-independent ERK1/2 activation by the beta2 adrenergic receptor. J Biol Chem 281: 1261–1273.

27. Kim J, Ahn S, Rajagopal K, Lefkowitz RJ (2009) Independent beta-arrestin2 and Gq/protein kinase Czeta pathways for ERK stimulated by angiotensin type 1A receptors in vascular smooth muscle cells converge on transactivation of the epidermal growth factor receptor. J Biol Chem 284: 11953–11962.

28. Noma T, Lemaire A, Naga Prasad SV, Barki-Harrington L, Tilley DG, et al. (2007) Beta-arrestin-mediated beta1-adrenergic receptor transactivation of the EGFR confers cardioprotection. J Clin Invest 117: 2445–2458.

29. Luttrell LM, Ferguson SS, Daaka Y, Miller WE, Maudsley S, et al. (1999) Beta-arrestin-dependent formation of beta2 adrenergic receptor-Src protein kinase complexes. Science 283: 655–661.

30. Miller WE, Maudsley S, Ahn S, Khan KD, Luttrell LM, et al. (2000) beta-arrestin1 interacts with the catalytic domain of the tyrosine kinase c-SRC. Role of beta-arrestin1-dependent targeting of c-SRC in receptor endocytosis. J Biol Chem 275: 11312–11319.

31. Komuro I, Kurabayashi M, Takaku F, Yazaki Y (1988) Expression of cellular oncogenes in the myocardium during the developmental stage and pressure-overloaded hypertrophy of the rat heart. Circ Res 62: 1075–1079.

32. Zhai P, Galeotti J, Liu J, Holle E, Yu X, et al. (2006) An angiotensin II type 1 receptor mutant lacking epidermal growth factor receptor transactivation does not induce angiotensin II-mediated cardiac hypertrophy. Circ Res 99: 528–536.

33. Yasuda N, Miura S, Akazawa H, Tanaka T, Qin Y, et al. (2008) Conformational switch of angiotensin II type 1 receptor underlying mechanical stress-induced activation. EMBO Rep 9: 179–186.

34. Zhang P, Xu D, Wang S, Fu H, Wang K, et al.(2011) Inhibition of aldehyde dehydrogenase 2 activity enhances antimycin-induced rat cardiomyocytes apoptosis through activation of MAPK signaling pathway. Biomed Pharmacother. 65:590–593.

13

IKKi Deficiency Promotes Pressure Overload-Induced Cardiac Hypertrophy and Fibrosis

Jia Dai[1,2,9], Di-Fei Shen[1,2,9], Zhou-Yan Bian[1,2,9], Heng Zhou[1,2], Hua-Wen Gan[1,2], Jing Zong[1,2], Wei Deng[1,2], Yuan Yuan[1,2], FangFang Li[1,2], Qing-Qing Wu[1,2], Lu Gao[3], Rui Zhang[1,2], Zhen-Guo Ma[1,2], Hong-Liang Li[1,2], Qi-Zhu Tang[1,2]*

1 Department of Cardiology, Renmin Hospital of Wuhan University, Wuhan, China, 2 Cardiovascular Research Institute of Wuhan University, Wuhan, China, 3 Department of Cardiology, Institute of Cardiovascular Disease, Union Hospital, Tongji Medical College, Huazhong University of Science and Technology, Wuhan, People's Republic of China

Abstract

The inducible IκB kinase (IKKi/IKKε) is a recently described serine-threonine IKK-related kinase. Previous studies have reported the role of IKKi in infectious diseases and cancer. However, its role in the cardiac response to pressure overload remains elusive. In this study, we investigated the effects of IKKi deficiency on the development of pathological cardiac hypertrophy using in vitro and in vivo models. First, we developed mouse models of pressure overload cardiac hypertrophy induced by pressure overload using aortic banding (AB). Four weeks after AB, cardiac function was then assessed through echocardiographic and hemodynamic measurements. Western blotting, real-time PCR and histological analyses were used to assess the pathological and molecular mechanisms. We observed that IKKi-deficient mice showed significantly enhanced cardiac hypertrophy, cardiac dysfunction, apoptosis and fibrosis compared with WT mice. Furthermore, we recently revealed that the IKKi-deficient mice spontaneously develop cardiac hypertrophy. Moreover, in vivo experiments showed that IKKi deficiency-induced cardiac hypertrophy was associated with the activation of the AKT and NF-κB signaling pathway in response to AB. In cultured cells, IKKi overexpression suppressed the activation of this pathway. In conclusion, we demonstrate that IKKi deficiency exacerbates cardiac hypertrophy by regulating the AKT and NF-κB signaling pathway.

Editor: Hiranmoy Das, Ohio State University Medical Center, United States of America

Funding: This research was supported by the National Natural Science Foundation of China (30901628 and 81000036) (http://www.nsfc.gov.cn/Portal0/default106.htm) and the Fundamental Research Funds for the Central Universities of China (No. 201130202020007) (http://www.gs.whu.edu.cn/newscenter/ReadNews.asp?NewsID=5728). The funders had the role in study design, data collection and analysis, decision to publish, or preparation of the manuscript.

Competing Interests: The authors have declared that no competing interests exist.

* E-mail: qztang@whu.edu.cn

⑨ These authors contributed equally to this work.

Introduction

Heart failure (HF) is a debilitating disease with a high prevalence, morbidity and mortality [1,2,3,4,5]. Pathological cardiac hypertrophy is an important predecessor of heart failure that is characterized by cardiac dysfunction, cell enlargement, reactivation of foetal gene expression, impaired myocardial vascularization, phenotypic changes in the extracellular matrix and hyperplasia of fibrosis [6,7,8,9]. Recent studies have shown that signaling pathways and their associated molecules play complex and pivotal roles in the development of cardiac hypertrophy,including mitogen activated protein kinases (MAPKs), phosphatidylinositol 3-kinase(PI3K)/AKT and calcineurin/nuclear factor of activated T cells (NFAT) [10]. However, effective blockade of the hypertrophy and prevention of transition to congestive heart failure remain a challenge. Thus, the identification of signals and pathways involved in pathological hypertrophy would open the door for the development of future therapeutic interventions for heart failure.

Nuclear factor-κB (NF-κB) plays a critical role in the immune response and influences gene expression events that affect cell survival, apoptosis, differentiation, proliferation, cancer progres-sion and development [11,12]. The NF-κB family of transcription factors includes five members, p50, p52, p65 (RelA), c-Rel, and RelB. These members share an N-terminal Rel homology domain (RHD),which is responsible for DNA binding and homo- and heterodimerization [11,12]. In the absence of a stimulus, NF-κB dimers normally combine with one of three typical IκB proteins, IκBα, IκBβ or IκBε, or the precursor protein p100. Stimulation with cytokines or other agonists results in the phosphorylation of IκB by the inhibitory-κB kinase (IKK) complex, which includes IKKα, IKKβ and IKKγ, triggering the degradation of IκB. Then, the freed NF-κB translocates to the nucleus, where it binds to and activates the promoters of the NFκB responsive genes [11,12].

Recent studies have shown that NF-κB directly exerts its role or alternatively involved in G protein-coupled receptor agonist- or tumour necrosis factor α(TNFα)-induced cardiac hypertrophy and pathological remodeling and fibrosis and NF-κB inhibition attenuates cardiac hypertrophy [13,14,15,16,17]. Furthermore, IKKβ-deficient mice exhibit cardiac dilation and dysfunction and lung congestion [18]. The inducible IκB kinase (IKKi/IKKε) a constitutively active serine-threonine IKK-related kinase shares 31% amino acid identity with IKKβ in the highly conserved N-terminal kinase domain but differs from IKKβ in several important aspects [19]. For example, IKKi is expressed in the cells and tissues of the immune system [19]. Recent studies have shown that human IKKi has two novel splice variants, IKKε-sv1 and IKKε-sv2, which have cell type- and stimulus-specific protein expression [20]. Some groups have described a role for IKKi in infectious diseases and cancer [21,22,23,24,25,26]. However, it has not been shown to be involved in cardiovascular disease. In this study, for the first time, we used IKKi-knockout (KO) mice to investigate the role of IKKi in cardiac hypertrophy induced by pressure overload. We demonstrate that IKKi deficiency in mice leads to cardiac hypertrophy, fibrosis, and cardiac dysfunction, indicating a crucial role for IKKi in regulating cardiac hypertrophy.

Materials and Methods

Animals and animal models

All animal procedures were performed in accordance with the *Guide for the Care and Use of Laboratory Animals*, which was published by the U.S. National Institutes of Health (NIH Publication No. 85-23, revised 1996) and approved by the Animal Care and Use Committee of the Renmin Hospital of Wuhan University (protocol number: 00020390).Male KO mice(C57BL/6 background; knockout mice were purchased from Jackson Laboratory, No. 006908) and their wild-type (WT) littermates, which ranged in age from 8 to 10 weeks, were subjected to aortic banding (AB) as described previously [27]. Each mouse was were anaesthetized with sodium pentobarbital (Sigma, 80 mg/kg, ip), and a horizontal skin incision was made at the level of 2–3 intercostal space. The descending aorta was isolated, and a 7.0 silk suture was wrapped around the aorta.A bent 26-gauge needle (for 25.5–27.5 g) or 27-gauge needle (for 23.5–25.5 g) was then placed next to the aorta, and the suture was tied snugly around the needle and the aorta. After ligation, the needle was quickly removed, the chest and skin were closed, and the mice were allowed to recover. Sham-operated mice underwent the same procedure without constriction. The adequacy of anesthesia was monitored during the surgical procedures by assessing the lack of the pedal withdrawal reflex, slow constant breathing, and no response to surgical manipulation. Buprenorphine (0.1 mg/kg, sc) was administered for post-operative analgesia. Four weeks after the operation, the hearts, lungs, and tibiae of the mice were dissected and weighed or measured to compare the heart weight (HW)/body weight (BW) (mg/g), HW/tibial length (TL) (mg/mm), and lung weight (LW)/BW (mg/g) ratios of the different groups.

Echocardiography and hemodynamic analyses

Echocardiography was performed on anesthetized (1.5% isoflurane) mice using a MyLab 30CV (ESAOTE S. P. A) with a 15 MHz linear array ultrasound transducer. The left ventricle (LV) dimensions were assessed in the parasternal short-axis view. End-systole and end-diastole were defined as the phases that were associated with the smallest and largest areas of the LV, respectively. The end-systolic (LVESD) and end-diastolic (LVEDD) LV internal diameters and posterior wall end-diastolic thickness (PWT) were measured from the LV M-mode tracing with a sweep speed of 50 mm/s at the mid-papillary muscle level. The percentage of fractional shortening (FS) was calculated as (LVEDD-LVESD)/LVEDD×100.

To perform the invasive hemodynamic measurements, we anesthetized the mice with 1.5% isoflurane, and a microtip transducer catheter (SPR-839, Millar Instruments, Houston, TX, USA) was inserted into the right carotid artery and advanced into the left ventricle. The pressure signals and heart rates were recorded continuously using a Millar Pressure-Volume System (MPVS-400, Millar Instruments, Houston, TX, USA), and the recordings were further analyzed using PVAN data analysis software.

Histological analysis and apoptotic cell assay

The hearts were excised, washed with PBS, arrested in diastole with 10% potassium chloride solution, weighed, placed in 10% formalin, and embedded in paraffin. They were then cut transversely and close to the apex to visualize the left and right ventricles. Several sections of each heart (4–5 μm thick) were prepared, stained with hematoxylin and eosin (H&E) for histopathology or picrosirius red (PSR) for collagen deposition by standard procedures and then visualized by light microscopy. For the myocyte cross-sectional area, sections were stained for membranes with FITC-conjugated WGA (Invitrogen) and for nuclei with DAPI. Single myocytes were measured using a quantitative digital image analysis system (Image Pro-Plus, version 6.0). The outlines of 100 myocytes were traced for each group. Cell death by apoptosis was evaluated using a TUNEL assay, which was performed on sections with In Situ Apoptosis Detection Kit (Roche, 11684817910) according to the manufacturer's recommendations.

Quantitative real-time RT-PCR

Real-time PCR was performed to detect the mRNA expression levels of hypertrophic and fibrotic markers. Total RNA was extracted from frozen pulverized mouse cardiac tissue using TRIzol (Invitrogen, 15596-026). The yields and purities were spectrophotometrically estimated using the A260/A280 and A230/260 ratios, as measured with a SmartSpec Plus Spectrophotometer (Bio-Rad). The RNA (2 μg of each sample) was reverse-transcribed into cDNA using oligo(DT) primers and the Transcriptor First Strand cDNA Synthesis Kit (Roche, 04896866001). The PCR amplifications were quantified using the LightCycler 480 SYBR Green 1 Master Mix (Roche,04707516001). The results were normalized against glyceraldehyde-3-phosphate dehydrogenase (GAPDH) gene expression.

Protein extraction and western blotting analyses

The left ventricles were harvested for western blotting analyses. They were first lysed in RIPA lysis buffer, and the protein concentrations were measured using the BCA Protein Assay Kit (Thermo, 23227) and an ELISA Reader(Synergy HT, Bio-Tek). The cell lysates (50 μg) were loaded into each lane and subjected to SDS-PAGE, and the proteins were then transferred onto Immobilon-FL transfer membranes (Millipore, IPFL00010). The membranes were incubated overnight at 4°C with primary antibodies against one of the following proteins: p-MEK1/2 (Cat#, 9154), T-MEK1/2 (Cat#,9122), p-ERK1/2 (Cat#,4370), T-ERK1/2 (Cat#,4695), p-P38 (Cat#,4511), T-P38 (Cat#,9212), p-JNK(Cat#,4668),T-JNK (Cat#,9258), p-PI3K(Cat#, 4228), T-PI3K (Cat#,4257), p-AKT (Cat#,4060), T-AKT (Cat#,4691), P-GSK3β (Cat#,9322), T-GSK3β (Cat#,9315), p-mTOR (Cat#,2971), T-mTOR (Cat#,2983), P-FOXO3A (Cat#,9465), T-FOXO3A (Cat#,2497), P-FOXO1 (Cat#,9461), T-FOXO1 (Cat#,2880), p-NFκB (Cat#,3033), T-NFκB (Cat#,4764), Bax (Cat#,2772), Bcl2(Cat#, 2870),Cleaved Caspase3(-Cat#,9661),GAPDH(Cat#,2118),and IKKi(Cat#,3416). All antibodies were purchased from Cell Signaling Technology.The membranes were then incubated with goat anti-rabbit IgG (LI-COR, 926-32211) for one hour IgG. The blots were scanned using a two-color infrared imaging system (Odyssey, LI-COR). Specific protein expression levels were normalized to the GAPDH protein for the total cell lysates and cytosolic proteins.

H9c2 cell culture and surface area

Cultures of H9c2 rat cardiomyocyte cells (ATCC, Rockville, MD, USA) were prepared as described previously [28]. H9c2 cells were seeded at a density of 1×10^6 cells/well onto 6-well culture plates in Dulbecco's modified Eagle's mediu-m (DMEM)/F12 1:1 medium mixed at a ratio of 1:1 (v/v) (Gibco,C11995) with 10% fetal bovine serum (FBS;Gibco,1133067), glutamine (2 mmol/L), penicillin (100 IU/ml), and streptomycin (100 mg/ml). After 48 hours, the culture medium was replaced with F10 medium containing 0.1% FBS,and the cells were infected with different adenoviruses followed by angiotensin II (Ang II; 1 μM) treatment.For the cell infections,cardiac myocytes were cultured in 6-well plates at a density of 1×10^6 cells/well and then exposed to 2×10^8 pfu of each virus in 1 ml of serum-free medium for 24 hours.The cells were then washed and incubated in serum-containing medium for 24 hours.The virus Ad-IKKi was used to overexpress IKKi, and the control virus AdGFP was used as a control.

To identify the cardiomyocytes and assess cardiomyocyte hypertrophy, we characterized the cells by analyzing their cardiac α-actinin expression using immunofluorescence.The cells were washed with PBS, fixed with RCL2 (ALPHELYS, RCL2-CS24L), permeabilized in 0.1%Triton X-100 in PBS, and stained with anti-α-actinin (Millipore, 05-384) at a dilution of 1:100 in 1% goat serum. The secondary antibody was Alexa Fluor® 488 goat anti-mouse IgG (Invitrogen, A11004). The myocytes on coverslips were mounted onto glass slides with SlowFade Gold antifade reagent with DAPI (Invitrogen, S36939).

Statistical analysis

Data are expressed as the means ± SEM. Differences among the groups were determined by a two-way ANOVA followed by a post hoc Tukey's test. Comparisons between two groups were performed using an unpaired Student's t-test. A p-value of <0.05 was considered to be statistically significant.

Results

IKKi expression is induced in hypertrophic hearts following AB

To investigate the potential role of IKKi in cardiac hypertrophy, we used the well-established cardiac hypertrophy model induced by AB. We found that IKKi protein and mRNA levels were slightly increased at 1 week but significantly up-regulated at 4 and 8 weeks after AB (Figure 1). These findings demonstrate that IKKi expression compensatorily increases during the development of cardiac hypertrophy.

IKKi deficiency induces severe and spontaneous hypertrophy

To evaluate alterations in cardiac structures and functions in IKKi-deficient mice, we harvested the hearts of 30-week-old mice and performed echocardiograms. It was documented that the HW, HW/BW, HW/TL, LVEDD, and LVESD were significantly increased and the FS was decreased compared with the WT mice (Table 1), which agrees with our hypothesis that the loss of IKKi leads to spontaneous cardiac hypertrophy and dysfunction.

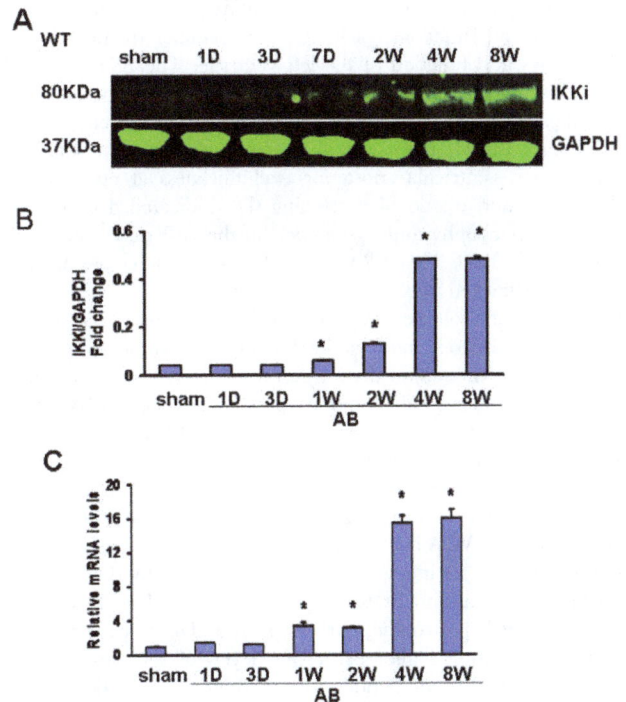

Figure 1. IKKi expression in the hypertrophic heart.A,Western blot analysis of the cardiac IKKi protein in WT mice after aortic banding at the time points indicated (n = 6). B, RT-PCR analysis of cardiac IKKi mRNA levels in WT mice after aortic banding at the time points indicated (n = 6). *P<0.05 vs. sham.

IKKi deficiency enhances cardiac hypertrophic and dysfunctional responses to pressure overload

To clarify the direct relationship between IKKi deficiency-mediated changes and cardiac hypertrophy, IKKi-KO mice and their WT littermates were subjected to cardiac pressure overload by AB or a sham surgery. The cumulative survival rate at 4 weeks after AB was strikingly decreased by IKKi deficiency (Figure 2E).

Table 1. Anatomic and echocardiographic analysis of 24- to 30 -week-old IKKi KO mice and WT mice.

Parameter	WT(n = 6)	IKKi KO(n = 6)
BW (g)	30.39±0.66	31.08±0.73
HW/BW(mg/g)	4.05±0.09	5.43±0.22*
LW/BW(mg/g)	4.67±0.15	4.44±0.16
HW/TL(mg/cm)	6.54±0.24	9.10±0.32*
HR (beats/min)	501±12	520±23
LVEDD(mm)	3.53±0.05	4.25±0.11*
LVESD(mm)	2.08±0.06	2.78±0.12*
LVPWD (mm)	0.72±0.01	0.73±0.02*
FS (%)	41.22±1.28	34±1.18*

BW,body weight;HW/BW,heart weight/body weight;LW/BW,lung weight/body weight; HW/TL,heart weight/tibial length; HR,heart rate; LVEDD,left ventricular end-diastolic dimension; LVESD,left ventricular end-systolic diameter; LVPWD,left ventricular posterior wall dimension; IVSD, Interventricular septal thickness at end-diastole; FS,fractional shortening.
*P<0.05 vs WT/KO.

Echocardiographic analyses were also utilized to evaluate cardiac structures and functions, including the chamber diameter, wall thicknesses and function of the left ventricle. The KO and WT mice that underwent sham surgery did not differ echocardiographically. However, the echocardiographic measurements of LVEDD, LVESD, interventricular septal thickness at end-diastole (IVSD), left ventricular posterior wall thickness at end-diastole (LVPWD), and fractional shortening (FS) indicated deteriorated cardiac hypertrophy and dysfunction in the KO mice compared with the WT mice (Figure 2A). The LV hemodynamic parameters of the anesthetized mice that were obtained during the acquisition of the pressure-volume (PV) loop further confirmed this significantly deteriorated hemodynamic dysfunction (volume and systolic and diastolic function) of the LV in the IKKi-KO mice as shown in Table 2. Under basal conditions, pressure-overloaded KO mice showed significantly increased ratios of HW/BW, HW/TL and LW/BW and cardiomyocyte cross-sectional area (CSA) compared with the WT mice. No significant differences were observed between the sham-operated groups (Figure 2B). The gross hearts and H&E and WGA staining results were also consistent with the role of IKKi as an inhibitor of cardiac hypertrophy (Figure 2C). Furthermore, real-time PCR was performed to analyze the mRNA expression of hypertrophic markers (Figure 2D). As expected, we found significantly higher expression levels of the cardiac fetal genes atrial natriuretic peptide (ANP), B-type natriuretic peptide (BNP), and β-myosin heavy chain (β-MHC) in the KO mice in response to AB. However, the mRNA expression levels of α-myosin heavy chain (α-MHC) and sarcoendoplasmic reticulum Ca^{2+}-ATPase (SERCA2α) were reduced. These results indicate that IKKi deficiency is responsible for the progressive hypertrophic effects and the impairment of cardiac function that is induced by pressure overload.

Forced IKKi expression attenuates the hypertrophic growth of myocytes in vitro

To specifically examine the role of IKKi in cardiomyocytes, we performed gain- of-function studies using cultured H9c2 rat cardiomyocytes. The H9c2 cells were serum-starved for 24 h in 0.5% FBS after infection with Ad-IKKi and then treated with 1 μM Ang II for the indicated times. Ad-IKKi infection led to a substantial increase in the level of IKKi protein in H9c2 rat cardiomyocytes. Further studies showed that the IKKi overexpression induced by Ad-IKKi infection attenuated Ang II-mediated cardiomyocyte hypertrophy, as measured by the cell surface area (Figure 3A). Moreover, RT-PCR showed that IKKi overexpression markedly decreased the mRNA levels of ANP and BNP induced by Ang II (Figure 3B). These in vitro data suggest the inhibitory effect of IKKi on cardiomyocyte hypertrophy.

IKKi deficiency significantly activates AKT/GSK3β/mTOR/ FOXO and NFκB signaling

To elucidate the molecular mechanism by which IKKi deficiency mediates the hypertrophic response, we examined the activation state of AKT and the expression of its downstream targets, including GSK3β, mTOR, forkhead box O3A (FOXO3A), forkhead box O1 (FOXO1) and NFκB using western blotting. The levels of phosphorylated AKT, GSK3β, mTOR, FOXO3A, FOXO1 and NF-κB were significantly increased in the hearts of the KO mice following pressure overload (Figures 4C, D). We then exposed cultured H9c2 cardiomyocytes infected with Ad-IKKi or Ad-GFP to 1 μM AngII. As shown in Figures 4E and F, AngII-stimulated AKT/GSK3β/mTOR/FOXO/NF-κB phosphorylation was attenuated by infection with Ad-IKKi. We further

investigated the role of MAPK, another important signaling molecule that regulates the development of hypertrophy. However, the levels of phosphorylated MEK-ERK1/2, JNK, p38 and PI3K were similar between the AB groups (Figures 4A, B).

Effects of IKKi deficiency on cardiac fibrosis induced by pressure overload

Fibrosis contributes to the phenotypic changes associated with the development of pathological cardiac hypertrophy. To detect the extent of fibrosis, we stained heart sections with PSR and found markedly increased perivascular and interstitial fibrosis and LV collagen volumes in the AB-induced KO and WT hearts compared with the sham-operated controls after 4 weeks. However, it should be noted that considerably increased cardiac fibrosis was also present in the KO mice (Figures 5A, B).

The observed interstitial fibrosis could be attributed to decreased collagen degradation or increased collagen synthesis. To evaluate the effect of IKKi on collagen synthesis, the mRNA expression levels of connective tissue growth factor (CTGF), transforming growth factor (TGF)-β1, TGF-β2, collagen I, collagen III, and fibronectin, which are known mediators of fibrosis, were analyzed. Increased expression levels of CTGF, TGF-β1, TGF-β2, collagen I, collagen III, and fibronectin were detected in the AB-induced KO mice (Figure 5C). These data suggest that IKKi deficiency promotes cardiac fibrosis.

IKKi deficiency enhances cardiac apoptosis induced by press-ure overload

To further explore the role of IKKi in hypertrophy, we assessed the apoptosis of myocytes after 4 weeks of AB using TUNEL assays. Apoptotic cells were detected in both KO and WT mice, and the fraction of apoptotic versus total cells was significantly higher in the pressure-overloaded hearts of the KO mice (Figures 6A,B). Furthermore, the levels of cleaved caspase 3, Bax (proapoptotic) and Bcl2 (antiapoptotic) proteins were assessed. The Bax protein level was increased and the Bcl2 protein level was decreased in the pressure-overloaded hearts of the KO mice, indicating a reduced Bcl2/Bax ratio. The level of cleaved caspase-3 was higher in the KO mice in response to AB (Figures 6C–E). These findings indicate that IKKi is involved in apoptosis in hypertrophic hearts subjected to pressure overload.

Discussion

Cardiac hypertrophy is characterized by the reactivation of fetal cardiac genes, increased cross-sectional areas of adult cardiomyocytes, and contractile dysfunction. In this study, we investigated the role of IKKi and its related molecular mechanisms in cardiac hypertrophy. The present study demonstrated that IKKi deficiency deteriorated cardiac hypertrophy and fibrosis. The important novel findings of our study are as follows: (1) IKKi expression is increased in AB-induced hypertrophic heart tissue; (2) IKKi deficiency provokes spontaneous hypertrophy; (3) IKKi deficiency promotes pathological hypertrophy and fibrosis; (4) IKKi overexpression markedly attenuates the hypertrophy of H9c2 rat cardiomyocytes induced by Ang II in vitro; (5) IKKi deficiency exacerbates cardiac remodeling by activating AKT and NF-κB signaling; and (6)IKKi deficiency is involved in apoptosis in hypertrophic hearts subjected to pressure overload

As a member of the IKK family, IKKi (inducible IκB kinase), which is also known as IKKε, is involved in the activation of transcription factors [25]. Although IKKi is constitutively expressed in T cells, its expression is mainly regulated by NF-κB in other cell types [26]. Our data demonstrate that IKKi

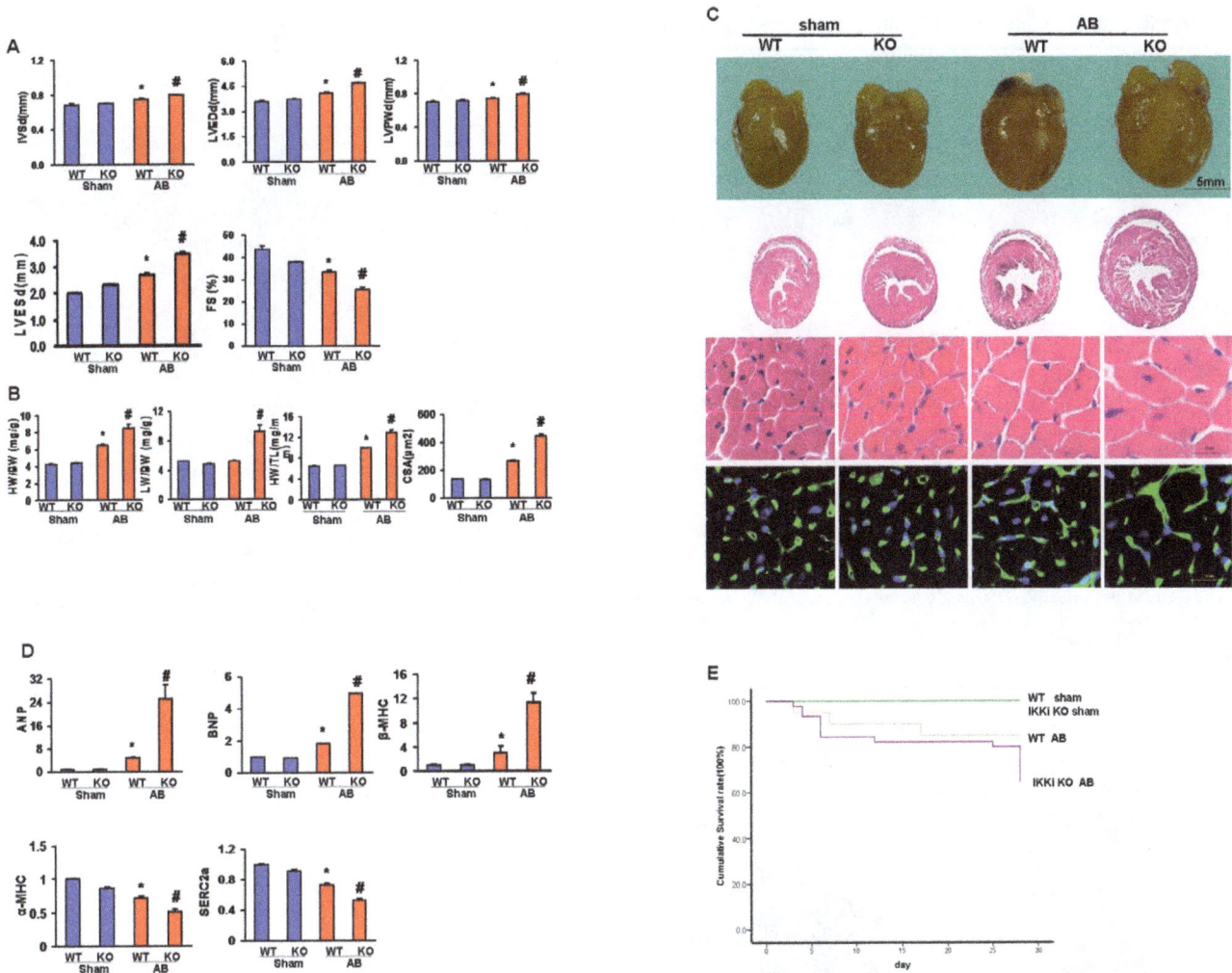

Figure 2. Effects of IKKi on cardiac hypertrophy. A, Echocardiographic results for the 4 groups of mice at 4 weeks following AB or sham surgery (n = 6). B, Statistical results of the HW/BW, LW/BW, and HW/TL ratios and myocyte cross-sectional areas of the indicated groups. C, Gross hearts, HE staining and WGA-FITC staining of the sham and AB mice at 4 weeks post-surgery. D, Expression levels of the transcripts of ANP, BNP, β-MHC, α-MHC and SERCA2α after AB were determined by RT-PCR analysis (n = 6). E. Kaplan-Meier curve depicting the survival of WT-sham, KO-sham, WT-AB, and KO-AB mice *$P < 0.05$ vs. WT/sham. # $P < 0.05$ vs. WT/AB following AB.

expression is significantly elevated in AB-induced hypertrophic heart tissues, which suggests that it is involved in promoting the development of cardiac hypertrophy and remodeling. This hypothesis is consistent with some studies involving other IKK family members, such as IKKβ [18].

The molecular mechanism by which IKKi affects cardiac remodeling remains unclear. To address this issue, we analyzed the activation of hypertrophic signaling pathways in AB mice. Pivotal signaling pathways that functioned in the pathogenesis of cardiac hypertrophy, including the mitogen-activated protein kinases (MAPKs) and AKT pathways, were assessed [10,27,29,30,31]. The downstream targets of AKT include GSK3β, mTOR,FOXO transcription factors and NFκB, all of which are involved in cardiac hypertrophy [10,27,29,30,31,32,33]. In this study,AKT phosphorylation was significantly enhanced in response to hypertrophic stimuli in the KO mice compared with WT mice. Consistent with the observed increase in AKT activity, hypertrophic stimuli caused increased levels of phosphorylated the GSK3β^{Ser9} and FOXO transcription factors at AKT phosphorylation sites (reducing their anti-

hypertrophic effects) and increased activation of mTOR in the IKKi-deficient mice compared with WT mice. However, IKKi did not influence the phosphorylation of ERK1/2, JNK1/2, p38, MAPK or PI3K. Therefore, our study demonstrates that the AKT and NF-κB signalling is a critical pathway by which IKKi influences cardiomyocyte growth. Furthermore, we demonstrated that IKKi overexpression markedly inhibited AKT and NF-κB signaling in cultured cardiomyocytes stimulated by Ang II.However, the mechanism by which IKKi specifically activates AKT signaling remains unknown. In accordance with our findings, TRAF-associated NFκB activator-binding kinase1 (TBK1), another IκB kinase-related kinase, which exhibits 49% identity and 65% similarity to IKKi, another member of the IKK family, has been shown to control the activation of AKT [34,35]. As a ligand for integrins, the absence of IKKi may be compensated for by TBK1,thus modulating integrin signaling or a specific integrin complex in a manner that specifically regulates AKT. Further experiments are needed to determine the molecular signaling mechanism by which IKKi regulates AKT. It is worth noting that the AKT pathway is a non-specific

Table 2. Anatomic and hemodynamic parameters in IKKi KO and WT mice at 4 weeks after surgery.

Parameter	Sham		AB	
	WT(n = 6)	IKKi KO(n = 6)	WT(n = 6)	IKKi KO(n = 6)
BW (g)	27.50±0.52	27.19±0.32	27.89±0.34	28.02±0.40
HW/BW(mg/g)	4.29±0.07	4.43±0.04	6.49±0.08*	8.53±0.42*#
LW/BW(mg/g)	5.20±0.05	4.90±0.10	5.19±0.13	9.33±0.76*#
HW/TL(mg/cm)	6.40±0.13	6.51±0.08	9.96±0.08*	12.83±0.48*#
HR (beats/min)	483±9	462±10	477±8	462±18
ESP (mmHg)	105.74±1.58	117.15±4.04	150.85±2.16*	149.25±2.30*
EDP (mmHg)	9.84±0.19	10.24±1.28	17.75±2.14*	24.31±1.84*#
ESV (ml)	10.09±0.44	10.51±1.46	23.58±1.93*	37.23±3.46*#
EDV (ml)	26.82±0.78	24.85±1.83	34.44±1.32*	48.37±3.29*#
dP/dt max (mmHg/s)	10585.47±540.98	10663.83±781.97	8171.17±326.82*	6694.33±306.38*#
dP/dt min (mmHg/s)	−9177.34±269.63	−8967.33±357.21	−7658.17±346.37*	−6578.17±416.63*#
EF(%)	65.60±1.35	64.02±2.66	39.18±2.40*	25.83±3.11*#

BW,body weight;HW/BW,heart weight/body weight;LW/BW,lung weight/body weight; HW/TL,heart weight/tibial length; HR,heart rate; ESP, end-systolic pressure; EDP, end-diastolic pressure; ESV, endsystolic volume; EDV, end-diastolic volume; EF, ejection fraction; dP/dtmax, maximal rate of pressure development; dP/dtmin, maximal rate of pressure decay.
*$P<0.05$ vs WT/sham;
#$P<0.05$ vs WT/AB after AB.

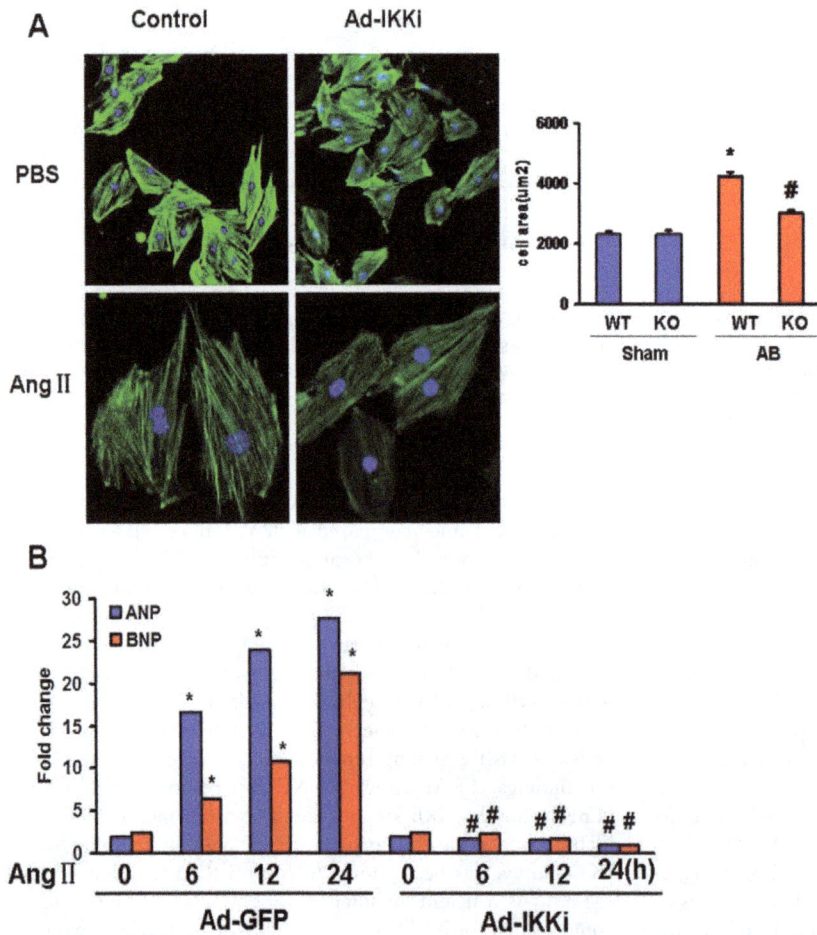

Figure 3. IKKi overexpression attenuates myocyte hypertrophy in vitro. A, The inhibitory effect of IKKi overexpression on the enlargement of myocyte induced by Ang II (1 μM for 48 h). B, RT-PCR analysis of the mRNA levels of ANP and BNP induced by Ang II at the time points indicated. * $P<0.05$ vs WT at the 0 time point. # $P<0.05$ vs WT at the same time point.

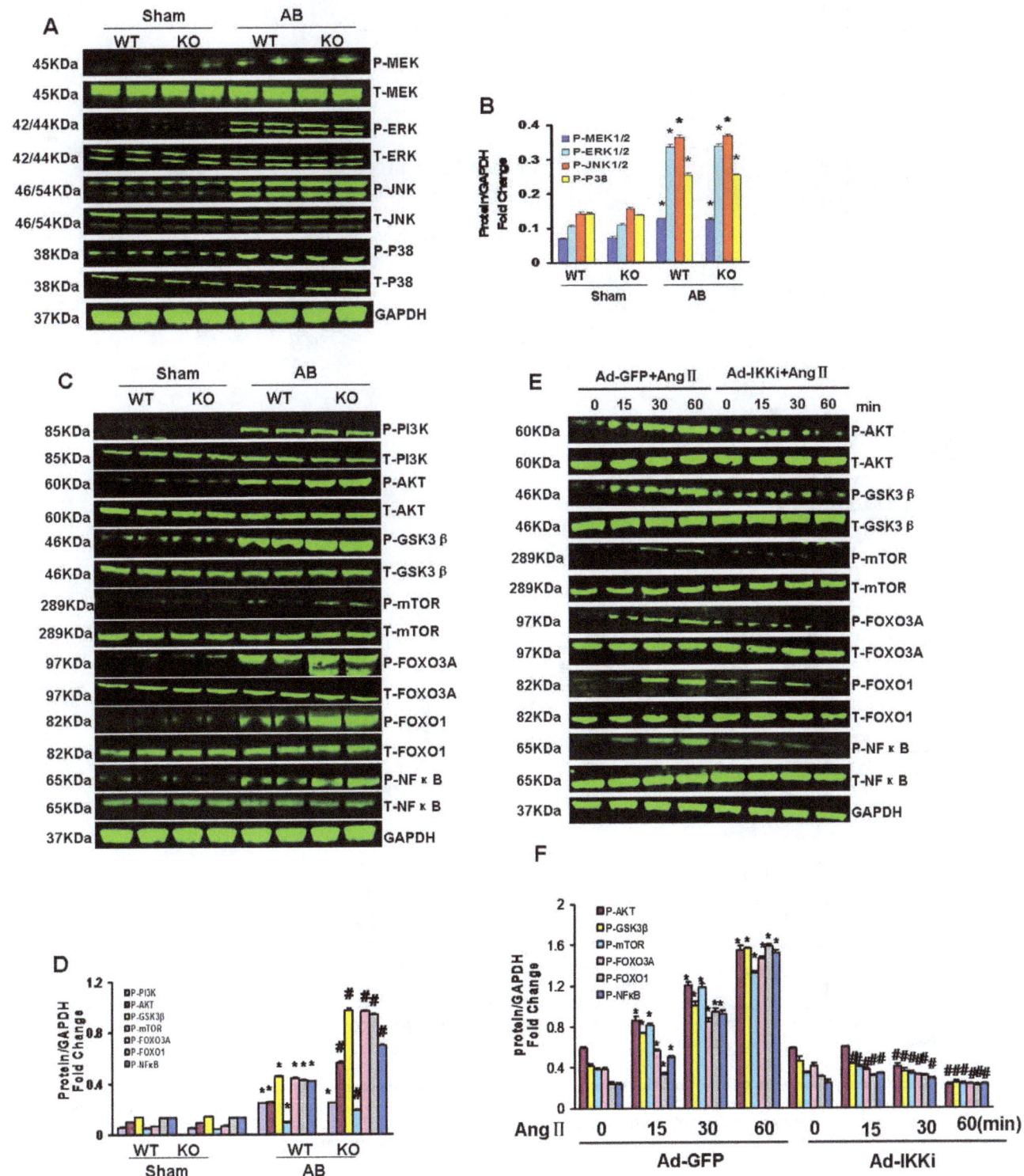

Figure 4. Effect of IKKi on the MAPK and AKT/GSK3β/mTOR/FOXO/NFκB signaling pathways. (A–D) Levels of total and phosphorylated MEK1/2, ERK1/2, JNK, P38PI3K, AKT, GSK3β, mTOR, FOXO and NFκB in the heart tissues of mice in the indicated groups (n = 6). A and C Representative blots. B and D Quantitative results. (E–F) Representative blots for total and phosphorylated AKT, GSK3β, mTOR, FOXO3A, FOXO1 and NFκB after treatment with Ang II for the indicated times in H9c2 rat cardiomyocytes infected with Ad-GFP or Ad-IKKi. E Representative blots. F, Quantitative results. *$P < 0.05$ vs. WT/sham; # $P < 0.05$ vs. WT/AB after AB.

pathways, and a change in the AKT pathway is likely to be an indicator rather than a true determinant and a pharmacological target.

Fibrosis is an important contributor to the development of cardiac dysfunction in diverse pathological conditions. Fibrosis involves the progressive over-accumulation of extracellular matrix

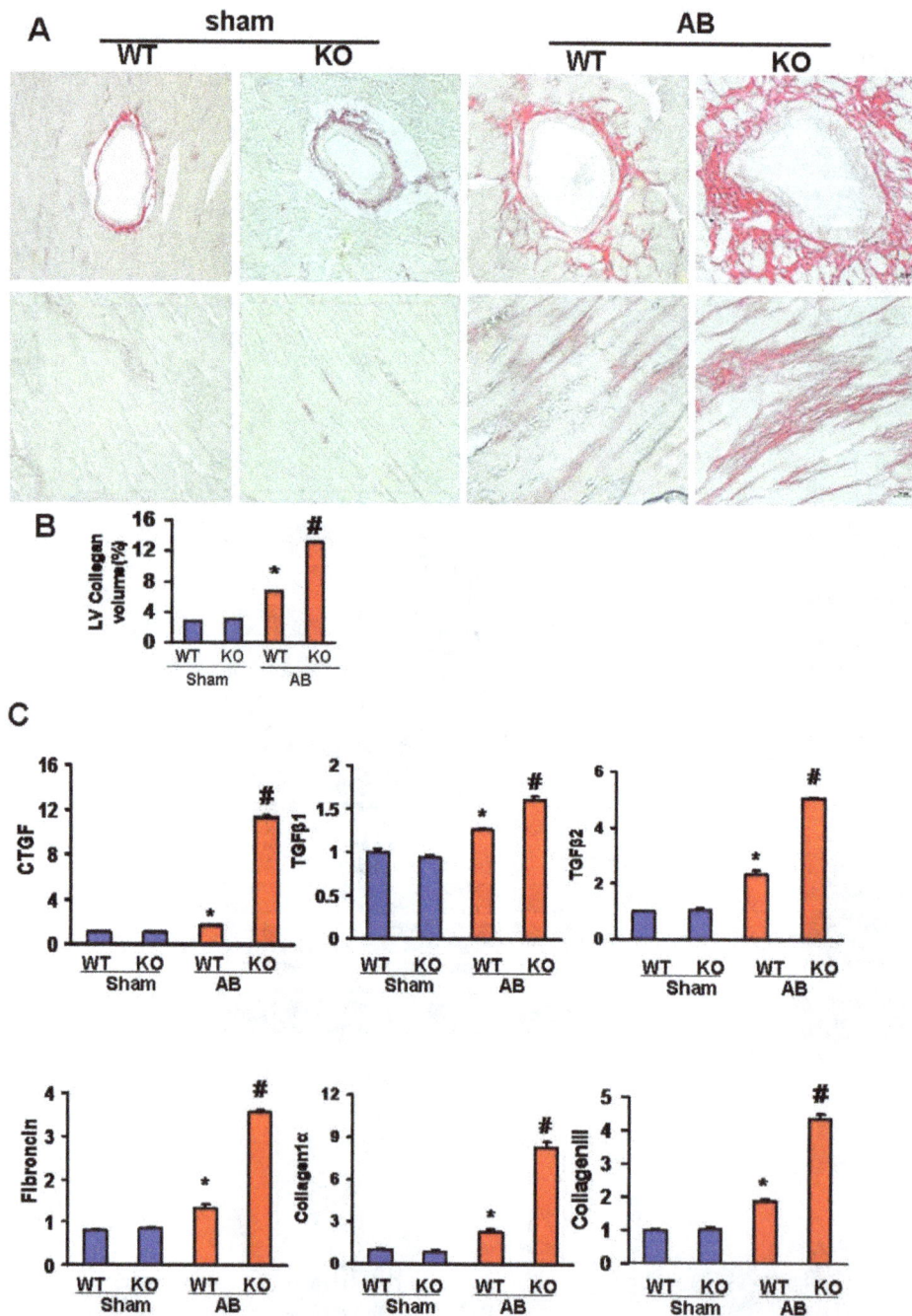

Figure 5. IKKi deficiency exacerbates the fibrotic response that is induced by pressure overload. A, Histological sections of the left ventricle were stained with picrosirius red in the indicated groups. B, The fibrotic areas from the histological sections were quantified using an image-analyzing system. C, The mRNA expression levels of collagen I, collagen III, fibronectin, TGF-β1, TGF-β2, and CTGF in the myocardium were obtained from the indicated groups using RT-PCR analysis. *$P<0.05$ vs. WT/sham; # $P<0.05$ vs. WT/AB after AB.

(ECM) (which surrounds and interconnects cells, is present in the myocardial wall and provides a scaffold for both myocytes and non-myocytes) components in cardiac muscle [36]. The major ECM proteins (type I and III collagens) are increasingly synthesized in the heart in response to pressure overload stimuli [36]. Moreover, the increased expression of TGF-β1 parallels the perivascular and myocardial interstitial fibrotic changes [37]. TGF-β and CTGF also modulate the proliferation of fibroblasts [30]. The present study has shown for the first time that IKKi deficiency leads to increased collagen deposition after AB and

increased mRNA levels of CTGF, TGFβ and collagen I and III mRNA. These results suggest that IKKi deficiency promotes fibrosis and cardiac remodeling by enhancing collagen synthesis and up-regulating fibrotic mediators.

Cardiac myocyte apoptosis is also a critical factor during the transition from compensatory cardiac hypertrophy in response to pressure overload to heart failure [38]. The present study showed increased apoptosis in the pressure-overloaded hearts of the KO mice compared with the WT mice. Furthermore, our results also demonstrated a significant increase in the of Bax-to-Bcl2

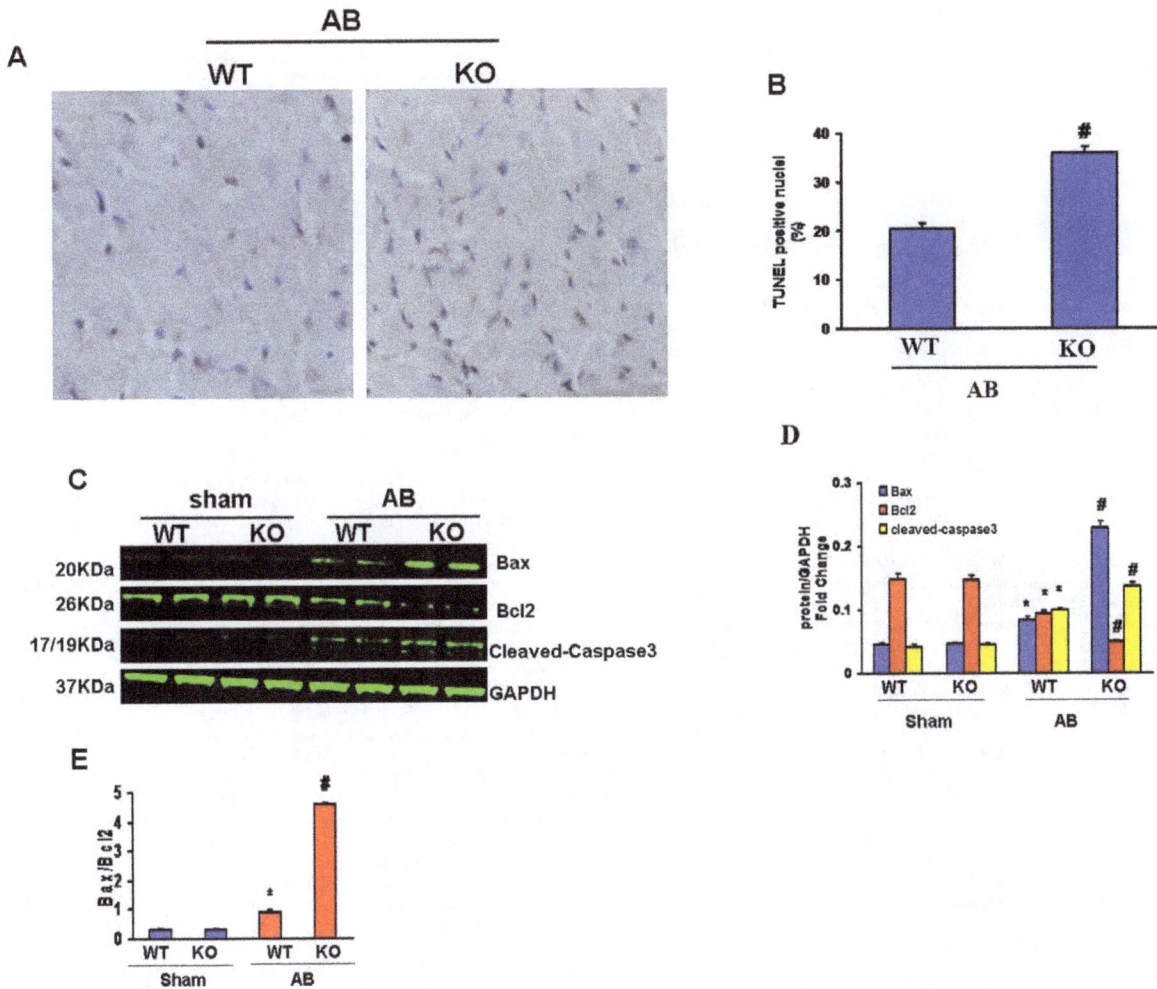

Figure 6. Effects of IKKi on cardiac apoptosis. A, TUNEL staining of AB mice at 4 weeks post-surgery. B, TUNEL-positive cells were quantified by the examination of 3000 nuclei from10 randomly selected fields per heart. # $P<0.05$ vs. WT/AB after AB.

expression ratio and the activation of caspase-3 in the hearts of the KO mice after AB. Taken together,these data indicate that IKKi deficiency could influence apoptosis by affecting apoptosis-regulating proteins.

The roles of IKKi in the cardiac hypertrophic response to pressure overload have not been described previously. We are one step closer to elucidating the IKKi-related mechanisms that are associated with the development of cardiac hypertrophy,fibrosis and apoptosis. IKKi protects against hypertrophy via negative feedback of the AKT and NF-κB signaling pathway and concurrently regulates collagen deposition and fibrotic mediators.

Taken together, our findings provide a rationale for further studies on the potential therapeutic benefits of IKKi in cardiovascular disease.

Author Contributions

Conceived and designed the experiments: QT JD DS ZB HL. Performed the experiments: JD DS ZB HZ HG JZ RZ. Analyzed the data: JD WD YY FL QW LG ZM. Contributed reagents/materials/analysis tools: QT HL. Wrote the paper: JD DS ZB HL QT.

References

1. Tamargo J, Lopez-Sendon J (2011) Novel therapeutic targets for the treatment of heart failure. Nat Rev Drug Discov 10: 536–555.
2. Dickstein K, Cohen-Solal A, Filippatos G, McMurray JJ, Ponikowski P, et al. (2008) ESC guidelines for the diagnosis and treatment of acute and chronic heart failure 2008: the Task Force for the diagnosis and treatment of acute and chronic heart failure 2008 of the European Society of Cardiology. Developed in collaboration with the Heart Failure Association of the ESC (HFA) and endorsed by the European Society of Intensive Care Medicine (ESICM). Eur J Heart Fail 10: 933–989.
3. Hunt SA, Abraham WT, Chin MH, Feldman AM, Francis GS, et al. (2009) 2009 Focused update incorporated into the ACC/AHA 2005 Guidelines for the Diagnosis and Management of Heart Failure in Adults A Report of the American College of Cardiology Foundation/American Heart Association Task Force on Practice Guidelines Developed in Collaboration With the International Society for Heart and Lung Transplantation. J Am Coll Cardiol 53: e1–e90.
4. Lloyd-Jones D, Adams RJ, Brown TM, Carnethon M, Dai S, et al. (2010) Executive summary: heart disease and stroke statistics–2010 update: a report from the American Heart Association. Circulation 121: 948–954.
5. Pazos-Lopez P, Peteiro-Vazquez J, Garcia-Campos A, Garcia-Bueno L, de Torres JP, et al. (2011) The causes, consequences, and treatment of left or right heart failure. Vasc Health Risk Manag 7: 237–254.
6. Iemitsu M, Miyauchi T, Maeda S, Sakai S, Kobayashi T, et al. (2001) Physiological and pathological cardiac hypertrophy induce different molecular phenotypes in the rat. Am J Physiol Regul Integr Comp Physiol 281: R2029–R2036.

7. De Boer RA, Pinto YM, Van Veldhuisen DJ (2003) The imbalance between oxygen demand and supply as a potential mechanism in the pathophysiology of heart failure: the role of microvascular growth and abnormalities. Microcirculation 10: 113–126.

8. Olson EN (2004) A decade of discoveries in cardiac biology. Nat Med 10: 467–474.

9. Thum T, Galuppo P, Wolf C, Fiedler J, Kneitz S, et al. (2007) MicroRNAs in the human heart: a clue to fetal gene reprogramming in heart failure. Circulation 116: 258–267.

10. Heineke J, Molkentin JD (2006) Regulation of cardiac hypertrophy by intracellular signalling pathways. Nat Rev Mol Cell Biol 7: 589–600.

11. Hayden MS, Ghosh S (2008) Shared principles in NF-kappaB signaling. Cell 132: 344–362.

12. Shih VF, Tsui R, Caldwell A, Hoffmann A (2011) A single NFkappaB system for both canonical and non-canonical signaling. Cell Res 21: 86–102.

13. Zelarayan L, Renger A, Noack C, Zafiriou MP, Gehrke C, et al. (2009) NF-kappaB activation is required for adaptive cardiac hypertrophy. Cardiovasc Res 84: 416–424.

14. Hirotani S, Otsu K, Nishida K, Higuchi Y, Morita T, et al. (2002) Involvement of nuclear factor-kappaB and apoptosis signal-regulating kinase 1 in G-protein-coupled receptor agonist-induced cardiomyocyte hypertrophy. Circulation 105: 509–515.

15. Higuchi Y, Otsu K, Nishida K, Hirotani S, Nakayama H, et al. (2002) Involvement of reactive oxygen species-mediated NF-kappa B activation in TNF-alpha-induced cardiomyocyte hypertrophy. J Mol Cell Cardiol 34: 233–240.

16. Liu Q, Chen Y, Auger-Messier M, Molkentin JD (2012) Interaction between NFkappaB and NFAT coordinates cardiac hypertrophy and pathological remodeling. Circ Res 110: 1077–1086.

17. Gaspar-Pereira S, Fullard N, Townsend PA, Banks PS, Ellis EL, et al. (2012) The NF-kappaB subunit c-Rel stimulates cardiac hypertrophy and fibrosis. Am J Pathol 180: 929–939.

18. Hikoso S, Yamaguchi O, Nakano Y, Takeda T, Omiya S, et al. (2009) The I{kappa}B kinase {beta}/nuclear factor {kappa}B signaling pathway protects the heart from hemodynamic stress mediated by the regulation of manganese superoxide dismutase expression. Circ Res 105: 70–79.

19. Wang N, Ahmed S, Haqqi TM (2005) Genomic structure and functional characterization of the promoter region of human IkappaB kinase-related kinase IKKi/IKKvarepsilon gene. Gene 353: 118–133.

20. Koop A, Lepenies I, Braum O, Davarnia P, Scherer G, et al. (2011) Novel splice variants of human IKKepsilon negatively regulate IKKepsilon-induced IRF3 and NF-kB activation. Eur J Immunol 41: 224–234.

21. Kravchenko VV, Mathison JC, Schwamborn K, Mercurio F, Ulevitch RJ (2003) IKKi/IKKepsilon plays a key role in integrating signals induced by pro-inflammatory stimuli. J Biol Chem 278: 26612–26619.

22. Shembade N, Harhaj EW (2011) IKKi: a novel regulator of Act1, IL-17 signaling and pulmonary inflammation. Cell Mol Immunol 8: 447–449.

23. Bulek K, Liu C, Swaidani S, Wang L, Page RC, et al. (2011) The inducible kinase IKKi is required for IL-17-dependent signaling associated with neutrophilia and pulmonary inflammation. Nat Immunol 12: 844–852.

24. Peant B, Forest V, Trudeau V, Latour M, Mes-Masson AM, et al. (2011) IkappaB-Kinase-epsilon (IKKepsilon/IKKi/IkappaBKepsilon) expression and localization in prostate cancer tissues. Prostate 71: 1131–1138.

25. Fitzgerald KA, McWhirter SM, Faia KL, Rowe DC, Latz E, et al. (2003) IKKepsilon and TBK1 are essential components of the IRF3 signaling pathway. Nat Immunol 4: 491–496.

26. Peters RT, Liao SM, Maniatis T (2000) IKKepsilon is part of a novel PMA-inducible IkappaB kinase complex. Mol Cell 5: 513–522.

27. Li H, He C, Feng J, Zhang Y, Tang Q, et al. (2010) Regulator of G protein signaling 5 protects against cardiac hypertrophy and fibrosis during biomechanical stress of pressure overload. Proc Natl Acad Sci U S A 107: 13818–13823.

28. Sambandam N, Steinmetz M, Chu A, Altarejos JY, Dyck JR, et al. (2004) Malonyl-CoA decarboxylase (MCD) is differentially regulated in subcellular compartments by 5′AMP-activated protein kinase (AMPK). Studies using H9c2 cells overexpressing MCD and AMPK by adenoviral gene transfer technique. Eur J Biochem 271: 2831–2840.

29. Bian ZY, Wei X, Deng S, Tang QZ, Feng J, et al. (2012) Disruption of mindin exacerbates cardiac hypertrophy and fibrosis. J Mol Med (Berl).

30. Zhou H, Shen DF, Bian ZY, Zong J, Deng W, et al. (2011) Activating transcription factor 3 deficiency promotes cardiac hypertrophy, dysfunction, and fibrosis induced by pressure overload. PLoS One 6: e26744.

31. Yan L, Wei X, Tang QZ, Feng J, Zhang Y, et al. (2011) Cardiac-specific mindin overexpression attenuates cardiac hypertrophy via AKT/GSK3beta and TGF-beta1-Smad signalling. Cardiovasc Res 92: 85–94.

32. Sun HZ, Yang TW, Zang WJ, Wu SF (2010) Dehydroepiandrosterone-induced proliferation of prostatic epithelial cell is mediated by NFKB via PI3K/AKT signaling pathway. J Endocrinol 204: 311–318.

33. Higuchi Y, Chan TO, Brown MA, Zhang J, DeGeorge BJ, et al. (2006) Cardioprotection afforded by NF-kappaB ablation is associated with activation of Akt in mice overexpressing TNF-alpha. Am J Physiol Heart Circ Physiol 290: H590–H598.

34. Chau TL, Gioia R, Gatot JS, Patrascu F, Carpentier I, et al. (2008) Are the IKKs and IKK-related kinases TBK1 and IKK-epsilon similarly activated? Trends Biochem Sci 33: 171–180.

35. Joung SM, Park ZY, Rani S, Takeuchi O, Akira S, et al. (2011) Akt contributes to activation of the TRIF-dependent signaling pathways of TLRs by interacting with TANK-binding kinase 1. J Immunol 186: 499–507.

36. Manabe I, Shindo T, Nagai R (2002) Gene expression in fibroblasts and fibrosis: involvement in cardiac hypertrophy. Circ Res 91: 1103–1113.

37. Yamazaki T, Yamashita N, Izumi Y, Nakamura Y, Shiota M, et al. (2012) The antifibrotic agent pirfenidone inhibits angiotensin II-induced cardiac hypertrophy in mice. Hypertens Res 35: 34–40.

38. Anilkumar N, Sirker A, Shah AM (2009) Redox sensitive signaling pathways in cardiac remodeling, hypertrophy and failure. Front Biosci 14: 3168–3187.

14

Pregnancy is Associated with Decreased Cardiac Proteasome Activity and Oxidative Stress in Mice

Andrea Iorga[1], Shannamar Dewey[2], Rod Partow-Navid[1], Aldrin V. Gomes[2], Mansoureh Eghbali[1]*

1 Department of Anesthesiology, Division of Molecular Medicine, David Geffen School of Medicine at University of California Los Angeles, Los Angeles, California, United States of America, **2** Department of Neurobiology, Physiology and Behavior, University of California Davis, Davis, California, United States of America

Abstract

During pregnancy, the heart develops physiological hypertrophy. Proteasomal degradation has been shown to be altered in various models of pathological cardiac hypertrophy. Since the molecular signature of pregnancy-induced heart hypertrophy differs significantly from that of pathological heart hypertrophy, we investigated whether the cardiac proteasomal proteolytic pathway is affected by pregnancy in mice. We measured the proteasome activity, expression of proteasome subunits, ubiquitination levels and reactive oxygen production in the hearts of four groups of female mice: i) non pregnant (NP) at diestrus stage, ii) late pregnant (LP), iii) one day post-partum (PP1) and iv) 7 days post-partum (PP7). The activities of the 26 S proteasome subunits $\beta 1$ (caspase-like), and $\beta 2$ (trypsin-like) were significantly decreased in LP ($\beta 1$:83.26±1.96%; $\beta 2$:74.74±1.7%, normalized to NP) whereas $\beta 5$ (chymotrypsin-like) activity was not altered by pregnancy but significantly decreased 1 day post-partum. Interestingly, all three proteolytic activities of the proteasome were restored to normal levels 7 days post-partum. The decrease in proteasome activity in LP was not due to the surge of estrogen as estrogen treatment of ovariectomized mice did not alter the 26 S proteasome activity. The transcript and protein levels of RPN2 and RPT4 (subunits of 19 S), $\beta 2$ and $\alpha 7$ (subunits of 20 S) as well as PA28α and $\beta 5$i (protein only) were not significantly different among the four groups. High resolution confocal microscopy revealed that nuclear localization of both core (20S) and RPT4 in LP is increased ~2-fold and is fully reversed in PP7. Pregnancy was also associated with decreased production of reactive oxygen species and ubiquitinated protein levels, while the de-ubiquitination activity was not altered by pregnancy or parturition. These results indicate that late pregnancy is associated with decreased ubiquitin-proteasome proteolytic activity and oxidative stress.

Editor: Yao Liang Tang, University of Cincinnati, United States of America

Funding: This work was supported by NIH grants T32GM065823 (A.I.), HL096819 (A.V.G), HL089876 and HL089876S1 (M.E). The funder had no role in study design, data collection and analysis, decision to publish, or preparation of the manuscript.

Competing Interests: The authors have declared that no competing interests exist.

* E-mail: meghbali@ucla.edu

Introduction

Cardiac hypertrophy, defined as an enlargement of the ventricles and cardiomyocytes, can be adaptive or maladaptive, and usually occurs in response to hemodynamic stress from volume or pressure overload. Sustained pressure overload leads to concentric hypertrophy, which is characterized by increased wall thickness without a concomitant chamber enlargement. However, in response to normal exercise or pregnancy, physiological or eccentric hypertrophy develops [1], which is characterized by an increase in cardiac pumping ability and muscle mass. Volume overload-induced hypertrophy is characterized by a proportional enlargement of the chamber size and the wall thickness [2] and is reversible without aberrant effects on cardiac function [3], [4], [5]. In these aspects, pregnancy- and exercise-induced hypertrophies are similar. However, pregnancy is also accompanied by acute changes in the mother's hormonal environment, and unlike exercise, the force demand placed on the heart is continuous as opposed to sporadic.

The ubiquitin-proteasome system (UPS) is the major pathway for protein degradation in the heart to remove damaged and misfolded proteins [6]. Regulation of proteasome function can occur through the association of the core 20 S proteasomal complex with different regulatory complexes such as 19 S or 11 S that affect proteasomal assembly and activity [6], [7], [8]. In general, the covalent binding of multiple ubiquitin molecules to the target protein dictates its degradation by the 26 S proteasome [9]. Following attachment of ubiquitin molecules to a target protein, the 19 S regulatory subunits recognize the polyubiquitin tags and transfer the protein substrate to the inner pore of the 20 S catalytic core where the polypeptide is degraded [10]. Proteasome dysfunction in the heart leads to accumulation of abnormal, damaged and misfolded proteins [11].

Altered ubiquitin-proteasome system regulation has been reported in different types of cardiac hypertrophy and myopathy [6], [12]. However, the precise role of the UPS in physiological heart hypertrophy during pregnancy is not yet known. To investigate the role of the UPS in the murine heart during pregnancy, we measured proteasome activity, proteasome subunit expression and subcellular distribution, ubiquitination and de-ubiquitination levels, as well as reactive oxygen production in four groups of female mouse hearts: i) non pregnant (NP) at diestrus stage, ii) late pregnant (LP), iii) one day post-partum (PP1) and iv) 7 days post-partum (PP7). We found that pregnancy is associated with decreased proteasome activity, protein ubiquitination, and oxidative stress.

Experimental Procedures

Animals and Treatment

Young adult female (3–4 months) mice (C57BL/6) in non pregnant (NP, at diestrus stage), late pregnant (LP, day 20 of pregnancy), 1 day post-partum (PP1), 7 days post-partum (PP7) as well as ovariectomized (OVX) mice were used. OVX mice were treated with a single subcutaneous 10-day continuous release 17β-estradiol (E2) pellet (0.012 mg/pellet, Innovative Research of America, Sarasota, FL), or placebo pellets (containing 5 compounds: cholesterol, lactose, cellulose, phosphates and cerates) as vehicle for E2. This study was carried out in strict accordance with the recommendations in the Guide for the Care and Use of Laboratory Animals of the National Institutes of Health. The protocol received approval from the Division of Laboratory Animal Medicine at the University of California, Los Angeles (Protocol Number: 2003-111-13).

Real Time PCR

Total RNA was isolated from hearts using Trizol (Invitrogen) and reverse transcribed with gene specific primers using the Omniscript RT kit (Qiagen). Controls were: (1) the reaction without reverse transcriptase and (2) H_2O instead of cDNA. The primer sequences used were as follows: RPN2 sense 5'-CAG CTC TCA TCA TGA TCC AAC AG-3' and anti-sense 5'-ACA GGT AGG AGT ATA AGC CAA TG-3', RPT4 sense 5'-TGA TCA TGG CTA CAA ACA GAC CA-3' and anti-sense 5'- CTC AGG TCT GCT CCA TTA AAG C -3', β2 sense 5'- AGC CAA GAA GCT AGT GAG TGA G-3'and anti-sense 5'- TAT CCA ACC ACC CAC AGC ACC -3', α7 sense 5'-AAA CAT CGA ACT TGC CGT CAT GA-3' and anti-sense 5'-GGC CCA CAG CAC CGA GGC T-3', and PA28α sense 5'-GGC CAC ACT GAG GGT CCA TC-3' and anti-sense 5'-ACA CAG GTC TTC ACG GAA CAC A-3'. GAPDH transcript levels were used as an internal control.

Western Blot

Whole heart cell lysates were prepared by homogenizing the hearts in: 50 mM Tris (pH 7.5), 1 mM EDTA, 5 mM $MgCl_2$, 150 mM NaCl, 1 mM DTT supplemented with Phosphatase and Protease Inhibitor cocktails (Roche). The samples were then centrifuged at 12,000 g for 10 min and the supernatants were collected. The protein concentrations were measured and 100 μg of protein was treated with SDS/DTT loading buffer prior to gel electrophoresis. The blots were probed with anti-RPN2, -RPT4 - α7, PA28α and −β5i (Enzo Life Sciences, 1:500) and with anti-mono- and polyubiquitinated conjugates (Enzo Life Sciences, clone FK2, 1:1000). Quantification of protein levels was achieved using the Metamorph software for protein levels of the proteasome subunits. For the quantification of ubiquitinated protein levels, 100 μg of protein was subjected to standard Western Blotting procedure and immunolabeled with anti-mono- and polyubiquitinated antibodies. The fluorescence intensity of the entire lane was assessed in each group using ImageJ software and average fluorescence intensities were normalized to NP levels.

Isolation of Cardiomyocytes

The hearts were quickly removed and perfused through the aorta with the following solutions: (i) Ca^{2+}-free Tyrode solution containing (in mM): 130 NaCl, 5.4 KCl, 1 $MgCl_2$, 0.33 NaH_2PO_4, 10 HEPES, 5.5 glucose (pH adjusted to 7.35–7.37 with NaOH) for 5 minutes, (ii) Ca^{2+}-free Tyrode solution containing 160.4 U/ml Collagenase Type II (Worthington) and 0.45 U/ml Protease Type XIV (Sigma) for ∼15 min; and (iii) Krebs solution containing (in

mM): 100 K-glutamate, 10 K-aspartate, 25 KCl, 10 KH_2PO_4, 2 $MgSO_4$, 20 taurine, 5 creatine base, 0.5 EGTA, 5 HEPES, 20 glucose (pH adjusted to 7.2 with KOH) for 5 minutes. The solutions were oxygenated with 5% CO_2 and 95% O_2 prior to use and were maintained at $37 \pm 1°C$.

Immunocytochemistry and Imaging

Freshly isolated cardiomyocytes were fixed in cold acetone for 10 min at $-20°C$. The isolated cells were incubated with 10% normal goat serum (NGS) to block the background and were then stained with anti-core and anti-RPT4 (Enzo Life Sciences, 1:200) primary antibodies in 1% NGS and 0.2% Triton X-100 in PBS at 4°C overnight. Cells were incubated with Alexa 488 goat anti-rabbit or Alexa 568 goat anti-mouse secondary antibodies. Images were acquired at 0.0575 nm per pixel with a confocal microscope (Olympus Fluoview). For dihydroethidium (DHE, Invitrogen) staining, whole hearts were excised, washed thoroughly with ice-cold PBS and frozen in O.C.T. compound. Fresh 6 μm sections were cut with a cryostat then incubated with 10 μM DHE in Krebs-HEPES buffer (containing in mM: 99 NaCl, 4.69 KCl, 25 $NaHCO_3$, 1.03 KH_2PO_4, 5.6 D-Glucose, 20 Na-HEPES, 2.5 $CaCl_2$ and 1.2 $MgSO_4$) for 1 hr and 15 min in the dark at room temperature. The sections were then washed 3 times for 1.5 hrs in the dark with Krebs-HEPES buffer, mounted with Prolong Antifade Reagent (Invitrogen) and visualized with a confocal microscope (Olympus Fluoview).

Proteasome Activity Assay

Heart cell lysates were prepared by homogenizing the hearts in: 50 mM Tris, 1 mM EDTA, 5 mM $MgCl_2$, 150 mM NaCl, 1 mM DTT, pH 7.5. The samples were then centrifuged at 12,000 g for 10 min and the supernatants were collected. Proteasome activity of heart homogenates (20 μg/sample) was measured with fluorescent substrates of Z-LLE-AMC (β1), Boc-LSTR-AMC (β2) and Suc-LLVY-AMC (β5) as previously described [13], [14]. The proteasome activity was measured in the presence and absence of proteasome inhibitors (40 μM Z-Pro-Nle-Asp-CHO for β1, 40 μM epoxomicin for β2, and 20 μM epoxomicin for β5). Assays were carried out in a total volume of 100 μl. The ATP-dependent 26 S proteasome activities were measured in the presence of 50 mM Tris, 1 mM EDTA, 150 mM NaCl, 10 mM $MgCl_2$, 0.1 mM ATP, pH 7.5. The ATP-independent 20 S proteolytic activity for β5 was carried out in 25 mM HEPES (pH 7.5), 0.5 mM EDTA, and 0.03% SDS. The buffer composition was 25 mM HEPES (pH 7.5), 0.5 mM EDTA, 0.05% Nonidet P-40, and 0.001% SDS for β1 and β5 20S activity measurements. These buffers used for 20 S proteasome activity were previously found to be optimal for proteasome activity in lysates from mouse heart tissue [13], [14]. Each assay was conducted in the absence and presence of a specific proteasome inhibitor ((40 μM Z-Pro-Nle-Asp-H for β1, 60 μM epoxomicin for β2 and 20 μM epoxomicin for β5) to determine proteasome-specific activity. Released AMC was measured using a Fluoroskan Ascent fluorometer (Thermo Electron) at an excitation wavelength of 390 nm and an emission wavelength of 460 nm.

De-ubiquitination Assay

De-ubiquitination activity was determined using 5 μg of protein in 50 mM Tris, 150 mM NaCl, 1 mM EDTA, 5 mM $MgCl_2$, 2 mM DTT, pH 7.5. All assays were carried out in a final volume of 100 μl. The reaction was initiated by adding 400nM ubiquitin-AMC (Enzo Life Sciences). Each assay was conducted in the absence and presence of a de-ubiquination inhibitor (10 mM N-ethylmaleimide (NEM)) to determine de-ubiquitination-specific activity. Released AMC was measured using a Thermo Fluoroskan Ascent fluorometer (Thermo Electron) at an excitation wavelength of 390 nm and an emission wavelength of 460 nm.

ELISA Assay

1µg of protein lysate was bound overnight at 4°C on a 96 well-ELISA plate, washed 4 times, and blocked with BSA. 100 µl of FK1 (1:1000 dilution) detection antibody (which only recognizes polyubiquitinated proteins and not monoubiquitinated or free ubiquitin) was added for 1 h, washed, and an anti-mouse HRP-conjugated secondary antibody was added for 1 hr. After washing the secondary antibody, 100 µl of Sureblue tetramethylbenzidine substrate (KPL Inc.) was added and incubated for 15 min. The reaction was stopped using 1 M HCl and absorbance was measured at 450 nm. Positive (pentaubiquitin chains, Enzo Life Sciences) and negative controls (BSA) were used to validate the assay.

Statistics

One-way ANOVA using SPSS SigmaStat 3.0 was used for statistical analysis. P values <0.05 were considered significant. Values are mean $\pm$ SEM.

Results

Proteasome Activity of 26S is Decreased in LP

During pregnancy, the heart develops physiological hypertrophy as a result of the natural volume overload (Fig. 1). However, the ratio of the heart weight to body weight decreases in LP due to a significant increase in body weight at the end of pregnancy as we reported previously [15]. Interestingly, the heart weight is reversed partially one day post partum (PP1) and fully one week post partum (PP7).

To examine whether the proteasome function is altered in the heart in late pregnancy, we measured the proteasome activity of total 26 S ATP-dependent as well as the 20 S ATP-independent proteasome. Regarding 26 S, the relative caspase-like catalytic β1 subunit activity was decreased from 100±6.82% in NP to 83.26±1.96% in late pregnancy, and was restored fully even one day post-partum (Fig. 2). The trypsin-like β2 subunit activity was also decreased in late pregnancy from 100±13.72% in NP to 74.74±1.7% in LP, and was only fully restored in PP7 (111.56±8.7%). Interestingly, the chymotrypsin-like β5 activity of the proteasome was significantly decreased 1 day post-partum (from 100±4.7% in NP to 69.62±4.5% in PP1). All three proteolytic activities of the 26 S proteasome were fully restored to normal levels 7 days after parturition (Fig. 2). Unlike 26 S, the proteasome activity of all three subunits of 20 S was not altered in LP (Fig. 2). However, the activity of β1 and β2 subunits was significantly lower 7 days after parturition (from 100±13.72% in NP to 64.69±3.89% in PP7 and from 100±13.35% in NP to 55.41±4.63% in PP7, respectively (Fig. 2).

Proteasome Activity is not Regulated by Estrogen Therapy

The levels of estrogen increases steadily during pregnancy and reach their maximum levels at the end of pregnancy. To elucidate whether decreased proteasome activity at the end of pregnancy was a result of the surge of estrogen, ovariectomized (OVX) mice were treated with E2 or placebo using continuous release pellets for 10 days. The 26 S ATP-dependent proteasome activity was not affected by estrogen treatment, as the activities of the three subunits were not significantly different between E2 and placebo groups (Fig. 3). Therefore, the reduced proteasome activity in late

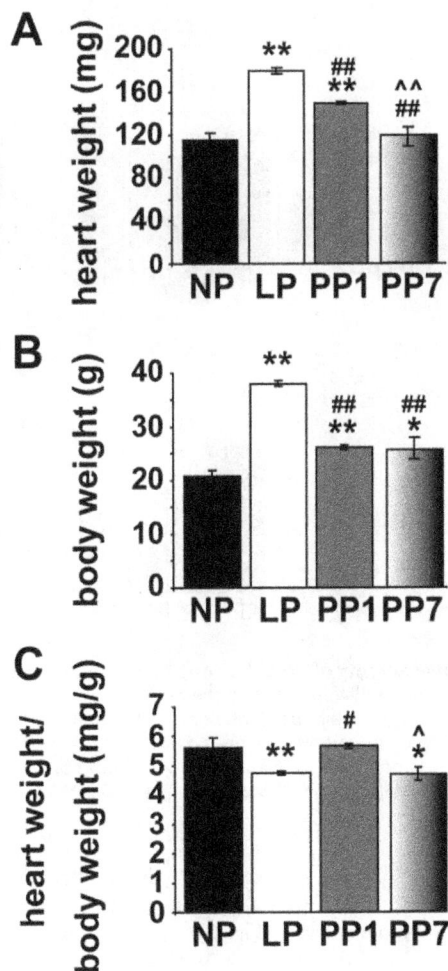

Figure 1. The increased in heart weight of LP mice is reversed post-partum. Heart weights (HW, A), body weights (BW, B) and HW/BW (C) in non-pregnant (NP, black bars, n = 8), late pregnant (LP, white bars, n = 11), one day post-partum (PP1, grey bars, n = 6) and seven days post-partum (PP7, shaded bars, n = 5) mice. Values are mean ± SEM, *p<0.05 and **p<0.001 vs. NP, #p<0.05 and ##p<0.001 vs. LP, ^p<0.05 and ^^p<0.001 vs. PP1.

pregnancy could not be explained by the rise of estrogen levels at the end of pregnancy.

The Transcript and Protein Levels of Proteasome Subunits are not Modified by Pregnancy

To elucidate whether the observed decrease in the proteasome proteolytic activity of 26 S in LP is due to decreased gene expression, we have performed Real-Time qPCR to quantify the transcript levels of the subunits of 19 S and 20 S. Because the 20 S proteasome can also associate with an 11S regulator (PA28) that can modulate proteolytic activity of the 26 S complex, we also examined the transcript levels of the PA28α subunit of the 11S/PA28 regulator. There were no significant differences in the transcript levels of these subunits neither with pregnancy nor up to one week after delivery (in PP1 and PP7, Fig. 4). Western Blot analysis also revealed no significant differences in the expression levels of RPN2 and RPT4 (subunits of 19 S, Fig. 5A–D), in α7 (a subunit of 20S, Fig. 5E–F), in PA28α (Fig. 5G–H) nor in β5i (Fig. 5I–J) with pregnancy or after partum in the four groups mentioned above. For β5i, the two bands labeled with 26kDa and

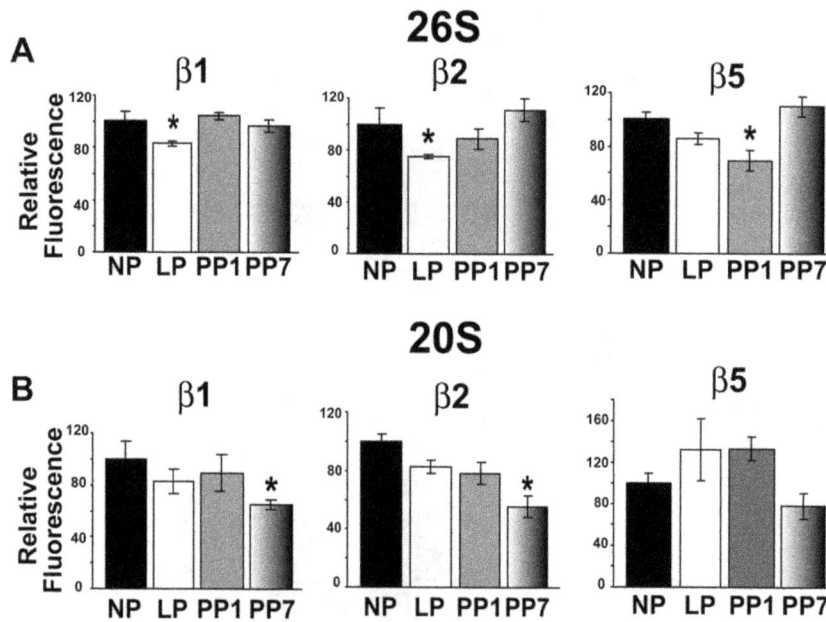

Figure 2. Proteasome activity of 26 S, but not 20 S is reduced in late pregnancy. Activity of different proteasomal beta subunits of the 26 S (A) and 20 S (B) was measured after initiating the reaction with: Z-LLE-AMC (β1), Boc-LSTR-AMC (β2) and Suc-LLVY-AMC (β5) for non pregnant (NP, black bars), late pregnant (LP, white bars), one day post-partum (PP1, grey bars) and seven days post-partum (PP7, shaded bars). The fluorescence values in arbitrary units are represented as mean ± SEM *p<0.05 vs. NP (n = 4 mice per group) and are normalized to NP levels. The raw proteasome activity values for the NP group are as follows (in nmol/min/mg protein): for the 26 S ATP-dependent activities, β1 was 0.11±0.01, β2 was 0.04±0.01 and β5 was 0.16±0.01, while for the 20 S activity, β1 was 0.21±0.03, β2 was 0.15±0.02 and β5 was 0.12±0.01.

30kDa, correspond to β5i and β5i containing its pro-peptide, respectively (Fig. 5I). Both bands were taken into consideration in the quantification of protein levels (Fig. 5J). Quantification of either band independent of the other also showed no difference between groups (data not shown).

Pregnancy is Associated with Increased Nuclear Labeling of 20S core and 19S RPT4 in Cardiomyocytes

To examine whether there are any changes in the subcellular distribution of proteasomal subunits in cardiomyocytes in LP, we have performed high resolution confocal microscopy. Fig. 6A shows typical examples of high resolution confocal images of cardiomyocytes co-labeled with anti-core (an antibody which

recognizes six 20S subunits: α5/7, β1, β5, β5i, and β7) and anti-RPT4 (a subunit of 19S) antibodies. In NP, the vast majority of the stained proteins resided in the t-tubules and the nuclear labeling was very weak (Fig. 6A). In late pregnancy however, there is increased nuclear localization of both core and RPT4, which was reversed one week after parturition. In fact, quantification of the nuclear labeling revealed approximately a 2-fold upregulation of nuclear labeling with pregnancy (from 1±0.04 to 1.97±0.20 for core and from 1±0.04 to 1.73±0.16 for RPT4). The increased nuclear labeling of both proteins was sustained one day post partum (1.95±0.17 for core and 1.73±0.06 for RPT4) and was only reversed back to NP levels seven days after delivery (to 0.88±0.06 for core and 1.15±0.07 for RPT4, Fig. 6B).

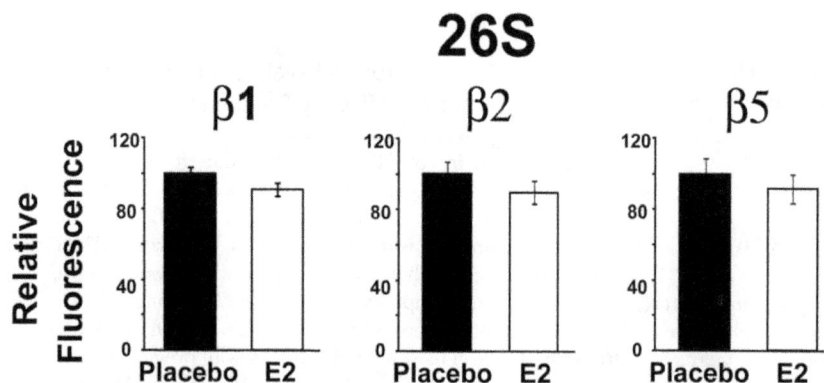

Figure 3. Proteasome activity of the 26S is unaffected by estrogen treatment. Activity of the different proteasomal beta subunits of the 26 S were measured after initiating the reaction with: Z-LLE-AMC (β1), Boc-LSTR-AMC (β2) and Suc-LLVY-AMC (β5) in ovariectomized female mice treated with placebo (Placebo, black bars) or with 17 β-estradiol for 10 days (E2, white bars). The fluorescence values in arbitrary units are normalized to Placebo levels and represented as mean ± SEM (n = 4 mice per group).

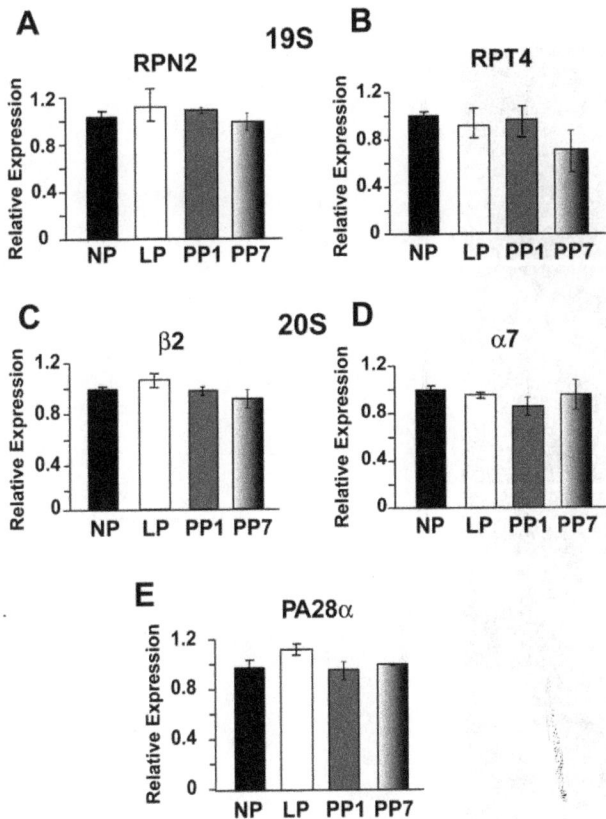

Figure 4. Transcript levels of proteasome 19S and 20S subunits, as well as the regulatory subunit PA28α, are not modified in late pregnancy. Relative transcript expression of the cardiac proteasome measured by Real-Time qPCR in non pregnant (NP, black bars), in late pregnancy (LP, white bars), 1 day post-partum (PP1, grey bars) and 7 days post-partum (PP7, shaded bars) for RPN2 and RPT4, which are subunits of 19 S (A–B), β2 and α7, which are subunits of 20 S (C–D) and the proteasome regulatory subunit PA28α (E). GAPDH was used as the internal reference gene (data not shown). Values are mean ± SEM as normalized to NP (n = 3–5 per group).

Figure 5. Protein levels of RPT4, RPN2, α7, PA28α and β5i are unaffected by pregnancy. Immunoblotting of whole heart lysates (100 μg) from non pregnant (NP, black bars), late pregnant (LP, white bars), 1 day post-partum (PP1, grey bars) and 7 days post-partum (PP7, shaded bars) with anti-RPN2 (A–B), -RPT4 (C–D), -α7 (E–F), -PA28α (G–H) and -β5i (I–J) antibodies. In (I), the upper 30 kDa band is the β5i containing the pro-peptide. The bar graphs represent the quantification of fluorescent signal intensity normalized to Vinculin. For β5i both bands were taken into consideration in the quantification of protein levels. Vinculin was used as the loading control (n = 4 per group). Values are mean ± SEM in arbitrary units.

Pregnancy is Associated with Decreased Production of Reactive Oxygen Species

Since the nuclear proteasome selectively degrades oxidatively-damaged histones in the nuclei of mammalian cells [16], we performed a qualitative dihydroethidium (DHE) staining of cardiac cross-sections to assess the levels of reactive oxygen species production. We have found that late pregnancy is associated with decreased levels of reactive oxygen species compared to NP, and these levels remain low up to one week after parturition (Fig. 7), as the average intensity of DHE staining normalized to NP levels is reduced about 5-fold and partially recovers only seven days post-partum (0.198±0.010 in LP, 0.213±0004 in PP1, and 0.405±0.030 in PP7, normalized to NP).

Pregnancy is Associated with Decreased Levels of Ubiquitinated Proteins

To further elucidate the underlying mechanism for the observed decrease of 26S proteasome activity in late pregnancy, we quantified polyubiquitinated proteins in the heart using two different methods. Western Blot analysis against mono- and polyubiquitinated proteins revealed that ubiquitinated protein levels are significantly decreased in late pregnancy from 1±0.05 in

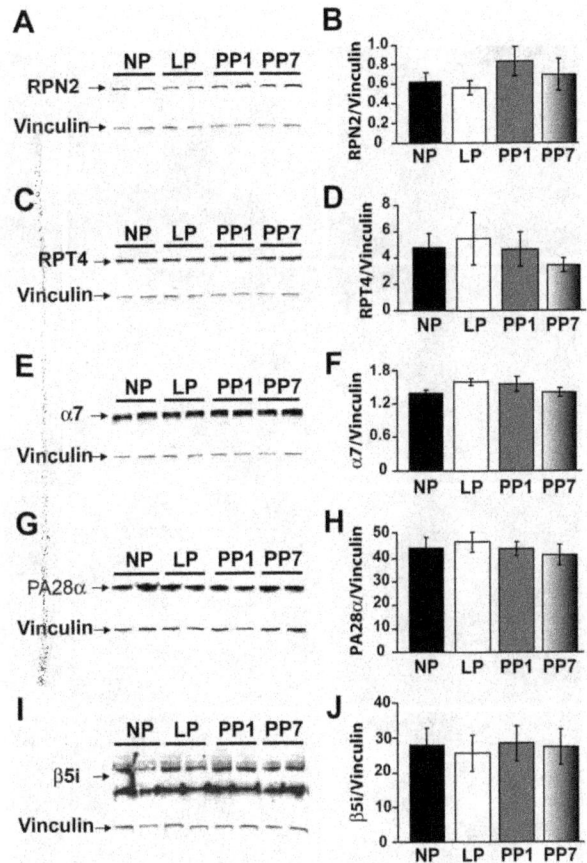

NP to 0.60±0.06 in LP, and they remain low 7 days post-partum (0.65±0.04, in arbitrary units normalized to NP, Fig. 8A–C). Reduced polyubiquitinated protein levels in LP were also confirmed by ELISA: the relative amount was significantly downregulated from 100±10.41% in NP to 66.68±3.69% in LP (Fig. 8D). In order to examine whether the observed decrease in the levels of ubiquitinated proteins is not due to an increase in de-ubiquitination activity, we have also performed a de-ubiquitination assay and found that there are no significant changes in this system with pregnancy and parturition (Fig. 8E).

Discussion

Characterization of cardiac physiological hypertrophy during pregnancy [15] led us to speculate that the late pregnant heart is "a better functioning heart," as contractile efficiency and capacity is enhanced in response to increased force and stretch demand [17]. Here we show for the first time that the activity of the total 26S ATP-dependent proteasome, polyubiquitinated protein levels as well as the production of reactive oxygen species are reduced at the end of pregnancy, all of which may support our previous

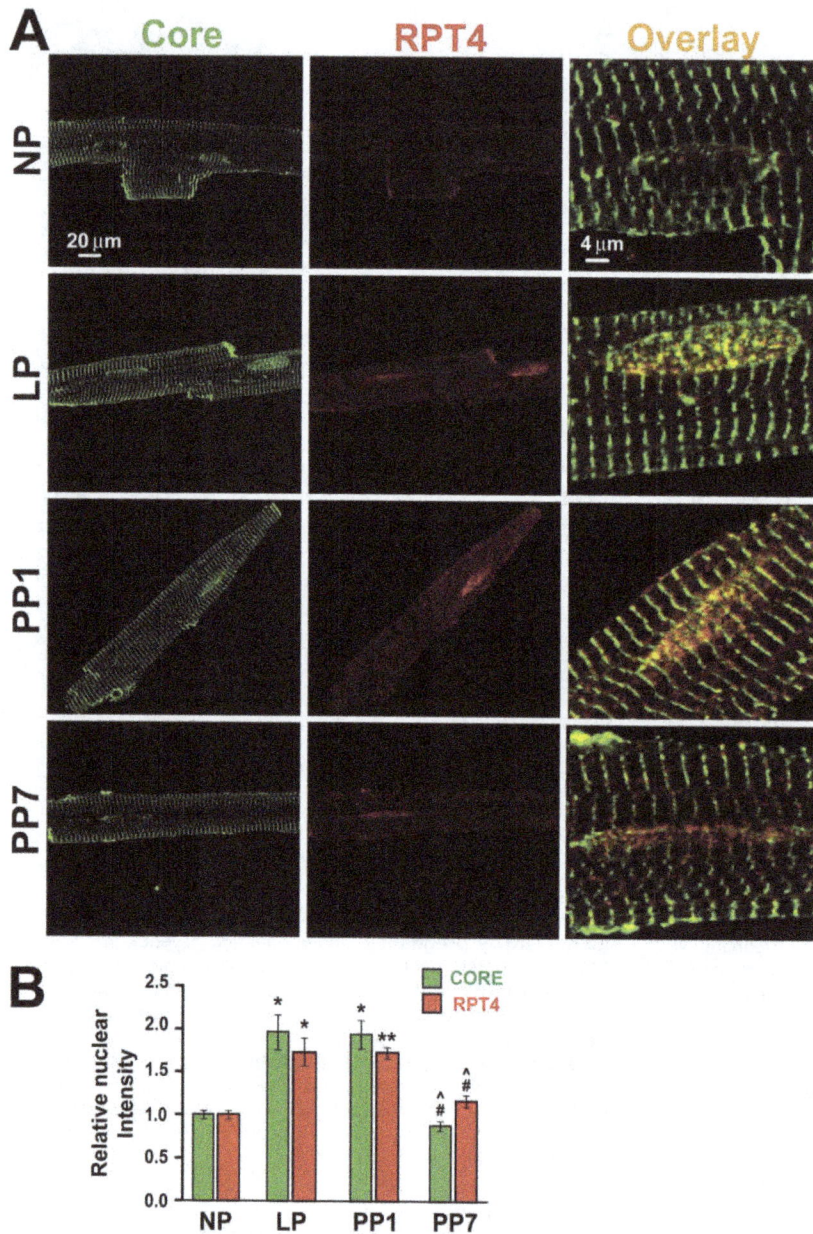

Figure 6. Increased nuclear labeling of core Subunits and RPT4 in late pregnancy was reversed one week postpartum. A. Representative single confocal sections of cardiomyocytes dissociated from non pregnant (NP), late pregnant (LP), one day post-partum (PP1) and seven days post-partum (PP7) are co-immunostained with anti-core (green) and -RPT4 (red) antibodies. The nuclear overlay of core and RPT4 are also shown at higher resolution. These results are representative of the labeling pattern observed in myocytes from 3 different animals in each group. B. Quantification of nuclear fluorescence labeling in the four groups mentioned above for core (green bars) and RPT4 (red bars) from at least 20–25 cells per group (n = 3 mice/group). Only the nucleus in the confocal plane of focus was taken into account. **denotes $p < 0.001$ *vs.* NP, #$p < 0.05$ *vs.* LP and ^$p < 0.05$ *vs.* PP1.

suggestion that a late pregnant heart is a better functioning heart. We also found that the activity of the 26S ATP-dependent proteasome was decreased in late pregnant hearts.

Proteasome Activity and Cardiac Hypertrophy

The heart is the only organ in the body that is constantly bearing a heavy workload and a high metabolic rate. As such, it is essential that cardiac cells maintain a very efficient and tightly controlled system for removal of misfolded or damaged proteins [18]. During cardiac hypertrophy, the increased protein synthesis in cardiomyocytes could potentially result in an increase of misfolded or aberrant proteins. An increase in 26S proteasomal degradation could result in the clearance of these aberrantly folded proteins. Alternatively, an increase in protein degradation by the proteasome could lead to tissue atrophy. Although decreased proteasome activities have been shown during the progression of cardiac dysfunction [19], many studies report increased proteasome activity in compensated heart hypertrophy induced by transaortic constriction (TAC) both in mouse and canine models [20], [21], while the proteasome inhibitor epoxomicin prevented the development of pre-existing hypertrophy and the further reduction in the ejection fraction [6], [19]. Both trypsin-like activity (β2) and

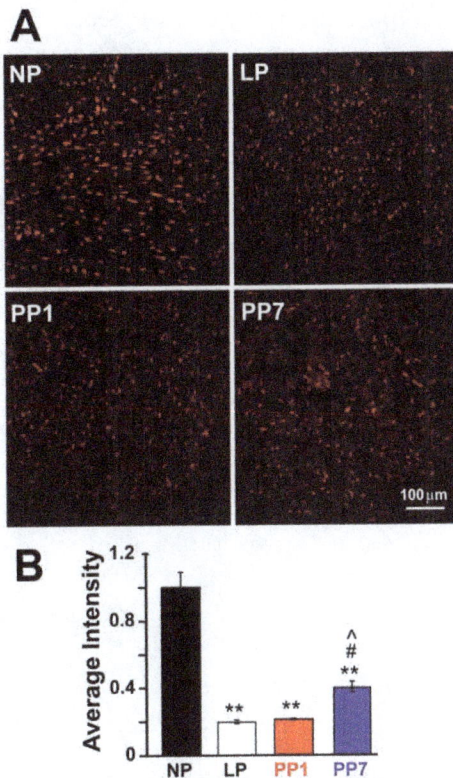

Figure 7. Superoxide production is decreased with pregnancy and remains low seven days after parturition. A. Representative dihydroethidium (DHE) staining of transverse heart sections in non pregnant (NP), late pregnant (LP), 1 day post-partum (PP1) and 7 days post-partum (PP7). Red staining indicates the presence of reactive oxygen species (ROS). B. Quantification of the DHE staining for detection of ROS in non pregnant (NP, black bar), late pregnant (LP, white bar), 1 day post-partum (PP1, grey bar) and 7 days post-partum (PP7, shaded bar). Values are mean ± SEM as normalized to NP (n = 3 per group), and **denotes $p < 0.001$ vs. NP, #$p < 0.05$ vs. LP and ^$p < 0.05$ vs. PP1.

chymotrypsin-like activities ($\beta 5$) were significantly increased in the subendocarium, which is subjected to the highest level of wall stress in a canine model of left-ventricular hypertrophy [20], [21]. In fact, increased proteasome activity has been suggested to be required for the development of compensated heart hypertrophy [20], [21]. Although during pregnancy the heart also develops compensated hypertrophy, the proteasome activity in this unique model of hypertrophy is not increased. In fact, the activity of the $\beta 1$ and $\beta 2$ subunits of the 26S proteasome is decreased in the LP heart. The decrease in 26S proteasome activity was not reflected by any changes in the inducible $\beta 5i$ subunit or in the PA28α subunit of the 11S/PA28 regulator. In contrast, in isoproterenol-induced cardiac hypertrophy, Drews et al. showed enhanced 26S proteasome activities, with a concomitant significant decrease in the caspase-like and trypsin-like 20S activities that may be due to a switch in proteasome subpopulations, altered expression and incorporation of the inducible β subunits [12].

Expression of Proteasome Subunits and Cardiac Hypertrophy

Some controversy regarding the expression of proteasome subunits at the mRNA and protein levels exists. Most reports show an increase in 26S proteasome expression in different models of

cardiomyopathy and hypertrophy. Otsuka et al. report an increase in 26S proteasome expression in patients suffering from dilated cardiomyopathy, possibly due to a compensatory mechanism in response to impaired proteasome activity [22]. Increased expression of the representative subunits of 19S (RPN2 and RPT11) and 20S ($\alpha 6$) have also been reported in the subendocarium of the canine model of left ventricular hypertrophy [20]. However, transcript levels of representative 20S subunits have been shown to be decreased in failing hearts [19], suggesting possible post-translational modifications. Here we did not observe any significant differences in the transcript or protein levels of $\alpha 7$ (a subunit of 20S), RPN2 and RPT4 (subunits of 19S) the regulatory subunit PA28α and the inducible subunit $\beta 5i$ (protein levels only) with pregnancy (Figs. 4, 5), further suggesting that pregnancy-induced hypertrophy has a molecular signature unlike all other models of hypertrophy that have previously been studied.

Pregnancy is Associated with Decreased Levels of Ubiquitinated Proteins

Proteins that are targeted for degradation by the proteasome must first initially be covalently tagged with ubiquitin molecules by the E2–E3 ligase complex [9]. These ubiquitin molecules are then recognized by the 19S regulatory particle of the 26S proteasome complex in an ATP-dependent binding [23]. Therefore, protein ubiquitination is one of the key mechanisms for targeting a peptide to be degraded by the proteasome's proteolytic pathway, and ubiquitnation levels are also important for the proteasome activity. Here, we have found that pregnancy is associated with decreased ubiquitinated protein levels (Fig. 8). Two independent methods (Western Blot and ELISA) were utilized to show that the levels of ubiquitination in the heart were decreased in late pregnancy relative to non pregnant mice. However, unlike pregnancy, immunocytochemical experiments previously revealed markedly increased expression levels of ubiquitin in patients with decompensated cardiomyopathy [22]. Increased ubiquitnation levels have also been reported in experimental models of pressure overload-induced left ventricular hypertrophy in murine and canine hearts [18], [19], [20]. Lower proteasome activity may conserve energy as less ATP would be needed for protein unfolding by the 19S complex and this may be beneficial to the heart. Changes in protein ubiquitination can occur from changes in proteasome activity, changes in de-ubiquitination activity or changes in the ubiquitin-conjugating activity system (E1, E2 and E3 enzymes). Lower proteasome activities are unlikely to cause lower polyubiquitination levels since the proteasome readily degrades polyubiquitinated proteins. Investigation of the de-ubiquitination activity showed that the total de-ubiquitination activity was not significantly affected by pregnancy. These results suggest that the ubiquitin-conjugating activity system may be lowered by pregnancy. It is possible that the proteasome has potentially less substrates (less polyubiquitinated proteins) to degrade post-translational modifications (which are known to affect the activity of the proteasome [13], [14]), which may be responsible for the reduced activity of the proteasome since the proteasomal gene and protein expression seems to be unchanged.

Reactive Oxygen Species Production and the 26S Proteasome

The proteasomal system has previously been shown to be the major proteolytic system involved in the removal of oxidized proteins, with the 26S proteasome being the most sensitive to oxidative stress [16]. Although the 26S proteasome generally functions as part of the ubiquitin-proteasome pathway, it also has

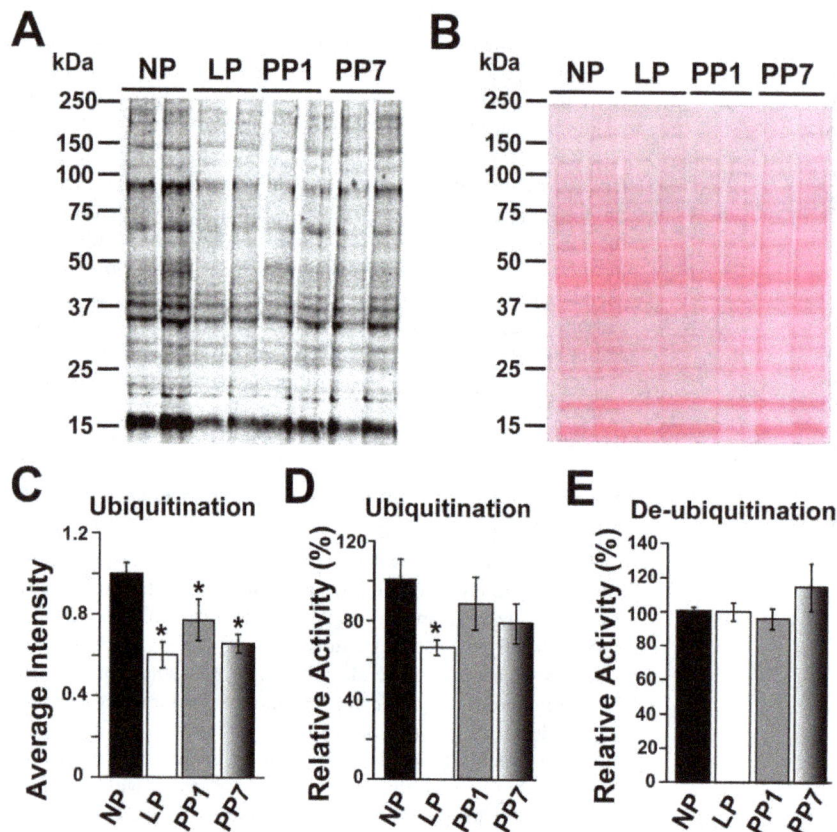

Figure 8. Pregnancy is associated with decreased polyubiquitinated protein levels, but not de-ubiquitination levels. A. Representative Western Blot of polyubiquitinated proteins (using the FK2 antibody) in whole heart lysates (100 µg) from non pregnant (NP), late pregnant (LP), 1 day post-partum (PP1) and 7 days post-partum (PP7). B. PonceauS was used as the loading control (n = 4 per group). C. Quantification of the polyubiquitinated proteins by Western Blot in non-pregnant (NP, black bar), late pregnant (LP, white bar), 1 day post-partum (PP1, grey bar) and 7 days post-partum (PP7, shaded bar). D. Polyubiquitination levels in NP, LP, PP1 and PP7 as determined by ELISA (using the FK1 antibody). E. De-ubiquitination activity levels in NP, LP, PP1 and PP7. Values are mean ± SEM and are normalized to NP, n = 4 per group and * denotes $p < 0.05$ vs. NP.

the capacity to degrade certain unfolded or damaged proteins, including "aged", denatured proteins, or proteins that have been oxidatively damaged, without initial ubiquitin tagging [13], [24]. We observed that the reactive oxygen species (ROS) generated in pregnancy is decreased and remains low one week after delivery (Fig. 6). ROS has been previously shown to increase the ubiquitin-conjugating activity and expression of genes for E3 enzymes (MuRF1 and MaFbx) in skeletal muscle myotubes [25]. Lower levels of ROS may account for the decreased polyubiquitination levels in the LP hearts.

Hormones and Proteasome Activity

It is also possible that estrogen may affect the proteasome, as interferon-induced oxidative stress has been shown to be associated with decreased proteasome amount and increased polyubiquitination [26]. Hormones, either directly or via the control of the metabolic status, can affect the ubiquitin-mediated control of protein degradation, as glucocorticoids have previously been shown to cause catabolic protein breakdown [27]. In skeletal muscle, degradation of cell proteins is of major physiological importance, and the size of a muscle cell is tightly regulated by the overall rate of proteolysis, a process precisely regulated by

hormones and cytokines [28]. Lastly, Genistein, a soy isoflavone with affinity for the estrogen receptor beta, has been shown to inhibit 20S proteasome activity in human prostate cancer cells [29]. The level of estrogen drastically increases at the end of pregnancy, but it is not clear whether estrogen treatment could regulate proteasome activity in the heart. Here we report for the first time that estrogen did not have any effect on the three proteolytic activities of the murine cardiac 26S proteasome. Thus, the changes in proteasome activity occurring in pregnancy cannot be attributed to the surge of estrogen.

Taken together, our results suggest that the ubiquitination, proteasome proteolytic pathway and the production of reactive oxygen species are affected by pregnancy. Late pregnancy is associated with a decrease in the polyubiquitination levels, which could be explained at least in part by reduced ROS production.

Author Contributions

Conceived and designed the experiments: AI AVG ME. Performed the experiments: AI SD RPN. Analyzed the data: AI SD RPN. Contributed reagents/materials/analysis tools: AI AVG ME. Wrote the paper: AI AVG ME.

References

1. Mone SM, Sanders SP, Colan SD (1996) Control mechanisms for physiological hypertrophy of pregnancy. Circulation 94: 667–72.
2. Dorn GW, Robbins J, Sugden PH (2003) Phenotyping hypertrophy: eschew obfuscation. Circ Res 92: 1171–5.
3. Daniels SR, Meyer RA, Liang YC, Bove KE (1988) Echocardiographically determined left ventricular mass index in normal children, adolescents and young adults. J Am Coll Cardiol 12: 703–8.
4. Pluim BM, Zwinderman AH, van der LA, van der Wall EE (2000) The athlete's heart. A meta-analysis of cardiac structure and function. Circulation 101: 336–44.
5. Schannwell CM, Zimmermann T, Schneppenheim M, Plehn G, Marx R, et al. (2002) Left ventricular hypertrophy and diastolic dysfunction in healthy pregnant women. Cardiology 97: 73–8.
6. Predmore JM, Wang P, Davis F, Bartolone S, Westfall MV, et al. (2010) Ubiquitin proteasome dysfunction in human hypertrophic and dilated cardiomyopathies. Circulation 121: 997–1004.
7. Glickman MH, Ciechanover A (2002) The ubiquitin-proteasome proteolytic pathway: destruction for the sake of construction. Physiol Rev 82: 373–428.
8. Glickman MH, Raveh D (2005) Proteasome plasticity. FEBS Lett 579: 3214–23.
9. Gomes AV, Zong C, Ping P (2006) Protein degradation by the 26S proteasome system in the normal and stressed myocardium. Antioxid Redox Signal 8: 1677–91.
10. Hochstrasser M (1996) Ubiquitin-dependent protein degradation. Annu Rev Genet 30: 405–39.
11. Mearini G, Schlossarek S, Willis MS, Carrier L (2008) The ubiquitin-proteasome system in cardiac dysfunction. Biochim Biophys Acta 1782: 749–63.
12. Drews O, Tsukamoto O, Liem D, Streicher J, Wang Y, et al. (2006) Differential regulation of proteasome function in isoproterenol-induced cardiac hypertrophy. Circ Res 107: 1094–101.
13. Zong C, Gomes AV, Drews O, Li X, Young GW, et al. (2006) Regulation of murine cardiac 20S proteasomes: role of associating partners. Circ Res 99: 372–80.
14. Gomes AV, Young GW, Wang Y, Zong C, Eghbali M, et al. (2009) Contrasting proteome biology and functional heterogeneity of the 20 S proteasome complexes in mammalian tissues. Mol Cell Proteomics 8: 302–15.
15. Eghbali M, Deva R, Alioua A, Minosyan TY, Ruan H, et al. (2005) Molecular and functional signature of heart hypertrophy during pregnancy. Circ Res 96: 1208–16.
16. Bader N, Grune T (2006) Protein oxidation and proteolysis. Biol Chem 387: 1351–5.
17. Eghbali M, Wang Y, Toro L, Stefani E (2006) Heart hypertrophy during pregnancy: a better functioning heart? Trends Cardiovasc Med 16: 285–91.
18. Li YF, Wang × (2011) The role of the proteasome in heart disease. Biochim Biophys Acta 1809: 141–9.
19. Tsukamoto O, Minamino T, Okada K, Shintani Y, Takashima S, et al. (2006) Depression of proteasome activities during the progression of cardiac dysfunction in pressure-overloaded heart of mice. Biochem Biophys Res Commun 340: 1125–33.
20. Depre C, Wang Q, Yan L, Hedhli N, Peter P, et al. (2006) Activation of the cardiac proteasome during pressure overload promotes ventricular hypertrophy. Circulation 114: 1821–8.
21. Hedhli N, Lizano P, Hong C, Fritzky LF, Dhar SK, et al. (2008) Proteasome inhibition decreases cardiac remodeling after initiation of pressure overload. Am J Physiol Heart Circ Physiol 295: H1385–H1393.
22. Otsuka K, Terasaki F, Shimomura H, Tsukada B, Horii T, et al. (2010) Enhanced expression of the ubiquitin-proteasome system in the myocardium from patients with dilated cardiomyopathy referred for left ventriculoplasty: an immunohistochemical study with special reference to oxidative stress. Heart Vessels 25: 474–84.
23. Liu CW, Li X, Thompson D, Wooding K, Chang TL, et al. (2006) ATP binding and ATP hydrolysis play distinct roles in the function of 26S proteasome. Mol Cell 24: 39–50.
24. Goldberg AL (2003) Protein degradation and protection against misfolded or damaged proteins. Nature 426: 895–9.
25. Li YP, Chen Y, Li AS, Reid MB (2003) Hydrogen peroxide stimulates ubiquitin-conjugating activity and expression of genes for specific E2 and E3 proteins in skeletal muscle myotubes. Am J Physiol Cell Physiol 285: C806–C812.
26. Seifert U, Bialy LP, Ebstein F, Bech-Otschir D, Voigt A, et al. (2010) Immunoproteasomes preserve protein homeostasis upon interferon-induced oxidative stress. Cell 142: 613–24.
27. Hamel FG, Fawcett J, Bennett RG, Duckworth WC (2004) Control of proteolysis: hormones, nutrients, and the changing role of the proteasome. Curr Opin Clin Nutr Metab Care 7: 255–8.
28. Lee DH, Goldberg AL (1998) Proteasome inhibitors: valuable new tools for cell biologists. Trends Cell Biol 8: 397–403.
29. Kazi A, Daniel KG, Smith DM, Kumar NB, Dou QP (2003) Inhibition of the proteasome activity, a novel mechanism associated with the tumor cell apoptosis-inducing ability of genistein. Biochem Pharmacol 66: 965–76.

15

EPC-Derived Microvesicles Protect Cardiomyocytes from Ang II-Induced Hypertrophy and Apoptosis

Shenhong Gu[1,2][9], Wei Zhang[3][9], Ji Chen[1,4][9], Ruilian Ma[1,3], Xiang Xiao[1], Xiaotang Ma[4], Zhen Yao[3]*[¶], Yanfang Chen[1,4]*[¶]

1 Department of Pharmacology and Toxicology, Boonshoft School of Medicine, Wright State University, Ohio, United States of America, 2 Department of Gerontology, the Affiliated Hospital of Hainan Medical College, Haikou, China, 3 Department of Cardiology, the People's Hospital of Sanya, Sanya, China, 4 Department of Neurology, the Affiliated Hospital of Guangdong Medical College, Zhanjiang, Guangdong, China

Abstract

Cell-released microvesicles (MVs) represent a novel way of cell-to-cell communication. Previous evidence indicates that endothelial progenitor cells (EPCs)-derived MVs can modulate endothelial cell survival and proliferation. In this study, we evaluated whether EPC-MVs protect cardiomyocytes (CMs) against angiotensin II (Ang II)-induced hypertrophy and apoptosis. The H9c2 CMs were exposed to Ang II in the presence or absence of EPC-MVs. Cell viability, apoptosis, surface area and β-myosin heavy chain (β-MHC) expression were analyzed. Meanwhile, reactive oxygen species (ROS), serine/threonine kinase (Akt), endothelial nitric oxide synthase (eNOS), and their phosphorylated proteins (p-Akt, p-eNOS) were measured. Phosphatidylinositol-3-kinase (PI3K) and NOS inhibitors were used for pathway verification. The role of MV-carried RNAs in mediating these effects was also explored. Results showed 1) EPC-MVs were able to protect CMs against Ang II-induced changes in cell viability, apoptosis, surface area, β-MHC expression and ROS over-production; 2) The effects were accompanied with the up-regulation of Akt/p-Akt and its downstream eNOS/p-eNOS, and were abolished by PI3K inhibition or partially blocked by NOS inhibition; 3) Depletion of RNAs from EPC-MVs partially or totally eliminated the effects of EPC-MVs. Our data indicate that EPC-MVs protect CMs from hypertrophy and apoptosis through activating the PI3K/Akt/eNOS pathway via the RNAs carried by EPC-MVs.

Editor: Gangjian Qin, Northwestern University, United States of America

Funding: This work was supported by the National Heart, Lung, and Blood Institute (HL-098637, YC), the American Heart Association (AHA, 13POST14780018 to JC) and the National Natural Science Foundation of China (NSFC, #81260060, #81300079). The funders had no role in study design, data collection and analysis, decision to publish, or preparation of the manuscript.

Competing Interests: The authors have declared that no competing interests exist.

* E-mail: yanfang.chen@wright.edu (YC); yao.zhen@126.com (ZY)

[9] These authors contributed equally to this work.

[¶] These authors also contributed equally to this work.

Introduction

Pathological cardiac hypertrophy leads to heart failure which remains the major cause of cardiovascular morbidity and mortality [1]. Its pathology is characterized by cardiomyocyte (CM) hypertrophy, apoptosis and inflammation [2,3]. It is well accepted that reactive oxygen species (ROS) plays an important role in the pathogenesis of cardiac hypertrophy [4]. Ang II-induced oxidative stress and inflammation have been demonstrated to contribute to the pathogenesis of cardiac hypertrophy [5,6]. Some signaling cascades such as phosphatidylinositol-3-kinase (PI3K) and serine/threonine kinase (Akt) pathways may inhibit CM hypertrophy [7,8]. The endothelial nitric oxide synthase (eNOS)/nitric oxide (NO) pathway, known as an important factor in regulating vascular function and one of the down-stream of Akt signaling, has also been shown to reduce ROS generation and exert anti-apoptotic effect on CMs [9,10].

Cellular microvesicles (MVs) released from various cell types in response to different stimuli represent a novel way of cell-to-cell communication. Cellular MVs are functional because they transfer or deliver proteins and gene messages such as mRNA and

microRNA (miRNA) to the target cells [11,12]. Cellular MVs have been shown to reverse endothelial injury probably through their dual effects on NO and ROS production [13,14]. It is suggested that bone marrow (BM)-derived endothelial progenitor cells (EPCs) could ameliorate cardiac hypertrophy [15,16]. Of notes, emerging evidence suggest that EPC-MVs have cell protective features. They can increase Akt/eNOS protein expression and phosphorylation, and induce the expression of the anti-apoptotic protein Bcl-xL in target endothelial cells (ECs) [11]. EPC-MVs are also shown to reprogram hypoxic resident renal cells to regenerate [17] and to activate an angiogenic process in islet endothelium [18]. However, the effects of EPC-MVs on CM hypertrophy and apoptosis remains unclear.

In this study, we first determined the effects of EPC-MVs on Ang II-induced CM hypertrophy, viability and apoptosis. Then, we explored whether the underling mechanisms are associated with ROS production and PI3K/Akt/eNOS signaling pathway. In addition, we examined whether the effects of EPC-MVs were mediated by MV- carried RNAs.

Materials and Methods

Ethics Statement

Adult C57BL/6J genetic background mice were used in the present study to obtain BM-derived EPCs. The strains were maintained in our laboratory (22°C) with a 12-hr light/dark cycle and fed with standard chow and drinking water ad libitum. All experimental procedures were approved by the Wright State University Laboratory Animal Care and Use Committee and were in accordance with the Guide for the Care and Use of Laboratory Animals issued by the National Institutes of Health (NIH).

Culture of Myocardial H9c2 Cell Line

H9c2 is a CM cell line (American Type Culture Collection, VA) derived from a clone of rat embryonic heart. Cells were cultured in Dulbecco's Modified Eagle Medium (DMEM) supplemented with 10% fetal bovine serum (FBS) containing 100 U/ml of penicillin G and 100 μg/ml of streptomycin, in a humidified atmosphere containing 5% CO_2 at 37°C. Before experimental intervention, confluent cultured cells were serum-starved for 12 h [9].

Concentration-response Studies of Ang II on CMs

Ang II (Sigma-Aldrich, St. Louis, MO) induced H9c2 injury model was produced as previously reported [19]. In brief, H9c2 CMs were seeded in 12-well plates (5×10^4 cells/well) or 96-well plate (5×10^3 cells/well) during the logarithmic growth phase. When the cells were nearly 80% confluent, cells were incubated with different concentrations of Ang II (0, 10^{-9}, 10^{-8}, 10^{-7} and 10^{-6} M) for 24 h. After co-incubation, cells were collected for analyses (cell surface areas, viabilities and apoptosis). Upon the completion of this study, we chose 10^{-6} M of Ang II for the following studies.

Culture of EPCs

The BM derived EPCs were cultured from adult (8–10 weeks of age, weight ranges from 25 g to 32 g) C57BL/6J genetic background mice as we previously described [20]. Mouse tibias and femurs were taken under deep anesthesia (pentobarbital, 150 mg/kg body weight) and BM was flushed out from tibias and femurs. BM mononuclear cells (MNCs) were isolated by using density gradient centrifuge method. After being washed with Phoshate-buffered saline (PBS), BM MNCs were counted and plated (1×10^7 cells) on a 25 cm² flask then grown in endothelial cell basal medium (EBM-2) supplemented with 5% FBS containing EPC growth cytokine cocktail (Lonza, Walkersville, MD). After 3 days in culture, non-adherent cells were removed by washing with PBS. Thereafter, culture medium was changed every 2 days.

Preparation of EPC-MVs and RNA-free EPC-MVs

After being cultured for 7 d, EPC cultures were washed with PBS, and incubated with serum-free medium overnight. The conditional medium which contained EPC secretions was collected and centrifuged (1,000 g, 15 min) at 4°C. Then the supernatant was ultracentrifuged (100,000 g, 60 min) at 4°C to pellet EPC-MVs [20]. For preparation of RNA-free EPC-MVs, we disrupted the EPC-MVs with ribonuclease A (RNase A) [21,22]. First, the EPC-MVs were incubated with 0.1% Triton X-100 (TX-100) for 5 min. Then the MV fraction was added in 200 U/ml of RNase A (Qiagen, CA) for 90 min at 37°C. After that, EPC-MVs were ultracentrifuged (100,000 g, 60 min) at 4°C to pellet the RNA deleted MVs (rdMVs) for the following experiments. To verify the effect of RNase A on MVs, the total RNAs were isolated from EPC-MVs and EPC-rdMVs using the RNA Isolation Kit (Ambion, NY), and the RNA concentrations were tested using quantitative assay (Thermo Scientific, Nanodrop 2000c, FL).

Concentration-response Studies of EPC-MVs on CM Viability

To determine the effective EPC-MV dose for increasing CM viability, CMs were treated with Ang II (10^{-6} M) and different doses (0, 12.5, 25 and 50 μg/ml) of EPC-MVs. After 24 h, CMs were harvested for viability analysis. The protein concentration of EPC-MVs was quantified by using Bradford assay (Bio-Rad, Hercules, CA).

Experimental Groups

Based on above studies, 10^{-6} M of Ang II and 50 μg/ml of EPC-MVs were used in the subsequent experiments. After reaching confluence, H9c2 CMs were randomly assigned to 4 different groups: serum-free medium (control), Ang II, Ang II+EPC-MVs, Ang II+drEPC-MVs. After incubation for 24 h, cells were harvested for analyses. For pathway blocking experiments, H9c2 CMs were pre-incubated with PI3K inhibitor (LY294002, 20 μM; Cayman Chemical, MI) or NOS inhibitor NG-nitro-arginine methyl ester (L-NAME, 100 μM; Sigma-Aldrich, St. Louis, MO) for 2 h [23].

Detection of EPC-MV Merging with H9c2 CMs

For observing whether EPC-MVs could merge with H9c2 CMs, a lipid membrane-intercalating fluorescent dye (PKH26) was used to label EPC-MVs before co-incubation. Briefly, 50 μg/ml EPC-MVs was mixed with 2 ml of PKH26 (2×10^{-6} M; Sigma-Aldrich, St. Louis, MO) at room temperature (RT) for 5 min. The labeled mixtures were dialyzed in 2 ml of 1% bovine serum albumin (BSA) and ultracentrifuged at 100,000 g for 60 min at 4°C to pellet the labeled MVs. After washed with EBM-2, the pellet was suspended with 1 ml of culture medium and added into H9c2 cells for 24 h incubation. The 4′, 6-diamidino-2 -phenylindole (DAPI, 1 ug/ml; Wako Pure Chemical Industries Ltd) was used for nuclear staining. Cell images were taken using an inverted microscope (EVOS, NY).

Measurement of Cell Surface Area

The surface area of CMs in different groups was measured according to the method of Simpson [24]. In brief, cell images were captured by a 20×magnification digital inverted microscope. Then the images of CMs were traced and the cell surface areas were analyzed by using Image J software (NIH, MA). The surface areas of CMs in 6 different fields were averaged. The surface area data in each treatment group was presented as the rate of that in control group.

Methyl Thiazolyl Tetrazolium (MTT) Assay

The viabilities of H9c2 CMs after different treatments were determined using the MTT Assay Kit (Invitrogen, NY) by following the manufacture's protocol. The CMs culture was replaced with 100 μl of fresh culture medium. Cells in 96-well plate were added in 10 μl of 12 mM MTT solution and incubated at 37°C for 4 h. Then 100 μl of the sodium dodecyl sulfate (SDS)-HCl solution was added to each well and incubated at 37°C for 4 h. Finally, the 96-well plate was read by a microtiterplate reader (Packard) at 535 nm. The percentage of viability was defined as the relative absorbance of the treated cells versus the untreated controls [19].

Flow Cytometry Analysis of Cell Apoptosis

The CM apoptosis was assessed by using an Apoptosis Assay Kit (Invitrogen, NY). The H9c2 CMs were collected by using 0.25% trypsin, and centrifuged at 200 g for 7 min. Cells were resuspended in 100 μl annexin-binding buffer, and incubated with 5 μl of annexin V-FITC and 1 μl of propidium iodide (PI) at RT in the dark for 15 min. Apoptotic cells were detected by a flow cytometer (Accuri C6 flow cytometer). The CMs stained with both annexin V and PI were considered to be late apoptotic CMs, and the cells stained only with annexin V were considered to be early apoptotic CMs [19].

Immunohistochemistry of β-myosin Heavy Chain (β-MHC)

H9c2 CMs were fixed with 2% paraformaldehyde at RT for 30 min and then permeated with 0.1% TX-100 at RT for 15 min. After being blocked with 1% BSA and 2% donkey serum for 1 h, the cells were incubated with β-MHC antibody (1:50; Millipore, MA) overnight at 4°C, and followed by incubation with Cy3-conjugated donkey anti-mouse antibody (1:250; Jackson, PA) at RT in the dark for 1 h. DAPI was used for nuclear stain. Images were obtained with an inverted microscope.

Intracellular ROS Detection

Intracellular ROS levels were determined by Dihydroethidium (DHE; Sigma-Aldrich, St. Louis, MO) staining [25,26]. Cells were incubated with the DHE working solution (2 μM) at 37°C for 2 h. After that, the solution was replaced with fresh culture medium, and the cells were observed under an inverted microscope. The cells were then trypsinized and collected by centrifugation (200 g, 7 min). The percentage of DHE positive cells was measured by using flow cytometry method.

Western Blot Analysis

After different treatments, proteins from H9c2 cells were obtained with lysis buffer (Thermo Scientific, FL) containing protease inhibitor. The proteins were subjected to electrophoresis and transferred onto nitrocellulose membranes. The membranes were blocked by incubating with 5% dry milk for 1 h, and then incubated with primary antibodies: against β-MHC (1:1000; Sigma-Aldrich, St. Louis, MO), Akt (1:500; Cell Signaling Technology, MA), p-Akt (Thr-308, 1:500; Cell Signaling Technology, MA), eNOS (1:500; Cell Signaling Technology, MA) or p-eNOS (ser-1177, 1:500; Cell Signaling Technology, MA), at 4°C overnight. β-actin (1:4000; Sigma-Aldrich, St. Louis, MO) was used to normalize protein loading. After being washed thoroughly, membranes were incubated with horseradish peroxidase (HRP) conjugated IgG (1:40000; Jackson ImmunoResearch Labs, INC. PA) for 1 h at RT. Blots were then developed with enhanced chemiluminescence developing solutions and quantified [27].

Statistical Analysis

Experimental data were expressed as the mean ± S.E, and were analyzed using one-way analysis of variance (ANOVA) followed by Bonferroni's t-test. Values of $P<0.05$ were considered to be statistical significance.

Results

Effects of Ang II on H9c2 CM Cell Surface Area, Viability and Apoptosis

To determine the effective dose of Ang II for inducing CM hypertrophy and apoptosis, H9c2 CM cells were treated with various concentrations (0, 10^{-9}, 10^{-8}, 10^{-7} or 10^{-6} M) of Ang II for 24 h. As seen in Figure 1A and 1B, Ang II dose-dependently increased cell surface area ($P<0.05$). The dose-dependent effects were also obtained in decreasing cell viability ($P<0.01$; Figure 1C) and in increasing cell apoptosis ($P<0.05$; Figure 1D). These results indicate the success of Ang II-induced CM hypertrophy and apoptosis model in H9c2 CMs. Based on these data, we chose 10^{-6} M Ang II for the following experiments.

Effective Dose of EPC-MVs for Preventing Ang II-induced Reduction in CM Viability

To determine the effective dose of EPC-MVs, we co-incubated different doses (0, 12.5, 25 or 50 μg/ml) of EPC-MVs and Ang II (10^{-6} M) with CMs for 24 h. We found that EPC-MVs at the dose of 50 μg/ml did not affect the survival of H9c2 cells, but significantly alleviated Ang II-induced reduction in CM viability ($P<0.01$; Figure 2). Thus, we chose 50 μg/ml EPC-MVs for the following experiments.

EPC-MVs Merge with H9c2 CMs after Co-incubation

The PKH26 labeled EPC-MVs were co-incubated with H9c2 CMs for 24 h. The PKH26 fluorescent was able to be detected in the cytoplasm of the H9c2 CMs, suggesting that EPC-MVs could merge with H9c2 CMs (Figure 3A).

RNase Treatment Effectively Depletes RNAs from EPC-MVs

To investigate the possible role of EPC-MV carried RNAs in MV function, we digested the total RNAs inside MVs by using RNAse A. As expected, we found that RNase A was able to deplete more than 80% of total RNAs in EPC-MVs (100±10.1% and 17.5±3.5%, $P<0.01$, MVs $vs.$ rdMVs; Figure 3B).

EPC-MVs Decrease Ang II-induced CM Hypertrophy via their Carried RNAs

Ang II induced CM hypertrophy is characterized by cell size increase and activation of fetal cardiac genes such as β-MHC [28]. Here, we found that EPC-MVs decreased Ang II-induced CM enlargement in cell surface area (1.9±0.4 and 2.7±0.2, Ang II+MVs $vs.$ Ang II, $P<0.01$; Figure 4A and 4B) and up-regulation in β-MHC expression ($P<0.01$; Figure 4A and 4C). In contrast, EPC-rdMVs totally blocked these effects ($P<0.01$; Figure 4).

EPC-MVs Protect CMs from Ang II-induced Decrease in Viability Partially via their Carried RNAs which Activate PI3K/NOS Pathway

Fig. 5 shows co-incubation of EPC-MVs prevented Ang II-induced decrease in cell viability (81.2±2.6% and 52.2±2.1%, Ang II+MVs $vs.$ Ang II, $P<0.01$). EPC-rdMVs were less effective on improving H9c2 cell viability compromised by Ang II (61.3±3.3% and 81.2±2.6%, Ang II+EPC-rdMVs $vs.$ Ang II+EPC-MVs, $P<0.01$), suggesting that the RNAs carried by EPC-MVs were partially required for the protective effect. In addition, LY294002 could abolish and L-NAME partially blocked the protective effect of EPC-MVs (52.8±3.7%, 65.7±4.6% and 81.2±2.6%, MVs+LY294002 or MVs+L-NAME $vs.$ MVs, $P<0.01$). These demonstrate the involvement of PI3K/NOS pathway in the protective effect of EPC-MVs.

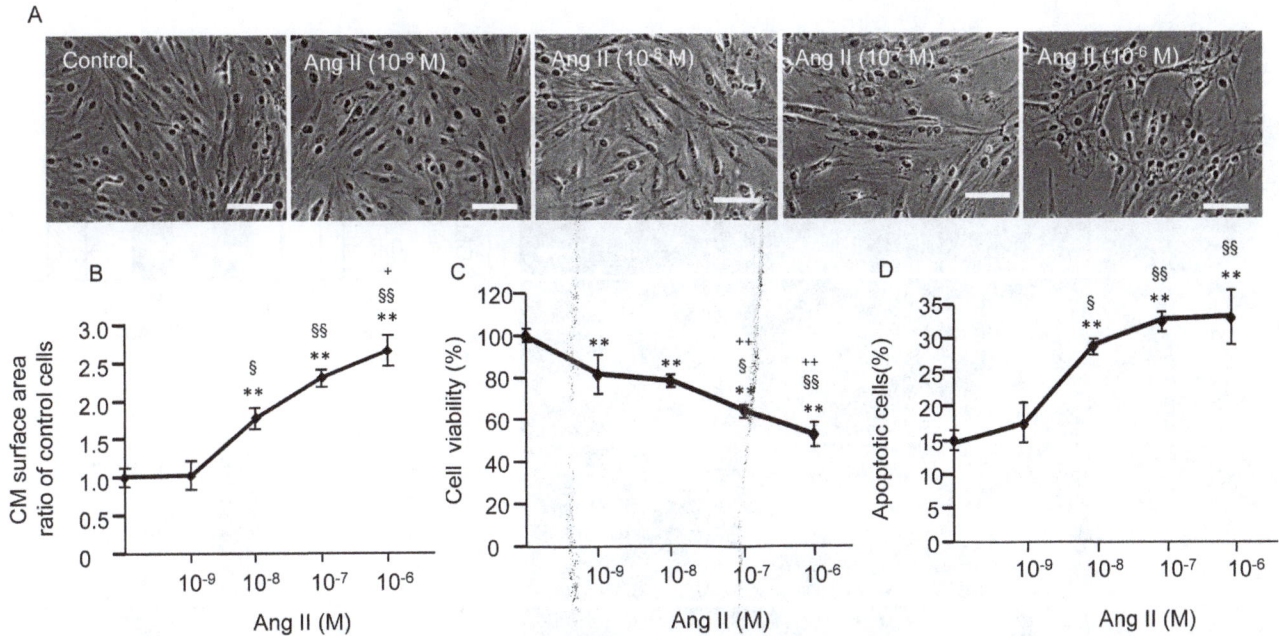

Figure 1. Concentration-response study of Ang II on H9c2 hypertrophy and apoptosis. (A) Representative images of H9c2 CMs. Scale bar, 100 µm. (B) Dose- dependent effect of Ang II on H9c2 cell surface area. (C) Dose-dependent effect of Ang II on H9c2 cell viability. (D) Dose-dependent effect of Ang II on H9c2 cell apoptosis. **$P<0.01$ vs. control; $^{§}P<0.05$, $^{§§}P<0.01$ vs. 10^{-9} M Ang II; $^{+}P<0.05$, $^{++}P<0.01$ vs. 10^{-8} M Ang II; n = 6/group.

EPC-MVs Protect CMs from Ang II-induced Apoptosis via their Carried RNAs which Activate the PI3K/NOS Pathway

As shown in Figure 6, EPC-MVs significantly decreased Ang II-induced CM apoptosis ($16.1\pm1.2\%$ and $32.8\pm4.5\%$, Ang II+MVs vs. Ang II, $P<0.01$). This effect was significantly reduced in the EPC-rdMV group ($22.1\pm1.6\%$ and $16.1\pm1.2\%$, Ang II+rdMVs vs. Ang II+MVs, $P<0.01$). Furthermore, LY294002 could abolish and L-NAME partially blocked the protective effect of EPC-MVs ($29.1\pm1.7\%$, $22.4\pm1.4\%$ and $16.1\pm1.2\%$, MVs+LY294002 or MVs+L-NAME vs. MVs, $P<0.01$).

EPC-MVs Inhibit Ang II-induced ROS Overproduction in CMs via their Carried RNAs which Activate PI3K/NOS Pathway

Oxidative stress is one of the main contributing factors that initiate hypertrophy and apoptosis in Ang II treated CMs [28]. We examined the role of EPC-MVs on ROS overproduction in CMs induced by Ang II. As shown in Figure 7A, Ang II induced an

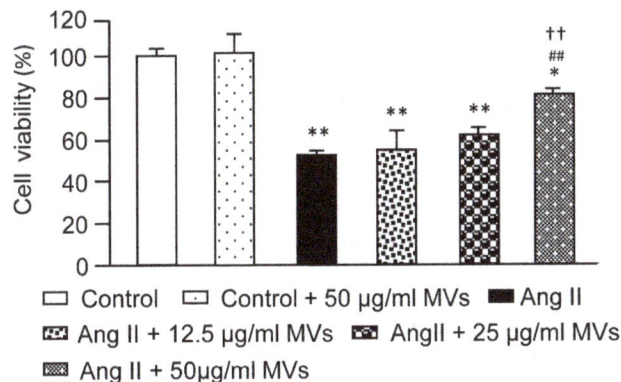

Figure 2. Dose-dependent effects of EPC-MVs on H9c2 viability. Summarized data on the effects of different EPC-MV doses on cell viabilities of H9c2 treated with 0 or 10^{-6} M Ang II. *$P<0.05$, **$P<0.01$ vs. control; $^{##}P<0.01$ vs. Ang II, $^{††}P<0.01$ vs. Ang II +25 µg/ml MVs; n = 6/group.

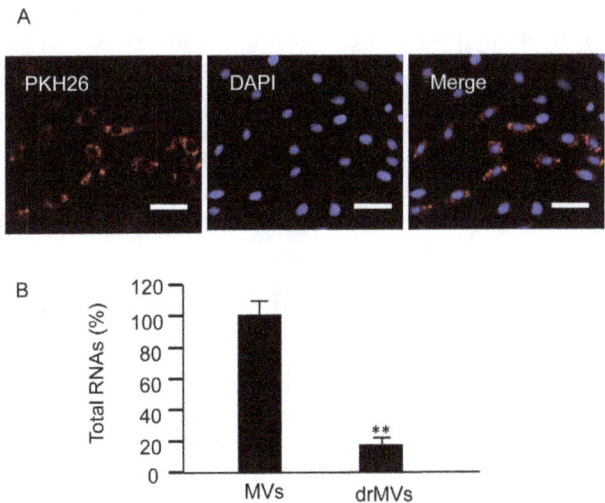

Figure 3. The incorporation of EPC-MVs with H9c2 and the RNAs depletion from EPC-MVs. (A) Representative images showing that EPC-MVs merge with H9c2 CMs. MVs were labeled with PKH26 (red). Nucleuses were labeled with DAPI (blue). Scale bar, 100 µm. (B) Summarized data of total RNAs in MVs and rdMVs. RNase treatment is effective in depleting RNAs from EPC-MVs. **$P<0.01$, EPC-rdMVs vs. EPC-MVs; n = 3/group. rdMVs: RNA deleted MVs.

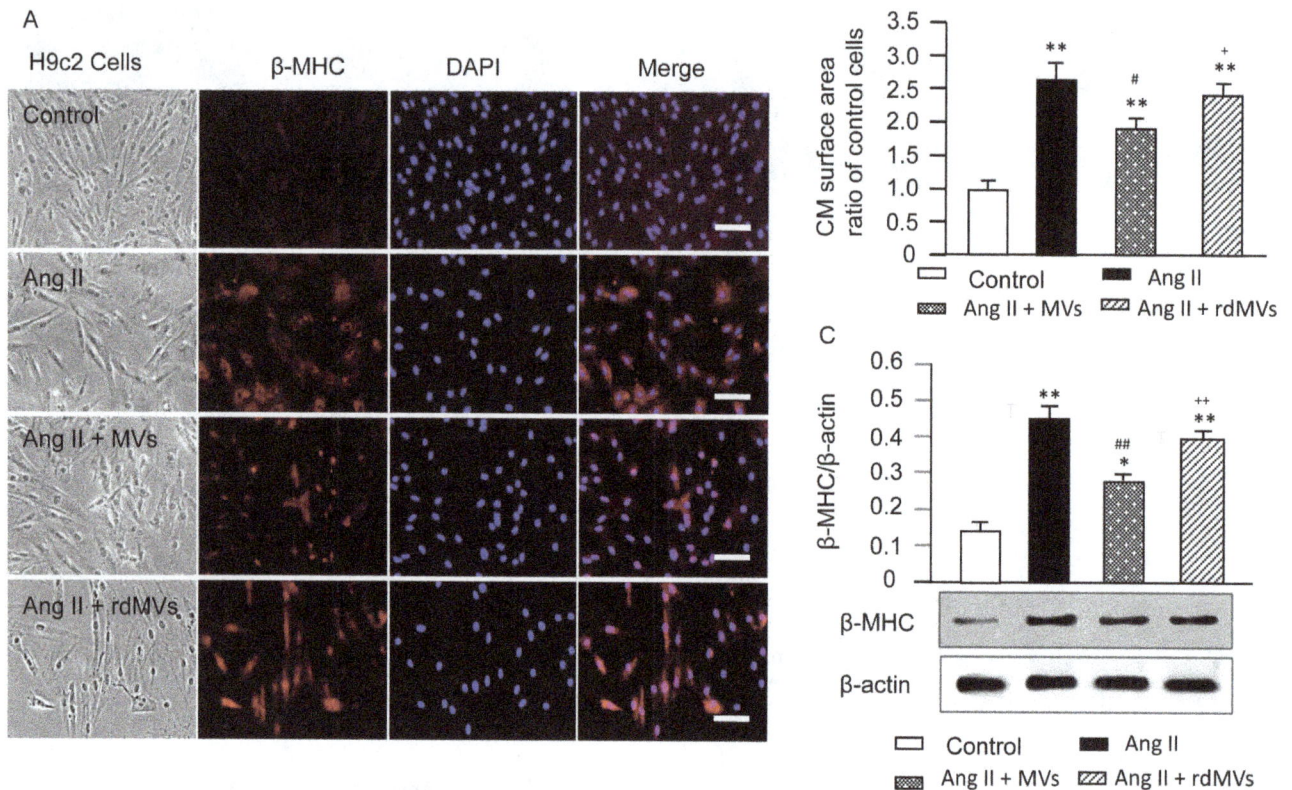

Figure 4. Effects of EPC-MVs on Ang II-induced CM hypertrophy and β-MHC protein expression. (A) Representative immunohistochemistry images of β-MHC expression in H9c2 CMs in each group. H9c2 CMs were labeled with β-MHC antibody (red), and DAPI (blue, for nucleus). Scale bar, 100 μm. (B) Summarized data of surface areas of CMs in each group. (C) Western blot bands and graphs showing the β-MHC expression in H9c2 CMs in different treatment groups. The molecular weights are 223 kDa for β-MHC and 43 kDa for β-actin. *$P<0.05$, **$P<0.01$ vs. control, #$P<0.05$, ##$P<0.01$ vs. Ang II, +$P<0.05$, ++$P<0.01$ vs. Ang II+ MVs; n = 4/group. rdMVs: RNA deleted MVs.

increase in DHE positive cells, which was suppressed by EPC-MVs. The flow cytometric data also showed that EPC-MVs significantly suppressed Ang II-induced intracellular ROS over-production (Figure 7B). EPC-rdMVs were less effective on reducing Ang II-induced ROS overproduction in CMs ($P<0.05$).

In addition, pre-incubation with LY294002 or L-NAME could abolish or partially block the protective effect of EPC-MVs ($P<0.01$; Figure 7).

EPC-MVs Activate PI3K/Akt/eNOS Signaling Pathway in CMs

Akt phosphorylation has been demonstrated to reflect Akt activation. EPC-MVs significantly increased the protein expression of p-Akt/Akt ($P<0.01$; Figure 8A) and p-eNOS/eNOS ($P<0.01$; Figure 8B) in CMs. EPC-rdMVs were less effective on up-regulating Akt, p-Akt, eNOS and p-eNOS ($P<0.05$ or 0.01; Figure 8).

Discussion

In this study, we demonstrated for the first time that EPC-MVs protect CMs from Ang II-induced hypertrophy and apoptosis. The underlying mechanism may partially rely on the RNAs carried by EPC-MVs which could inhibit ROS overproduction and activate the PI3K/Akt/eNOS signaling pathway.

MVs were first described about 30 years ago and considered to be membrane nano-fragments (0.05–1 μm) [13]. MVs are shed from the cell surface upon activation, stress or apoptosis. It can be derived from various cell types, such as platelets, endothelial cells, EPCs and leukocytes, etc [29,30]. They express different cell surface markers, which vary according to their cell origin, and the process of MV formation. Therefore, MVs can be used as

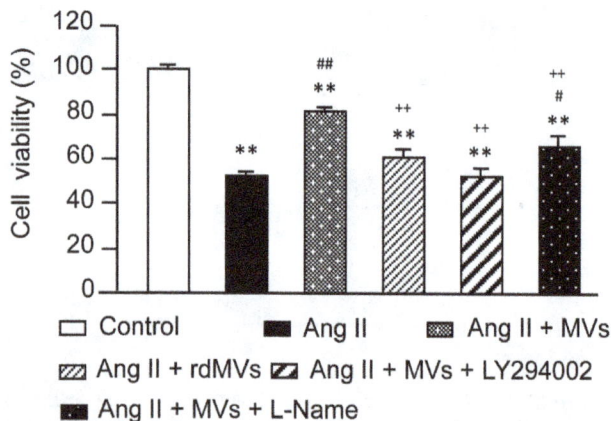

Figure 5. Effect of EPC-MVs on cell viability of Ang II-treated H9c2 CMs. Summarized data on H9c2 CM viability in each group. **$P<0.01$ vs. control; #$P<0.05$, ##$P<0.01$ vs. Ang II; ++$P<0.01$ vs. Ang II+EPC-MVs; n = 6/group. rdMVs: RNA deleted MVs.

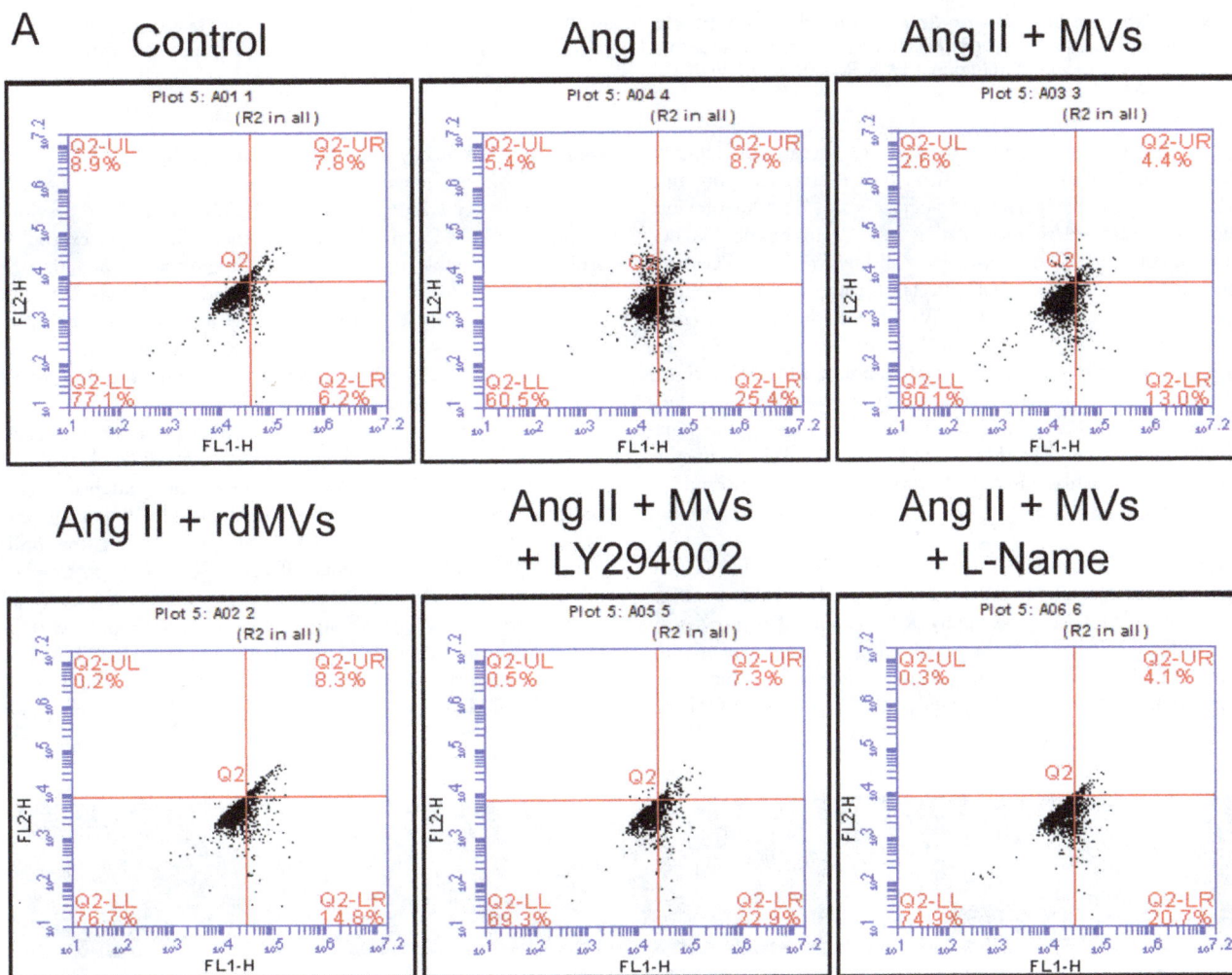

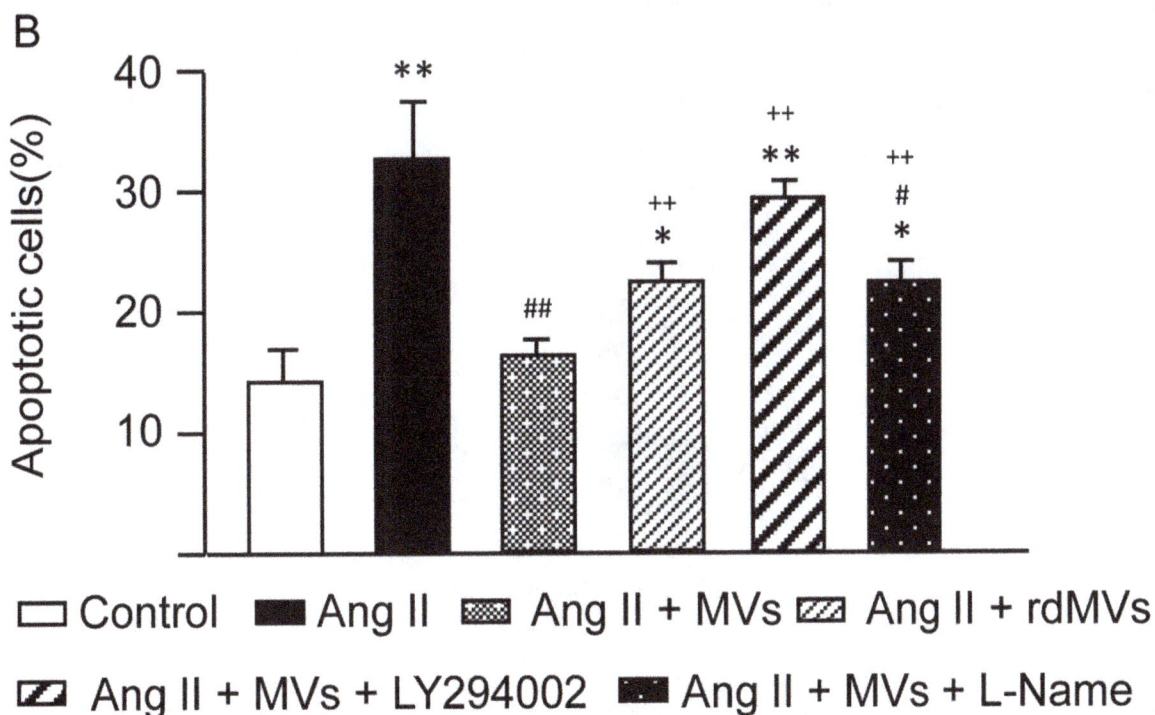

Figure 6. Effect of EPC-MVs on Ang II-induced CM apoptosis. (A) Representative flow cytometric plots of H9c2 CM apoptosis in different treatment groups. (B) Summarized data on the percentage of apoptotic H9c2 CMs in each group. **$P<0.01$ vs. control, [#]$P<0.05$, [##]$P<0.01$ vs. Ang II, [++]$P<0.01$ vs. Ang II+MVs; n = 6/group. rdMVs: RNA deleted MVs.

biomarkers for disease and indicators for therapeutic efficacy. More recently, studies showed that MVs exert effects on anti-inflammatory, anticoagulant and angiogenesis [31]. Our previous study demonstrated that circulating MVs from db/db diabetic mice impair the EPC function *in vitro* and *in vivo* [20]. EPCs have been shown to have beneficial effects on cardiovascular regeneration and protection [32–34]. MVs released from EPCs could carry their parent cell biological information and thus are functional to the target cells [13]. For examples, EPC-MVs trigger a repair program to injured tissues such as vasculatures, kidney and pancreatic islets [11,17,18]. Therefore, targeting the functional properties of EPC-MVs could open a novel therapeutic approach for vascular disease. However, there is no information regarding the effects of EPC-MVs on cardiac hypertrophy and apoptosis.

For testing our hypothesis that EPC-MVs play a protective role in cardiac hypertrophy and apoptosis, we produced the model of Ang II-induced CM hypertrophy and apoptosis as previously reported [35,36]. As we expected, Ang II dose-dependently induced CM hypertrophy and apoptosis, suggesting a success of model reproduce. After co-incubation of EPC-MVs with CM, we

found that EPC-MVs can effectively incorporate into CMs. This finding is in agreement with previous reports showing that the MVs can merge with CMs or ECs [11,37]. Most of the previous studies on EPC-MVs are focusing on angiogenesis. For examples, EPC-MVs are able to trigger *in vivo* angiogenesis in a murine model of hindlimb ischemia [11]. Incubation of EPC-MVs with HUVECs promotes EC survival, proliferation and *in vitro* formation of capillary-like structures [11]. Here, we demonstrate for the first time that EPC-MVs prevent CMs from Ang II-induced hypertrophy and apoptosis.

The underlying mechanisms of EPC-MVs' protective effects on CMs might involve oxidative stress and PI3K/Akt/eNOS signaling pathway. Firstly, ROS overproduction has been demonstrated in Ang II-treated CMs by others [36,38] and in our present study. Meanwhile, our results reveal that the anti-hypertrophic and anti-apoptotic effects of EPC-MVs are correlated with the inhibition of ROS overproduction. Secondly, we found in this study that EPC-MVs up-regulate Akt/eNOS and p-Akt/p-eNOS expression in CM hypertrophy model. The PI3K/Akt signaling pathway has been shown to play a crucial role in protecting CMs from Ang II-induced hypertrophy and apoptosis

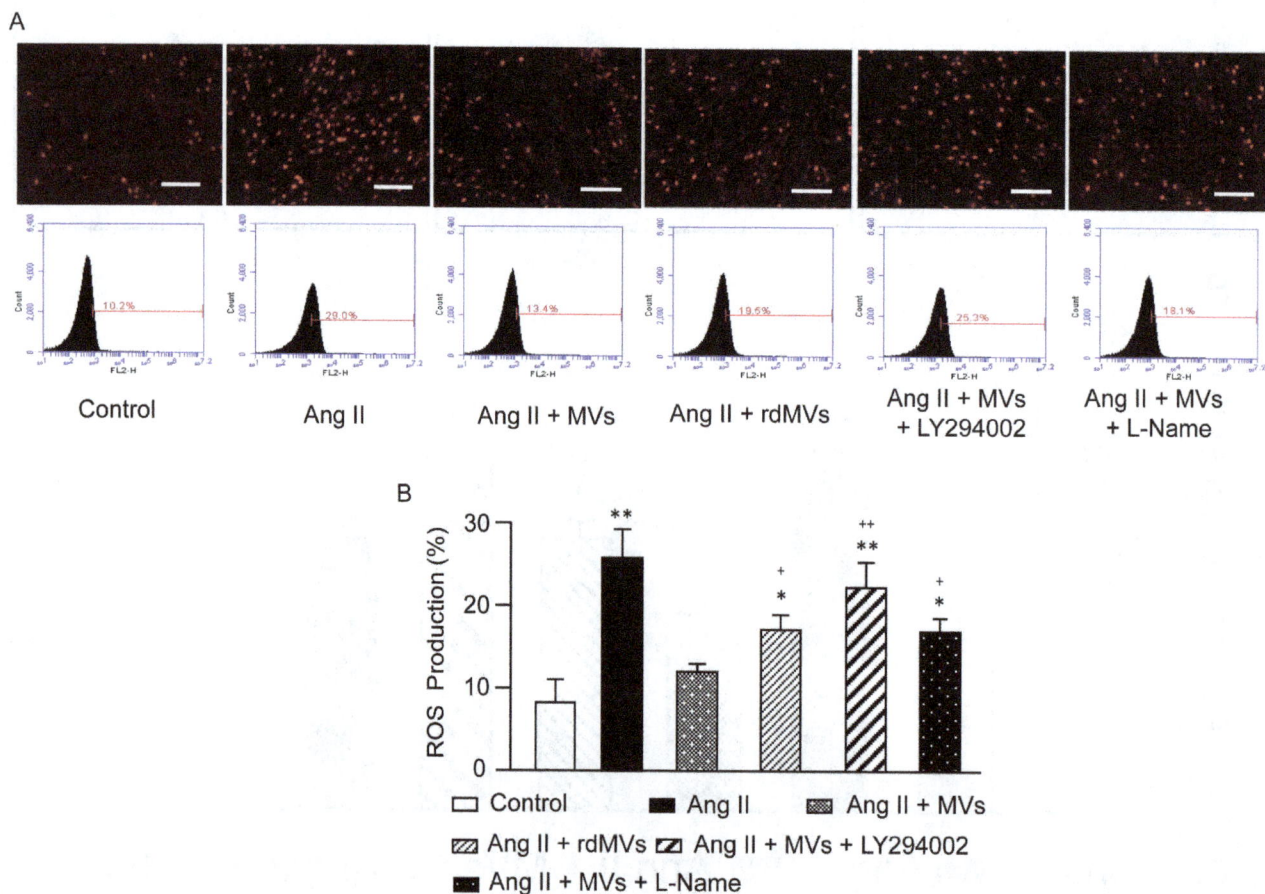

Figure 7. Effect of EPC-MVs on intracellular ROS production of Ang II-treated H9c2 CMs. (A) Representative images of intracellular DHE staining and flow traces in different groups. Scale bar, 200 μm. (B) Summarized data on the measurement of ROS production in H9c2 CMs in different groups. *$P<0.05$, ** $P<0.01$ vs. control, [##]$P<0.01$ vs. Ang II, [+]$P<0.05$, [++]$P<0.01$ vs. Ang II+MVs; n = 6/group. rdMVs: RNA deleted MVs.

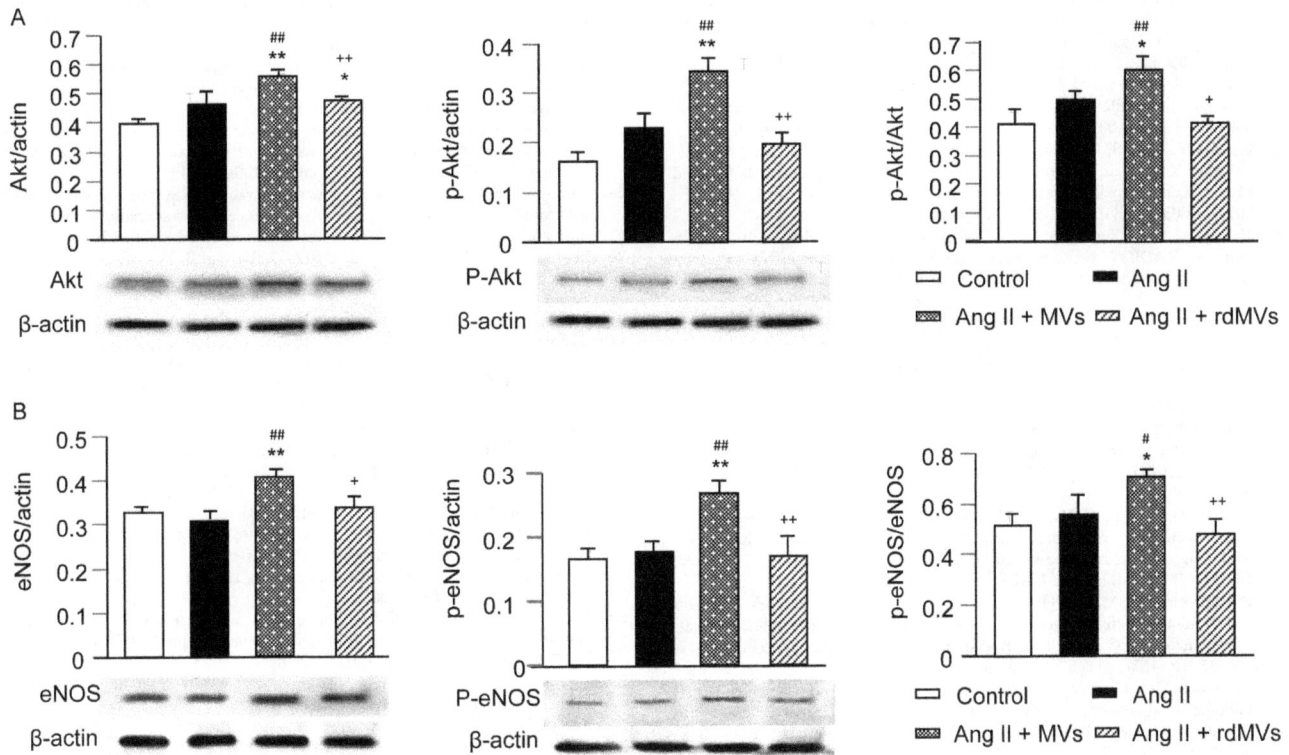

Figure 8. EPC-MVs up-regulate Akt/eNOS activation in Ang II-treated H9c2 CMs. Representative Western blot bands showing Akt/p-Akt (A), and eNOS/p-eNOS (B) expression of CMs in different treatment groups. The molecular weights are 60 kDa for Akt and p-Akt, and 140 kDa for eNOS and p-eNOS. Summarized data on Akt/p-Akt (A) and eNOS/p-eNOS (B) expression in CMs in different treatment groups. *$P<0.05$, **$P<0.01$ vs. control, #$P<0.05$, ##$P<0.01$ vs. Ang II, +$P<0.05$, ++$P<0.01$ vs. Ang II+MVs; n = 4/group. rdMVs: RNA deleted MVs.

[39,40]. In particular, it is indicated that EPC-MVs are involved in the angiogenic and anti-apoptotic program by shuttling specific RNAs associated with PI3K/Akt and eNOS pathways [11]. Supported by these previous studies, our data suggest that activation of PI3K/Akt/eNOS pathway could be responsible for the effects of EPC-MVs on preventing CMs from Ang II-induced hypertrophy and apoptosis. Thirdly, activation of eNOS/NO production scavenges superoxide anion to prevent ROS overproduction [41,42]. These studies provide mechanism explanations for our novel findings that EPC-MVs activate eNOS and reduce ROS production in Ang II-treated H9c2 CMs. Finally and most importantly, we have applied the pathway inhibitors to verify the role of PI3K/Akt/eNOS pathway in EPC-MVs' protective effects. We found that the pathway blockers partially (L-NAME) or totally (LY294002) inhibit the protective effects of EPC-MVs on Ang II-induced CM hypertrophy, apoptosis and oxidative stress. Taken together, our results demonstrate that EPC-MVs could trigger the PI3K/Akt/eNOS signaling cascades to reduce ROS production, and consequently to inhibit Ang II-induced hypertrophy and apoptosis.

MVs exert different functions depending on their composition, such as protein, receptor, mRNA and miRNA. A recent report suggests that RNAs in MVs have led to the genetic communication between cells, and the mRNAs in these RNAs could be translated into proteins after being taken up by the cells [37]. Deregibus et al showed that EPC-MVs activate angiogenic program in ECs by a horizontal transfer of mRNA [11]. In the present study, we investigated the role of EPC-MVs carried RNAs in the effects of EPC-MVs. Interestingly, our data showed that the protective effects of EPC-MVs on CM apoptosis, cell viability and ROS production could be partially blocked by RNA depletion. Depletion of RNAs abolished EPC-MVs' effects on hypertrophy and modulating Akt/eNOS signaling pathway, suggesting that the other mechanisms such as their carried protein components might also be involved. Our findings suggest that the beneficial effects of EPC-MVs are partly mediated by their carried RNAs. Nevertheless more detailed mechanisms, such as the responsive miRNAs, mRNAs and/or proteins, await future exploration.

Author Contributions

Conceived and designed the experiments: SG JC ZY YC. Performed the experiments: SG WZ JC RM XM XX. Analyzed the data: SG WZ JC RM XX XM. Contributed reagents/materials/analysis tools: SG JC RM YC. Wrote the paper: SG JC ZY YC.

References

1. Wang S, Han HM, Pan ZW, Hang PZ, Sun LH, et al (2012) Choline inhibits angiotensin II-induced cardiac hypertrophy by intracellular calcium signal and p38 MAPK pathway. Naunyn Schmiedebergs Arch Pharmacol 385: 823–831. 10.1007/s00210-012-0740-4 [doi].

2. Bernardo BC, Weeks KL, Pretorius L, McMullen JR (2010) Molecular distinction between physiological and pathological cardiac hypertrophy: experimental findings and therapeutic strategies. Pharmacol Ther 128: 191–227. S0163-7258(10)00079-3 [pii];10.1016/j.pharmthera.2010.04.005 [doi].

3. Levy D, Garrison RJ, Savage DD, Kannel WB, Castelli WP (1990) Prognostic implications of echocardiographically determined left ventricular mass in the Framingham Heart Study. N Engl J Med 322: 1561–1566. 10.1056/NEJM199005313222203 [doi].

4. Canton M, Menazza S, Sheeran FL, Polverino de LP, Di LF, et al (2011) Oxidation of myofibrillar proteins in human heart failure. J Am Coll Cardiol 57: 300–309. S0735-1097(10)04462-1 [pii];10.1016/j.jacc.2010.06.058 [doi].

5. Izumiya Y, Araki S, Usuku H, Rokutanda T, Hanatani S, et al (2012) Chronic C-Type Natriuretic Peptide Infusion Attenuates Angiotensin II-Induced Myocardial Superoxide Production and Cardiac Remodeling. Int J Vasc Med 2012: 246058. 10.1155/2012/246058 [doi].

6. Valente AJ, Clark RA, Siddesha JM, Siebenlist U, Chandrasekar B (2012) CIKS (Act1 or TRAF3IP2) mediates Angiotensin-II-induced Interleukin-18 expression, and Nox2-dependent cardiomyocyte hypertrophy. J Mol Cell Cardiol 53: 113–124. S0022-2828(12)00156-3 [pii];10.1016/j.yjmcc.2012.04.009 [doi].

7. McMullen JR, Amirahmadi F, Woodcock EA, Schinke-Braun M, Bouwman RD, et al (2007) Protective effects of exercise and phosphoinositide 3-kinase(p110alpha) signaling in dilated and hypertrophic cardiomyopathy. Proc Natl Acad Sci U S A 104: 612–617. 0606663104 [pii];10.1073/pnas.0606663104 [doi].

8. DeBosch B, Treskov I, Lupu TS, Weinheimer C, Kovacs A, et al (2006) Akt1 is required for physiological cardiac growth. Circulation 113: 2097–2104. CIRCULATIONAHA.105.595231 [pii];10.1161/CIRCULATIO-NAHA.105.595231 [doi].

9. Liou SF, Hsu JH, Liang JC, Ke HJ, Chen IJ, wt al (2012) San-Huang-Xie-Xin-Tang protects cardiomyocytes against hypoxia/reoxygenation injury via inhibition of oxidative stress-induced apoptosis. J Nat Med 66: 311–320. 10.1007/s11418-011-0592-0 [doi].

10. Wu Y, Xia ZY, Meng QT, Zhu J, Lei S, et al (2011) Shen-Fu injection preconditioning inhibits myocardial ischemia-reperfusion injury in diabetic rats: activation of eNOS via the PI3K/Akt pathway. J Biomed Biotechnol 2011: 384627. 10.1155/2011/384627 [doi].

11. Deregibus MC, Cantaluppi V, Calogero R, Lo IM, Tetta C, et al (2007) Endothelial progenitor cell derived microvesicles activate an angiogenic program in endothelial cells by a horizontal transfer of mRNA. Blood 110: 2440–2448. blood-2007-03-078709 [pii];10.1182/blood-2007-03-078709 [doi].

12. Morel O, Toti F, Hugel B, Freyssinet JM (2004) Cellular microparticles: a disseminated storage pool of bioactive vascular effectors. Curr Opin Hematol 11: 156–164. 00062752-200405000-00004 [pii].

13. Meziani F, Tesse A, Andriantsitohaina R (2008) Microparticles are vectors of paradoxical information in vascular cells including the endothelium: role in health and diseases. Pharmacol Rep 60: 75–84.

14. Agouni A, Mostefai HA, Porro C, Carusio N, Favre J, et al (2007) Sonic hedgehog carried by microparticles corrects endothelial injury through nitric oxide release. FASEB J 21: 2735–2741. fj.07-8079com [pii];10.1096/fj.07-8079com [doi].

15. Ruetten H, Dimmeler S, Gehring D, Ihling C, Zeiher AM (2005) Concentric left ventricular remodeling in endothelial nitric oxide synthase knockout mice by chronic pressure overload. Cardiovasc Res 66: 444–453. S0008-6363(05)00069-6 [pii];10.1016/j.cardiores.2005.01.021 [doi].

16. Buys ES, Raher MJ, Blake SL, Neilan TG, Graveline AR, et al (2007) Cardiomyocyte-restricted restoration of nitric oxide synthase 3 attenuates left ventricular remodeling after chronic pressure overload. Am J Physiol Heart Circ Physiol 293: H620–H627. 01236.2006 [pii];10.1152/ajpheart.01236.2006 [doi].

17. Cantaluppi V, Gatti S, Medica D, Figliolini F, Bruno S, et al (2012) Microvesicles derived from endothelial progenitor cells protect the kidney from ischemia-reperfusion injury by microRNA-dependent reprogramming of resident renal cells. Kidney Int 82: 412–427. ki2012105 [pii];10.1038/ki.2012.105 [doi].

18. Cantaluppi V, Biancone L, Figliolini F, Beltramo S, Medica D, et al (2012) Microvesicles derived from endothelial progenitor cells enhance neoangiogenesis of human pancreatic islets. Cell Transplant 21: 1305–1320. ct0360cantaluppi [pii];10.3727/096368911X627534 [doi].

19. Yang C, Wang Y, Liu H, Li N, Sun Y, et al (2012) Ghrelin protects H9c2 cardiomyocytes from angiotensin II-induced apoptosis through the endoplasmic reticulum stress pathway. J Cardiovasc Pharmacol 59: 465–471. 10.1097/FJC.0b013e31824a7b60 [doi].

20. Chen J, Chen S, Chen Y, Zhang C, Wang J, et al (2011) Circulating endothelial progenitor cells and cellular membrane microparticles in db/db diabetic mouse: possible implications in cerebral ischemic damage. Am J Physiol Endocrinol Metab 301: E62–E71. ajpendo.00026.2011 [pii];10.1152/ajpendo.00026.2011 [doi].

21. Li L, Zhu D, Huang L, Zhang J, Bian Z, Chen X, et al (2012) Argonaute 2 complexes selectively protect the circulating microRNAs in cell-secreted microvesicles. PLoS One 7: e46957. 10.1371/journal.pone.0046957 [doi];-PONE-D-12-15623 [pii].

22. Ullal AJ, Pisetsky DS, Reich CF, III (2010) Use of SYTO 13, a fluorescent dye binding nucleic acids, for the detection of microparticles in in vitro systems. Cytometry A 77: 294–301. 10.1002/cyto.a.20833 [doi].

23. Liu AH, Cao YN, Liu HT, Zhang WW, Liu Y, et al (2008) DIDS attenuates staurosporine-induced cardiomyocyte apoptosis by PI3K/Akt signaling pathway: activation of eNOS/NO and inhibition of Bax translocation. Cell Physiol Biochem 22: 177–186. 000149795 [pii];10.1159/000149795 [doi].

24. Simpson P, Savion S (1982) Differentiation of rat myocytes in single cell cultures with and without proliferating nonmyocardial cells. Cross-striations, ultrastructure, and chronotropic response to isoproterenol. Circ Res 50: 101–116.

25. Shanmugam P, Valente AJ, Prabhu SD, Venkatesan B, Yoshida T, et al (2011) Angiotensin-II type 1 receptor and NOX2 mediate TCF/LEF and CREB dependent WISP1 induction and cardiomyocyte hypertrophy. J Mol Cell Cardiol 50: 928–938. S0022-2828(11)00089-7 [pii];10.1016/j.yjmcc.2011.02.012 [doi].

26. Venkatachalam K, Prabhu SD, Reddy VS, Boylston WH, Valente AJ, et al (2009) Neutralization of interleukin-18 ameliorates ischemia/reperfusion-induced myocardial injury. J Biol Chem 284: 7853–7865. M808824200 [pii];10.1074/jbc.M808824200 [doi].

27. Chen J, Chen J, Chen S, Zhang C, Zhang L, et al (2012) Transfusion of CXCR4-primed endothelial progenitor cells reduces cerebral ischemic damage and repair in db/db diabetic mice. PLoS One 7: e50105. 10.1371/journal.pone.0050105 [doi];PONE-D-12-23137 [pii].

28. Singh VP, Le B, Khode R, Baker KM, Kumar R (2008) Intracellular angiotensin II production in diabetic rats is correlated with cardiomyocyte apoptosis, oxidative stress, and cardiac fibrosis. Diabetes 57: 3297–3306. db08-0805 [pii];10.2337/db08-0805 [doi].

29. Lee Y, El AS, Wood MJ (2012) Exosomes and microvesicles: extracellular vesicles for genetic information transfer and gene therapy. Hum Mol Genet 21: R125–R134. dds317 [pii];10.1093/hmg/dds317 [doi].

30. Martinez MC, Tesse A, Zobairi F, Andriantsitohaina R (2005) Shed membrane microparticles from circulating and vascular cells in regulating vascular function. Am J Physiol Heart Circ Physiol 288: H1004–H1009. 288/3/H1004 [pii];10.1152/ajpheart.00842.2004 [doi].

31. McVey M, Tabuchi A, Kuebler WM (2012) Microparticles and acute lung injury. Am J Physiol Lung Cell Mol Physiol 303: L364–L381. ajplung.00354.2011 [pii];10.1152/ajplung.00354.2011 [doi].

32. Asahara T, Murohara T, Sullivan A, Silver M, van der Zee R, et al (1997) Isolation of putative progenitor endothelial cells for angiogenesis. Science 275: 964–967.

33. Fan Y, Shen F, Frenzel T, Zhu W, Ye J, et al (2010) Endothelial progenitor cell transplantation improves long-term stroke outcome in mice. Ann Neurol 67: 488–497. 10.1002/ana.21919 [doi].

34. Sen S, McDonald SP, Coates PT, Bonder CS (2011) Endothelial progenitor cells: novel biomarker and promising cell therapy for cardiovascular disease. Clin Sci (Lond) 120: 263–283. CS20100429 [pii];10.1042/CS20100429 [doi].

35. Liu JJ, Li DL, Zhou J, Sun L, Zhao M, et al (2011) Acetylcholine prevents angiotensin II-induced oxidative stress and apoptosis in H9c2 cells. Apoptosis 16: 94–103. 10.1007/s10495-010-0549-x [doi].

36. Qin F, Patel R, Yan C, Liu W (2006) NADPH oxidase is involved in angiotensin II-induced apoptosis in H9C2 cardiac muscle cells: effects of apocynin. Free Radic Biol Med 40: 236–246. S0891-5849(05)00452-1 [pii];10.1016/j.freeradbiomed.2005.08.010 [doi].

37. Chen TS, Lai RC, Lee MM, Choo AB, Lee CN, et al (2010) Mesenchymal stem cell secretes microparticles enriched in pre-microRNAs. Nucleic Acids Res 38: 215–224. gkp857 [pii];10.1093/nar/gkp857 [doi].

38. Nakagami H, Takemoto M, Liao JK (2003) NADPH oxidase-derived superoxide anion mediates angiotensin II-induced cardiac hypertrophy. J Mol Cell Cardiol 35: 851–859. S0022282803001457 [pii].

39. Wen Y, Zhang XJ, Ma YX, Xu XJ, Hong LF, et al (2009) Erythropoietin attenuates hypertrophy of neonatal rat cardiac myocytes induced by angiotensin-II in vitro. Scand J Clin Lab Invest 69: 518–525. 910211769 [pii];10.1080/00365510902802286 [doi].

40. Hong HJ, Liu JC, Cheng Th, Chan P (2010) Tanshinone IIA attenuates angiotensin II-induced apoptosis via Akt pathway in neonatal rat cardiomyocytes. Acta Pharmacol Sin 31: 1569–1575. aps2010176 [pii];10.1038/aps.2010.176 [doi].

41. Chavakis E, Dernbach E, Hermann C, Mondorf UF, Zeiher AM, et al (2001) Oxidized LDL inhibits vascular endothelial growth factor-induced endothelial cell migration by an inhibitory effect on the Akt/endothelial nitric oxide synthase pathway. Circulation 103: 2102–2107.

42. Huie RE, Padmaja S (1993) The reaction of no with superoxide. Free Radic Res Commun 18: 195–199.

16

Postnatal Ablation of Foxm1 from Cardiomyocytes Causes Late Onset Cardiac Hypertrophy and Fibrosis without Exacerbating Pressure Overload-Induced Cardiac Remodeling

Craig Bolte[1]*, Yufang Zhang[1], Allen York[2], Tanya V. Kalin[1], Jo El J. Schultz[3], Jeffery D. Molkentin[2], Vladimir V. Kalinichenko[1]*

1 Division of Pulmonary Biology, Cincinnati Children's Hospital Research Foundation, Cincinnati, Ohio, United States of America, 2 Molecular Cardiovascular Biology, Cincinnati Children's Hospital Research Foundation, Cincinnati, Ohio, United States of America, 3 Department of Pharmacology and Cell Biophysics, University of Cincinnati College of Medicine, Cincinnati, Ohio, United States of America

Abstract

Heart disease remains a leading cause of morbidity and mortality in the industrialized world. Hypertrophic cardiomyopathy is the most common genetic cardiovascular disorder and the most common cause of sudden cardiac death. Foxm1 transcription factor (also known as HFH-11B, Trident, Win or MPP2) plays an important role in the pathogenesis of various cancers and is a critical mediator of post-injury repair in multiple organs. Foxm1 has been previously shown to be essential for heart development and proliferation of embryonic cardiomyocytes. However, the role of Foxm1 in postnatal heart development and in cardiac injury has not been evaluated. To delete *Foxm1* in postnatal cardiomyocytes, *αMHC-Cre/Foxm1*^{fl/fl} mice were generated. Surprisingly, *αMHC-Cre/Foxm1*^{fl/fl} mice exhibited normal cardiomyocyte proliferation at postnatal day seven and had no defects in cardiac structure or function but developed cardiac hypertrophy and fibrosis late in life. The development of cardiomyocyte hypertrophy and cardiac fibrosis in aged Foxm1-deficient mice was associated with reduced expression of Hey2, an important regulator of cardiac homeostasis, and increased expression of genes critical for cardiac remodeling, including MMP9, αSMA, fibronectin and vimentin. We also found that following aortic constriction Foxm1 mRNA and protein were induced in cardiomyocytes. However, *Foxm1* deletion did not exacerbate cardiac hypertrophy or fibrosis following chronic pressure overload. Our results demonstrate that Foxm1 regulates genes critical for age-induced cardiomyocyte hypertrophy and cardiac fibrosis.

Editor: Robert Dettman, Northwestern University, United States of America

Funding: These studies were supported by National Institute of Health grant RO1HL84151 (VVK). The funders had no role in study design, data collection and analysis, decision to publish, or preparation of the manuscript.

Competing Interests: The authors have declared that no competing interests exist.

* E-mail: Vladimir.Kalinichenko@cchmc.org (VVK); Craig.Bolte@cchmc.org (CB)

Introduction

Cardiac hypertrophy can result from increased hemodynamic load, myocardial infarction, extreme athletic training, aging, chronic respiratory diseases or can be seemingly idiopathic. Hypertrophy following an increased hemodynamic load is a compensatory mechanism to maintain perfusion of the peripheral tissues and prevent cardiac insufficiency. However, cardiac remodeling is only compensatory in the short term and leads to heart failure when either the chamber walls become too thin and weak to effectively expel blood (systolic dysfunction) or when thickening of the myocardium decreases the lumen of the chamber to the point the heart can no longer fill properly (diastolic dysfunction). Both outcomes are irreversible and require surgical intervention. Idiopathic cardiac hypertrophy typically manifests from a genetic predisposition and is known as hypertrophic cardiomyopathy. Hypertrophic cardiomyopathy (HCM) is defined as hypertrophy of the myocardium in the absence of sufficient external force [1,2]. Hundreds of mutations in at least 13 known

genes, mostly sarcomeric proteins, have been linked to HCM [2]; however, mutations in genes encoding proteins of the extracellular matrix can produce a similar phenotype [3–5]. With a frequency of 1 in 500 in the general population, HCM is the most common genetic cardiovascular disorder [2] and also the most common cause of sudden cardiac death in individuals under 35 years of age [2]. In the absence of family history HCM often goes undiagnosed until cardiac arrhythmias occur, potentially culminating in sudden cardiac death. In many cases HCM is discovered by electrocardiography for another indication, with echocardiography remaining the best means to evaluate the extent and track the progression of HCM [2].

Foxm1 (formerly known as HFH-11B, Trident, Win or MPP2) is a member of the Forkhead Box (Fox) family of transcription factors that share homology in the winged helix/forkhead DNA binding domain. Foxm1 is highly expressed in proliferating cells, but expression wanes postnatally and Foxm1 protein can only be detected in intestinal crypts, testes and thymus in the adult [6,7]. Foxm1 expression in human fibroblasts has been previously shown

Table 1. TaqMan gene expression assays (Applied Biosystems) used for qRT-PCR analysis.

Mouse α-SMA	Mm00702100_s1
Mouse β-actin	Mm00607939_s1
Mouse BMP4	Mm01321704_m1
Mouse CaMKIIδ	Mm00499266_m1
Mouse CDC25B	Mm00499136_m1
Mouse collagen 1α1	Mm00801666_g1
Mouse collagen 3α1	Mm00802331_m1
Mouse CXCR4	Mm01292123_m1
Mouse Cyclin B₁	Mm00838401_g1
Mouse Fibronectin	Mm01256744_m1
Mouse Foxm1	Mm00514924_m1
Mouse Fsp-1	Mm00724330_m1
Mouse Hey2	Mm00469280_m1
Mouse IL-1β	Mm01336189_m1
Mouse IL-1R	Mm01337566_m1
Mouse IκBKB	Mm01222247_m1
Mouse MMP2	Mm00439498_m1
Mouse MMP9	Mm00442991_m1
Mouse Myocardin	Mm00455051_m1
Mouse NFATc3	Mm01249200_m1
Mouse NFκB	Mm00479807_m1
Mouse nMyc	Mm00476449_m1
Mouse p21^{cip1}	Mm01303209_m1
Mouse Plk-1	Mm00440924_g1
Mouse TGF-β1	Mm01178820_m1
Mouse TIMP1	Mm00441818_m1
Mouse TNFα	Mm00443258_m1
Mouse Vimentin	Mm00449201_m1

to decrease with advancing age and to be decreased in Progeria syndrome, which is characterized by premature aging [8]. Overexpression of Foxm1 in transgenic mice prevented age-related defects during liver repair, implicating Foxm1 in regulation of the aging process [9]. We have previously shown that Foxm1 plays an essential role in embryonic cardiac development [10,11]. Ablation of *Foxm1* from all cell types (*Foxm1*$^{-/-}$) [11,12] or cardiomyocyte-specific deletion of Foxm1 (*Nkx2.5-Cre/Foxm1*$^{fl/fl}$) [10] is embryonic lethal due to defects in cardiomyocyte proliferation. Cardiomyocytes from *Foxm1*$^{-/-}$ and *Nkx2.5-Cre/Foxm1*$^{fl/fl}$ mice were enlarged and the percentage of proliferating cardiomyocytes was decreased. Deletion of *Foxm1* in embryonic cardiomyocytes caused early withdrawal from the cell cycle, resulting in premature entrance into the hypertrophic phase of cardiac growth. Due to embryonic lethality in *Foxm1*$^{-/-}$ and *Nkx2.5-Cre/Foxm1*$^{fl/fl}$ mice, the role of Foxm1 in postnatal cardiac development and cardiac injury remains unknown.

In this study, we generated a new mouse line with cardiomyocyte-specific Foxm1 deletion after birth (*αMHC-Cre/Foxm1*$^{fl/fl}$). Surprisingly, hearts from these mice were structurally and functionally normal, indicating that Foxm1 is dispensable for postnatal heart development. *αMHC-Cre/Foxm1*$^{fl/fl}$ mice developed cardiac hypertrophy and fibrosis after aging. The development of cardiac fibrosis and cardiomyocyte hypertrophy in aged

αMHC-Cre/Foxm1$^{fl/fl}$ mice was associated with reduced expression of Hey2, a critical regulator of cardiac homeostasis [13]. Given the vital role Foxm1 plays during cardiac embryogenesis as well as the predisposition for end of life cardiac hypertrophy in *αMHC-Cre/Foxm1*$^{fl/fl}$ mice, we also investigated the importance of Foxm1 in cardiac pathology using a mouse model of cardiac hypertrophy induced by aortic banding. Although Foxm1 protein and message were increased following transaortic constriction, deletion of Foxm1 from cardiomyocytes did not affect survival, the development of cardiac hypertrophy or the degree of cardiac remodeling. Thus, Foxm1 expression in cardiomyocytes is critical for age-related cardiac hypertrophy but dispensable for pressure overload-induced cardiomyocyte hypertrophy.

Materials and Methods

Mice

We have previously described the generation of *Foxm1* LoxP/LoxP (*Foxm1*$^{fl/fl}$) mice, in which LoxP sequences flank exons 4 through 7 of the *Foxm1* gene that encode the DNA binding and transcriptional activation domains of the FOXM1 protein [14]. *Foxm1*$^{fl/fl}$ mice were bred with *αMHC-Cre* mice [15] to generate *αMHC-Cre/Foxm1*$^{fl/fl}$ mice, resulting in postnatal cardiomyocyte-specific deletion of *Foxm1*. *αMHC-Cre/Foxm1*$^{fl/fl}$ mice were bred with *Foxm1*$^{fl/fl}$ mice to generate litters with an expected 1:1 ratio of *αMHC-Cre/Foxm1*$^{fl/fl}$ mice to *Foxm1*$^{fl/fl}$ control mice.

Ethics statement

Animal studies were reviewed and approved by the Animal Care and Use Committee of Cincinnati Children's Hospital Research Foundation (protocol # 0D08057).

Evaluation of cardiac function

In vivo cardiac function was determined in *αMHC-Cre/Foxm1*$^{fl/fl}$ and control mice not undergoing surgery by Millar catheterization as described [16]. Briefly, following anesthesia a 2F Millar Catheter was inserted into the lumen of the carotid artery and advanced until it reached the left ventricle of the heart. Once inside the left ventricle, the catheter was held in place with suture. Interventricular pressure was recorded with a DigiMed system recorder. A 3-point EKG was attached to the mouse and sinus rhythm recorded with DigiMed software.

Aortic banding

Cardiac hypertrophy was induced in *αMHC-Cre/Foxm1*$^{fl/fl}$ and control *Foxm1*$^{fl/fl}$ mice by aortic banding as described [17]. Banding was performed on mice of both sexes at 8 to 10 weeks of age. No differences were observed between males and females. Mice were sedated with 3% isoflurane and 600 mL/min O₂. Subsequently, mice were intubated to maintain pulmonary pressure, the sternum split, ribs retracted and the left portion of the thymus removed to allow aortic visualization. To ensure a reproducible degree of aortic constriction, suture was secured around a bent 27G needle between the 1st and 2nd branches of the aortic arch. Once the suture was in place, the needle was removed, the thoracic cavity was closed and the chest evacuated to prevent a pneumothorax.

Echocardiography

Progression of cardiac hypertrophy was monitored by echocardiography as described [17]. Mice from all genotypes and treatment groups were anesthetized with isoflurane and echocardiography was performed using a SONOS 5500 instrument (Hewlett Packard) with a 15-MHz microprobe. Echocardiographic

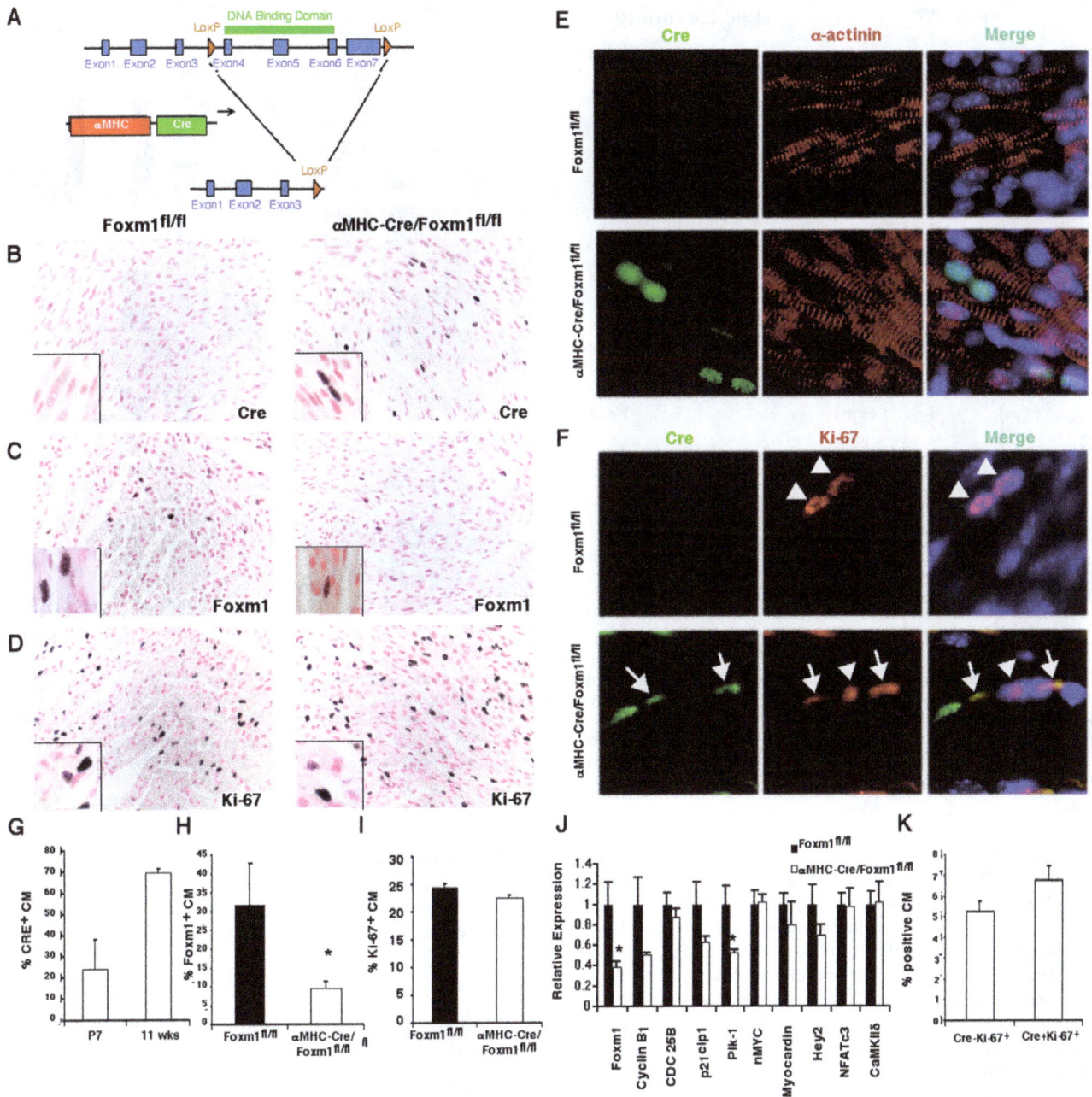

Figure 1. Cardiomyocyte proliferation unaltered at P7 in α*MHC-Cre/Foxm1*^{fl/fl} mice. The Cre-LoxP system was utilized to conditionally delete *Foxm1* from cardiomyocytes (CM). Mice homozygous for the *Foxm1*^{fl/fl} allele (in which LoxP sites flank exons 4 through 7 of the *Foxm1* gene) were mated to mice expressing α*MHC-Cre* to generate mice with a conditional deletion of *Foxm1* from cardiomyocytes (α*MHC-Cre/Foxm1*^{fl/fl}) (A). Cre expression was observed in approximately 25% of cardiomyocytes at postnatal day 7 (P7) in α*MHC-Cre/Foxm1*^{fl/fl} mice (G). Cre was not detected in control hearts (B, E). The number of FOXM1-positive cardiomyocytes was higher in *Foxm1*^{fl/fl} than in α*MHC-Cre/Foxm1*^{fl/fl} mice at P7 (C, H). Ki-67 staining was similar in α*MHC-Cre/Foxm1*^{fl/fl} and control hearts (D, I). There was no difference in the percentage of α*MHC-Cre/Foxm1*^{fl/fl} cardiomyocytes positive for Ki-67 (Cre⁻Ki-67⁺) (arrow heads) and those double positive for Ki-67 and Cre (Cre⁺Ki-67⁺) (arrows) (F, K). Foxm1 mRNA was decreased in α*MHC-Cre/Foxm1*^{fl/fl} hearts as was Plk-1. Cyclin B₁, CDC 25B, p21^{cip1}, nMYC, myocardin, Hey2, NFATc3 and CaMKIIδ mRNAs were unaltered (J). Significant differences ($p < 0.05$) were indicated by asterisk. "N" was 4 for all groups. Magnifications were 40x (B–D), 400x (insets B–D) and 200x (E–F).

measurements were taken on M-mode in triplicate for each mouse at the level of the papillary muscle. Pressure gradients across the constriction were measured by Doppler echocardiography. Fractional shortening was calculated as ([LVEDdLVEDs]/LVEDd)×100, (%) [18].

Immunohistochemical staining

Hearts from α*MHC-Cre/Foxm1*^{fl/fl} and control *Foxm1*^{fl/fl} mice were collected at postnatal day 7 (P7), 11 weeks of age and 16 months of age. Aortic constriction was performed on 8–10 week old mice and mice were harvested 18 weeks after aortic banding. Hearts were fixed in 4% paraformaldehyde overnight and embedded into paraffin blocks. Paraffin sections of 5 μm were

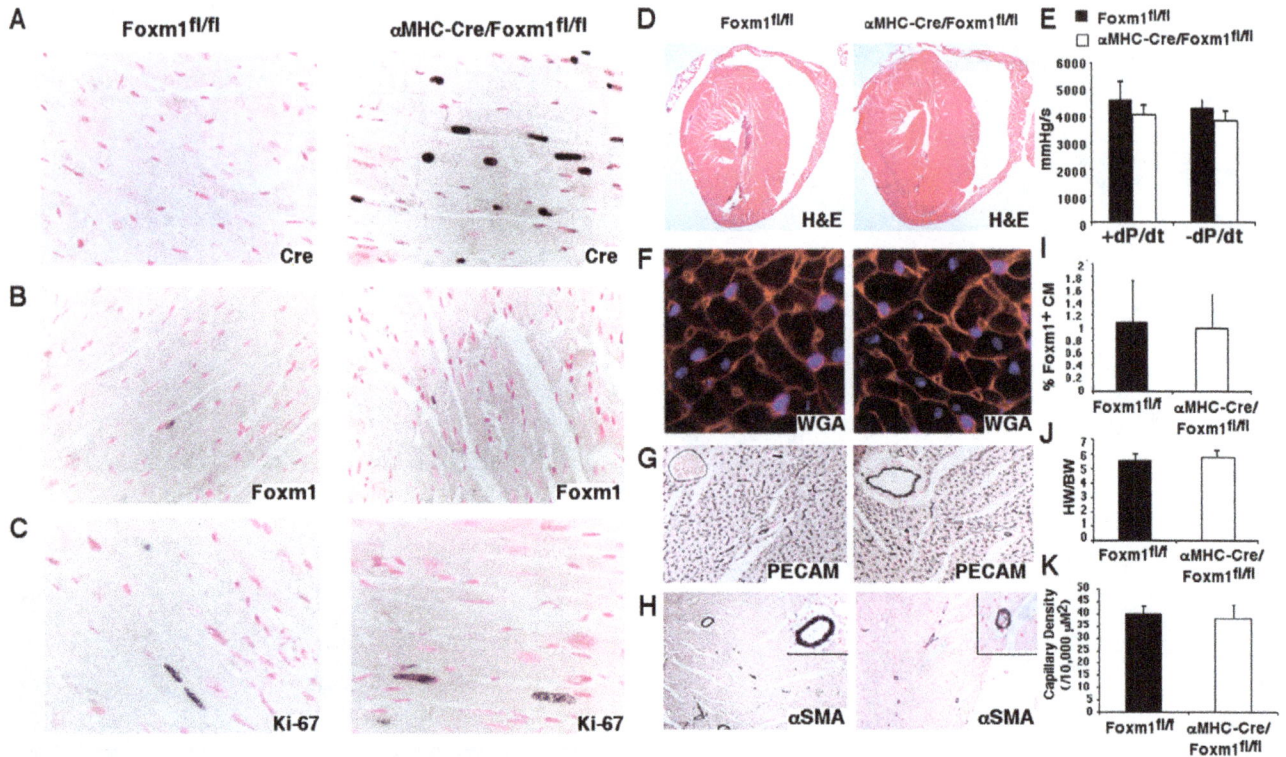

Figure 2. Postnatal deletion of Foxm1 does not alter cardiac morphology or function. Immunohistochemistry showed Cre protein in adult $\alpha MHC\text{-}Cre/Foxm1^{fl/fl}$ cardiomyocytes (A). FOXM1-positive cardiomyocytes were rare in adult $\alpha MHC\text{-}Cre/Foxm1^{fl/fl}$ and control mice (B, I), as were Ki-67-positive cells (C). Hearts from adult $\alpha MHC\text{-}Cre/Foxm1^{fl/fl}$ mice were similar in size to $Foxm1^{fl/fl}$ control mice (D, J) and had similar cardiac inotropy (+dP/dt) and lusitropy ($-$dP/dt) (E). There was no change in cardiomyocyte size as indicated by WGA staining (F), capillary density as shown by PECAM-1 staining (G, K) or coronary artery formation as visualized by αSMA staining (H). "N" was 5 control and 6 $\alpha MHC\text{-}Cre/Foxm1^{fl/fl}$ mice. Magnifications were (A–C, F, inset H) 40x, (G & H) 20x and (D) 5x.

immunostained for FOXM1 (1:500; k-19; Santa Cruz), Cre (1:5000; 7 Hills Biotech), PECAM-1 (1:10,000; Pharminogen), α-smooth muscle actin (αSMA; 1:10,000; Sigma-Aldrich) or Ki-67 (1:10,000; Dako). Antibody-antigen complexes were detected using biotinylated secondary antibody followed by avidin-HRP complex and DAB substrate (Vector Labs, Burlingame, CA), as previously described [11,19–21]. Sections were counterstained with nuclear fast red. Co-localization studies were performed using primary antibodies against α-actinin (1:100; Sigma-Aldrich), Ki-67 (1:400), FOXM1 (1:50) and Cre (1:500) followed by secondary antibodies labeled with fluorescein isothiocynate (FITC) or Texas Red. Slides were counterstained with DAPI to detect cell nuclei (Vector Labs). Heart sections were also stained with hematoxylin and eosin (H&E) to evaluate cardiac morphology, wheat-germ agglutinin to measure cardiomyocyte size or Masson's Trichrome to detect cardiac fibrosis. Slides were photographed using a Zeiss Axioplan2 microscope and Axiovision Rel 4.8 software.

Quantitative real-time RT-PCR (qRT-PCR)

Total cardiac RNA was prepared from individual $\alpha MHC\text{-}Cre/Foxm1^{fl/fl}$ and control $Foxm1^{fl/fl}$ hearts using RNA-STAT-60 (Tel-Test "B" Inc. Friendswood, TX). cDNA was generated using the Applied Biosystems High Capacity cDNA Reverse Transcription kit (Applied Biosystems, Foster City, CA). Evaluation of expression levels of specific genes was performed by qRT-PCR using Taqman probes (Table 1) and the StepOnePlus Real-Time PCR system (Applied Biosystems, Foster City, CA), as previously described [19,22,23].

Statistical analysis

Student's T-test was used to determine statistical significance. P values <0.05 were considered significant. Values for all measurements were expressed as mean $\pm$ standard error of mean (SEM).

Results

Cardiomyocyte proliferation unaltered at P7 in $\alpha MHC\text{-}Cre/Foxm1^{fl/fl}$ mice

$\alpha MHC\text{-}Cre$ transgenic mice [15] were bred with $Foxm1^{fl/fl}$ mice [14] to produce $\alpha MHC\text{-}Cre/Foxm1^{fl/fl}$ mice. In these mice, exons 4–7 encoding the DNA binding and transcriptional activation domains of the FOXM1 protein were deleted specifically from postnatal cardiomyocytes (Figure 1A). At P7, approximately 25% of cardiomyocytes in $\alpha MHC\text{-}Cre/Foxm1^{fl/fl}$ mice were positive for Cre protein (Figure 1B & G). Cre-expressing cardiomyocytes maintained expression of α-actinin, a sarcomeric marker (Figure 1E). Decreased expression of Foxm1 mRNA (Figure 1J) as well as less FOXM1-positive cardiomyocytes was observed in $\alpha MHC\text{-}Cre/Foxm1^{fl/fl}$ hearts at P7 when compared to age-matched controls (Figure 1C & H). Despite decreased FOXM1 protein and mRNA in juvenile cardiomyocytes, there was no difference in the percentage of Ki-67-positive cells at P7 (Figure 1D & I). Co-localization experiments showed that cardiomyocytes positive for Cre expressed the proliferation-specific protein Ki-67 (Figure 1F), indicating they undergo the cell cycle. The percentage of proliferating cells was similar in Cre-positive and Cre-negative subsets of $\alpha MHC\text{-}Cre/Foxm1^{fl/fl}$ cardiomyocytes (Figure 1F & K).

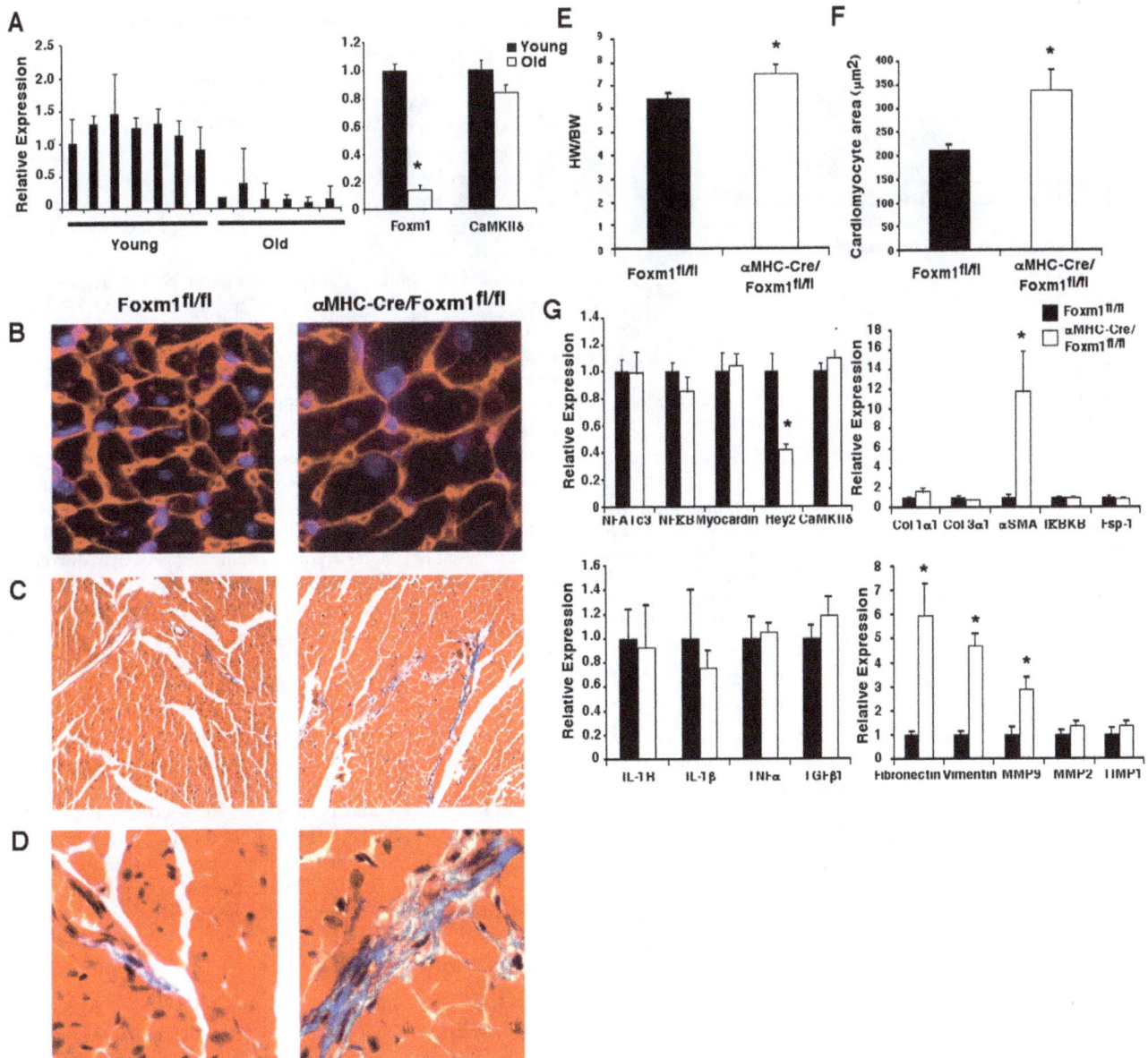

Figure 3. Cardiac hypertrophy and fibrosis in aged α*MHC-Cre/Foxm1*^fl/fl^ **mice.** Foxm1 mRNA was significantly decreased, while CaMKIIδ mRNA was unaltered, in hearts of old WT mice compared to young mice as shown by qRT-PCR (A). Old α*MHC-Cre/Foxm1*^fl/fl^ mice had significant cardiac hypertrophy as indicated by increased heart weight-to-body weight ratios (E) and increased cardiomyocyte area (F). Cardiomyocyte area was visualized and measured in WGA stained sections using 50 cardiomyocytes from random fields (B). Cardiac fibrosis was increased in old α*MHC-Cre/Foxm1*^fl/fl^ mice as shown by Masson's Trichrome staining (C, D). qRT-PCR analysis showed increased αSMA, fibronectin, vimentin and MMP9 and decreased Hey2 mRNA levels in hearts of old α*MHC-Cre/Foxm1*^fl/fl^ mice compared to age-matched control mice (G). Significant differences (p<0.05) were indicated by asterisk. "N" was 7 young and 6 old wildtype mice (A) and 6 control and 4 α*MHC-Cre/Foxm1*^fl/fl^ mice (E–G). Magnifications were 40x (B, D) and 10x (C).

Deletion of *Foxm1* in postnatal cardiomyocytes reduced mRNA of Plk-1, a known Foxm1 target gene [10,24], but did not significantly influence mRNA levels of cyclin B$_1$, CDC 25B, p21^cip1^, nMYC, myocardin, Hey2, NFATc3 or CaMKIIδ (Figure 1J). Thus *Foxm1* deletion in α*MHC-Cre/Foxm1*^fl/fl^ mice does not influence proliferation of cardiomyocytes in P7 hearts.

Normal cardiac morphology and function in adult α*MHC-Cre/Foxm1*^fl/fl^ mice

Cre expression was considerably higher in cardiomyocytes from adult (10–13 weeks) α*MHC-Cre/Foxm1*^fl/fl^ mice compared to P7

mice (Figures 1B & G & 2A). Few cardiomyocytes stained positively for FOXM1 in either line at this time point (Figure 2B & I), and there was no change in cardiomyocyte proliferation as demonstrated by Ki-67 staining (Figure 2C). Histological evaluation of α*MHC-Cre/Foxm1*^fl/fl^ mice showed no gross morphological alterations in right or left ventricular anatomy compared to control *Foxm1*^fl/fl^ littermates (Figure 2D) and heart weight-to-body weight ratios were similar (Figure 2J). Cardiomyocyte size (Figure 2F), capillary density (Figure 2G & K) and coronary vessel formation (Figure 2H) were also normal in α*MHC-Cre/Foxm1*^fl/fl^ mice.

A

B

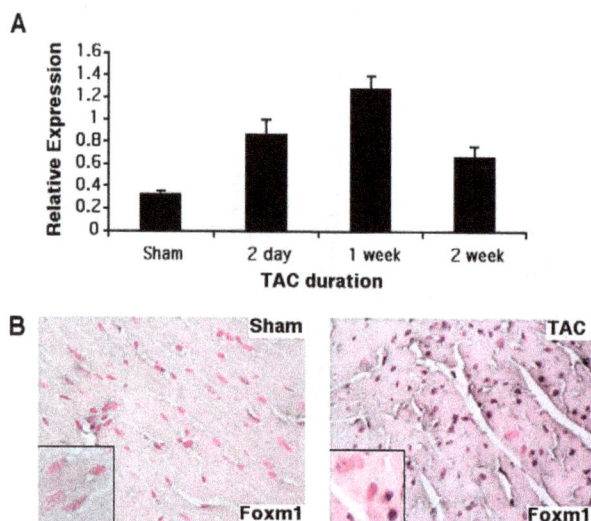

Figure 4. Foxm1 mRNA and protein increased following aortic banding. qRT-PCR showed increased whole-heart Foxm1 mRNA expression as early as 2 days after TAC surgery with levels peaking around a week post-surgery and remaining elevated for at least 2 weeks (A). The incidence of FOXM1-positive cardiomyocytes was increased 2 weeks after aortic banding as shown by immunostaining with FOXM1-specific antibodies (B). Magnifications were 40x (B) and 400x (B insets).

Furthermore, *in vivo* parameters of cardiac inotropy (+dP/dt) and lusitropy (−dP/dt) were indistinguishable between adult *αMHC-Cre/Foxm1$^{fl/fl}$* and control mice (Figure 2E). Nor was there a difference in sinus rhythm or greater occurrence of arrhythmia in *αMHC-Cre/Foxm1$^{fl/fl}$* compared to control mice (data not shown). Thus, postnatal deletion of *Foxm1* does not influence heart structure or function in adult mice.

Late onset cardiac hypertrophy in old *αMHC-Cre/Foxm1$^{fl/fl}$* mice

Foxm1 mRNA levels decreased in hearts of old (16 month) WT mice compared to young adult mice, while CaMKIIδ remained constant (Figure 3A). Cardiac structure was altered in old *αMHC-Cre/Foxm1$^{fl/fl}$* mice. Consistent with late onset cardiac hypertrophy, old *αMHC-Cre/Foxm1$^{fl/fl}$* mice had a significant increase in heart weight-to-body weight ratio compared to control mice (Figure 3E). Cardiomyocyte size in both ventricles in *Foxm1*-deficient hearts was increased by 60% as demonstrated by staining of heart sections with wheat-germ agglutinin (Figure 3B & F). In addition, increased myocardial fibrosis was observed by Masson's Trichrome staining in old *αMHC-Cre/Foxm1$^{fl/fl}$* hearts compared to age-matched controls (Figure 3C & D). Real-time RT-PCR analysis showed a decrease in Hey2 mRNA (Figure 3G), a transcription factor implicated in the development of cardiomyocyte hypertrophy [25,26]. Expression of genes critical for cardiac fibrosis, such as αSMA, fibronectin, vimentin and MMP9 was significantly increased in old *αMHC-Cre/Foxm1$^{fl/fl}$* hearts compared to age-matched controls. mRNAs of NFκB, NFATc3, myocardin, IL-1β, IL-1Rα, TNFα, TGFβ, MMP2, TIMP1, Fsp-1, IκBKB and CaMKIIδ were unaltered (Figure 3G). Thus Foxm1 is critical for proper maintenance of myocardial structure during aging.

Foxm1 expression in cardiomyocytes is not critical for TAC-induced cardiac hypertrophy

Experiments were performed to examine Foxm1 expression during pathological cardiac hypertrophy. Following aortic constriction in young WT mice, increased Foxm1 mRNA was observed as soon as 2 days and elevated levels were maintained for 14 days after injury (Figure 4A). FOXM1 protein was increased in several cell types including cardiomyocytes, endothelial and inflammatory cells 2 weeks after banding (Figure 4B and data not shown).

We next determined the specific role of Foxm1 in cardiomyocytes during TAC-mediated hypertrophy. *αMHC-Cre/Foxm1$^{fl/fl}$* and control mice at 8–10 weeks old were subjected to echocardiography prior to aortic banding as well as serially throughout the subsequent progression of cardiac hypertrophy. Based on echocardiography, there were no differences in left ventricular (LV) mass or fractional shortening between *αMHC-Cre/Foxm1$^{fl/fl}$* and control mice prior to aortic banding (Figure 5A & B). Aortic banding caused a significant increase in minimum and maximum aortic pressure in all mice, with no difference between control and *αMHC-Cre/Foxm1$^{fl/fl}$* mice (58.6±6.2 mmHg vs. 48.4±4.9 mmHg pressure gradient across constriction, respectively). Increased aortic pressure equally induced cardiac hypertrophy in both groups of mice, as evidenced by increased LV mass (Figure 5C & E), and decreased cardiac function, indicated by fractional shortening (Figure 5D & F). Heart weight-to-tibia length ratios (Figure 6D) and cardiomyocyte area (Figure 6C & E) were similar in *αMHC-Cre/Foxm1$^{fl/fl}$* and control mice. Cardiac fibrosis, as shown by Masson's Trichrome staining, was also similar between *Foxm1*-deficient and control mice (Figure 6A and B). *Foxm1* deletion did not alter mRNA expression of genes critical for cardiac hypertrophy and fibrosis such as α-SMA, collagen 1α1, CaMKIIδ, TNFα, BMP4, MMP9, CXCR4 and Hey2 (Figure 6F). Altogether, our results demonstrate that *Foxm1* expression in cardiomyocytes is critical for age-induced cardiac hypertrophy but it is not required for TAC-induced hypertrophy.

Discussion

We have previously shown that *Foxm1* is a critical mediator of heart development and cardiomyocyte proliferation. Total ablation of *Foxm1* in *Foxm1$^{-/-}$* mice [11] or conditional deletion in *Nkx2.5-Cre/Foxm1$^{fl/fl}$* mice [10] caused ventricular hypoplasia and embryonic lethality. However, the postnatal regulation of cardiac development by Foxm1 has not been investigated. In the present study, we generated a novel mouse line utilizing the Cre-LoxP system to selectively delete *Foxm1* from cardiomyocytes in the late postnatal period using the α-myosin heavy chain Cre (αMHC-Cre) [15]. *αMHC-Cre/Foxm1$^{fl/fl}$* mice were viable and healthy, displaying no heart abnormalities until old age. Despite a 70% decrease in Foxm1 mRNA and protein at P7, there was no change in the percentage of Ki-67-positive cardiomyocytes in *αMHC-Cre/Foxm1$^{fl/fl}$* hearts. Furthermore, the proliferation of Cre-positive and Cre-negative cardiomyocytes was similar, suggesting that Foxm1 does not regulate cardiomyocyte proliferation in the postnatal heart at P7. Consistent with this hypothesis, we found no differences between control and *αMHC-Cre/Foxm1$^{fl/fl}$* hearts in mRNA levels of cell cycle regulators such as cyclin B$_1$, CDC 25B, p21^{cip1} or nMYC. Interestingly, there was a significant decrease in Plk-1, a cell cycle regulator known to be transcriptionally regulated by Foxm1 [10,24]. Reduced expression of Plk-1 was insufficient to cause proliferation defects in *αMHC-Cre/Foxm1$^{fl/fl}$* hearts. As

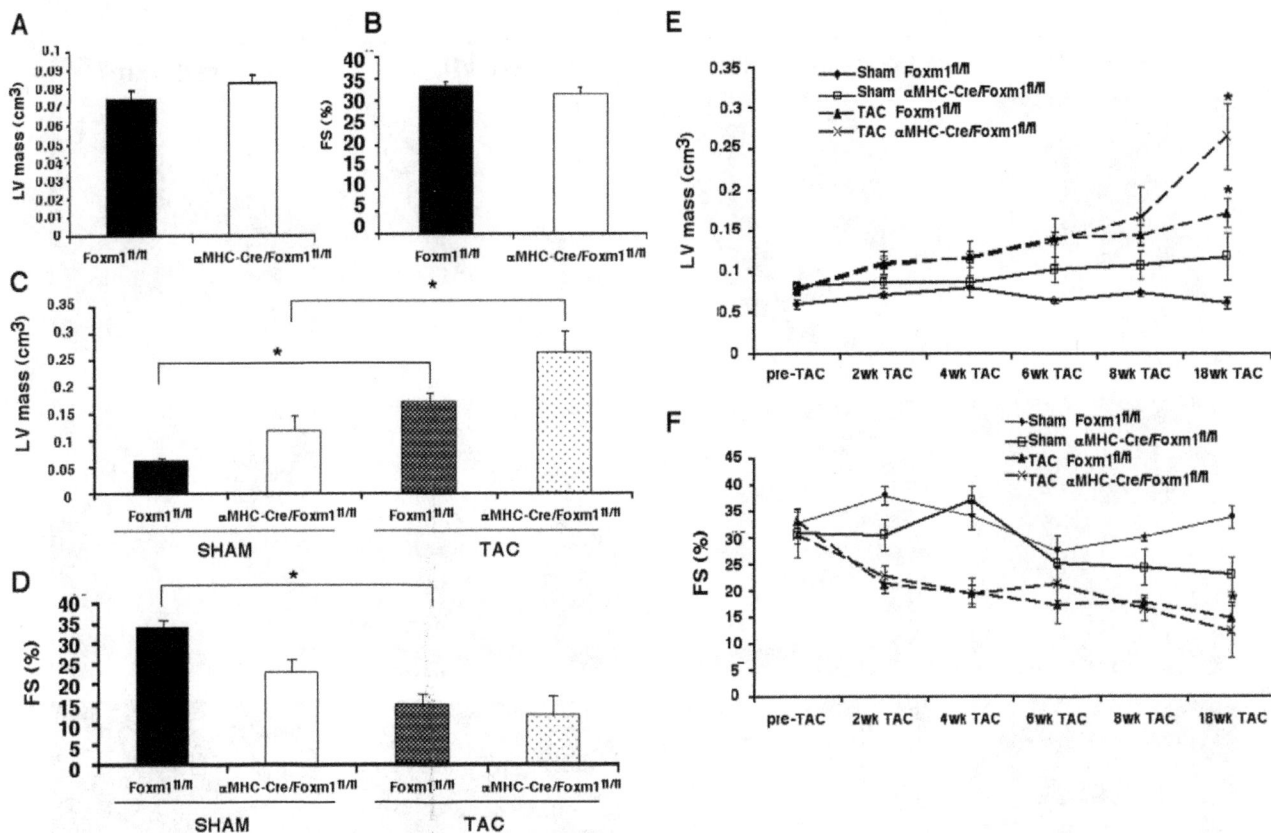

Figure 5. Foxm1 deficiency does not affect TAC-induced cardiac hypertrophy. *Foxm1$^{fl/fl}$* and *αMHC-Cre/Foxm1$^{fl/fl}$* mice were evaluated by echocardiography prior to aortic banding and serially throughout the development of cardiac hypertrophy. There was no difference between *Foxm1$^{fl/fl}$* and *αMHC-Cre/Foxm1$^{fl/fl}$* mice in LV mass (A) or fractional shortening (FS) prior to aortic banding (B). Aortic banding caused a significant increase in LV mass in mice from both lines without a difference between *Foxm1$^{fl/fl}$* and *αMHC-Cre/Foxm1$^{fl/fl}$* mice (C, E). Fractional shortening was decreased following aortic banding with no difference between lines (D, F). Sham surgery mice were used as control. Significant differences between TAC and Sham treated mice ($p<0.05$) were indicated by asterisk. "N" was 3 for all groups.

αMHC-Cre expression is low in the early postnatal period (P1-7) [15,27], our studies do not rule out the possibility that Foxm1 may be important for cardiomyocyte proliferation in the early postnatal period. Our results suggest different requirements for Foxm1 function between embryonic and postnatal cardiomyocytes.

Young adult *αMHC-Cre/Foxm1$^{fl/fl}$* mice had normal cardiac morphology and function; yet old age *αMHC-Cre/Foxm1$^{fl/fl}$* mice had a significant increase in heart weight-to-body weight ratios and cardiomyocyte size as well as myocardial fibrosis. Foxm1 expression has been previously shown to progressively decrease in fibroblasts from adult humans and to be down-regulated in fibroblasts from patients with Progeria syndrome, a rare disorder in which individuals prematurely show signs of aging including cardiovascular disease [8]. We showed here that Foxm1 expression was decreased in the hearts of old mice when compared to young adults. Cardiomyocyte hypertrophy in old *αMHC-Cre/Foxm1$^{fl/fl}$* mice was associated with decreased expression of Hey2, an important transcriptional regulator in cardiomyocytes [13,26,28,29]. We previously showed decreased Hey2 mRNA in *Nkx2.5-Cre/Foxm1$^{fl/fl}$* embryonic hearts which had enlarged cardiomyocytes [10]. These data indicate a genetic link between *Foxm1* and Hey2 that is persistent in the embryonic and adult heart. Since hearts of Hey2-deficient mice exhibited cardiomyocyte hypertrophy [13], decreased Hey2 expression may contribute to cardiac abnormalities in Foxm1-deficient myocardium. Our data also demonstrates that cardiomyocyte-derived Foxm1 is

dispensable for cardiac development in the late postnatal period, yet Foxm1 plays a critical role in cardiac maintenance in the older heart.

Given the essential role Foxm1 plays in embryonic cardiac development as well as the propensity for late onset cardiac hypertrophy in mice with cardiomyocyte-specific Foxm1 deletion, we investigated a potential role for Foxm1 in pressure overload-induced cardiac remodeling in young mice. Although aortic constriction increased Foxm1 mRNA and protein in cardiomyocytes of WT mice, there was no difference in cardiac hypertrophy or remodeling between *αMHC-Cre/Foxm1$^{fl/fl}$* and control mice. The gene expression profile was also unaltered between groups following prolonged pressure overload. Thus, Foxm1 expression in cardiomyocytes is not critical for pressure overload-induced cardiac hypertrophy in young mice.

Foxm1 is a known regulator of embryogenesis and has been shown to play tissue- and cell-type specific roles in different organs [7,14,19,30–37]. In this study, using *αMHC-Cre/Foxm1$^{fl/fl}$* mice we demonstrated that *Foxm1* is not essential for cardiac development in the late postnatal period into adulthood. Decreased Foxm1 expression at P7 did not alter cardiomyocyte proliferation as did embryonic deletion of Foxm1 from cardiomyocytes [10], suggesting an alternative role for Foxm1 in postnatal compared to embryonic cardiomyocytes. *αMHC-Cre/Foxm1$^{fl/fl}$* mice developed normally into adulthood with normal cardiac morphology and function; however, late in life these mice developed cardiac

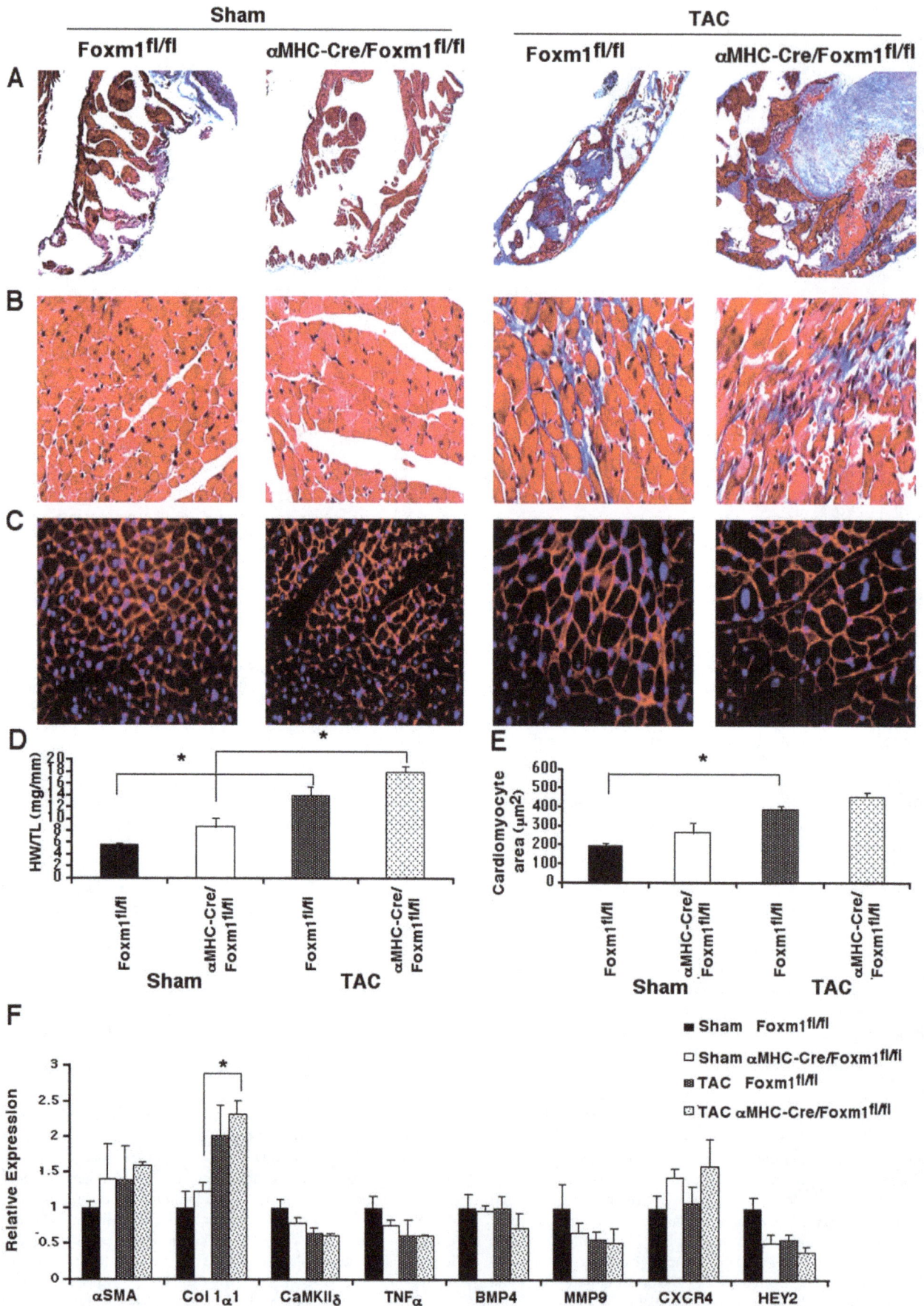

Figure 6. Cardiac remodeling is unaltered following TAC surgery in α*MHC-Cre/Foxm1*$^{fl/fl}$ mice. Masson's Trichrome staining of mice 18 weeks after aortic banding indicated fibrotic deposition in the atria (A) and ventricles (B) was similar between α*MHC-Cre/Foxm1*$^{fl/fl}$ and control mice. WGA staining showed cardiomyocyte size significantly increased following aortic banding with no difference between mouse lines (C, E). Heart weight-to-tibia length ratios were unaltered between α*MHC-Cre/Foxm1*$^{fl/fl}$ and control mice following TAC surgery (D). qRT-PCR showed an increase in collagen 1α1 mRNA following TAC (F). mRNA levels of αSMA, CaMKIIδ, TNFα, BMP4, MMP9, CXCR4 and Hey2 were unaltered. Significant differences ($p<0.05$) were indicated by asterisk. "N" was 3 for all groups. Magnifications were (A) 5x and (B, C) 20x.

hypertrophy and fibrosis. These results suggest that Foxm1 is essential for long-term maintenance of cardiac structure and function, as has been previously indicated in patients with Progeria syndrome [8]. It is becoming increasingly evident that cardiomyopathies can manifest at any developmental time point [38–41]. In fact, familial hypertrophic cardiomyopathy of known origin can result in strikingly different phenotypes and time of onset within a single family [39]. These findings indicate the heterogeneous nature of the disease and make it evident that multiple factors are involved in disease progression. However, mutations associated with the latest onset of disease phenotype are primarily in genes involved in sarcomere structure and not function [39,42]. These genes include the myosin binding protein C, troponin I [40], and members of the sarcoglycan family, particularly δ-sarcoglycan [42]. Furthermore, a number of muscular dystrophies have also been shown to present with cardiac abnormalities [3,4] and defects in other extracellular matrix proteins can result in cardiac aberrations similar to those observed here [4,5]. Therefore, it is quite possible that Foxm1 may regulate the transcription of a cardiac structural protein or extracellular matrix protein in the heart, the deficiency of which in α*MHC-Cre/Foxm1*$^{fl/fl}$ mice may not manifest structural or functional consequences until late in life. Alternatively, Foxm1 may be required for proliferation or differentiation of endogenous cardiac progenitor cells. This hypothesis is consistent with expression of Foxm1 in rare populations of cells in the adult heart. In the absence of Foxm1,

cardiac progenitors may not be able to compensate for the normal attrition of cardiomyocytes during the lifetime of the heart. As cells die and cannot be replaced by new cardiomyocytes the existing myocytes compensate by hypertrophying and the deficit between cardiomyocyte loss and existing cardiomyocyte hypertrophy is balanced by scar formation. The absence of Foxm1 may lead to impairment in cardiac maintenance, causing hypertrophy and fibrosis during aging. Despite a propensity for aging-mediated cardiac hypertrophy when cardiomyocyte-derived Foxm1 is absent, Foxm1 is not a mediator of the timeline or extent of cardiac hypertrophy or remodeling following aortic banding.

In summary, Foxm1 is not essential for postnatal cardiac development or cardiomyocyte proliferation after postnatal day 7 but plays an important role in maintenance of cardiac structure during aging. Mice with cardiomyocyte-specific deletion of *Foxm1* develop cardiac hypertrophy and fibrosis late in life. Our results demonstrate that Foxm1 function in cardiomyocytes is dependent on age and disease state.

Author Contributions

Conceived and designed the experiments: CB VVK. Performed the experiments: CB YZ AY JEJS. Analyzed the data: CB AY TVK JEJS VVK. Contributed reagents/materials/analysis tools: JDM TVK VVK. Wrote the paper: CB VVK.

References

1. Raju H, Alberg C, Sagoo GS, Burton H, Behr ER (2011) Inherited cardiomyopathies. BMJ 343: d6966.
2. Semsarian C (2011) Guidelines for the diagnosis and management of hypertrophic cardiomyopathy. Heart Lung Circ 20: 688–690.
3. Bowles NE, Towbin JA (1998) Molecular aspects of myocarditis. Curr Opin Cardiol 13: 179–184.
4. Gaschen L, Lang J, Lin S, Ade-Damilano M, Busato A, et al. (1999) Cardiomyopathy in dystrophin-deficient hypertrophic feline muscular dystrophy. J Vet Intern Med 13: 346–356.
5. Kapelko VI (2001) Extracellular matrix alterations in cardiomyopathy: The possible crucial role in the dilative form. Exp Clin Cardiol 6: 41–49.
6. Korver W, Roose J, Clevers H (1997) The winged-helix transcription factor Trident is expressed in cycling cells. Nucleic Acids Res 25: 1715–1719.
7. Ye H, Holterman AX, Yoo KW, Franks RR, Costa RH (1999) Premature expression of the winged helix transcription factor HFH-11B in regenerating mouse liver accelerates hepatocyte entry into S phase. Mol Cell Biol 19: 8570–8580.
8. Ly DH, Lockhart DJ, Lerner RA, Schultz PG (2000) Mitotic misregulation and human aging. Science 287: 2486–2492.
9. Wang X, Quail E, Hung NJ, Tan Y, Ye H, et al. (2001) Increased levels of forkhead box M1B transcription factor in transgenic mouse hepatocytes prevent age-related proliferation defects in regenerating liver. Proc Natl Acad Sci U S A 98: 11468–11473.
10. Bolte C, Zhang Y, Wang IC, Kalin TV, Molkentin JD, et al. (2011) Expression of Foxm1 transcription factor in cardiomyocytes is required for myocardial development. PLoS One 6: e22217.
11. Ramakrishna S, Kim IM, Petrovic V, Malin D, Wang IC, et al. (2007) Myocardium defects and ventricular hypoplasia in mice homozygous null for the Forkhead Box M1 transcription factor. Dev Dyn 236: 1000–1013.
12. Korver W, Schilham MW, Moerer P, van den Hoff MJ, Dam K, et al. (1998) Uncoupling of S phase and mitosis in cardiomyocytes and hepatocytes lacking the winged-helix transcription factor Trident. Curr Biol 8: 1327–1330.
13. Kokubo H, Miyagawa-Tomita S, Tomimatsu H, Nakashima Y, Nakazawa M, et al. (2004) Targeted disruption of hesr2 results in atrioventricular valve anomalies that lead to heart dysfunction. Circ Res 95: 540–547.
14. Krupczak-Hollis K, Wang X, Kalinichenko VV, Gusarova GA, Wang IC, et al. (2004) The mouse Forkhead Box m1 transcription factor is essential for

hepatoblast mitosis and development of intrahepatic bile ducts and vessels during liver morphogenesis. Dev Biol 276: 74–88.
15. Palermo J, Gulick J, Colbert M, Fewell J, Robbins J (1996) Transgenic remodeling of the contractile apparatus in the mammalian heart. Circ Res 78: 504–509.
16. Schultz Jel J, Witt SA, Glascock BJ, Nieman ML, Reiser PJ, et al. (2002) TGF-beta1 mediates the hypertrophic cardiomyocyte growth induced by angiotensin II. J Clin Invest 109: 787–796.
17. Nakayama H, Wilkin BJ, Bodi I, Molkentin JD (2006) Calcineurin-dependent cardiomyopathy is activated by TRPC in the adult mouse heart. FASEB J 20: 1660–1670.
18. Oka T, Maillet M, Watt AJ, Schwartz RJ, Aronow BJ, et al. (2006) Cardiac-specific deletion of Gata4 reveals its requirement for hypertrophy, compensation, and myocyte viability. Circ Res 98: 837–845.
19. Kalin TV, Wang IC, Meliton L, Zhang Y, Wert SE, et al. (2008) Forkhead Box m1 transcription factor is required for perinatal lung function. Proc Natl Acad Sci U S A 105: 19330–19335.
20. Kim IM, Zhou Y, Ramakrishna S, Hughes DE, Solway J, et al. (2005) Functional characterization of evolutionarily conserved DNA regions in forkhead box f1 gene locus. J Biol Chem 280: 37908–37916.
21. Kim IM, Ramakrishna S, Gusarova GA, Yoder HM, Costa RH, et al. (2005) The forkhead box m1 transcription factor is essential for embryonic development of pulmonary vasculature. J Biol Chem 280: 22278–22286.
22. Ustiyan V, Wang IC, Ren X, Zhang Y, Snyder J, et al. (2009) Forkhead box M1 transcriptional factor is required for smooth muscle cells during embryonic development of blood vessels and esophagus. Dev Biol 336: 266–279.
23. Wang IC, Meliton L, Ren X, Zhang Y, Balli D, et al. (2009) Deletion of Forkhead Box M1 transcription factor from respiratory epithelial cells inhibits pulmonary tumorigenesis. PLoS One 4: e6609.
24. Murakami H, Aiba H, Nakanishi M, Murakami-Tonami Y (2010) Regulation of yeast forkhead transcription factors and FoxM1 by cyclin-dependent and polo-like kinases. Cell Cycle 9: 3233–3242.
25. Liu Y, Yu M, Wu L, Chin MT (2010) The bHLH transcription factor CHF1/Hey2 regulates susceptibility to apoptosis and heart failure after pressure overload. Am J Physiol Heart Circ Physiol 298: H2082–2092.
26. Yu M, Liu Y, Xiang F, Li Y, Cullen D, et al. (2009) CHF1/Hey2 promotes physiological hypertrophy in response to pressure overload through selective

repression and activation of specific transcriptional pathways. OMICS 13: 501–511.

27. Ng WA, Grupp IL, Subramaniam A, Robbins J (1991) Cardiac myosin heavy chain mRNA expression and myocardial function in the mouse heart. Circ Res 68: 1742–1750.

28. Sakata Y, Koibuchi N, Xiang F, Youngblood JM, Kamei CN, et al. (2006) The spectrum of cardiovascular anomalies in CHF1/Hey2 deficient mice reveals roles in endocardial cushion, myocardial and vascular maturation. J Mol Cell Cardiol 40: 267–273.

29. Niessen K, Karsan A (2008) Notch signaling in cardiac development. Circ Res 102: 1169–1181.

30. Kalinichenko VV, Gusarova GA, Tan Y, Wang IC, Major ML, et al. (2003) Ubiquitous expression of the forkhead box M1B transgene accelerates proliferation of distinct pulmonary cell types following lung injury. J Biol Chem 278: 37888–37894.

31. Kalinichenko VV, Lim L, Shin B, Costa RH (2001) Differential expression of forkhead box transcription factors following butylated hydroxytoluene lung injury. Am J Physiol Lung Cell Mol Physiol 280: L695–704.

32. Ren X, Zhang Y, Snyder J, Cross ER, Shah TA, et al. (2010) Forkhead box M1 transcription factor is required for macrophage recruitment during liver repair. Mol Cell Biol 30: 5381–5393.

33. Schuller U, Zhao Q, Godinho SA, Heine VM, Medema RH, et al. (2007) Forkhead transcription factor FoxM1 regulates mitotic entry and prevents spindle defects in cerebellar granule neuron precursors. Mol Cell Biol 27: 8259–8270.

34. Xue L, Chiang L, He B, Zhao YY, Winoto A (2010) FoxM1, a forkhead transcription factor is a master cell cycle regulator for mouse mature T cells but not double positive thymocytes. PLoS One 5: e9229.

35. Zhang H, Ackermann AM, Gusarova GA, Lowe D, Feng X, et al. (2006) The FoxM1 transcription factor is required to maintain pancreatic beta-cell mass. Mol Endocrinol 20: 1853–1866.

36. Zhang H, Zhang J, Pope CF, Crawford LA, Vasavada RC, et al. (2010) Gestational diabetes mellitus resulting from impaired beta-cell compensation in the absence of FoxM1, a novel downstream effector of placental lactogen. Diabetes 59: 143–152.

37. Zhao YY, Gao XP, Zhao YD, Mirza MK, Frey RS, et al. (2006) Endothelial cell-restricted disruption of FoxM1 impairs endothelial repair following LPS-induced vascular injury. J Clin Invest 116: 2333–2343.

38. Maron BJ, Casey SA, Hauser RG, Aeppli DM (2003) Clinical course of hypertrophic cardiomyopathy with survival to advanced age. J Am Coll Cardiol 42: 882–888.

39. Niimura H, Bachinski LL, Sangwatanaroj S, Watkins H, Chudley AE, et al. (1998) Mutations in the gene for cardiac myosin-binding protein C and late-onset familial hypertrophic cardiomyopathy. N Engl J Med 338: 1248–1257.

40. Kubo T, Kitaoka H, Okawa M, Nishinaga M, Doi YL (2010) Hypertrophic cardiomyopathy in the elderly. Geriatr Gerontol Int 10: 9–16.

41. Ommen SR (2011) Hypertrophic cardiomyopathy. Curr Probl Cardiol 36: 409–453.

42. Sakamoto A, Ono K, Abe M, Jasmin G, Eki T, et al. (1997) Both hypertrophic and dilated cardiomyopathies are caused by mutation of the same gene, delta-sarcoglycan, in hamster: an animal model of disrupted dystrophin-associated glycoprotein complex. Proc Natl Acad Sci U S A 94: 13873–13878.

17

Garlic Attenuates Cardiac Oxidative Stress via Activation of PI3K/AKT/Nrf2-Keap1 Pathway in Fructose-Fed Diabetic Rat

Raju Padiya[1], Debabrata Chowdhury[2], Roshan Borkar[3], R. Srinivas[3], Manika Pal Bhadra[2], Sanjay K. Banerjee[1]*

[1] Division of Medicinal Chemistry and Pharmacology, Indian Institute of Chemical Technology, Hyderabad, India, [2] Division of Chemical Biology, Indian Institute of Chemical Technology, Hyderabad, India, [3] National Centre for Mass Spectrometry, Indian Institute of Chemical Technology, Hyderabad, India

Abstract

Background: Cardiovascular complication due to diabetes has remained a major cause of death. There is an urgent need to intervene the cardiac complications in diabetes by nutritional or pharmacological agents. Thus the present study was designed to find out the effectiveness of garlic on cardiac complications in insulin-resistant diabetic rats.

Methods and Results: SD rats were fed high fructose (65%) diet alone or along with raw garlic homogenate (250 mg/kg/day) or nutrient-matched (65% corn starch) control diet for 8 weeks. Fructose-fed diabetic rats showed cardiac hypertrophy, increased NFkB activity and increased oxidative stress. Administration of garlic significantly decreased ($p < 0.05$) cardiac hypertrophy, NFkB activity and oxidative stress. Although we did not observe any changes in myocardial catalase, GSH and GPx in diabetic heart, garlic administration showed significant ($p < 0.05$) increase in all three antioxidant/enzymes levels. Increased endogenous antioxidant enzymes and gene expression in garlic treated diabetic heart are associated with higher protein expression of Nrf2. Increased myocardial H_2S levels, activation of PI3K/Akt pathway and decreased Keap levels in fructose-fed heart after garlic administration might be responsible for higher Nrf2 levels.

Conclusion: Our study demonstrates that raw garlic homogenate is effective in reducing cardiac hypertrophy and fructose-induced myocardial oxidative stress through PI3K/AKT/Nrf2-Keap1 dependent pathway.

Editor: Tianqing Peng, University of Western Ontario, Canada

Funding: Financial support was provided by Department of Science and Technology (SR/S0/AS-18/2011), Ramalingaswami Fellowship, and CSIR (UNDO, BSC0103). The funders had no role in study design, data collection and analysis, decision to publish, or preparation of the manuscript.

Competing Interests: The authors have declared that no competing interests exist.

* E-mail: banerjees74@hotmail.com

Introduction

Type 2 diabetes mellitus is a major lifestyle disorder of the 21st century and associated with cardiac complications. Coronary artery diseases and hypertension are leading cause of death in diabetic patients. However, along with micro- and macro-vascular complication, heart failure due to cardiac dysfunction is very common with diabetes [1]. The pathogenesis of cardiac dysfunction associated with diabetes is due to insulin resistance and changes in different metabolic parameters. It is a big challenge for the researchers to investigate the molecular defects underling the cardiac changes and to find a way to prevent it,

High blood levels of insulin, free fatty acid and glucose as well as oxidative stress can alter important signalling pathways and may increase cardiovascular risk [2]. In our previous study we confirmed that high-fructose diet leads to insulin resistance and increased hepatic oxidative stress [3]. Metabolic complication and insulin resistance in fructose-fed rats can lead to cardiac complications such as oxidative stress and hypertrophy, and alter cellular structure and function. Cardiac hypertrophy and oxidative

stress has been observed previously in response to fructose feeding [4]. A causal role for oxidative stress in the development of cardiovascular complications in diabetes is increasingly recognized [5]. Similarly, a specific link between oxidative stress and insulin resistance is also well established [6].

Despite the availability of anti-diabetic drugs for the management of diabetes, cardiovascular complication is the leading cause of death in diabetic patients. Thus there is an urgent need to intervene the cardiac complications by nutritional or pharmacological agents. The anti-diabetic effect of garlic is well established in different animal models of type I as well as type II diabetes [7]. Despite the promising evidence of effectiveness of raw garlic in reducing hyperglycemia, little is known about its effectiveness for ameliorating cardiac complications in insulin-resistance diabetic animals.

Thus the present study was designed to investigate whether raw garlic can attenuate pathological changes on fructose fed type 2 diabetic heart and to find the molecular signalling pathway responsible for this beneficial effect.

Materials and Methods

Chemicals and antibodies

Garlic was purchased from local market Hyderabad, India. Antibodies like Anti-GAPDH, (IMG6665A) is from Imgenes, Anti-NFkB p50 (251563), Anti-NFkB p65 (C22B4) and Anti-Nrf2 (251445) are from Abbiotec, Anti- AKT (9272S), phospho-Akt (9271S), Anti-PI3K class III (D4E2) (3358S), Keap1 (8047S) are from Cell Signaling, phospho-PI3K (3332R) from Bioss and Anti-Lamin A MAB3540 from Millipore, Anti-Rabbit IgG-HRP and Anti-mouse IgG-HRP are from Santa Cruz. All other chemicals were obtained from Sigma, USA.

Preparation of garlic Homogenate

Garlic was purchased from local market Hyderabad, India. Individual bulbs were put in a grinder to form a juicy paste as described. The garlic homogenate was prepared freshly each day.

Determination of garlic constituent by LC/MS

The supernatant of garlic homogenate were filtered through 0.45 μm glass filter and diluted further to make appropriate solution. 20 μL was injected in LC-MS. The analysis was carried out on an Agilent 1200 series HPLC instrument (Agilent Technologies, USA) equipped with a quaternary pump (G13311A, USA), a de-gasser (G1322A, USA), a diode-array detector (G1315D, USA), an auto sampler (G1329A, USA) and a column compartment (G1316A, USA). Mass spectrometric detection was carried out on a quadrupole time-of-flight (Q-TOF) mass spectrometer (Q-TOF LC/MS 6510 series classic G6510A, Agilent Technologies, USA) equipped with an ESI source. The data acquisition was under the control of Mass Hunter workstation software. The typical operating source conditions for MS scan in positive ion ESI mode were optimized as follows; the fragmentor voltage was set at, 80 V; the capillary at, 3000–3500 V; the skimmer at, 60 V; nitrogen was used as the drying (300°C; 9 L/min) and nebulizing (45 psi) gas. For full scan MS mode, the mass range was set at m/z 100–2000. All the spectra were recorded under identical experimental conditions and are average of 20–25 scans.

Animals and Treatment

All animal experiments were undertaken with the approval of Institutional Animal Ethical Committee of Indian Institute of Chemical Technology (IICT), Hyderabad (Approval no. IICT/PHARM/SKB/11/08/10). Male Sprague-Dawley rats (200–250 gms) were purchased from the National Institute of Nutrition (NIN), Hyderabad, India. The animals were housed in BIOSAFE, an animal quarantine facility of the Indian Institute of Chemical Technology (IICT), Hyderabad, India. The animal house is maintained at temperature $22\pm2°C$ with relative humidity $50\pm15\%$ and 12 hour dark/light cycle throughout the study. Rats were randomly divided into three groups (n = 7). Control group (Control) was fed 65% corn starch diet (Research diet, USA), whereas diabetic group (Diabetic) was fed 65% fructose diet (Research diet, USA) for the induction of diabetes and associated metabolic [3]. The third group (Dia+Garl) was fed 65% fructose diet along with raw garlic homogenate (250 mg/kg) for a period of 8 weeks.

Sample collection and biochemical assay

The animals of all three groups were sacrificed after 8 weeks of study. Cardiac tissues were collected and stored at −80°C for further biochemical evaluation. Each heart tissue was homogenized with 20 times volume of heart weight in ice cold 0.05 M potassium phosphate buffer (pH-7.4) and treated separately for different measurements.

Estimation of heart weight/body weight ratio

In each group, heart weight/body weight ratio was measured on the day of sacrifice. Heart weight was measured after keeping the heart in ice cold saline and squeezing out the blood.

TBARS, Conjugated dienes and Nitric oxide

The extent of lipid peroxidation in hearts was determined by measuring malondialdehyde (MDA), conjugated dienes and nitric oxide. Malondialdehyde (MDA) content was determined according to modified method based on the reaction with thiobarbituric acid [8]. Data were expressed as nanomoles per gm heart weight using extinction co-efficient of 1.56×10^{-5} M^{-1} cm^{-1}. Conjugated dienes was also measured as a marker of lipid peroxidation by a biochemical method [8]. Nitric oxide, another marker of oxidative stress, was determined by a commercially available kit (Assay design, USA). Assay is based on reduction of NO_3^- into NO_2^- using nitrate reductase. The azo dye is produced by diazotization of sulfanilic acid (Griss Reagent-1) with NO_2^- and then subsequent coupling with N-(1-napthyl)-ethylene diamine (Griss Reagent-2). The azo dye was measured calorimetrically at 540 nm. NO level was expressed as μmol/gm heart.

Measurement of ROS

Reactive oxygen species (ROS) was measured fluorometrically in heart tissue homogenates using 2,7-dichlorofluorescein diacetate (DCF-DA). Briefly 100 μM of DCF-DA and tissue homogenate was incubated for 30 min at room temperature in dark. After incubation, the volume of the reaction was adjusted with phosphate buffer saline (PBS, 0.1 M, pH-7.4) and fluorescence was measured at 488 nm excitation and 525 nm emission wavelength. The data obtained was expressed as percentage of control [9].

NFkB Activity

The cardiac NFkB activity was determined by the kit obtained from Cayman Chemical (Cat. 10007889). This is a non-radioactive and sensitive method for detecting DNA-binding activity of NFkB obtained from tissue extracts.

Catalase, SOD, GSH and GPx

Catalase, GSH and GPx were measured by biochemical methods as described [10]. SOD activity in the myocardial homogenate was determined according to the standard assay kit (Fluka Analytical, Switzerland, Catalog No. 19160).

Hydrogen Sulphide (H₂S) and Protein estimation

H_2S concentration was measured as described earlier [3]. Briefly, 0.1 ml supernatant was added into a test tube containing 0.125 ml 1% zinc acetate and 0.15 ml distilled water. Then 0.067 ml 20 mM N, N-dimethyl-phenylene diamine dihydro chloride in 7.2M HCL was added. This was followed by addition of 0.067 ml 30 mM $FeCl_3$ in 1.2 M HCL. The absorbance of resulting solution was measured with a spectrophotometer at a wavelength of 670 nm. The H_2S concentration in a solution was calculated according to the calibration curve of sodium hydrogen sulphide (NaHS: 3.12–400 μmol) and data were expressed as H_2S concentration in μmol/gm heart. Protein concentrations were measured from heart supernatant [3].

Table 1. List of primer sequences for RT-PCR.

Gene	Primers	Sequence
ANP	Forward	5-GAGAAGATGCCGGTAGAAGA-3
	Reverse	5-AGAGCACCTCCATCTCTCTG-3
β-MHC	Forward	5-TGGAGCTGATGCACCTGTAG-3
	Reverse	5-ACTTCGTCTCATTGGGGATG-3
Nrf2	Forward	5-CAGTCTTCACCACCCCTGAT-3
	Reverse	5-GGTAGTCTCAGCCTGCTGCT-3
MnSOD	Forward	5-GAACCACAGGCCTTATTCCA-3
	Reverse	5-GGGCTTCACTTCACTTCTTGCAAAC-3
RPL32	Forward	5-AGATTCAAGGGCCAGATCCT-3
	Reverse	5-CGATGGCTTTTCGGTTCTTA-3

Gene expression

Total RNA was extracted from a piece of 0.2 g heart with Trizol (Sigma). Gene expression of ANP, β-MHC, Nrf2, KEAP and MnSOD were performed [8]. Briefly, cDNA was prepared from RNA and PCR was performed in a 0.2 ml tube containing 2 µl cDNA, 1 µl of (10 pmol) each forward and reverse primers, 2.0 µl of dNTP (1.25 mM each nucleotide), 2.5 µl of 10× PCR Buffer, 0.25 µl of Taq polymerase and 11.25 µl of dH_2O. After denaturizing at 95°C for 5 min, the whole mixture underwent PCR at 95°C for 60 seconds, 61°C (annealing temperature) for 60

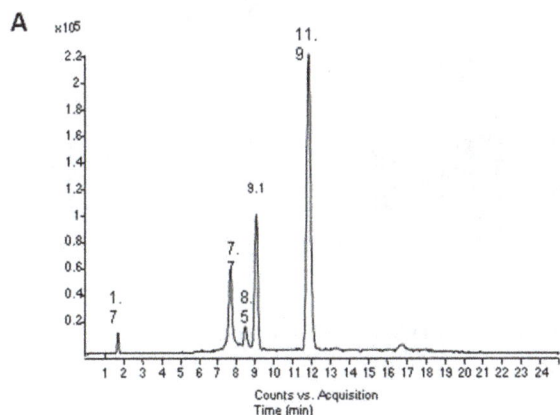

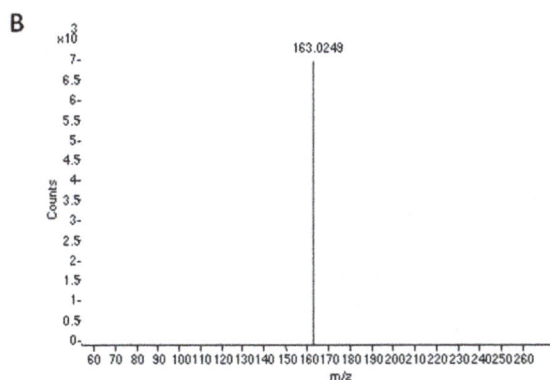

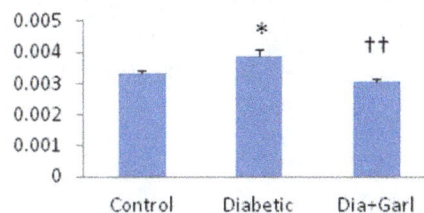

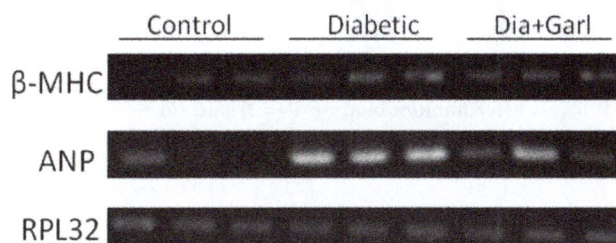

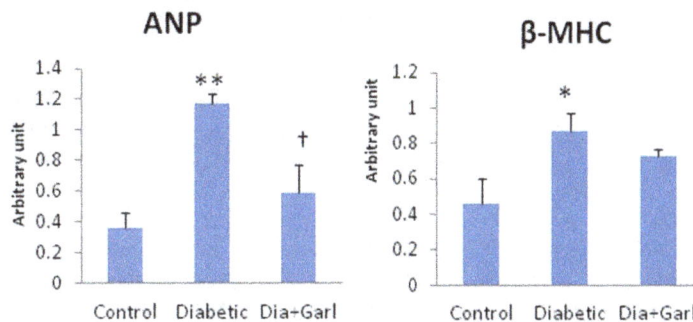

Figure 1. (A) LC-ESI-MS total ion chromatogram (TIC) of garlic extract (B) positive ion ESI-MS spectra of Allicin (m/z 163, Rt = 11.9 min). (C) Effect of garlic on heart weight body weight ratio (N = 7) and (D) β-MHC and ANP levels. (N = 3) *p<0.05, **p<0.01 vs. Control group; †p<0.05, ††p<0.01 vs. Diabetic group.

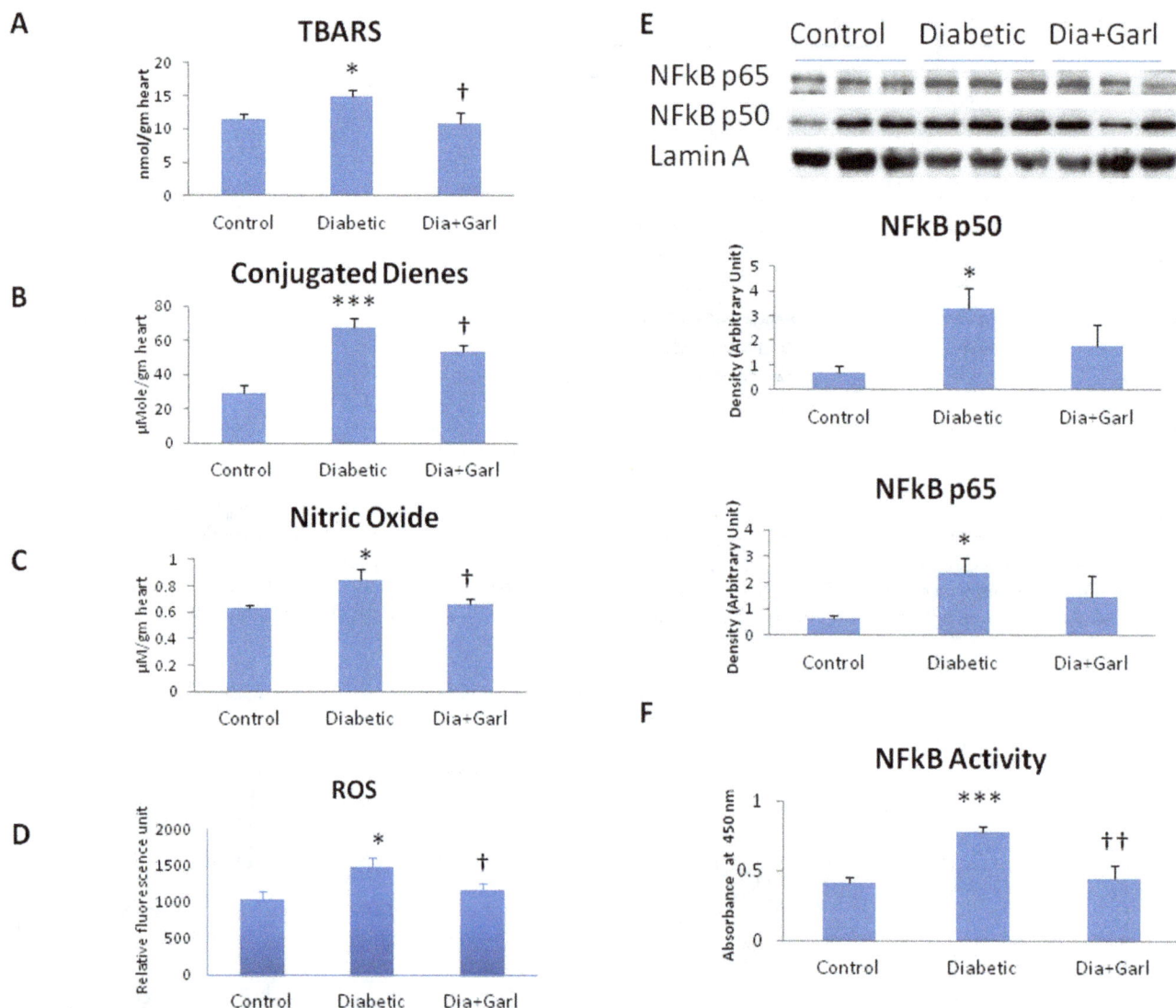

Figure 2. Effect of garlic on (A) TBARS levels, (B) Conjugated diens levels, (C) Nitric oxide levels (D) ROS generation (E) Nuclear NFkB levels after immunoblotting (N = 3) and (F) NFkB activity. (N = 7) *p<0.05, ***p<0.001 vs. Control group; †p<0.05, ††p<0.01 vs. Diabetic group.

seconds, 72°C for 60 seconds for 32 cycles. The PCR products were separated on 2% agarose gel stained with ethidium bromide. The optical density of bands was measured by using the Gel Documentation System. The analysis was based on reference gene RPL32. The sequence of the primers are summarised in Table 1.

Immunoblotting analysis

Separation of nuclear and cytoplasmic fraction was done by using Nuclear and Cytoplasmic Extraction Kit (Thermo Scientific) and whole heart protein for immunoblotting was prepared as described by Banerjee et al., 2010 [11]. Briefly, quantity of protein was measured by Bradford method. An equal amount (50 μg) of protein was separated by sodium dodecyl sulfate polyacrylamide gel electrophoresis (SDS-PAGE). After electrophoresis, protein was transferred to PVDF membranes (Amersham Biosciences). The membranes were then blocked by 5% non-fat dry milk in Tris-buffered saline Tween-20 (TBS-T; 10 mM Tris, pH 7.5, 150 Mm NaCl, 0.05% Tween-20) for 1 h, and subsequently washed and incubated with primary antibody p50NFkB and p65NFkB (1:1000

dilution, Abbiotec) in TBS-T and 5% non-fat dry milk at 4°C overnight. After washing with TBS-T, membranes were incubated with anti-rabbit horseradish peroxidase conjugated secondary antibody (1:1500 dilutions, Amersham) for 1 h. Signal was detected by chemiluminescence using the ECL detection system (Amersham). The same procedure was repeated for P-PI3K (1:1000, Bioss), PI3K (1:1000, Cell signalling), P-AKT (1:1000, Cell Signaling), AKT (1:1000, Cell Signalling), Nrf2 (1:300 dilution, Abbiotec), Keap1 (1:1000, Cell Signaling), Lamin A 1:500 (Millipore) and GAPDH (1:1000, Imgenes). Gel staining with coomassie blue was used as an internal control for equal loading of protein. Quantification of bands was performed using Image J Software (NIH).

Statistical analysis

All values are expressed as mean ± SEM. Data were statistically analysed using one way ANOVA for multiple group comparison, followed by student unpaired 't' test for group wise comparison. Significance was set at P<0.05.

A

Catalase level

B

SOD activity

C

GSH level

D

GPx level

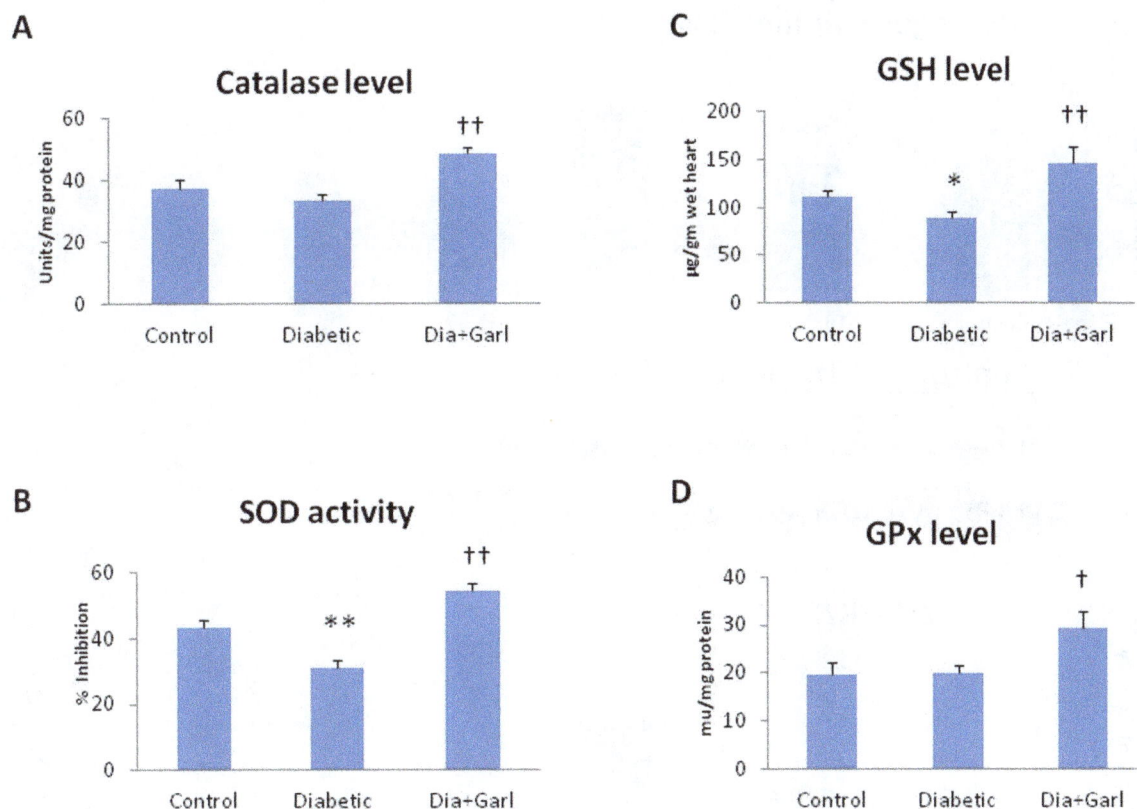

Figure 3. Effect of garlic on myocardial (A) Catalase activity, (B) SOD activity, (C) GSH levels and (D) GPx activity. (N = 7) *p<0.05, **p<0.01 vs. Control group; †p<0.05, ††p<0.01 vs. Diabetic group.

Results

Determination of allicin and other garlic constituent by LC/MS

The separated components of garlic are γ-glutamyl-S-allyl-L-cysteine (Rt1.7 min, 291 m/z); Alliin (Rt 7.7 min, 178 m/z); S-Allyl-l-cysteine, deoxyalliin (Rt 8.5 min, 162 m/z); Vinyldithiin (Rt 9.1 min, 145 m/z); Allicin (Rt 11.9 min, 163 m/z) (Fig. 1A). The total ion chromatogram (TIC) and MS/MS spectrum of protonated allicin are given in Figs. 1A and 1B respectively.

Cardiac Hypertrophy

A significant (p<0.05) increase in heart/body weight ratio as well as β-MHC and ANP gene expression was observed in diabetic group compared to control group. However, significant (p<0.05) decrease in heart/body weight ratio and ANP gene expression was observed in garlic treated (Dia+Garl) group compared to diabetic group (Fig.1C & 1D).

TBARS, Conjugated dienes and Nitric Oxide

A significant (p<0.05) increase in TBARS, conjugated dienes and nitric oxide levels was observed in diabetic group in comparison to control group. However, significant (p<0.05) decrease in all three oxidative stress parameters was observed in garlic treated diabetic (Dia+Garl) group (Fig.2A, 2B, 2C).

ROS Generation

A significant (p<0.05) increase in ROS levels was observed in diabetic group in comparison to control group. However,

significant (p<0.05) decrease in ROS levels was observed in garlic treated diabetic (Dia+Garl) group (Fig.2D).

Protein expression and activity of NFkB

A significant (p<0.05) increase in p50 and p65 subunit of NFkB levels was observed in diabetic group in comparison to control group. Although, decrease in NFkB levels was observed in garlic treated diabetic (Dia+Garl) group compared to diabetic group, it was not significant (Fig.2E). However, enhanced NFkB activity that observed in diabetic heart was decreased significantly (p<0.05) in garlic treated diabetic (Dia+Garl) group (Fig. 2F).

Catalase, SOD, GSH, GPx and H₂S

There was no change in myocardial catalase and GPx activity in diabetic group compared to control group. However, a significant (p<0.05) increase in myocardial catalase and GPx activity was observed in garlic treated diabetic (Dia+Garl) group compared to diabetic group (Fig. 3A & 3D).

A significant (p<0.05) decrease in myocardial SOD activity, GSH and H₂S levels was observed in diabetic group compared to control group. However, there was significant (p<0.01) increase in all parameters observed in garlic treated diabetic (Dia+Garl) group compared to diabetic group (Fig. 3B, 3C & 4A).

Gene expression

Although an increase in Nrf2 expression was observed in both diabetic and garlic treated diabetic (Dia+Garl) group in comparison to control group but it was not significant. A significant (p<0.05) increase in MnSOD expression was observed in diabetic group compared to control group. Further increase (p<0.05) in

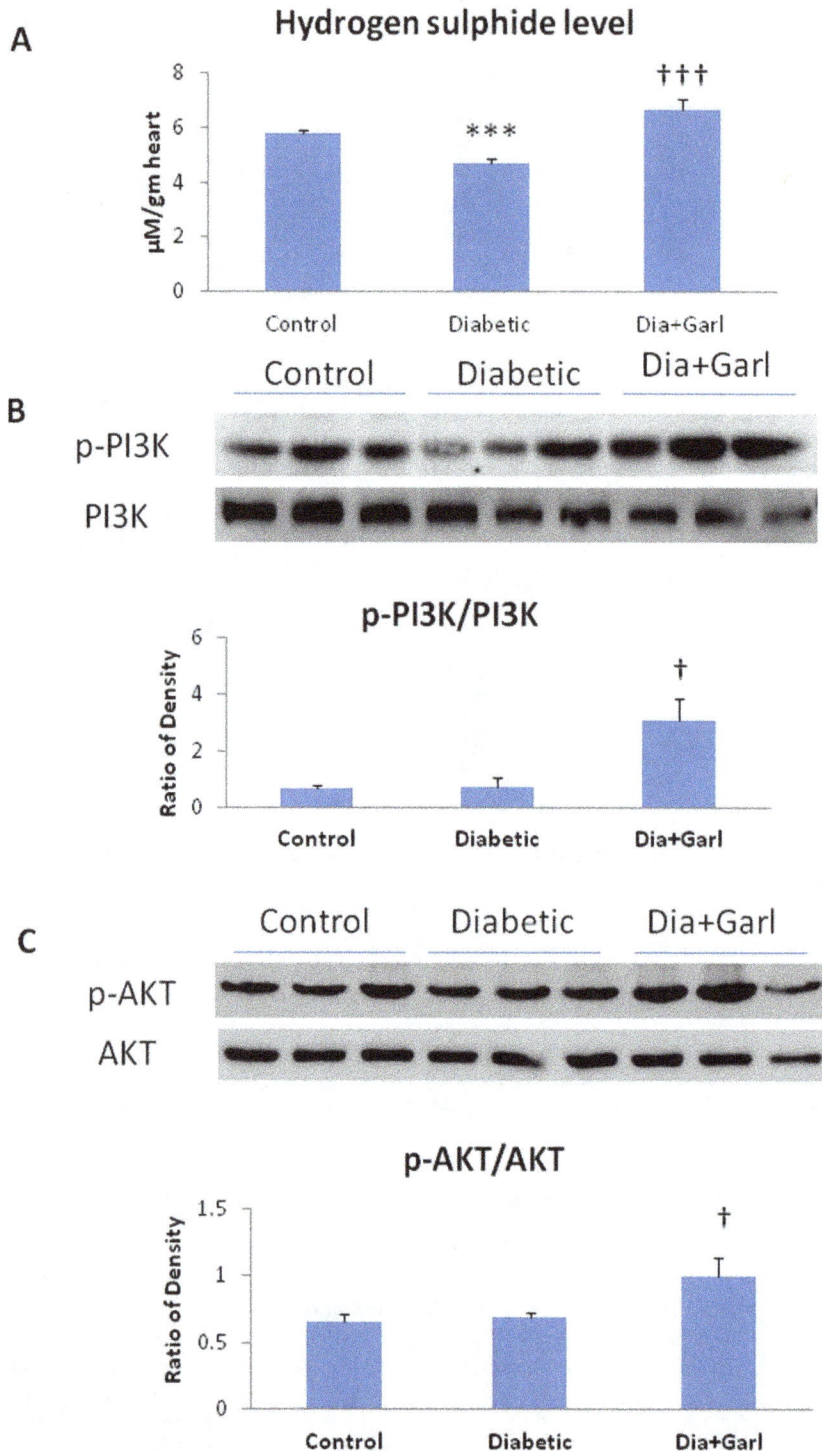

Figure 4. Effect of garlic on (A) myocardial H₂S levels (N = 7), (B) Immunoblotting of p-PI3K and PI3K, and their ratio (N = 3) (C) immunoblotting of p-AKT and total AKT, and their ratio (N = 3). ***p<0.001 vs. Control group; †p<0.05, †††p<0.001 vs. Diabetic group.

MnSOD expression was observed in garlic treated diabetic (Dia+Garl) group compared to diabetic group (Fig. 5B).

Immunoblotting

Although the ratio of p-PI3K/PI3K and p-AKT/AKT were not changed in diabetic group compared to control group, significant (p<0.05) increase in both ratio was observed in garlic treated (Dia+Garl) group compared to diabetic group (Fig. 4B & 4C). Nrf2 protein levels were significantly (p<0.01) increased in both diabetic and garlic treated (Dia+Garl) groups compared to control group (Fig. 5A). Keap1 protein levels were increased (p< 0.05) in diabetic group compared to control group and decreased in garlic treated diabetic (Dia+Garl) group compared to diabetic group (Fig. 5A).

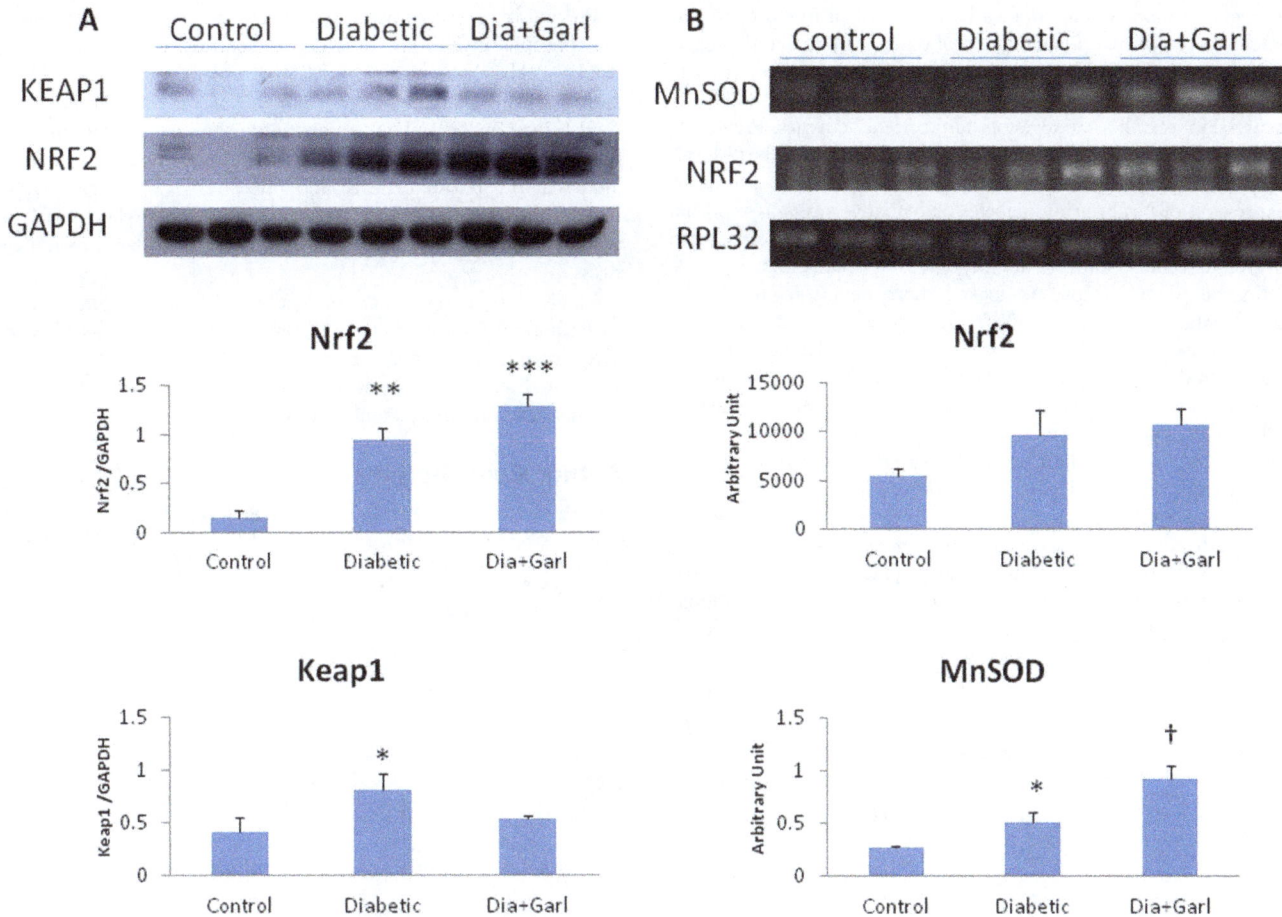

Figure 5. Effect of garlic on (A) immunoblotting of Nrf2 and Keap1, and (B) gene expression of Nrf2 and MnSOD. (N = 3) *p<0.05, **p<0.01, ***p<0.001 vs. Control group; †p<0.05 vs. Diabetic group.

Discussion

High fructose-induced insulin resistance is associated with an overproduction of superoxide anion in aorta and heart, and promotes cardiovascular alterations such as hypertension, vascular disorder and cardiac hypertrophy [12]. Vascular and cardiac hypertrophy was associated with ROS generation at different times after the initiation of fructose-enriched diet [13]. We observed significant increase in heart weight and body weight ratio, and higher expression of ANP and β-MHC in fructose fed diabetic rat heart. However, administration of raw garlic (rich with allicin) in fructose-fed rats normalised the cardiac hypertrophy along with hypertrophic gene expression. To confirm the presence of allicin we have done LC-MS study. Our data indicated that the raw garlic homogenate that used for the present study was rich with allicin and other compounds like γ-glutamyl-S-allyl-L-cysteine, Alliin, S-Allyl-l-cysteine, deoxyalliin and Vinyldithiin. Previously, allicin, γ-glutamyl-S-allyl-L-cysteine and S-allyl cysteine were reported to have antioxidant property by direct or indirect effect [14]. However, the molecular mechanism behind the beneficial/antioxidant effect of raw garlic was not investigated in heart.

In the present study, high fructose feeding increased oxidative stress as evidenced by elevation of myocardial conjugated dienes, TBARS and cardiac nitric oxide levels, and reduced the myocardial endogenous antioxidants like GSH and SOD.

Increased myocardial oxidative stress in fructose-fed rats may also responsible for increased NFkB activity. Increased activity of NFkB provides a molecular mechanism responsible for inflammation and insulin resistance in type 2 diabetes mellitus under basal conditions [15]. Similarly, we also observed increased NFkB activity along with significant increase in nuclear p50 and p65 NFkB protein in diabetic heart. However, administration of raw garlic extract reduced the NFkB activity as well as p50 and p65 NFkB protein levels in diabetic heart.

The present study showed that freshly prepared homogenate of garlic increased H_2S levels and reverses cardiac pathological changes in fructose-fed insulin resistance rats. Previously, it has been shown that fresh raw garlic homogenate generates H_2S after interaction with in cellular proteins [16]. It has already been reported that H_2S scavenge ROS directly, and activates endogenous antioxidant defences [17]. H_2S reduced oxidative stress in the heart through Nrf2-dependent pathway [18]. Nrf2 is a transcription factors, modulates the gene expression of a number of enzymes including Mn-superoxide dismutase (Mn-SOD) and GPx that serve to detoxify pro-oxidative stressors [18]. Our present study showed that garlic administration increased myocardial Nrf2 expression in fructose fed rat. Increased Nrf2 was also associated with increased myocardial MnSOD expression. Along with Mn-SOD gene expression, garlic administration significantly increased myocardial GSH levels and myocardial SOD, catalase and GPx activity. We believe that increased Nrf2 levels along with endogenous antioxidant after garlic treatment in fructose-fed rats might be responsible for reduction of oxidative stress and cardiac hypertrophy. Although, Nrf2 expression was slightly increased in fructose-fed heart, there was no increase in myocardial Mn-SOD expression as well as endogenous antioxidant activities. Previously it was reported that mild injury or stress can augment Nrf2 levels without increasing antioxidant status [19]. Thus increased expression of Nrf2 during diabetes or oxidative stress as reported previously and in the present study is an adaptive change to overcome cellular damage at early stages of cellular injury.

In the present study, we looked more details regarding the translocation mechanism of Nrf2. In response to oxidative stress, Nrf2 easily dissociates from its repressor protein-Keap, translocates into the nucleus, binds to antioxidant response elements and transactivates the genes of detoxifying and antioxidant enzymes [20]. Significant increase in keap1 expression was observed in fructose fed rat heart. This indicates that Nrf2 was more associated with Keap1 and thus less translocation of Nrf2 in the nucleus to activate antioxidant gene expression. However, administration of raw garlic decreased the keap1 protein expression along with higher Nrf2 expression. Both effects together may increase the nuclear translocation of Nrf2, enhance the expression of antioxidant gene (MnSOD) and increase the endogenous antioxidant activities.

Previously, garlic showed neuroprotective effect by activating the phosphatidylinositol 3-kinase–dependent pathway (PI3K/AKT) [21]. The phosphatidylinositol 3-kinase (PI3K)/AKT pathway plays a major role in cell survival and also required for Nrf2 activation [22]. The present study showed that administration of garlic homogenate in fructose fed rats significantly increased the phospho-PI3K and phospho-AKT protein levels. Increased ratio of p-AKT/AKT might phosphorylate Nrf2 to activate its antioxidant activity and protect heart from oxidative stress.

In conclusion, our study showed that administration of raw garlic homogenate in insulin resistance fructose fed rat activated myocardial Nrf2 through H_2S and PI3K/AKT pathway, and attenuated cardiac hypertrophy and oxidative stress through augmentation of antioxidant defense system.

Author Contributions

Conceived and designed the experiments: SKB RS MPB. Performed the experiments: RP DC RB. Analyzed the data: RP RB RS MPB SKB. Contributed reagents/materials/analysis tools: RS MPB SKB. Wrote the paper: RP SKB.

References

1. Rubler S, Dlugash J, Yuceoglu YZ, Kumral T, Branwood AW, et al. (1972) New type of cardiomyopathy associated with diabetic glomerulosclerosis. *Am J Cardiol*; 30: 595–602.
2. Ceriello A, Quagliaro L, D'Amico M, Di Filippo C, Marfella R, et al. (2002) Acute hyperglycemia induces nitrotyrosine formationand apoptosis in perfused heart from rat. *Diabetes*; 51: 1076–82.
3. Padiya R, Khatua TN, Bagul PK, Kuncha M, Banerjee SK (2011) Garlic improves insulin sensitivity and associated metabolic syndromes in fructose fed rats. *Nutr Metab*; 8: 53.
4. Delbosc S, Paizanis E, Magous R, Araiz C, Dimo T, et al. (2005) Involvement of oxidative stress and NADPH oxidase activation in the development of cardiovascular complications in a model of insulin resistance, the fructose-fed rat. *Atherosclerosis*; 179: 43–49.
5. Jay D, Hitomi H, Griendling KK (2006) Oxidative stress and diabetic cardiovascular complications. *Free Radic Biol Med*; 40: 183–92.
6. Giacco F, Brownlee M (2010) Oxidative stress and diabetic complications. *Circ Res*; 107: 1058–70.
7. Padiya R, Banerjee SK (2013) Garlic as an anti-diabetic agent: recent progress and patent reviews. Recent Pat Food Nutr Agric; 5: 105–27.
8. Bagul PK, Middela H, Matapally S, Padiya R, Bastia T, et al. (2012) Attenuation of insulin resistance, metabolic syndrome and hepatic oxidative stress by resveratrol in fructose-fed rats. *Pharmacol Res*; 66: 260–68.
9. Maity P, Bindu S, Dey S, Goyal M, Alam A, et al. (2009) Indomethacin, a non-steroidal anti-inflammatory drug, develops gastropathy by inducing reactive oxygen species-mediated mitochondrial pathology and associated apoptosis in gastric mucosa: a novel role of mitochondrial aconitase oxidation. *J Biol Chem*. 284: 3058–68.
10. Banerjee SK, Dinda AK, Manchanda SC, Maulik SK (2002) Chronic garlic administration protects rat heart against oxidative stress induced by ischemic reperfusion injury. BMC Pharmacol; 16; 2: 16.
11. Banerjee SK, Wang DW, Alzamora R, Huang XN, Pastor-Soler NM, et al. (2010) SGLT1, a novel cardiac glucose transporter, mediates increased glucose uptake in PRKAG2 cardiomyopathy. *J Mol Cell Cardiol*; 49: 683–92.
12. Delbosc S, Paizanis E, Magous R, Araiz C, Dimo T, et al. (2005) Involvement of oxidative stress and NADPH oxidase activation in the development of cardiovascular complications in a model of insulin resistance, the fructose-fed rat. *Atherosclerosis*; 179: 43–49.
13. Zhang J, Zhang BH, Yu YR, Tang CS, Qi YF (2011) Adrenomedullin protects against fructose-induced insulin resistance and myocardial hypertrophy in rats. *Peptides*; 32: 1415–21.
14. Banerjee SK, Mukherjee PK, Maulik SK (2003) The antioxidant effect of garlic. The good, the bad and the ugly. *Phytotherapy Res*. 17: 1–10.
15. Zhang X, Dong F, Ren J, Driscoll MJ, Culver B (2005) High dietary fat induces NADPH oxidase-associated oxidative stress and inflammation in rat cerebral cortex. *Exp Neurol*; 191: 318–25.
16. Das DK (2007) Hydrogen sulfide preconditioning by garlic when it starts to smell. *Am J Physiol Heart Circ Physiol*; 293:H2629–30.
17. Calvert JW, Coetzee WA, Lefer DJ (2010) Novel insights in to hydrogen sulfide-mediated cytoprotection. *Antioxid Redox Signal*; 12: 1203–17.
18. Calvert JW, Jha S, Gundewar S, Elrod JW, Ramachandran A, et al. (2009) Hydrogen sulfide mediates cardioprotection through Nrf2 signaling. *Circ Res*; 105: 365–74.
19. Erejuwa OO, Sulaiman SA, AbWahab MS, Sirajudeen KN, Salleh S, et al. (2012) Honey supplementation in spontaneously hypertensive rats elicits antihypertensive effect via amelioration of renal oxidative stress. *Oxid Med Cell Longev*; 2012: 374037.
20. Palsamy P, Subramanian S (2011) Resveratrol protects diabetic kidney by attenuating hyperglycemia-mediated oxidative stress and renal inflammatory cytokines via Nrf2–Keap1 signaling. *Biochim Biophys Acta*; 1812: 719–31.
21. Milner JA (2006) Preclinical perspectives on garlic and cancer. *J Nutr*; 136: 827S–831S.
22. Wang L, Chen Y, Sternberg P, Cai J (2008) Essential roles of the PI3 kinase/Akt pathway in regulating Nrf2-dependent antioxidant functions in the RPE. *Invest Ophthalmol Vis Sci*; 49: 1671-78.

18

The Huntington's Disease-Related Cardiomyopathy Prevents a Hypertrophic Response in the R6/2 Mouse Model

Michal Mielcarek*, Marie K. Bondulich, Linda Inuabasi, Sophie A. Franklin, Thomas Muller¤, Gillian P. Bates*

Department of Medical and Molecular Genetics, King's College London, London, United Kingdom

Abstract

Huntington's disease (HD) is neurodegenerative disorder for which the mutation results in an extra-long tract of glutamines that causes the huntingtin protein to aggregate. It is characterized by neurological symptoms and brain pathology that is associated with nuclear and cytoplasmic aggregates and with transcriptional deregulation. Despite the fact that HD has been recognized principally as a neurological disease, there are multiple epidemiological studies showing that HD patients exhibit a high rate of cardiovascular events leading to heart failure. To unravel the mechanistic basis of cardiac dysfunction in HD, we employed a wide range of molecular techniques using the well-established genetic R6/2 mouse model that develop a considerable degree of the cardiac atrophy at end stage disease. We found that chronic treatment with isoproterenol, a potent beta-adrenoreceptor agonist, did not change the overall gross morphology of the HD murine hearts. However, there was a partial response to the beta-adrenergic stimulation by the further re-expression of foetal genes. In addition we have profiled the expression level of *Hdacs* in the R6/2 murine hearts and found that the isoproterenol stimulation of *Hdac* expression was partially blocked. For the first time we established the *Hdac* transcriptional profile under hypertrophic conditions and found 10 out of 18 *Hdacs* to be markedly deregulated. Therefore, we conclude that R6/2 murine hearts are not able to respond to the chronic isoproterenol treatment to the same degree as wild type hearts and some of the hypertrophic signals are likely attenuated in the symptomatic HD animals.

Editor: Xiao-Jiang Li, Emory University, United States of America

Funding: This work was supported by the CHDI Foundation, a not-for-profit biomedical research organization exclusively dedicated to discovering and developing therapeutics that slow the progression of Huntington's disease. Research conducted at King's College London was performed in collaboration with and funded by the CHDI Foundation. In these cases, the funder, through CHDI Management, fully participated in study design, data collection and analysis, the decision to publish, and preparation of the manuscript. TM is currently an employee of Affimed Therapeutics AG. Affimed Therapeutics AG provided no support for this work. They did not provide salary support for TM when he was working at King's College London and they did not have any role in the study design, data collection and analysis, decision to publish, or preparation of the manuscript. The specific roles of the authors is articulated in the 'author contributions' section.

Competing Interests: TM is an employee of Affimed Therapeutics AG. There are no patents, products in development, or marketed products to declare.

* Email: michal.mielcarek@kcl.ac.uk (MM); gillian.bates@kacl.ac.uk (GPB)

¤ Current address: Affimed Therapeutics AG, Heidelberg, Germany

Introduction

Huntington's disease (HD) is an inherited neurodegenerative disorder caused by the expansion of a polyglutamine (polyQ) stretch within the huntingtin protein (HTT) [1]. The core features of HD are mainly neurological with a wide-spread brain pathology that is associated with the accumulation of toxic mutant huntingtin aggregate species [2]. In addition, HD is also characterised by peripheral pathological processes such as cardiac failure, weight loss and skeletal muscle atrophy [3,4]. This might be explained by the ubiquitous expression of HTT and its fundamental biological functions in many cellular processes [2,5,6]. HTT is predicted to form an elongated superhelical solenoid structure due to a large number of HEAT motifs suggesting that it plays a scaffolding role for protein complex formation [6]. More than 200 HTT interaction partners have been identified which can be classified based on their function and include proteins that are involved in gene transcription, intracellular signalling, trafficking, endocytosis, and metabolism [7].

There are a number of factors to indicate that HD patients experience an HD-related heart pathology reviewed by Sassone et al [3]. This has been supported by multiple epidemiological studies that identified heart disease as the second cause of death in patients with HD [8–10]. A proof of concept study with an artificial transgenic mouse model expressing either a mutant polyQ peptide of 83 glutamines (PQ83) or a control peptide of 19 glutamines (PQ19), under the control of the α-myosin heavy chain promoter (MyHC) to drive cardiomyocyte-specific expression, showed a severe cardiac dysfunction and dilation leading to a reduced lifespan [11]. HD mouse models include the R6/2 and R6/1 lines, that are transgenic for a mutated N-terminal exon 1 HTT fragment [12] and the *Hdh*Q150 line in which an expanded

CAG repeat has been knocked into the mouse *Htt* gene [13,14]. Many pre-clinical studies have supported the hypothesis that mouse models of HD do indeed develop a cardiac dysfunction [15–18]. It has been demonstrated that R6/2 mice developed cardiac dysfunction by 8 weeks of age progressing to severe heart failure at 12 weeks with significant alterations in mitochondrial ultrastructure and increased levels of cardiac lysine acetylation [16]. In the HD symptomatic animals, pronounced functional changes have been previously showed by cardiac MRI revealing a contractile dysfunction, which might be a part of dilated cardiomyopathy (DCM). This was accompanied by the re-expression of foetal genes, apoptotic cardiomyocyte loss and a moderate degree of interstitial fibrosis but occurred in the absence of either mutant HTT aggregates in cardiac tissue or an HD-specific transcriptional deregulation.

R6/1 mice have also been shown to develop unstable R–R intervals that were reversed following atropine treatment, suggesting parasympathetic nervous activation, as well as brady- and tachyarrhythmias, including paroxysmal atrial fibrillation and sudden death. Collectively, R6/1 mice exhibited profound cardiac dysfunction related to autonomic nervous system that may be related to altered central autonomic pathways [17]. A recent study in the R6/2 and *Hdh*Q150 knock-in mouse models showed that the HD-related cardiomyopathy is caused by altered central autonomic pathways and was not due to the accumulation of toxic HTT aggregates as had previously been anticipated [11,18].

In this study, we took advantage of the well-characterised beta-adrenergic agonist, isoproterenol. Chronic administration isoproterenol has been used in animals to study the mechanism of cardiac hypertrophy and failure [19]. Chronic infusion of isoproterenol has been reported to induce left ventricular hypertrophy accompanied by myocardial necrosis, apoptosis and fibrosis. Chronic isoproterenol infusion elicits alterations in cardiac gene expression that are consistent with the development of myocyte hypertrophy [20,21]. Sympathetic nervous activation is a crucial compensatory mechanism in heart failure. However, excess catecholamine may induce cardiac dysfunction and beta-adrenergic desensitization [20,21]. Altered alpha- and beta-adrenergic receptor signalling is associated with cardiac hypertrophy and failure. One of the main heart-related phenotypes in the R6/2 mouse model is a severe cardiac atrophy which may lead to cardiac failure [15]. Isoproterenol, a beta-adrenergic receptor (AR) agonist is known to induce myocardial hypertrophy and might prevent the HD-related cardiac phenotype [19–21]. We explored the importance of the HD axis in an isoproterenol-induced model of heart failure and tested the hypothesis that in pre-clinical settings, HD murine hearts might be resistant to isoproterenol action.

Results

We tested the hypothesis that induction of myocardial hypertrophy might be prevented by the HD-related cardiac phenotypes. We administered isoproterenol (Iso) to symptomatic R6/2 mice from 10 weeks of age for two weeks. The wild type (WT) and R6/2 mice had comparable body weights at both the start (Figure 1A) and end of the trial (Figure 1B) and comparable tibia length at 12 weeks of age (Figure 1C). As expected, the heart weight was significantly increased in the WT (Iso) group but surprisingly not in the R6/2 (Iso) mice (Figure 1D). Consequently, the HW/TL index (heart weight to tibia Length) was significantly increased in the WT (Iso) group in comparison to the WT vehicle (veh) group but there was no significant change between R6/2 (Iso) and R6/2 (veh) groups (Figure 1E). Next, to determine

whether isoproterenol treatment triggered an increased in heart rate, we examined electrocardiogram (ECG) recordings in conscious mice at the end of trial. We found that, WT (Iso) but not R6/2 (Iso) treated mice had a significantly higher heart rate in comparison to their respective vehicle groups (Figure 1F). We conclude from this morphometric analysis that R6/2 mice do not respond to chronic isoproterenol treatment. This was supported by the visualisation of cardiomyocyte gross morphology with phalloidin staining as shown in Figure 2. We have previously described the cardiomyocyte loss in the hearts of R6/2 mice [15] and the phalloidin staining indicated that isoptroterenol treatment of R6/2 mice does not lead to an improvement in cardiomyocyte disarray or to an increase in cardiomyocytes size (Figure 2).

It is well established that chronic treatment with isoproterenol may lead to increased fibrosis. As we previously reported, R6/2 mice develop an interstitial type of fibrosis [15] and this has can be visualised in (Figure 3A). As expected WT (iso) mice displayed a higher degree of fibrosis than their vehicle controls, while R6/2 (Iso) mice did not develop further fibrotic deposits in comparison to the R6/2 vehicle group (Figure 3B).

Pathological changes in the heart are often associated with the reactivation of a foetal gene programme and therefore, we assessed the expression levels of genes known to be changed as a consequence of cardiac hypertrophy or dilated cardiomyopathy (DCM). We found *Anp* (atrial natriuretic peptide) and *Bnp* (brain natriuretic peptide) to be up-regulated in WT (Iso) mice as well in the R6/2 (Iso) animals in comparison to their respective vehicle groups (Figure 4). Two members of the four and half only LIM family, namely *Fhl1* and *Fhl2*, are also typically reactivated foetally-expressed genes. Both transcripts showed a significant up-regulation in the R6/2 and WT isoproterenol treated mice (Figure 4). To further examine the degree of heart pathology, we determined the expression levels of additional genes that are typically altered in the HD diseased hearts. The multifunctional Ca^{2+}-binding protein *S100A4* has been shown to be up regulated in the R6/2 mice [15]. However, isoproterenol treatment did not cause a further up-regulation of *S100A4* transcripts while a 50% fold induction has been observed in WT (Iso) animals (Figure 5A). *Vgl-4* (vestigial related factor 4) and *Vgl-3* (vestigial related factor 3) are vital co-activators of the TEF (transcription enhancer family) and have been anticipated to be markers of cardiac hypertrophy [22–25]. *Vgl-3* mRNA was significantly up-regulated in both WT and R6/2 isoproterenol treated mice and in R6/2 mice in comparison to WT littermates (Figure 5A), while *Vgl-4* transcripts were only elevated in the WT (Iso) group but not in R6/2 (Figure 5A). As previously shown *Vgl-4* transcripts were up-regulated in the R6/2 mice in comparison to WT animals (Figure 5A) [15].

Bdnf (brain derived neutrophic factor) is down-regulated in the brain of HD mouse models [26] and we previously found that its transcripts were decreased in the hearts of R6/2 mice [15]. Isoproterenol treatment caused a significant reduction of *Bdnf* mRNA in WT animals but no further reduction has been observed in the R6/2 (Iso) group (Figure 5A). A similar profile of transcriptional deregulation was observed for *Mck* (muscle creatinine kinase) (Figure 5A). Transcriptional enhancer family (TEFs) members' (TEAD) have been described to be involved in the development of cardiac hypertrophy in rodents [27–29]. In the isoproterenol treated WT animals a significant induction of their transcripts was detected for *Tead-1* and *Tead-3* (Figure 5B). None of four TEF members was found to be deregulated in the symptomatic R6/2 mice (Figure 5B). Only *Tead-3* showed a significant further up-regulation upon isoproterenol treatment in the hearts of R6/2 animals (Figure 5B).

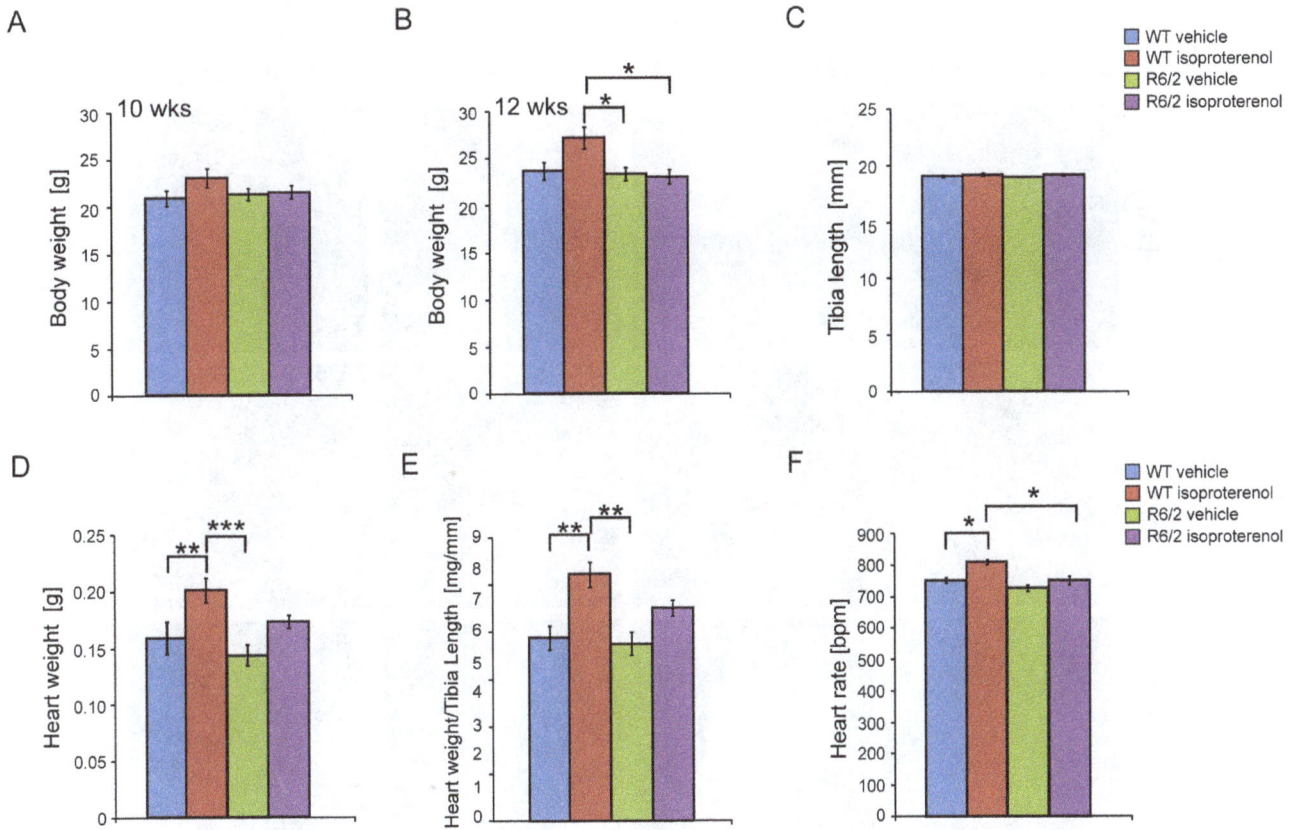

Figure 1. Morphometric analysis of the isoproterenol treated mice. (A) Body weight at 10 weeks of age prior to implantation of the alzet pumps. (B) Body weight (C) tibia length (D) heart weight (E) heart weight to tibia length index (F) heart rate were measured at 12 weeks of age. The gender-combined analysis of body weight did not detect a decrease in the R6/2 group, which may be because of a gender imbalance between the R6/2 and WT groups. All values are mean $\pm$ SEM ($n = 8$ WTveh, $n = 9$ WTiso, $n = 14$ R6/2veh, $n = 14$ R6/2iso). One-way ANOVA with Bonferroni *post-hoc* test: *$p < 0.05$, **$p < 0.01$, ***$p < 0.001$.

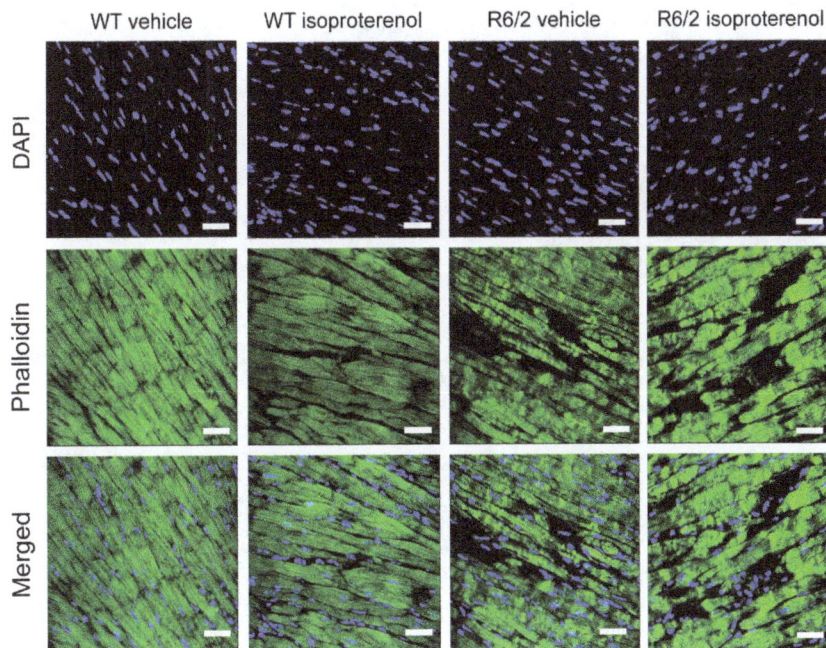

Figure 2. Gross cardiac morphology of the hearts treated with isoproterenol. Representative phalloidin staining (green) shows left ventricle myocyte hypertrophy in WT mice but not in 12 week old R6/2 mice. Nuclei (blue) were visualized with DAPI. Scale bar 30 µm.

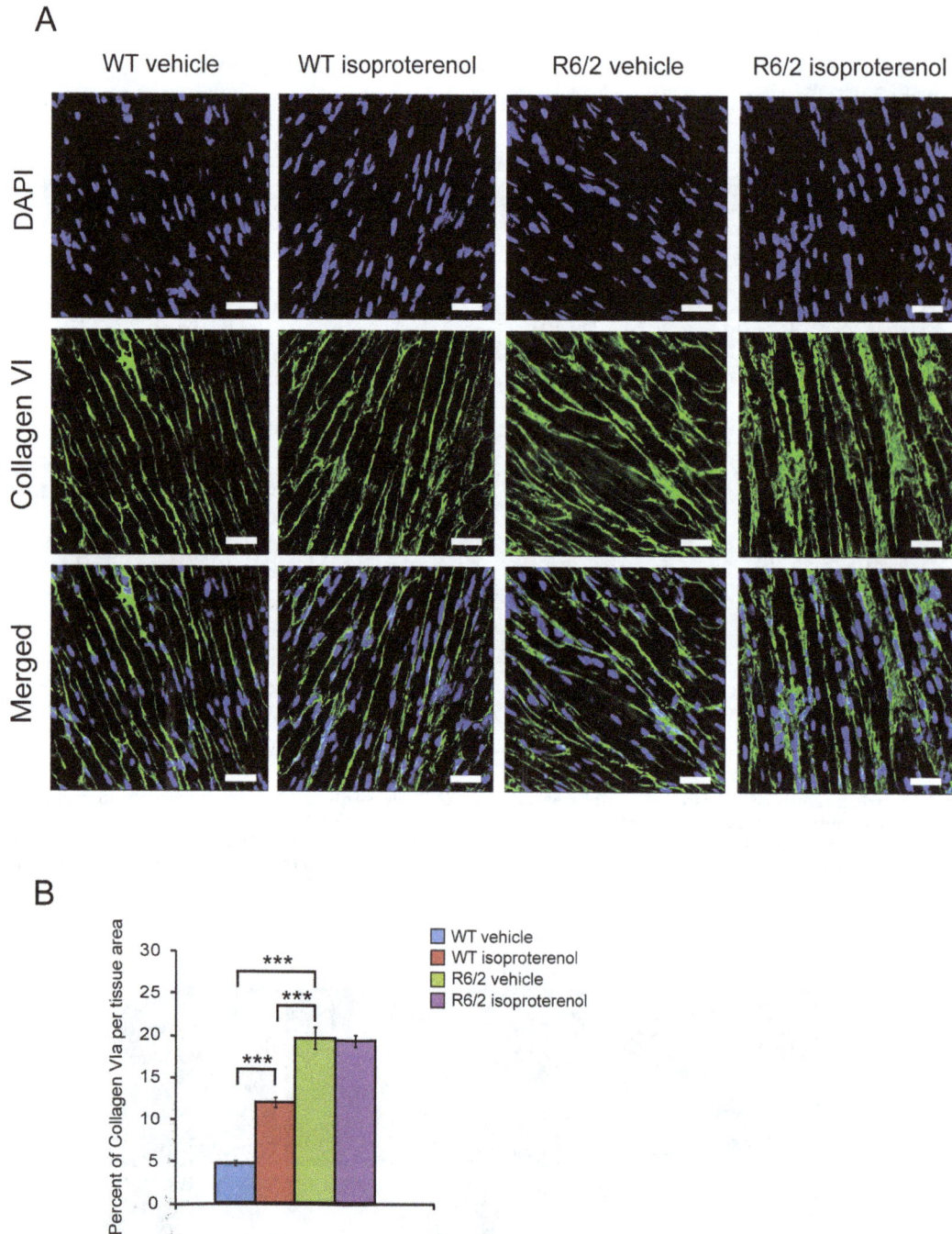

Figure 3. Moderate fibrosis level based on collagen VI deposits is not attenuated in the hearts of R6/2 mice. (A) Representative confocal pictograms of whole heart sections from 12 week old WT and R6/2 mice. (B) Quantification of the collagen VI staining area. Fibrosis was detected with the anti-collagen VI antibody (green) and nuclei (blue) were visualised with DAPI. Scale bar 30 μm. Values are mean ± SEM ($n=3$). Student's t test: *$p<0.05$, ***$p<0.001$.

The heart responds to pathological stresses by remodelling in a manner that is associated with myocyte hypertrophy and recent studies suggest key roles for histone deacetylases (HDACs) in the control of pathological cardiac remodelling [30–32]. Hence, first we sought to monitor the transcriptional profile of *Hdacs* and *Sirtuins* in the R6/2 mouse model. We performed a longitudinal study in the R6/2 mouse model from 4 weeks of age (presymptomatic) to 15 weeks (symptomatic) to evaluate the transcriptional changes of 11 *Hdacs* (Figure S1) and 7 *Sirtuins*

(Figure S2). *Hdac 3* and *Hdac9* were dysregulated in 4 week old R6/2 hearts (Figure S1A), but by 8 weeks of age the expression level of all *Hdacs* was comparable to WT. (Figure S1B). However, in the symptomatic R6/2 animals at 12 and 15 weeks of age, we found a significant up-regulation of *Hdac1*, *Hdac4*, *Hdac5*, *Hdac6* and *Hdac8* while *Hdac3* mRNA was markedly decreased (Figure S1C and D). Of the 7 *Sirtuins*, *Sirt 6* and *Sirt 7* transcripts were upregulated at 8 weeks of age, *Sirt 1* at 12 weeks and *Sirt4* and

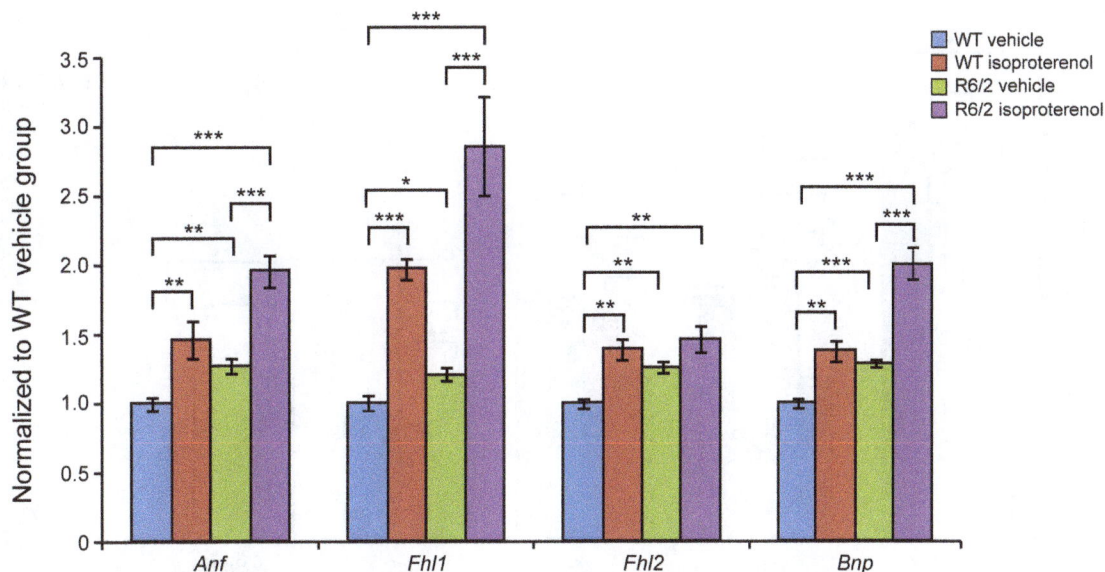

Figure 4. Partial re-activation of foetal gene markers in the hearts of R6/2 treated with isoproterenol. *Anp* (atrial natriuretic peptide), *Bnp* (brain natriuretic protein) and members of the four and half LIM family *Fhl1* and *Fhl2 were* elevated in the heart of WT and R6/2 mice. All Taqman qPCR values were normalized to the geometric mean of three housekeeping genes: *Actb*, *Cyc1* and *Gapdh*. Error bars are SEM (n = 6). Two-way ANOVA with Bonferroni *post-hoc* test: *$p<0.05$, **$p<0.01$; ***$p<0.001$.

Sirt6 at the end stage of disease in R6/2 mouse models hearts (Figure S2).

For the first time, we showed that chronic isoproterenol treatment caused up-regulation of *Hdac1*, *Hdac2*, *Hdac4*, *Hdac6*, *Hdac7* and *Hdac8* transcripts and down-regulation of *Hdac3* mRNA in WT mice (Figure 6A). In the R6/2 isoproterenol treated mice, we only found a significant deregulation of *Hdac4* and *Hdac6* (Figure 6A). *Sirtuins* showed a minor degree of transcriptional changes with a significant down-regulation of *Sirt1* and *Sirt2*, while transcripts of *Sirt3* and *Sirt5* were significantly up-regulated in the WT animals (Figure 6B). Only *Sirt1* mRNA was significantly down-regulated in the hearts of R6/2 isoproterenol treated mice (Figure 6B). Overall, one might conclude that chronic stimulation of beta-adrenergic receptors in the hearts of WT mice led to a significant deregulation of specific *Hdacs* and *Sirtuins*.

Discussion

Cardiac hypertrophy represents a critical compensatory mechanism to hemodynamic stress or injury. HD-related cardiomyopathy has been recently characterised by aberrant gap junction channel expression and a significant deregulation of hypertrophic markers that may predispose them to arrhythmia and an overall change in cardiac function. These changes were accompanied by the re-expression of foetal genes, apoptotic cardiomyocyte loss and a moderate degree of interstitial fibrosis in the symptomatic animals [15].

It has been previously reported that the heart rate response to the maximal single dose of isoproterenol was attenuated in the symptomatic R6/1 HD mouse model but not in pre-symptomatic animals in comparison to the WT littermates [17] and this might indicate that the hypertrophic response in HD hearts is attenuated. One of the strategies to unravel the mechanism of cardiac hypertrophy and failure is a chronic administration of the beta-adrenergic receptor agonist isoproterenol [19]. Chronic infusion of Iso has been reported to induce left ventricular systolic and

diastolic dysfunction and left ventricular hypertrophy accompanied by myocardial apoptosis and necrosis [20,21]. As heart atrophy and hypertrophy are governed by similar pathways, a better understanding of the cross talk between them may also contribute to an elucidation of the mechanism of HD-related cardiomyopathy. Since the proliferative capacity of adult cardiomyocytes is rather limited, the regulation of heart size is based on hypertrophy and atrophy at the cellular level. Interestingly the beta-adrenergic receptor densities were not altered in the R6/2 animals based on immunohistochemistry as has been shown previously [16].

In this study we aimed to provide a broad spectrum of experimental insights into the hypertrophic response in the hearts of R6/2 mouse model of HD. A cardiac morphometry revealed that HD hearts were not responsive to hypertrophic stimuli in the symptomatic animals while WT animals had developed all of the typical characteristics of hypertrophic hearts including increased heart weight, HW/TL index and increased heart rate in comparison to vehicle groups. Similarly, based on immunohistochemistry, we did not find an increased fibrosis in the hearts of R6/2 (Iso) mice while WT animals developed a significantly higher level of fibrotic deposits. In addition, cardiac gross morphology did not change upon isoproterenol treatment and there was no obvious cardiomyocyte hypertrophy, although the pronounced cardiomyocyte disarray was still observed in the Iso treated hearts of R6/2 mice. In contrast to the morphometry and immunohistochemistry analysis, we found further re-activation of foetal genes such as *Anf*, *Fhl1* and *Bnp* but not *Fhl2* in the isoproterenol treated R6/2 hearts. This might suggest that the HD hearts were able to respond at least partially to beta-adrenergic stimulation. It has to be noted that the WT animals responded as expected and the levels of all examined transcripts were significantly increased.

In addition, we analysed the expression pattern of transcripts known to be deregulated in HD mouse models [15]. We noted that chronic administration of Isoproterenol did not further modify expression of *S100A4*, *Vgl-4*, *Vgl-3*, *Mck* and *Bdnf*. In

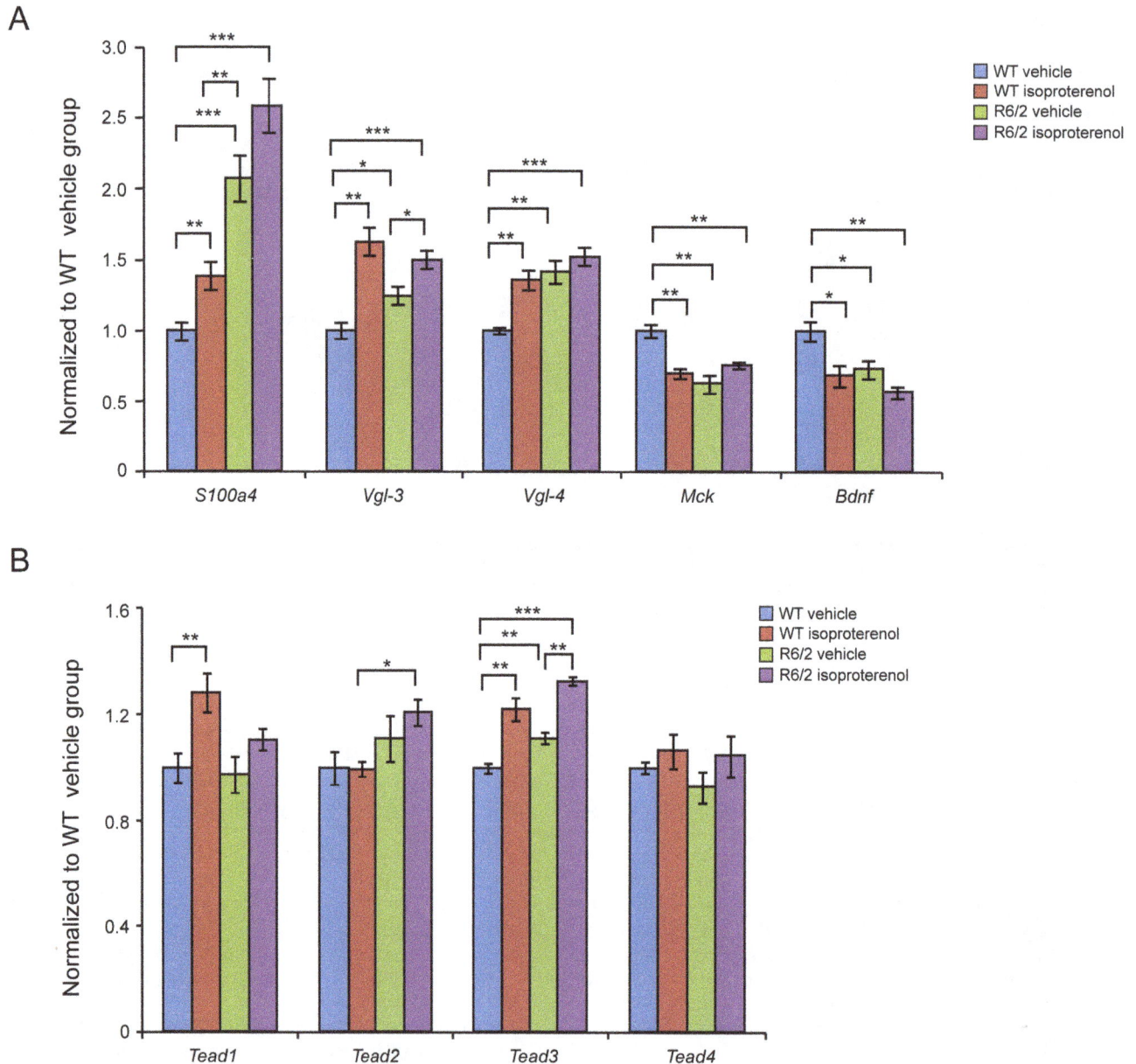

Figure 5. Transcriptional deregulation of HD markers involved in heart failure. (A) *S100A4* (S100 calcium binding protein A4), Vgl-3 (vestigial related factor 3), *Vgl-4* (vestigial related factor 4) were up-regulated while *Mck* (muscle creatine kinase) and *Bdnf* (brain derived neurotophic factor) transcripts were significantly decreased in the heart of R6/2 mice. (B) Transcripts of Transcriptional Enhancer Family members (TEAD or TEFs) were significantly deregulated in isoproterenol treated mice. All Taqman qPCR values were normalized to the geometric mean of three housekeeping genes: *Actb*, *Cyc1* and *Gapdh*. Error bars are SEM (n = 6). Two-way ANOVA with Bonferroni *post-hoc* test: *$p < 0.05$, **$p < 0.01$; ***$p < 0.001$.

addition, we found for the first time that beta adrenergic stimulation was sufficient to modulate the expression levels of *S100a4*, *Vgl-3*, *Vgl-4* in WT animals, underlining their function in heart hypertrophy. It has been previously proposed that TEA domain transcription factor-1 (TEAD-1) is essential for proper heart development. It is implicated in cardiac specific gene expression and the hypertrophic response of primary cardiomyocytes to hormonal and mechanical stimuli, and its activity increases in the pressure-overloaded hypertrophied hearts. Hence, TEAD family members have been proposed to play a crucial role in the hypertrophic response [28]. For the first time we identified that *Tead-1* and *Tead-3* are the major players in the hypertrophic response as their transcripts levels were significantly increased in

WT animals treated with isoproterenol. In the R6/2 mice there was no further up-regulation of all 4 isoforms of the TEAD family. However, only *Tead-3* was clearly significantly up-regulated in the R6/2 mice treated with isoproterenol. Also the expression pattern of *Mck* and *Bdnf* transcripts in R6/2 hearts was similar to that in WT animals treated with isoproterenol and was not further modified in the R6/2 Iso treated mice.

Global protein acetylation was found to be increased in the symptomatic R6/2 hearts based on immunohistochemistry [16] and it is well know that epigenetic remodelling is crucial for cellular differentiation and development. HDACs in the heart control events such as hypertrophy [33,34], fibrosis [35], contractility [36] and energy metabolism [37]. Global HDAC

A

B

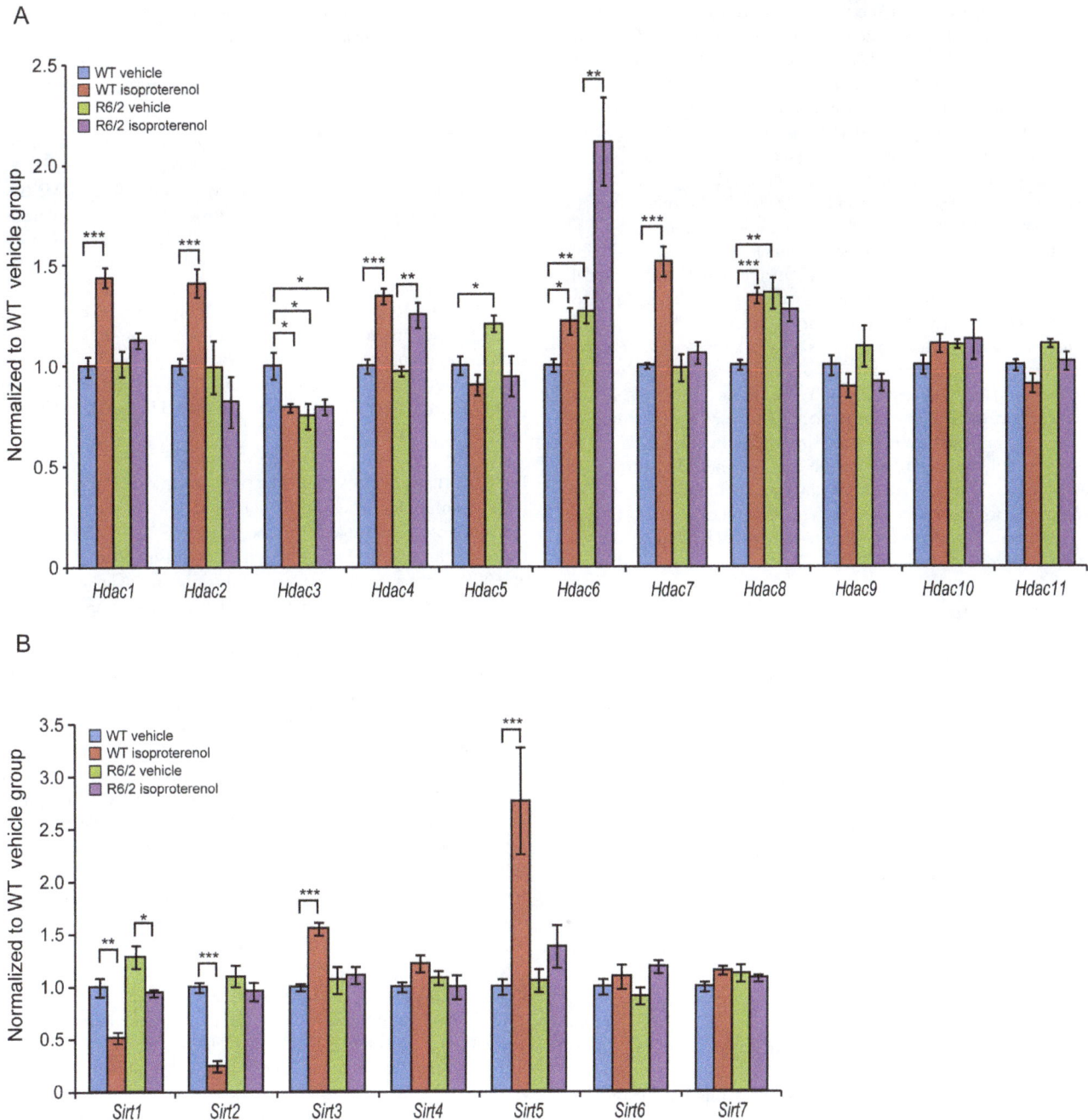

Figure 6. Chronic administration of isoproterenol causes a significant transcriptional deregulation of many *Hdacs* **and** *Sirtuins*. (A) *Hdac1, Hdac2, Hdac4, Hdac6, Hdac7* and *Hdac8* transcript levels were increased while *Hdac3* mRNA was significantly reduced in the heart of WT mice treated with Isoproterenol. Only *Hdac4* and *Hdac6* were significantly increased in the hearts of R6/2 mice. (B) *Sirt3* and *Sirt5* transcript levels were significantly increased in the heart of WT mice treated with Isoproterenol. *Sirt 1* and *Sirt 2* were decreased in the hearts of WT mice, but only *Sirt2* was decreased in the hearts of R6/2 mice. All Taqman qPCR values were normalized to the geometric mean of three housekeeping genes: *Actb, Cyc1* and *Gapdh*. Error bars are SEM (n = 6). Two-way ANOVA with Bonferroni *post-hoc* test: *$p<0.05$, **$p<0.01$; ***$p<0.001$.

activity is increased in the hypertrophic rat hearts [38] and in a model of cardiac ischemia-reperfusion injury [39]. The mechanisms by which HDAC inhibitors suppress pathological cardiac hypertrophy are still being elucidated. Previous studies has shown that HDAC inhibitors can reduce cardiac hypertrophy under pathological conditions [34,38] and may also attenuate structural remodelling after myocardial infarction [40]. Hence, we were interested in profiling the expression pattern of all 18 HDACs in

the R6/2 hearts. We found that *Hdac1, Hdac3, Hdac4, Hdac5, Hdac6* and *Hdac8* were significantly deregulated in the murine R6/2 hearts at the end stage of disease. Our longitudal analysis clearly showed that there was no difference in the expression of all *Hdacs* in early symptomatic animals. Similarly we found that *Sirt4* and *Sirt6* transcripts were significantly up-regulated in the fully symptomatic animals.

In addition, we found the following *Hdacs* to be significantly deregulated in the isoproterenol treated murine WT hearts: *Hdac1, Hdac2, Hdac3, Hdac4, Hdac6, Hdac7, Hdac8, Sirt1, Sirt2, Sirt3* and *Sirt5*. Some of the findings are in line with a previous study and confirmed a role for *Hdacs* in hypertrophic signalling. For example, it has been shown that *Hdac2* over-expression provokes severe cardiac hypertrophy [41]. *Hdac3* over-expression in the heart resulted in cardiomyocyte hyperplasia [41]. Silencing of *Hdac5* [42] and *Hdac9* [43] resulted in an exaggerated hypertrophic response to the pressure overload and spontaneous hypertrophy in older animals while *Sirt1* inhibition resulted in enhanced apoptosis [44]. In the R6/2 mouse model, chronic isoproterenol treatment caused a further deregulation of *Hdac4, Hdac6* and *Sirt1* while the expression profile of others *Hdacs* remained unchanged. This might indicate that chronic treatment with isoproterenol was able to partially replicate the expression pattern observed in the WT animals and it is likely that some hypertrophic pathways are altered in the HD mouse models. In conclusion, our present work shed light on mutant HTT as novel modulator of cardiac function. Given that beta-adrenergic signalling is a vital regulator of myocardial function, it will be important to elucidate and explore new pathways to further understand this complex cardiac response in HD mouse models and potentially in clinical settings.

Materials and Methods

Ethics statement

All experimental procedures performed on mice were conducted under a project licence from the Home Office and approved by the King's College London Ethical Review Process Committee.

Mouse maintenance and breeding

Hemizygous R6/2 mice were bred by backcrossing R6/2 males to (CBA x C57BL/6) F1 females (B6CBAF1/OlaHsd, Harlan Olac, Bicester, UK). All animals had unlimited access to water and breeding chow (Special Diet Services, Witham, UK), and housing conditions and environmental enrichment were as previously described [45]. Mice were subject to a 12-h light/dark cycle. All experimental procedures were performed according to Home Office regulations.

Genotyping

Genomic DNA was isolated from an ear-punch. R6/2 mice were genotyped by PCR and the CAG repeat length was measured as previously described [46] and listed in Table S1. Dissected tissues were snap frozen in liquid nitrogen or embedded in OCT and stored at $-80°C$ until further analysis.

Chronic treatment with Isoproterenol

Isoproterenol hydrochloride was prepared fresh, diluted in PBS (SIGMA, I6504-1G lot 018K5003). Mini osmotic pumps (Alzet pumps Model 2002, Charles River 0000296) were loaded with 200 µl of either vehicle or isoproterenol at a dose of 220 µg/g/day to allow diffusion at 0.5 µl/hour for 14 days. Animals were initially anesthetized with 5% isoflurane, and then anaesthesia was maintained at ~1.5% isoflurane throughout the surgical procedure. Alzet pumps were implanted subcutaneously onto the back of the mouse and the skin was stapled together using wound clippers. After 14 days the mice were culled and their hearts taken for analysis. Mice were randomised from litters born as closely matched as possible. Body weight was measured at the beginning and the end of the trial.

RNA extraction and Taqman real-time PCR expression analysis

Total RNA from whole hearts was extracted with the mini-RNA kit according to manufacturer's instructions (Qiagen). The reverse transcription reaction (RT) was performed using MMLV superscript reverse transcriptase (Invitrogen) and random hexamers (Operon) as described elsewhere [47]. The final RT reaction was diluted 10-fold in nuclease free water (Sigma). All Taqman qPCR reactions were performed as described previously [48] using the Chromo4 Real-Time PCR Detector (BioRad). Estimation of mRNA copy number was determined in triplicate for each RNA sample by comparison to the geometric mean of three endogenous housekeeping genes (Primer Design) as described [49]. Primer and probe sets for genes of interest were purchased from Primer Design or ABI.

Immunohistochemistry and confocal microscopy

For immunohistochemical studies, hearts were snap frozen in liquid nitrogen, or frozen in isopentane at $-50°C$, or incubated overnight in 4% PFA followed by overnight incubations in 20% and 30% sucrose in PBS, prior to embedding in OCT and storage at $-80°C$. 10–15 µm sections were cut using a cryostat (Bright instruments), air dried and immersed in 4% PFA in PBS or in acetone at $-20°C$ for 15 min and washed for 3×5 min in 0.1% PBS-Triton X-100. Blocking was achieved by incubation with 5% BSA-C (Aurion) in 0.1% PBS-Triton X-100 for at least 30 min at RT. Immunolabeling with primary antibodies was performed in 0.1% PBS-Triton X-100, 1% BSA-C overnight in a humidity box at 4°C as described previously [15]. Sections were washed 3× in PBS, incubated for 60 min at RT in a dark box with the anti-rabbit (FITC Invitrogen 1:1000 in PBS), washed 3× in PBS and counterstained with DAPI (Invitrogen). Sections were mounted in Vectashield mounting medium (Vector Laboratories). Sections were examined using the Leica TCS SP4 laser scanning confocal microscope and analysed with Leica Application Suite (LAS) v5 (Leica Microsystems, Heidelberg, Germany).

ECG evaluation in conscious mice

Heart rate was monitored using the ECGenie apparatus (Mouse Specifics, Inc., Boston, MA, USA). This device is a PowerLab-based system that acquires signal through disposable footpad electrodes located in the floor of a 6.5 cm by 7 cm recording platform. Heart rate was determined from the average of the RR interval.

Statistical analysis

All data were analysed with Microsoft Office Excel and Student's *t*-test (two tailed) or TWO-WAY ANOVA with Bonferroni *post-hoc* test SPSS (IBM).

Supporting Information

Figure S1 Longitude changes in *Hdac* gene expression in the hearts of R6/2 mice. Transcript levels of 11 *Hdacs* were monitored in the hearts of pre- and symptomatic R6/2 mice at (A) 4 weeks, (B) 8 weeks, (C) 12 weeks and (D) 15 week of age. All Taqman qPCR values were normalized to the geometric mean of three housekeeping genes: *Actb*, *Cyc1* and *Gapdh*. Error bars are SEM (n = 6). Student *t-test*: *p<0.05, **p<0.01; ***p<0.001.

Figure S2 Longitude changes in the *Sirtuin* expression in the hearts of R6/2 mice. Transcript levels of 7 *Sirtuins* were monitored in the hearts of pre- and symptomatic R6/2 mice at (A) 4 weeks, (B) 8 weeks, (C) 12 weeks and (D) 15 weeks od age. All Taqman qPCR values were normalized to the geometric mean of three housekeeping genes: *Actb*, *Cyc1* and *Gapdh*. Error bars are SEM (n = 6). Student *t-test*: *p<0.05, **p<0.01; ***p<0.001.

Table S1 Summary of the number of mice per genotype used in all studies and their CAG repeat sizes. SD = standard deviation.

Author Contributions

Conceived and designed the experiments: MM. Performed the experiments: MM MKB SAF LI TM. Analyzed the data: MM. Contributed reagents/materials/analysis tools: GPB. Wrote the paper: MM GPB.

References

1. Bates GP, Tabrizi SJ, Jones AL (2014) Huntington's Disease. New York: Oxford University Press.
2. Strong TV, Tagle DA, Valdes JM, Elmer LW, Boehm K, et al. (1993) Widespread expression of the human and rat Huntington's disease gene in brain and nonneural tissues. Nat Genet 5: 259–265.
3. Sassone J, Colciago C, Cislaghi G, Silani V, Ciammola A (2009) Huntington's disease: the current state of research with peripheral tissues. Exp Neurol 219: 385–397.
4. van der Burg JM, Bjorkqvist M, Brundin P (2009) Beyond the brain: widespread pathology in Huntington's disease. Lancet Neurol 8: 765–774.
5. Li SH, Schilling G, Young WS 3rd, Li XJ, Margolis RL, et al. (1993) Huntington's disease gene (IT15) is widely expressed in human and rat tissues. Neuron 11: 985–993.
6. Li W, Serpell LC, Carter WJ, Rubinsztein DC, Huntington JA (2006) Expression and characterization of full-length human huntingtin, an elongated HEAT repeat protein. J Biol Chem 281: 15916–15922.
7. Harjes P, Wanker EE (2003) The hunt for huntingtin function: interaction partners tell many different stories. Trends Biochem Sci 28: 425–433.
8. Sorensen SA, Fenger K (1992) Causes of death in patients with Huntington's disease and in unaffected first degree relatives. J Med Genet 29: 911–914.
9. Chiu E, Alexander L (1982) Causes of death in Huntington's disease. Med J Aust 1: 153.
10. Lanska DJ, Lavine L, Lanska MJ, Schoenberg BS (1988) Huntington's disease mortality in the United States. Neurology 38: 769–772.
11. Pattison JS, Sanbe A, Maloyan A, Osinska H, Klevitsky R, et al. (2008) Cardiomyocyte expression of a polyglutamine preamyloid oligomer causes heart failure. Circulation 117: 2743–2751.
12. Mangiarini L, Sathasivam K, Seller M, Cozens B, Harper A, et al. (1996) Exon 1 of the HD gene with an expanded CAG repeat is sufficient to cause a progressive neurological phenotype in transgenic mice. Cell 87: 493–506.
13. Lin CH, Tallaksen-Greene S, Chien WM, Cearley JA, Jackson WS, et al. (2001) Neurological abnormalities in a knock-in mouse model of Huntington's disease. Hum Mol Genet 10: 137–144.
14. Woodman B, Butler R, Landles C, Lupton MK, Tse J, et al. (2007) The Hdh(Q150/Q150) knock-in mouse model of HD and the R6/2 exon 1 model develop comparable and widespread molecular phenotypes. Brain Res Bull 72: 83–97.
15. Mielcarek M, Inuabasi L, Bondulich MK, Muller T, Osborne GF, et al. (2014) Dysfunction of the CNS-Heart Axis in Mouse Models of Huntington's Disease. PLoS Genet 10: e1004550.
16. Mihm MJ, Amann DM, Schanbacher BL, Altschuld RA, Bauer JA, et al. (2007) Cardiac dysfunction in the R6/2 mouse model of Huntington's disease. Neurobiol Dis 25: 297–308.
17. Kiriazis H, Jennings NL, Davern P, Lambert G, Su Y, et al. (2012) Neurocardiac dysregulation and neurogenic arrhythmias in a transgenic mouse model of Huntington's disease. J Physiol 590: 5845–5860.
18. Melkani GC, Trujillo AS, Ramos R, Bodmer R, Bernstein SI, et al. (2013) Huntington's disease induced cardiac amyloidosis is reversed by modulating protein folding and oxidative stress pathways in the Drosophila heart. PLoS Genet 9: e1004024.
19. Boluyt MO, Long X, Eschenhagen T, Mende U, Schmitz W, et al. (1995) Isoproterenol infusion induces alterations in expression of hypertrophy-associated genes in rat heart. Am J Physiol 269: H638–647.
20. Grimm D, Elsner D, Schunkert H, Pfeifer M, Griese D, et al. (1998) Development of heart failure following isoproterenol administration in the rat: role of the renin-angiotensin system. Cardiovasc Res 37: 91–100.
21. Jin YT, Hasebe N, Matsusaka T, Natori S, Ohta T, et al. (2007) Magnesium attenuates isoproterenol-induced acute cardiac dysfunction and beta-adrenergic desensitization. Am J Physiol Heart Circ Physiol 292: H1593–1599.
22. Chen HH, Mullett SJ, Stewart AF (2004) Vgl-4, a novel member of the vestigial-like family of transcription cofactors, regulates alpha1-adrenergic activation of gene expression in cardiac myocytes. J Biol Chem 279: 30800–30806.
23. Mielcarek M, Piotrowska I, Schneider A, Gunther S, Braun T (2009) VITO-2, a new SID domain protein, is expressed in the myogenic lineage during early mouse embryonic development. Gene Expr Patterns 9: 129–137.
24. Gunther S, Mielcarek M, Kruger M, Braun T (2004) VITO-1 is an essential cofactor of TEF1-dependent muscle-specific gene regulation. Nucleic Acids Res 32: 791–802.
25. Mielcarek M, Gunther S, Kruger M, Braun T (2002) VITO-1, a novel vestigial related protein is predominantly expressed in the skeletal muscle lineage. Mech Dev 119 Suppl 1: S269–274.
26. Benn CL, Fox H, Bates GP (2008) Optimisation of region-specific reference gene selection and relative gene expression analysis methods for pre-clinical trials of Huntington's disease. Mol Neurodegener 3: 17.
27. Stewart AF, Suzow J, Kubota T, Ueyama T, Chen HH (1998) Transcription factor RTEF-1 mediates alpha1-adrenergic reactivation of the fetal gene program in cardiac myocytes. Circ Res 83: 43–49.
28. Tsika RW, Ma L, Kehat I, Schramm C, Simmer G, et al. (2010) TEAD-1 overexpression in the mouse heart promotes an age-dependent heart dysfunction. J Biol Chem 285: 13721–13735.
29. McLean BG, Lee KS, Simpson PC, Farrance IK (2003) Basal and alpha1-adrenergic-induced activity of minimal rat betaMHC promoters in cardiac myocytes requires multiple TEF-1 but not NFAT binding sites. J Mol Cell Cardiol 35: 461–471.
30. Colussi C, Illi B, Rosati J, Spallotta F, Farsetti A, et al. (2010) Histone deacetylase inhibitors: keeping momentum for neuromuscular and cardiovascular diseases treatment. Pharmacol Res 62: 3–10.
31. McKinsey TA (2012) Therapeutic potential for HDAC inhibitors in the heart. Annu Rev Pharmacol Toxicol 52: 303–319.
32. Bush EW, McKinsey TA (2009) Targeting histone deacetylases for heart failure. Expert Opin Ther Targets 13: 767–784.
33. Antos CL, McKinsey TA, Dreitz M, Hollingsworth LM, Zhang CL, et al. (2003) Dose-dependent blockade to cardiomyocyte hypertrophy by histone deacetylase inhibitors. J Biol Chem 278: 28930–28937.
34. Kook H, Lepore JJ, Gitler AD, Lu MM, Wing-Man Yung W, et al. (2003) Cardiac hypertrophy and histone deacetylase-dependent transcriptional repression mediated by the atypical homeodomain protein Hop. J Clin Invest 112: 863–871.
35. Kee HJ, Sohn IS, Nam KI, Park JE, Qian YR, et al. (2006) Inhibition of histone deacetylation blocks cardiac hypertrophy induced by angiotensin II infusion and aortic banding. Circulation 113: 51–59.
36. Gupta MP, Samant SA, Smith SH, Shroff SG (2008) HDAC4 and PCAF bind to cardiac sarcomeres and play a role in regulating myofilament contractile activity. J Biol Chem 283: 10135–10146.
37. Montgomery RL, Potthoff MJ, Haberland M, Qi X, Matsuzaki S, et al. (2008) Maintenance of cardiac energy metabolism by histone deacetylase 3 in mice. J Clin Invest 118: 3588–3597.
38. Cardinale JP, Sriramula S, Pariaut R, Guggilam A, Mariappan N, et al. (2010) HDAC inhibition attenuates inflammatory, hypertrophic, and hypertensive responses in spontaneously hypertensive rats. Hypertension 56: 437–444.
39. Granger A, Abdullah I, Huebner F, Stout A, Wang T, et al. (2008) Histone deacetylase inhibition reduces myocardial ischemia-reperfusion injury in mice. FASEB J 22: 3549–3560.
40. Lee TM, Lin MS, Chang NC (2007) Inhibition of histone deacetylase on ventricular remodeling in infarcted rats. Am J Physiol Heart Circ Physiol 293: H968–977.
41. Trivedi CM, Lu MM, Wang Q, Epstein JA (2008) Transgenic overexpression of Hdac3 in the heart produces increased postnatal cardiac myocyte proliferation but does not induce hypertrophy. J Biol Chem 283: 26484–26489.
42. Chang S, McKinsey TA, Zhang CL, Richardson JA, Hill JA, et al. (2004) Histone deacetylases 5 and 9 govern responsiveness of the heart to a subset of stress signals and play redundant roles in heart development. Mol Cell Biol 24: 8467–8476.
43. Zhang CL, McKinsey TA, Chang S, Antos CL, Hill JA, et al. (2002) Class II histone deacetylases act as signal-responsive repressors of cardiac hypertrophy. Cell 110: 479–488.
44. Alcendor RR, Kirshenbaum LA, Imai S, Vatner SF, Sadoshima J (2004) Silent information regulator 2alpha, a longevity factor and class III histone deacetylase, is an essential endogenous apoptosis inhibitor in cardiac myocytes. Circ Res 95: 971–980.

45. Hockly E, Woodman B, Mahal A, Lewis CM, Bates G (2003) Standardization and statistical approaches to therapeutic trials in the R6/2 mouse. Brain Res Bull 61: 469–479.

46. Sathasivam K, Lane A, Legleiter J, Warley A, Woodman B, et al. (2010) Identical oligomeric and fibrillar structures captured from the brains of R6/2 and knock-in mouse models of Huntington's disease. Hum Mol Genet 19: 65–78.

47. Mielcarek M, Seredenina T, Stokes MP, Osborne GF, Landles C, et al. (2013) HDAC4 does not act as a protein deacetylase in the postnatal murine brain in vivo. PLoS One 8: e80849.

48. Mielcarek M, Landles C, Weiss A, Bradaia A, Seredenina T, et al. (2013) HDAC4 reduction: a novel therapeutic strategy to target cytoplasmic huntingtin and ameliorate neurodegeneration. PLoS Biol 11: e1001717.

49. Mielcarek M, Benn CL, Franklin SA, Smith DL, Woodman B, et al. (2011) SAHA decreases HDAC 2 and 4 levels in vivo and improves molecular phenotypes in the R6/2 mouse model of Huntington's disease. PLoS One 6: e27746.

19

Determinants and Improvement of Electrocardiographic Diagnosis of Left Ventricular Hypertrophy

Ahmadou M. Jingi[1], Jean Jacques N. Noubiap[2]*, Philippe Kamdem[3], Samuel Kingue[1,4]

1 Department of Internal Medicine and Specialties, Faculty of Medicine and Biomedical Sciences, University of Yaoundé I, Yaoundé, Cameroon, **2** Internal Medicine Unit, Edéa Regional Hospital, Edéa, Cameroon, **3** Centre Médical de la Trinité, Bafoussam, Cameroon, **4** Department of Internal Medicine, Yaoundé General Hospital, Yaoundé, Cameroon

Abstract

Background: Left ventricular hypertrophy (LVH) is a major cardiovascular risk factor. The electrocardiogram (ECG) has been shown to be a poor tool in detecting LVH due to cardiac and extracardiac factors. We studied the determinants and possibility of improving the test performance of the ECG in a group of Black Africans.

Methods: We studied echocardiograms and electrocardiograms of 182 Cameroonian patients among whom 113 (62.1%) were having an echocardiographic LVH. Echocardiographic LVH was defined as Left Ventricular Mass Indexed to height $^{2.7}$ (LVMI) >48 g/m$^{2.7}$ in men, and >44 g/m$^{2.7}$ in women or Body Surface Area ≥ 116 g/m^2 in men, and ≥ 96 g/m^2 in women. Test performances were calculated for 6 classic ECG criteria Sokolow-Lyon, Cornell, Cornell product, Gubner-Ungerleiger, amplitudes of R in aVL, V_5 and V_6.

Results: The most sensitive criteria were Cornell (37.2%) and Sokolow-Lyon index (26.5%). The most specific criteria were Gubner (98.6%), RaVL (97.1%), RV$_5$/V$_6$ (95.7%) and Cornell product (94.2%). The performance of the ECG in diagnosing LVH significantly increased with the severity of LVH for Cornell index ($r = 0.420$, $p < 0.0001$) and Sokolow index ($r = 0.212$, $p = 0.002$). It decreased with body habitus ($r = -0.248$, $p = 0.001$) for Sokolow-Lyon index. Cornell index was less affected (age $p = 0.766$; body habitus: $p = 0.209$). After sex-specific adjustment for BMI, Cornell BMI sensitivity increased from 37.2% to 69% ($r = 0.472$, $p < 0.0001$), and Sokolow-Lyon BMI sensitivity increased from 26.5% to 58.4% ($r = 0.270$, $p < 0.001$).

Conclusion: The test performance of the ECG in diagnosing LVH is low in this Black African population, due to extracardiac factors such as age, sex, body habitus, and cardiac factors such as LVH severity and geometry. However, this performance is improved after adjustment for extracardiac factors.

Editor: Larisa G. Tereshchenko, Johns Hopkins University SOM, United States of America

Funding: The authors have no support or funding to report.

Competing Interests: The authors have declared that no competing interests exist.

* E-mail: noubiapjj@yahoo.fr

Introduction

Increased left ventricular mass (LVM) is an adaptation of the heart to increased hemodynamic burden, and alters cardiac functioning. It is often associated with hypertension and has been shown to be an independent cardiovascular risk factor [1]. Methods of diagnosing left ventricular hypertrophy (LVH) with increasing performance include a comprehensive clinical assessment, chest X-ray, electrocardiography (ECG), Cardiac ultrasound, CT scan, Nuclear Magnetic Resonance imaging (NMR). The ECG is the most cost-effective and is recommended for routine use in assessing LVH [2,3]. The test performance of the ECG has been shown to be influenced by race, gender, age and body habitus [4,5]. Adjustment of ECG LVH criteria for body mass index (BMI) and age has been shown to improve the classification accuracy in Caucasians [6]. Such studies are scarce in Sub-Saharan Africa and mostly looked at the test performance of the ECG [7,8]. Our objective was to study the test performance and determinants of some classic easy to use ECG criteria and the possibility of improvement.

Methods

Ethical Considerations

The study was granted ethical approval by the Institutional Review Board of the Health Science Foundation, Cameroon, and was performed in accordance with the guidelines of the Helsinki Declaration. Written informed consent was obtained from all the participants.

Study Design and Setting

The study was conducted between April and December 2011 in the "Centre Medical de la Trinité", one of the two cardiologic clinics in the West Region of Cameroon.

Study Population and Sampling

We included patients aged 18 years or more seen during the study period, consenting to participate, who underwent a Doppler echocardiography and an ECG on the same day. Eligible patients had to fulfil one of these criteria: **i)** normal LV size (Left Ventricular chamber size in end diastole (LVEDd) ≤59 mm and indexed LVEDd to BSA (indexed LVEDd) ≤31 mm/m² in men or ≤32 mm/m² in women) with normal LV or concentric LV remodeling or concentric LV hypertrophy; **ii)** minimally dilated LV (LVEDd ≤59 mm and indexed LVEDd >31 mm/m² in men or >32 mm/m² in women) with normal LV or concentric LV remodeling or concentric LV hypertrophy; **iii)** apparently dilated LV (LVEDd >59 mm and indexed LV ≤31 mm/m² in men or ≤ 32 mm/m² in women) with normal LV or concentric LV remodeling or concentric LV hypertrophy.

We excluded patients with: **i)** markedly dilated LV, LVEDd > 70 mm and indexed LVEDd >31 mm/m² in men or >32 mm/m² in women) as in LV aneurysm and dilated cardiomyopathy; **ii)** chronic obstructive pulmonary disease (COPD); **iii)** septal dyskinesia; **iv)** asymmetric septal hypertrophy (septum/posterior wall ratio >1.3); **v)** technically difficult echocardiography; **vi)** pericardial effusion; **vii)** chest deformity; **viii)** incomplete data (missing weight or height), discordant timing of tests (Echo/ECG).

A sample size of 90 patients was required, assuming the prevalence of 6.25% of LVH among patients with hypertension in Cameroon, a 5% margin of error and a 95% confidence level. The assumption of prevalence of 6.25% among was based on the prevalence of 25% of hypertension in Cameroon [9,10] and the prevalence of 25% of LVH among patients with hypertension [1].

Procedure

First, ECG was performed by a trained technician at rest in the supine position with a Mac 500 GE apparatus using standard procedure (speed and voltage regulation of 25 mm/s and 1 mV/ 10 mm respectively). Secondly, blinded to the ECG, the transthoracic echocardiography was performed with the patient in the left lateral decubitus position by an experienced cardiologist using commercially available echocardiography equipment (HP Sonos 2000 Color Doppler ver. A.2, HP Color) and a 4–7 Megahertz transducer.

Measurements

Subject identity (name, age, sex) were collected by a nurse. The blood pressure (BP) was measured with a mercury sphygmomanometer, the height measured with a stadiometer, and the weight with a clinical scale balance. The body surface area (BSA) was automatically calculated by the echocardiograph to nearest two decimals. The body mass index (BMI) calculated as Weight (kg)/ height² (m²) to nearest one decimal. Left ventricular measurements were done on long parasternal long axis 2-D guided M-mode using the ASE recommendations [11]. The LVM was calculated using the formula:

$$LVM = 0.8\left(1.04\left[(IVSd + LVPWd + LVEDd)^3 - LVEDd^3\right]\right) + 0.6g$$

LVM: Left Ventricular Mass
IVSd: Septal thickness in end diastole
LVPWd: Posterior wall thickness in end diastole

LVEDd: Left Ventricular chamber size in end diastole

LVH was defined based on ASE recommendations [11] as Indexed LVM (LVM per m² of BSA or LVM per m²·⁷ of height) >115 g/m² (BSA) or >48 g/m²·⁷ (height in case of obesity) in men and Indexed LVM >95 g/m² or >44 g/m²·⁷ in women. The severity of Left Ventricular Mass (LVM) indexed to BSA was classified according to ASE recommendations as [11]:

- Mild (LVM: 116–132 g/m² in men and 96–109 g/m² in women)
- Moderate (LVM: 133–149 g/m² in men and 110–122 g/m² in women)
- Severe (LVM >149 g/m² in men and 122 g/m² in women).

The relative wall thickness (RWT) was calculated using the formula:

$$RWT = (IVSd + LVPWd)/LVEDd$$

The cut off 0.42 was used to define the LV geometry as:

- Normal: normal LVM and RWT ≤0.42
- Concentric remodeling: normal LVM and RWT >0.42
- Eccentric LVH: LVH and RWT ≤0.42
- Concentric LVH: LVH and RWT >0.42.

The ECG was then interpreted by the same cardiologist (PK). Voltage amplitude was measured to the nearest 0.05 mV and time to the nearest 0.02 s. The following voltage index criteria were evaluated.

- Sokolow-Lyon: SV1+ RV5 or RV6≥3.5 mV
- Cornell voltage index: RaVL+SV3≥2.8 mV in men and 2.0 mV in women
- Cornell product: (RaVL+SV3)×QRSd ≥0.244 mV.s
- Gubner index: RD1+ SD3≥2.5 mV.
- RaVL ≥1.1 mV
- RV5 or RV6≥2.7 mV.

Adjustment for body habitus was done by multiplying the voltage criteria and the BSA or BMI based on previous findings that body habitus has an inverse relationship with ECG voltage criteria.

Data Analysis

Data was coded, entered and analyzed using the Statistical Package for Social Science (SPSS) version 16.0 for Windows (SPSS, Chicago, Illinois, USA). We described continuous variables using means with standard deviations, and categorical variables using their frequencies and percentages. Pearson's correlation coefficient was used to associate LVMI (Left Ventricular Mass Index) and the several criteria that were analyzed. Sensitivity and specificity were calculated using 2×2 tables (Classifying ECG LVH as against Echo LVH as the standard). We calculated the specificity as true negatives divided by the sum of true negatives and false positives. Similarly, we calculated the sensitivity as true positives divided by the sum of true positives and false negatives. Regression lines were used to determine cut offs for the BSA or BMI adjusted criteria for two selected voltage criteria (Sokolow-Lyon and Cornell) when the LVM indexed to BSA ≥116 g/m2 for men, and ≥96 g/m2 for women). Mean values of demographic, electrocardiographic and echocardiographic variables were compared using 2-way ANOVA. The chi-square test or its equivalent was used to compare qualitative variables and a p value less than 0.05 was considered statistically significant.

Results

Clinical, ECG, and echocardiographic data were available and adequate for analysis in 182 patients aged 18 to 99 years with a mean age of 63 years (SD = 15.9). There was no significant age difference between sexes (males 61.7±15.8 years and females 64.1±16 years, p = 0.301). Most of the participants (81.9%) were aged ≥50 years. The most represented age groups were the 70 to 79 years (25.8%) and 60 to 69 years (24.2%) age groups (Figure 1). Fifty four point nine percent of patients (95% CI: 47.4–62) were females and 45.1% (95% CI: 37.7–52.6) were males. The prevalence of echocardiographic LVH was 62.1% (95% CI: 54.6–69.2) for LVM indexed to BSA (LVM ≥116 g/m2 for men, and ≥96 g/m2 for women). The prevalence of LVH when the LVM is indexed to height $^{2.7}$ (LVM >48 g/m$^{2.7}$ in men, and >44 g/m$^{2.7}$ in women) was 72.5% (95% CI: 65.4–78.9%). The concordance between indexing to BSA and height$^{2.7}$ was 87.4% (95% CI: 81.6–91.8). This was comparable between sexes and ages above or below 55 years. The LVH severity when the LVM is indexed to BSA is shown in figure 2. The proportions in the study population and mean values for the different LV geometry types are shown in table 1 and table 2 respectively.

Determinants of Test Performance

Table 3 shows the ECG voltage test performances with the severity of LVH. The sensitivity increased with the degree of LVH without a major decrease in the specificity. This was especially seen with the Cornell voltage criterion. Table 4 shows some other possible factors that could determine the test performance of the Sokolow-Lyon and Cornell voltage indices. The Sokolow-Lyon criterion is more sensitive in males though to a lesser extent than the Cornell criterion, which is more sensitive in females. Overall, Cornell voltage criterion performed better in both sexes. The test performance of the Sokolow-Lyon criterion significantly decreased with age (r = −0.159, p = 0.032), while the Cornell criterion showed a non-significant increase with age (r = 0.082, p = 0.766). The body habitus generally showed a significant negative effect on the Sokolow-Lyon criterion (r = −0.248, p = 0.001) while the Cornell criterion showed a non-significant positive effect (r = 0.094, p = 0.209). A positive effect was shown with the LV geometric pattern concordant with the pathologic evolution in both the Sokolow – Lyon and Cornell criteria.

Test Performances after Adjusting for Sex and Body Habitus

Table 5 shows the test performances of the un-adjusted and adjusted Sokolow-Lyon and Cornell indices with thresholds determined from regression equations at LV mass index ≥ 116 g/m^2 in males and ≥96 g/m^2 in females. The sensitivity doubled with both criteria with a decrease in the specificity by half and by a third with both the Sokolow-Lyon and Cornell criteria respectively. The test accuracy was better in the adjusted criteria.

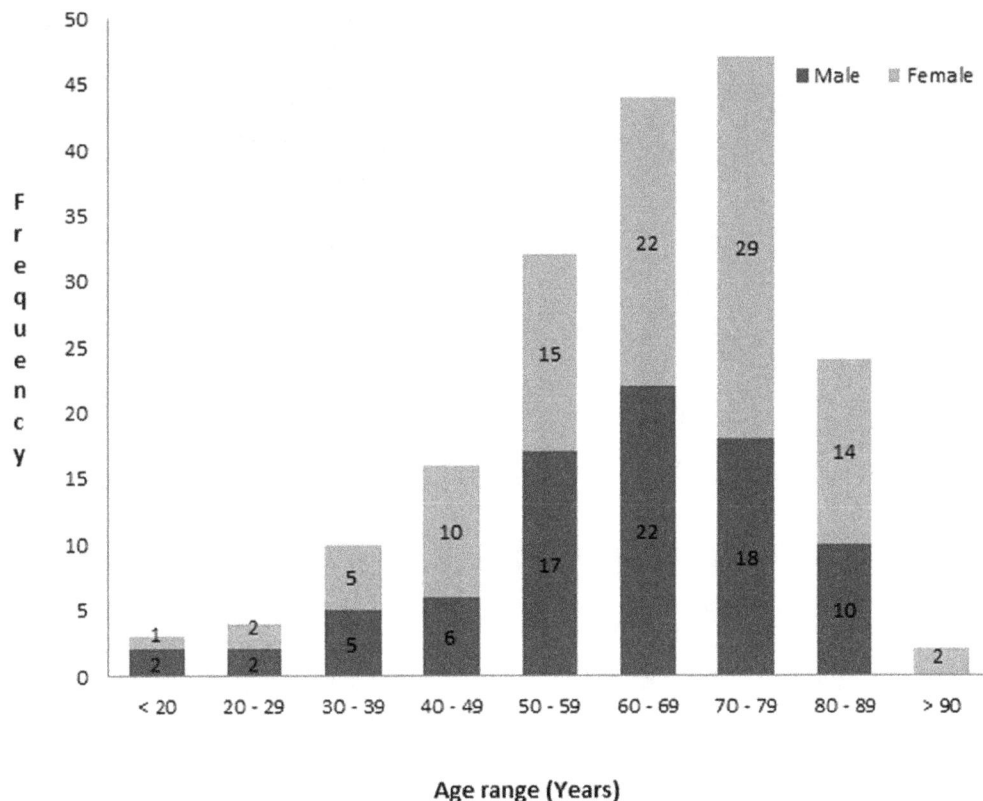

Figure 1. Age distribution of the study population.

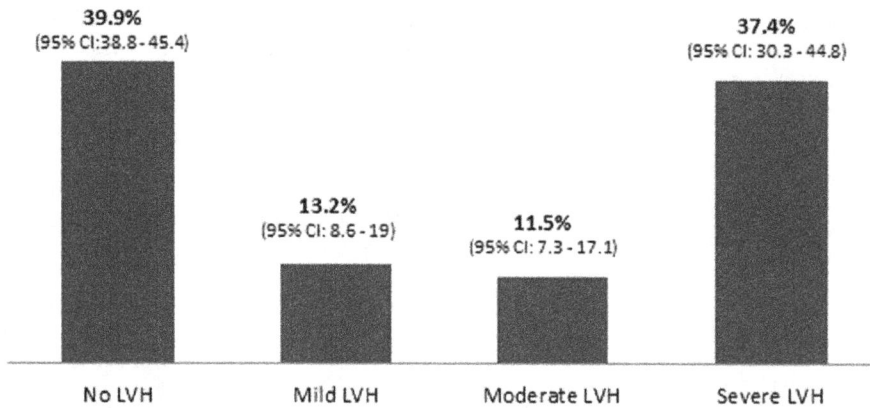

Figure 2. Left ventricular hypertrophy (LVH) severity when the left ventricular mass is indexed to the body surface area.

Table 1. Clinical, echocardiographic and electrocardiographic criteria (N = 182).

Characteristic	Frequency (%)
Body habitus (BMI)	
Underweight	7 (3.3)
Normal	66 (36.3)
Overweight	55 (30.2)
Obesity	54 (29.7)
Systolic blood pressure >140 mmHg	140 (76.9)
Diastolic blood pressure >90 mmHg	133 (73.1)
LV Chamber size	
Dilated	35 (19.2)
Normal	147 (80.8)
Pulmonary pressure >30 mmHg	61 (35.5)
LVH*	113 (62.1)
LVH**	132 (72.5)
LV Geometry	
Normal	13 (7.1)
Concentric remodeling	43 (23.6)
Concentric hypertrophy	96 (52.7)
Eccentric hypertrophy	30 (16.5)
Ejection fraction >50%	116 (63.7)
Heart rhythm	
Sinus	172 (94.5)
Atrial fibrillation	10 (5.5)
Sokolow LVH	44 (22.5)
Cornell LVH	51 (28)
Cornell product LVH	27 (14.8)
Gubner LVH	11 (6)
RaVL LVH	16 (8.8)
RV_5/RV_6 LVH	6 (3.3)

*(LVM Indexed to BSA $\geq$116 g/m^2 in men and $\geq$96 g/m^2 in women).
**(LVM Indexed to Height $\geq$49 g/m$^{2.7}$ in men and $\geq$45 g/m$^{2.7}$ in women).

Table 2. Clinical, electrocardiographic and echocardiographic characteristics comparing mean values relative to the left ventricular geometry type.

Characteristics	Normal N=13	Concentric remodeling N=43	Concentric hypertrophy N=96	Eccentric hypertrophy N=29	p value	Total	Range
Clinical							
Age (SD) years	49.9 (19.4)	60.1 (18.1)	66(13.7)	62.9(14.9)	0.003	62.98(15.9)	18–99
Systolic BP (SD)mmHg	147.9(24.6)	155.6(30.4)	169.5(33.1)	146.6(30.7)	<0.0001	160.45(33)	90–260
Diastolic BP(SD)mmHg	92.6(17.2)	94.3(15.9)	99(20.8)	89.2(19.5)	0.09	95.8(19.5)	50–177
BMI (SD) g/m²	27.1(6.3)	26.8(5.7)	27.9(5.8)	25.7(5.6)	0.315	27.2(5.8)	16.3–43
BSA (SD) m²	1.94(0.38)	1.89(0.26)	1.92(0.32)	1.84(0.32)	0.68	1.9(0.3)	1.27–2.89
Electrocardiogram							
Heart rate (SD): beats/min	75.5(11.4)	80.7(21)	76(19.1)	87.3(24)	0.057	78.9(20.3)	45–150
P wave duration (SD) s	0.1(0.01)	0.1(0.02)	0.1(0.02)	0.11(0.02)	0.283	0.10(0.02)	0.08–0.14
P-R (SD) s	0.17(0.03)	0.17(0.02)	0.17(0.03)	0.18(0.03)	0.428	0.17(0.03)	0.12–0.24
QRS							
Duration (s)	0.09 (0.02)	0.08(0.01)	0.08(0.01)	0.10(0.03)	<0.0001	0.08(0.02)	0.06–0.16
Axis	20.3(37.8)	31.5(42.6)	19.3(32)	10.4(36.1)	0.114	20.9	−46–120
QTc (s)	0.39(0.02)	0.39(0.03)	0.39(0.03)	0.38(0.04)	0.004	0.39 (0.03)	0.32–0.48
RaVL (mV)	0.54(0.26)	0.43(0.32)	0.65(0.42)	0.73(0.43)	0.004		
Sokolow (mV)	2.73(0.7)	2.55(0.79)	2.96(0.87)	3.02(0.97)	0.038	28.7(8.7)	6–55
Cornell (mV)	1.36(0.58)	1.49(0.54)	1.95(0.72)	2.65(0.88)	<0.0001	19.2(8)	4–42
Cornell product (mV.s)	0.113(0.042)	0.115(0.045)	0.161(0.07)	0.261(0.129)	<0.0001	1.64(0.91)	0.32–6.72
Gubner - Ungerleiger(mV)	1.07(0.41)	0.96(0.56)	1.36(0.77)	1.51(0.79)	0.713	12.7(7.3)	0–42
Echocardiogram							
LA (cm)	3.6(0.8)	3.3(0.6)	4.1(0.9)	4.6(0.8)	<0.0001	3.97(0.88)	1.92–6.56
LVPWd (cm)	0.95(0.12)	1.09(0.13)	1.32(0.21)	1.15(0.15)	<0.0001	1.21(0.21)	0.79–2.2
IVSd (cm)	0.92(0.12)	1.17(0.12)	1.41(0.19)	1.15(0.15)	<0.0001	1.28(0.23)	0.74–2.11
DTDVg Index (cm/m²)	2.59(0.3)	2.15(0.4)	2.49(0.5)	3.48(0.5)	<0.0001	2.58(0.63)	1.39–4.62
EF (%)	63.6(12.3)	63.4(12.1)	57(13.3)	37.5(14.4)	<0.0001	55.76(15.6)	14–88
LVM Index (g/m²)	80.72(16)	80.95(16.9)	136.26(38.2)	178.68(43.97)	<0.0001	126.22(48)	52.4–280.6
RVSP mmHg	34(10.7)	38.2(15.9)	43.9(17.6)	44.2(20.6)	0.485	42.3(17.5)	14–90

Table 3. Sensitivity and specificity at different thresholds for Left Ventricular Hypertrophy Mass Indexed to Body Surface Area (ASE).

Index	Mild LVH* (N=24)		Moderate LVH** (N=21)		Severe LVH*** (N=68)		r	p value
	Sensitivity	Specificity	Sensitivity	Specificity	Sensitivity	Specificity		
Sokolow-Lyon	26.5%	84.1%	27.8%	82.6%	28.4%	80.9%	0.212	0.004
Cornell	37.2%	87%	42.2%	85.9%	49.3%	84.3%	0.420	<0.0001
Cornell product	20.4%	94.2%	23.3%	93.5%	31.3%	94.8%	0.419	<0.0001
Gubner-Ungerleiger	8.8%	98.6%	6.7%	93.5%	6%	93.9%	0.165	0.027
RaVL	11.5%	95.7%	4.9%	91.3%	10.4%	92.2%	0.179	0.016
RV$_5$/V$_6$	3.5%	97.1%	1.6%	97.8%	4.5%	97.4%	0.082	0.269
All combined	55.8%	73.9%	60%	70.7%	67.2%	68.7%	NA	NA

Mild LVH*: For at least LVM $\geq$116 g/m^2 for men and $\geq$96 g/m^2 for women.
Moderate LVH**: For at least LVM $\geq$133 g/m^2 for men and $\geq$110 g/m^2 for women.
Severe LVH***: For at least LVM $\geq$149 g/m^2 for men and $\geq$122 g/m^2 for women.

Discussion

These findings demonstrate that the test performance of the ECG in diagnosing LVH is low in this Black African population. This is affected by a number of extracardiac factors such as age, sex, body habitus, and cardiac factors such as LVH severity and geometry. Sex specific adjustment to body habitus improves the test sensitivity. Dzudie et al. reported a similar finding of performance in a similar population [7]. Dada et al. reported a high test performance in a neighboring community [8]. The poor performance of the ECG in detecting LVH has been shown in several studies [4,12,13,14].

ECG and Sex

Sex is a major determinant of body structure and function. The Sokolow-Lyon criterion performed better in males. This could be attributed to the fixed voltage criterion that does not take account of structural body difference. Levy et al. reported an overall better performance in males where most indices used are non-sex specific [4]. Cornell criterion had an overall better performance especially in females. Rodrigues et al. reported a similar finding [14].

ECG and Age

Sokolow-Lyon and Cornell indices test performance decreased with advancing age. This was particularly significant with the Sokolow-Lyon criterion. The Cornell criterion showed a very weak but non-significant positive trend with age. Left axis shift and precordial voltages have been shown to decrease with age in men and left axis shift in women [15]. This could explain the trend observed with both criteria. Sokolow-Lyon index depends only on precordial leads while Cornell index depends on a precordial and limb leads. Left axis shift might lead to a higher R voltage in the augmented unipolar left limb lead used in Cornell index, thus a positive but non-significant trend. Aging is associated with physical changes such as a reduction in height. The enlarged heart then deviates to the left with changes in the cardiac vector as explained by Levy et al. [15]. Voltage changes associated with age cancel out with the Cornell index, thus less affected by age. The overall lower sensitivity with age could be attributed to lower tissue conductance, a point for further investigations.

ECG and Body Habitus

Sokolow-Lyon index showed a significant negative trend with increasing body size while Cornell index showed a non-significant positive trend. Levy et al. reported an overall negative trend [4]. Compared with normal weight patients, overweight and obese patients had a higher sensitivity and specificity with the Cornell index. This shows that the Cornell index is more accurate in diagnosing LVH in overweight and obese patients than Sokolow-Lyon index. Okin et al. reported a similar finding [5,16]. This could be explained by the high prevalence of LVH with obesity and attenuating effects of obesity on precordial voltages [17]. The less affected augmented limb lead in Cornell index will pull the voltage towards higher values for LVH. Sokolow-Lyon criterion depends on the precordial leads that undergo significant attenuation in overweight and obese patients, thus a decrease in its sensitivity.

ECG and LV Geometry

The sensitivity progressively increased with the severity of LVH and with the pathologic evolution of the LV with both indices. This was higher with the Cornell index. Levy et al. and Schillaci et al. reported a similar finding of increased sensitivity with LVH [4,13].

Table 4. Factors influencing the specificity and sensitivity for two selected index criteria: Sokolow-Lyon and Cornell indices.

Index	Sokolow-Lyon				Cornell			
	Sensitivity	Specificity	r	p value	Sensitivity	Specificity	r	p value
Sex								
Male	27.6%	83.3%	NA	NA	23.1%	90%	NA	NA
Female	24.3%	88.5%	–	–	49.2%	84.6%	–	–
Age								
≤55 years	35%	82.6%	-0.160	0.032	47.2%	87.1%	0.082	0.766
>55 years	26%	88.9%	–	–	32.5%	86.8%	–	–
Body habitus								
Underweight	40%	–	-0.248	0.001	20%	–	0.094	0.209
Normal	31.8%	72.7%	–	–	27.3%	86.4%	–	–
Overweight	29%	91.7%	–	–	45.2%	83.3%	–	–
Obesity1	15.6%	90.9%	–	–	28.1%	90.9%	–	–
LV geometry								
Normal	–	84.6%	0.172	0.020	–	100%	0.472	<0.0001
Remodeling	–	87.4%	–	–	–	87.8%	–	–
Concentric LVH	25.9%	73%	–	–	30.9%	73.4%	–	–
Eccentric LVH	30%	–	–	–	56.7%	–	–	–

NA: not applicable.

Table 5. Test performance of unadjusted and adjusted indices when the Left Ventricular Mass is indexed to the Body Surface Area.

Index	Threshold (Male/Female)	Sensitivity	Specificity	PPV	NPV	Accuracy	Likelihood ratio	r	p value
Sokolow-Lyon									
Unadjusted (mV)	3.5	26.5%	84.1%	73.2%	41.1%	48.4%	1.66	0.162	0.029
Adjusted to BSA (mV.m²)	5.17/5.1	55.8%	46.4%	63%	39%	52.2%	1.04	0.283	<0.001
Adjusted to BMI (mV.Kg/m²)	72.82/71.49	58.4%	40.6%	61.7%	37.8%	51.7%	0.98	0.270	<0.001
Cornell									
Unadjusted (mV)	2.8/2.0	37.2%	87%	82.4%	45.8%	56%	2.86	0.424	<0.0001
Adjusted to BSA (mV.m²)	3.11/3.02	68.1%	52.2%	70%	50%	62.1%	1.43	0.501	<0.0001
Adjusted to BMI (mV.Kg/m²)	44.23/42.74	69%	49.3%	69%	50%	61.5%	1.36	0.472	<0.0001
Combined indices									
Unadjusted	NA	50.4%	76.8%	78.1%	48.6%	60.4%	2.08	NA	NA
Adjusted to BSA	NA	77%	38.1%	62.1%	38.1%	56.6%	1.24	NA	NA
Adjusted to BMI	NA	79.6%	23.1%	62.9%	39.5%	57.7%	1.04	NA	NA

PPV: positive predictive value; NPV: negative predictive value; NA: not applicable.

Unadjusted and Adjusted Criteria

Sex specific adjustment to body habitus markedly increased the sensitivity by 2 fold with both Sokolow-Lyon and Cornell indices, with a fall in the specificity by a third and by half with Cornell and Sokolow-Lyon criteria. The highest increase was noted with Cornell index or combined indices adjusted to body mass index. With a fall in specificity, the predictive values were comparable (Table 5). Okin et al. and Norman et al. reported similar effects [5,6]. We used thresholds estimated from regression equations, which are considered to be the mean in the measured parameters. Sensitivity and specificity move in opposite directions [18]. Specificity increases with the set threshold, with a concomitant decrease in the sensitivity. Concomitant high sensitivity and specificity are seen in measurements with less spread about the mean (very strong correlation). This is however difficult to achieve with biological measurements especially when reproducibility is not perfect. Biological parameters have a high variability and are less reproducible. This gives sensitivities and specificities wide apart. The cut-off point between normal and abnormal of a test may therefore be varied to increase sensitivity or specificity (with concomitant decrease in the other) according to what we are using the test for [19]. LVH has been shown to be an independent cardiovascular risk factor and as well treatable [1,16]. It is best not to miss the diagnosis thus, the need for a test with a high sensitivity as the sex specific adjusted criteria [19]. Rodrigues et al. proposed a lower sex specific threshold for the Cornell index with the aim of improving the sensitivity [14]. This will be particularly useful in high risk patients. Further analysis using the ROC curve will give a clearer view of the situation with optimal cut-offs.

One of the limitations of our study is that only a single observer made the diagnosis of LVH both in the echocardiography and ECG. Echocardiography measurements are observer-dependent and no agreement test was carried out. The study was a specialist clinic based with selection bias of patients with heart disease. There is the risk of generalizing our findings. The echocardiography was used for comparison instead of more accurate tools like the CT scan and MRI. These are however very expensive, highly technical and not widely available. The echocardiography is widely available and user friendly, and has been shown to have a strong correlation with autopsy findings [20]. Not all possible determinants of electrocardiographic diagnosis of LVH were studied such as the cardiovascular risk factors and ethnicity. Moreover, our study is limited by the small number of subjects aged less than 40 years, as there is a significant difference in voltage between this younger age group and the more elderly. Hence the relationship between age and ECG test performance should be considered with caution. Notwithstanding, our work has some implications. We have contributed in paving the way for the ECG to be more accurate, since it is widely available and more user friendly than the echocardiography, and more accurate than the clinical method and X-ray in diagnosing LVH. Similar studies need to be carried out in the general population. A combined adjustment for age, sex, and body habitus with optimal cut-offs derived from the ROC curve is necessary for a clearer view of the possibility of improving the ECG. Fewer ECG criteria were studied further. Our choices were motivated by their better performance and are easier to use in routine clinical practice.

Conclusion

These findings demonstrate that the test performance of the ECG in diagnosing LVH is low in this black African population. This is affected by a number of extracardiac factors such as age, sex, body habitus, and cardiac factors such as LVH severity and geometry. Cornell voltage criteria had a higher performance and less affected than the Sokolow-Lyon voltage criteria. Sex specific adjustment to body habitus improves the test sensitivity by two fold and a fall in the specificity.

References

1. Levy D, Garrison RJ, Savage DD, Kannel WB, Castelli WP (1990) Prognostic implication of echocardiographically determined left ventricular mass in the Framingham Heart Study. N Engl J Med 322: 1561–1566.
2. National High Blood Pressure Education Program (1998) The sixth report of the Joint National Committee on Prevention, Detection, Evaluation, and Treatment of High Blood Pressure. Arch Intern Med 157: 241–46.
3. Chobanian AV, Bakris GL, Black HR, Cushman WC, Green LA, et al. (2003) The Seventh Report of the Joint Committee on Prevention, Detection, Evaluation, and Treatment of High Blood Pressure: the JNC 7 report. JAMA 289 (19): 2560–72.
4. Levy D, Labib SB, Anderson KM, Christianson JC, Kannel WB, et al. (1990) Determinants of Sensitivity and Specificity of Electrocardiographic Criteria for Left Ventricular Hypertrophy. Circulation 81: 815–820.
5. Okin PM, Roman MJ, Devereux RB, Kligfield P (1996) ECG identification of left ventricular hypertrophy. Relationship of test performance to body habitus. J Electrocardiol 29 Suppl: 256–61.
6. Norman JE Jr, Levy D (1996) Adjustment of ECG left ventricular hypertrophy criteria for body mass index and age improves classification accuracy. The effects of hypertension and obesity. J Electrocardiol 29 suppl: 241–7.
7. Dzudie A, Muna W, Kingue S, Akono M, Ouankou M, et al. (2006) Electrocardiograms to assess left ventricular hypertrophy in black African hypertensives. Abstract 005. First PanAfrican congress on hypertension organized by International Forum for Hypertension Prevention and Control in Africa (IFHA).
8. Dada A, Adebiyi AA, Aje A, Oladapo OO, Falase AO (2005) Standard Electrocardiogrphic Criteria for Left Ventricular Hypertrophy in Nigerian Hypertensives. Ethn Dis 15(4): 578–84.
9. Mbanya JCN, Minkoulou EM, Salah JN, Balkau B (1998) The prevalence of hypertension in rural and urban Cameroon. Int J Epidem 27: 181–185.
10. Kingue S, Befidi-Mengue R, Angwafo F III, Abbenyi AS, Wansi E, et al. (2000) Prevalence of hypertension in Cameroon. Preliminary results of the Cameroon National Health Survey (Abstract). Proc 12th Natn Med Conf Cameroon, Yaounde.
11. Lang RM, Biering M, Devereux RB, Flachskampf FA, Foster E, et al. (2005) Recommendations for chamber quantification: a report from the American Society of Echocardiography's guidelines and standards committee and the Chamber quantification writing group, developed in conjunction the European Association of Echocardiography, a branch of the European Society of Cardiology. J Am Soc Echocardiogr 18: 1440–63.
12. Verdecchia P, Dovellini EV, Gorini M, Gozzelino G, Milletich A, et al. (2000) Comparison of eletrocardiographic criteria for diagnosis of left venricular hypertrophy in hypertension: the MAVI study. Ital Heart J 1(3): 207–15.
13. Schillaci G, Verdecchia P, Borgioni C, Ciucci A, Guerrieri M, et al. (1994) Improved electrocardiogrphic diagnosis of left ventricular hypertrophy. Am J Cardiol 74 (7): 714–9.
14. Rodrigues SL, D'Angelo L, Pereira AC, Krieger JE, Mill JG (2008) Revision of the Sokolow-Lyon-Raappaport and Cornell voltage criteria for left ventricular hypertrophy. Arq Bras Cardiol 90(1): 46–53.
15. Levy D, Bailey JJ, Garrison RJ, Horton MR, Bak SM, et al. (1987) Electrocardiographic changes with advancing age. A cross-sectional study of the association of age with QRS axis, duration and voltage. J Electrocardiol 20 Suppl: 44–7.
16. Okin PM, Jern S, Devereux RB, Kieldsen SE, Dahlof B, et al. (2000) Effect of Obesity on Electrocardiographic Left Ventricular Hypertrophy in Hypertensive Patients: the Losartan Intervention For Endpoint (LIFE) reduction in hypertension study. Hypertension 35(1pt 1): 13–8.
17. De Simone G, Devereux RB, Roman MJ, Aliderman MH, Laragh JH (1994) Relation of obesity and gender to left ventricular hypertrophy in normotensive and hypertensive adults. Hypertension 23: 600–606.
18. Akobeng AK (2007) Understanding diagnostic tests 1: Sensitivity, Specificity, and Predictive values. Acta Paediatr 96(3): 338–41.
19. Akobeng AK (2007) Understanding diagnostic tests 3: Receiver Operating Characteristics curves. Acta Paediatr 96(5): 644–7.
20. Devereux RB, Alonso DR, Lutas EM, Gottlieb GJ, Campo E, et al. (1986) Echocardiographic assessment of left ventricular hypertrophy: comparison to necropsy findings. Am J Cardiol 57: 450–80.

Author Contributions

Conceived and designed the experiments: AMJ JJNN. Performed the experiments: AMJ PK. Analyzed the data: AMJ JJNN. Contributed reagents/materials/analysis tools: AMJ JJNN SK. Wrote the paper: AMJ JJNN. Revised the manuscript: JJNN AMJ SK.

20

Cytosolic CARP Promotes Angiotensin II- or Pressure Overload-Induced Cardiomyocyte Hypertrophy through Calcineurin Accumulation

Ci Chen[1], Liang Shen[1], Shiping Cao[1]*, Xixian Li[1], Wanling Xuan[1], Jingwen Zhang[1], Xiaobo Huang[1], Jianping Bin[1], Dingli Xu[1], Guofeng Li[2], Masafumi Kitakaze[1,3], Yulin Liao[1]*

1 State Key Laboratory of Organ Failure Research, Department of Cardiology, Nanfang Hospital, Southern Medical University, Guangzhou, China, **2** Department of Pharmacy, Nanfang Hospital, Southern Medical University, Guangzhou, China, **3** Cardiovascular Division of the Department of Medicine, National Cerebral and Cardiovascular Center, Osaka, Japan

Abstract

The gene ankyrin repeat domain 1 (Ankrd1) is an enigmatic gene and may exert pleiotropic function dependent on its expression level, subcellular localization and even types of pathological stress, but it remains unclear how these factors influence the fate of cardiomyocytes. Here we attempted to investigate the role of CARP on cardiomyocyte hypertrophy. In neonatal rat ventricular cardiomyocytes (NRVCs), angiotensin II (Ang II) increased the expression of both calpain 1 and CARP, and also induced cytosolic translocation of CARP, which was abrogated by a calpain inhibitor. In the presence of Ang-II in NRVCs, infection with a recombinant adenovirus containing rat Ankrd1 cDNA (Ad-Ankrd1) enhanced myocyte hypertrophy, the upregulation of atrial natriuretic peptide and β-myosin heavy chain genes and calcineurin proteins as well as nuclear translocation of nuclear factor of activated T cells. Cyclosporin A attenuated Ad-Ankrd1-enhanced cardiomyocyte hypertrophy. Intra-myocardial injection of Ad-Ankrd1 in mice with transverse aortic constriction (TAC) markedly increased the cytosolic CARP level, the heart weight/body weight ratio, while short hairpin RNA targeting Ankrd1 inhibited TAC-induced hypertrophy. The expression of calcineurin was also significantly increased in Ad-Ankrd1-infected TAC mice. Olmesartan (an Ang II receptor antagonist) prevented the upregulation of CARP in both Ang II-stimulated NRVCs and hearts with pressure overload. These findings indicate that overexpression of Ankrd1 exacerbates pathological cardiac remodeling through the enhancement of cytosolic translocation of CARP and upregulation of calcineurin.

Editor: Ryuichi Morishita, Osaka University Graduate School of Medicine, Japan

Funding: This work was supported by grants from the National Natural Science Foundation of China (81170146, 31271513 to Y.L.), the Team Program of Natural Science Foundation of Guangdong Province, China (S2011030003134, to Y.L. and B.J.). The funders had no role in study design, data collection and analysis, decision to publish, or preparation of the manuscript.

Competing Interests: The authors have declared that no competing interests exist.

* Email: liao18@msn.com (YL); csp2012@126.com (SC)

Introduction

Cardiac ankyrin repeat protein (CARP) binds to various proteins, such as titin/connectin, myopalladin [1], and calsequestrin [2], and it plays a critical role in the maintenance of sarcomere integrity, stretch sensing, and excitation-contraction coupling under physiological and pathological conditions. Similar to the genes for natriuretic peptides and β-myosin heavy chain (β-MHC), the gene for CARP (termed ankyrin repeat domain 1: Ankrd1) was also identified as a fetal gene, expression of which is augmented in both animals and humans with cardiac hypertrophy [3,4] and heart failure (HF) [5,6]. Natriuretic peptides have been shown to have cardioprotective effect [7]. In contrast, the role of Ankrd1/CARP in cell growth remains controversial. Although there is clinical evidence that Ankrd1 mutations are involved in the pathogenesis of hypertrophic and dilated cardiomyopathy [8–10], there is no consensus about whether CARP enhances or attenuates cardiac hypertrophy.

Subcellular distribution of CARP is thought to be associated with its different function [11], while the cytosolic protease calpain 3 has been reported to be responsible for cytosolic retention of CARP [12]. It appears that Ankrd1/CARP can function as pro-hypertrophic gene in the myofibril by gain of function and as an anti-hypertrophic gene in the nucleus by suppression of cardiac genes expression [11,13]. A recent study revealed that hypertrophic cardiomyopathy (HCM) associated mutations in Ankrd1 (P52A, T123M, and I280V) have an increased binding ability of CARP to titin and myopalladin [9], while overexpression of either wildtype or HCM related mutant Ankrd1 (P52A or I280V) in cardiomyocytes reduced myocyte contractility [14]. In addition, it has been proposed that calpains influence signaling pathways that are involved in myocardial hypertrophy, including those for calcineurin [15,16]. Therefore, we postulated that an increased cytosolic translocation of CARP could be a mediator of calpain-related signal transduction processes. Moreover, CARP is involved in calcium-dependent signaling [2], while increased binding of CARP to titin and myopalladin has been suggested to induce

Table 1. Sequences of primers for regular PCR.

Transcripts	Forward primer (5′–3′)	Reverse primer (5′–3′)	Product size (bp)
ANP (rat)	GGCTCCTTCTCCATCACCAA	TGTTATCTTCGGTACCG	458
ANKRED1 (rat)	CGGGATCCATGATGGTTTTTCGAGTAGAGG	GGCCTCGAGTCAGAACGTAGCTATGCGC	960
Egr-1 (rat)	AGCCTTCGCTCACTCCACTA	GACTCAACAGGGCAAGCATAC	184
GAPDH (rat)	ACCAACTGCTTAGCCCCCC	GCATGTCAGATCCACAACGG	281

myocardial hypertrophy [9]. These findings suggest the hypothesis that CARP might accelerate the progression of cardiac hypertrophy.

Although substantial evidence indicates that evaluation of Ankrd1/CARP expression may be helpful for diagnostic or prognostic assessment of cardiac hypertrophy, it is unknown whether Ankrd1/CARP could also be a therapeutic target. Considering that overproduction of angiotensin II (Ang II) is responsible for cardiac hypertrophy and upregulation of Ankrd1/CARP, it seems reasonable for Ankrd1/CARP to be a potential target of Ang II receptor 1 blockers (ARB). Accordingly, we used Ang II-stimulated cultured cardiomyocytes and mice with transverse aortic constriction (TAC) to examine the following issues: (1) the influence of Ankrd1/CARP on cardiac hypertrophy; (2) whether Ankrd1/CARP modulates calcineurin and nuclear factor of activated T cells (NFAT) and (3) whether the ARB olmesartan medoxomil prevents the upregulation of Ankrd1/CARP in response to Ang II or pressure overload.

Materials and Methods

All procedures were performed in accordance with our Institutional Guidelines for Animal Research and the investigation conformed to the Guide for the Care and Use of Laboratory Animals published by the US National Institutes of Health (NIH Publication No. 85-23, revised in 1996). The study was approved by the ethics review board of Southern Medical University. The concentrations or dose of olmesartan and its active form RNH-6270 were decided according to previous reports [17] and our preliminary experiments.

Cell culture

The neonatal rats were sacrificed by 2% isoflurane inhalation and cervical dislocation. Isolation and culture of ventricular cardiomyocytes was performed as described previously [18]. The confirmation of cell type was performed using immunochemistry assay (antimyoactin antibody, Wuhan Boster Biological Technology., LTD, China). Cells were cultured for 4 days and then treated with 0.1–1 μM Ang II or 1 μM calpain inhibitor 1 (Sigma Aldrich), or RNH-6270 1 μM (RNH, active metabolite of olmesartan, provided by Daiichi Sankyo, Tokyo), or recombinant adenovirus containing the rat Ankrd1 cDNA (Ad-Ankrd1) or adeno-associate virus (AAV) carrying short hairpin RNA targeting Ankrd1 (sh-Ankrd1). Cell surface area was also measured by staining with rhodamine phalloidin and diamidino-2-phenylindole dihydrochloride (DAPI). Briefly, the cells were fixed with 4.0% paraformaldehyde in PBS, permeabilized in 0.1% Triton X-100 in PBS, and stained with rhodamine phalloidin (5 μg/ml, Invitrogen) and DAPI (5 mg/mL, Beyotime) by standard immunocytochemical techniques. At least 30 random cells from each group were measured by the Image J software.

Construction of recombinant adenovirus carrying Ankrd1 or AAV containing silenced Ankrd1

The full-length cDNA of rat Ankrd1 was inserted into the vector pUC57, and then subcloned into the shuttle vector pDC316-mCMV-EGFP. The Ankrd1 cDNA clones were sequenced completely to confirm the absence of cloning artifacts and mutation. The Ad-MAX system was used for the generation of recombinant adenovirus carrying Ankrd1 cDNA or empty vector (pEGFP). Briefly, pDC316-mCMV-EGFP-Ankrd1 and virus backbone plasmid pBHGloxdelIE13cre were co-transfected into cultured HEK293 cells by using lipofectamine 2000 (Invitrogen), then the recombinant adenovirus were collected and amplified in HEK293. The overexpression of Ankrd1 was achieved by transfecting cultured neonatal rat ventricular cardiomyocytes (NRVCs) with the recombinant adenovirus (multiplicity of infection (MOI) = 10) or by myocardial injection of 5×10^{11} adenovirus particles containing Ankrd1 or control vector into three points of the left ventricular wall.

Table 2. Sequences of primers for real-time PCR.

Transcripts	Forward primer (5′–3′)	Reverse primer (5′–3′)	Product size (bp)
β-MHC (rat)	GCTACCCAACCCTAAGGATGC	TCTGCCTAAGGTGCTGTTTCA	196
ANP (rat)	CTCCGATAGATCTGCCCTCTTGAA	GGTACCGGAAGCTGTTGCAGCCTA	216
β-actin (rat)	ATCGTGCGGGACATCAAGG	CAGGAAGGAGGGCTGGAACA	180
ANP (mouse)	CGGTGTCCAACACAGATC	TCTTCTACCGGCATCTTTC	71
β-actin (mouse)	TGGACAGTGAGGCAAGGATAG	TACTGCCCTGGCTCCTAGCA	121
Calpain 1 (rat)	TGCCATGTTCCGTGCTTTCA	GACCGTAAAAACGTGGCTGC	178
GAPDH (rat)	GATGCCCCCATGTTTGTGAT	GGTCATGAGCCCTTCCACAAT	216

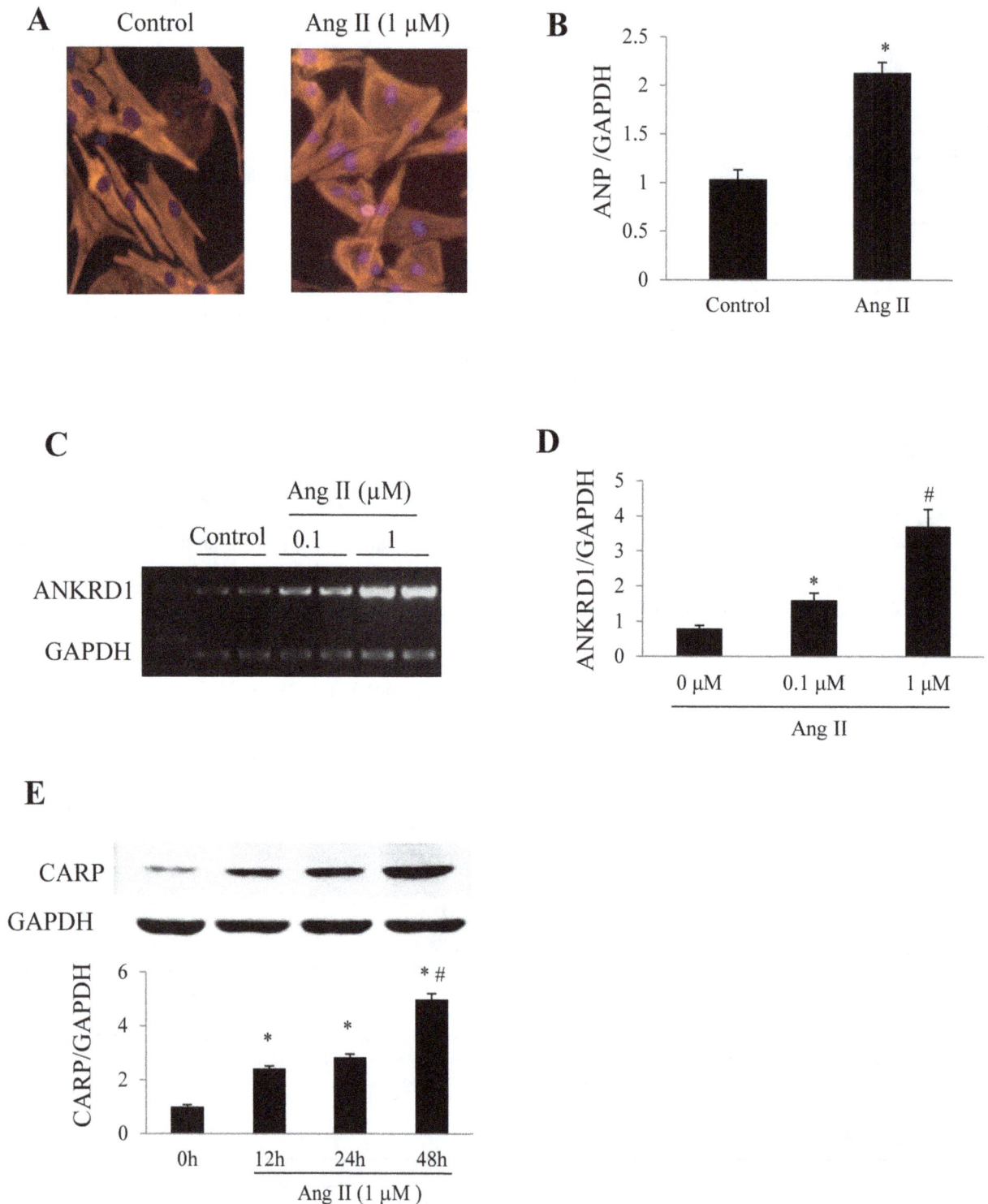

Figure 1. Ankrd1/CARP upregulation in response to Angiotensin II stimulation. *(A)* Representative images of cultured neonatal rat ventricular cardiomyocytes (NRVCs) stained with rhodamine phalloidin and 4′, 6-diamidino-2-phenylindole dihydrochloride (DAPI), and the cell size increased when treated with Angiotensin II (Ang II 1 μM) for 24h. *(B)* Hypertrophic marker atrial natriuretic peptide (ANP) detected by Real-time PCR using GAPDH as an internal control (*$P<0.05$ vs. the control group). Expression changes of Ankrd1 in response to Ang II in cultured NRVCs were detected by PCR *(C)* or real-time PCR *(D)*. *(E)* Western blot analysis of time-dependent changes of CARP expression in NRVCs exposed to Ang II. *$P<0.05$ vs. Ang II-untreated group, #$P<0.01$ vs. Ang II 24 h group. Repeat times n = 3. Data are mean ± SEM.

AAV-mediated gene delivery was also employed. pAAV2/9-CMV-ZsGreen vectors carrying short hairpin RNA targeting Ankrd1 (sh-Ankrd1) or scramble were created by a professional company (Biowit, Shenzheng, China). For in vitro transfection, pAAV2/9-CMV-ZsGreen-shAnkrd1 or scramble virus particles (5×10^5 viral genomes/cell) were added in cultured NRVCs. After

A

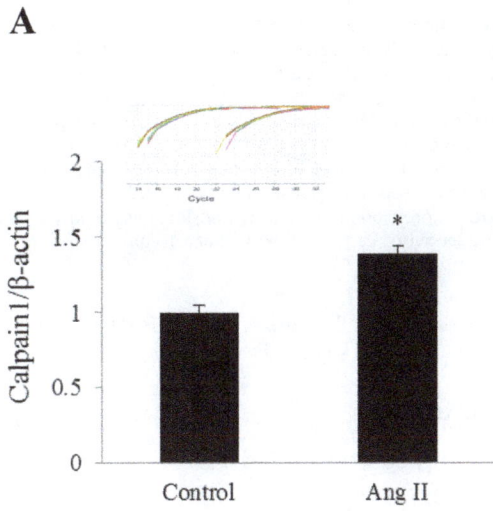

B

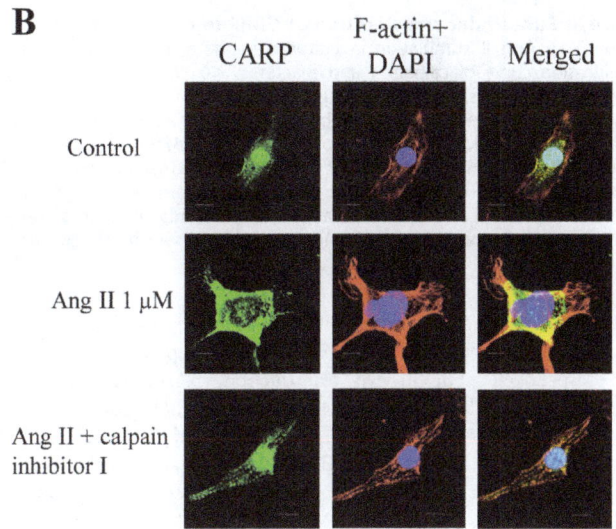

C

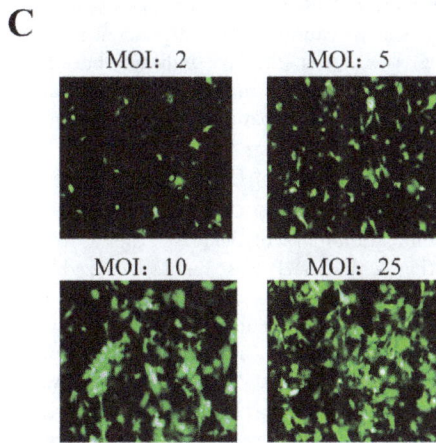

D

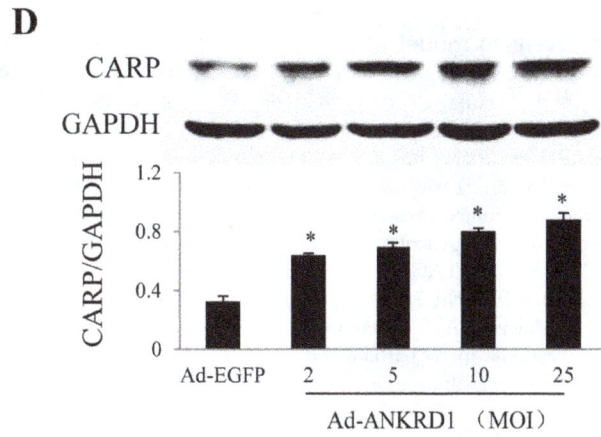

E

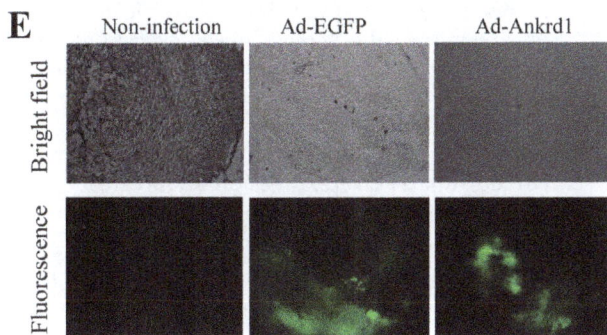

F

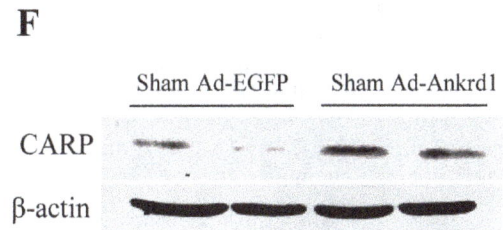

G

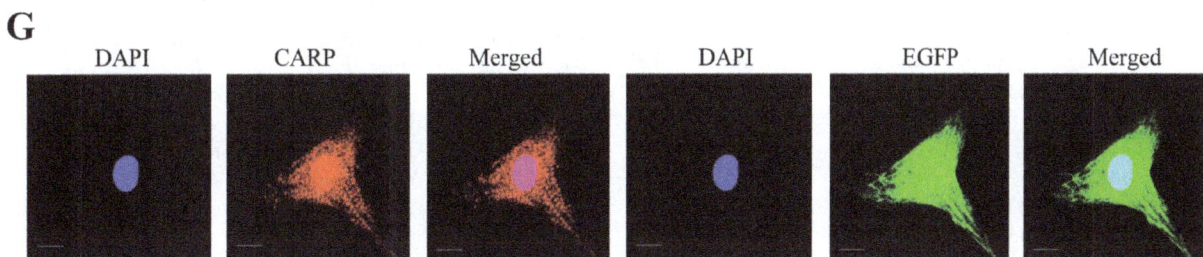

Figure 2. Subcellular translocation of CARP in response to treatment with Ang II or Ad-Ankrd1. *(A)* Expression changes of calpain 1 in response to Ang II stimulation in cultured neonatal rat ventricular cardiomyocytes (NRVCs) detected by real-time PCR, the insert represents amplification curve of calpain 1 and β-actin, *P<0.05. *(B)* Confocal microscopic subcellular distribution of CARP (green) in response to Ang II stimulation in NRVCs. Immunostaining with F-actin (red) was used to confirm the cardiomyocytes, and DAPI (blue) was used to stain the nuclei. Bar = 10 μm. *(C)* Dose-dependent infective efficiency of Ad-Ankrd1 in cultured NRVCs detected by the green fluorescence of co-expressed EGFP. MOI: multiplicity of infection. *(D)* Western blot analysis of CARP protein levels in response to different dose of Ad-Ankrd1 infection (*P<0.01 vs. Ad-EGFP group, n = 3). *(E)* Representative EGFP fluorescence microscopic photos of LV myocardium at 1 week after intramyocardial injection of vehicle (non-transfection), Ad-EGFP or Ad-Ankrd1 delivery. *(F)* Western blot analysis of CARP protein levels in response to intramyocardial injection of Ad-EGFP or Ad-Ankrd1 at 1 week after sham operation. *(G)* Subcellular location of forced Ankrd1 expression in Ad-Ankrd1 transfected cardiomyocytes. The green fluorescence was emitted from the report gene EGFP which was constructed in adenovirus carrying Ankrd1. Bar = 10 μm.

transfection for ninety-six hours, infection efficiency and silencing effect were evaluated using a fluorescence microscopy and western blot, respectively. For in vivo transduction, pAAV2/9-CMV-ZsGreen-sh-Ankrd1 or scramble virus particles (1×10^{11} viral genomes/ml) were administered by direct injection in the left ventricular free wall (2 sites, 10 μl/site) in mice at 4 weeks old using a syringe with a 30-gauge needle, and four weeks later, sham or TAC surgery was performed.

Transduction efficiency of in vivo gene transfer by adenovirus or AAV was assessed by EGFP fluorescence (510 nm) in cryosectioned heart slices using a fluorescence microscopy.

Pressure overload model

C57BL/6 male mice (8–10 weeks old, weighing 22–25 g, provided by the Animal Center of Southern Medical University) were anesthetized with a mixture of xylazine (5 mg/kg, intraperitoneally) and ketamine (100 mg/kg, intraperitoneally), and the adequacy of anesthesia was monitored from the disappearance of pedal withdrawal reflex. Pressure overload model was created by transverse aortic constriction (TAC) as described elsewhere [18,19]. Some of the TAC mice were randomized to treatment with olmesartan (Daiichi Sankyo, Tokyo, 10 mg/kg/d added in the food) or vehicle alone for 4 weeks. The mice were sacrificed by overdose anesthesia (pentobarbital sodium 150 mg/kg intraperitoneally) and cervical dislocation.

Polymerase chain reaction analysis (PCR) and Western blot

Total RNA of homogenized murine whole heart or cultured cardiomyocytes was isolated using Total RNA Kit II (Omega) according to the protocol provided by the manufacturer. Conventional or quantitative real-time PCR using a Quantitect SYBR Green RT-PCR kit (QIAGEN) and an Applied Biosystems 7500 system targeting the genes of Ankrd1, ANP, β-MHC, calpain 1, early growth response 1 (egr-1), β-actin and GAPDH, was performed. Primers were showed in Table 1 and 2.

Proteins were extracted from the cultured cardiomyocytes or their mitochondria, or the murine heart. Immunoblotting was performed by using antibodies against CARP (Santa Cruz), calcineurin (Abcam). Blotting of β-actin or GAPDH (Santa Cruz) was used as a loading control.

Immunofluorescence assay

Immunofluorescence staining was used to examine the cellular distribution of the CARP proteins and NFAT. Location of CARP and NFAT (Abcam) in the cardiomyocytes was detected with a confocal microscopy.

Statistical analysis

Data are expressed as the mean ± SEM. Statistical significance was analyzed using Student's unpaired *t*-test or one-way ANOVA, followed by Bonferroni's correction for post hoc multiple

comparisons. In all analyses, *P* values<0.05 were considered to indicate statistical significance.

Results

Ang II upregulates Ankrd1/CARP in cultured cardiomyocytes

In cultured NRVCs, stimulation with Ang II for 24 h increased the cell surface area and upregulated ANP (Fig. 1 A and B). Ang II stimulation markedly increased the expression of Ankrd1 mRNA detected by routine PCR (Fig. 1C) and quantitative real-time PCR (Fig. 1D), as well as causing a time-dependent increase of CARP protein (Fig. 1E). These findings indicate that the myocardial expression pattern of Ankrd1/CARP is similar to that of natriuretic peptides during pathological stimulation.

Cytosolic translocation of CARP in response to Ang II or infection of Ad-Ankrd1 in cultured NRVCs

Ang II stimulation markedly increased the expression of calpain 1 mRNA (Fig. 2A). CARP was mainly localized to the nucleus under basal conditions, cytoplasmic translocation of CARP was noted when Ang II treatment for 24 h in NRVCs, which was abolished by a calpain 1 inhibitor (Fig. 2B), suggesting that cytosolic retention of CARP contributes to Ang II-induced cardiomyocyte hypertrophy. Then we infected NRVCs with Ad-Ankrd1. After incubation for 48 h, the transfection efficiency of Ad-Ankrd1 or Ad-EGFP and the subcellular localization of Ankrd1 in cultured cardiomyocytes were evaluated by confocal fluorescence microscopy. It was found that the number of Ad-Ankrd1-transfected cells (Fig. 2B) and the level of CARP protein (Fig. 2C) both increased in a MOI-dependent fashion. We noted that the forced overexpression of Ankrd1 was detected in both the cytoplasm and the nucleus (Fig. 2G).

Forced Ankrd1 overexpression aggravates cardiomyocyte hypertrophy in response to Ang II stimulation

The hypertrophy-associated fetal genes ANP and β-MHC were significantly upregulated in Ad-Ankrd1 infected cardiomyocytes both in the absence and the presence of Ang II stimulation (Fig. 3A and B). In addition, overexpression of Ankrd1 significantly enhanced the Ang II-stimulated increase of cell surface area (Fig. 3C). CARP was reported to upregulate egr-1 [20] which participates calcineurin-NFAT signal pathway [21]. It has been well documented that the calcineurin/NFAT pathway plays a pivotal role in myocardial hypertrophy [22]. Therefore, we examined erg-1 mRNA, calcineurin and NFAT protein levels. We noted that Ankrd1 overexpression significantly upregulated erg-1 (Fig. 3 D). Western blot analysis showed that overexpression of Ankrd1 led to a significant increase of calcineurin (Fig. 3E) and to an increased expression and nuclear translocation of NFAT (Fig. 3F) even in the absence of Ang-II stimulation. The increase of

A

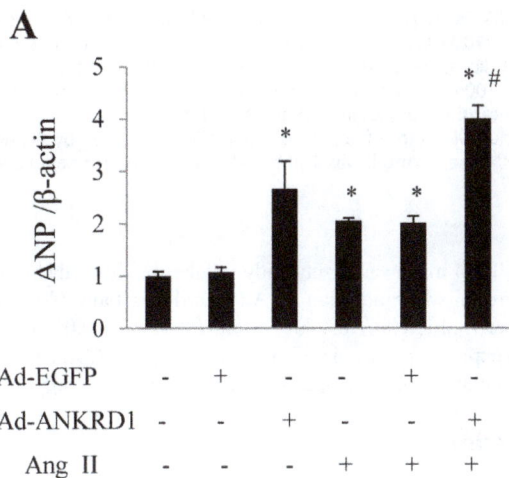

Ad-EGFP	-	+	-	-	+	-
Ad-ANKRD1	-	-	+	-	-	+
Ang II	-	-	-	+	+	+

B

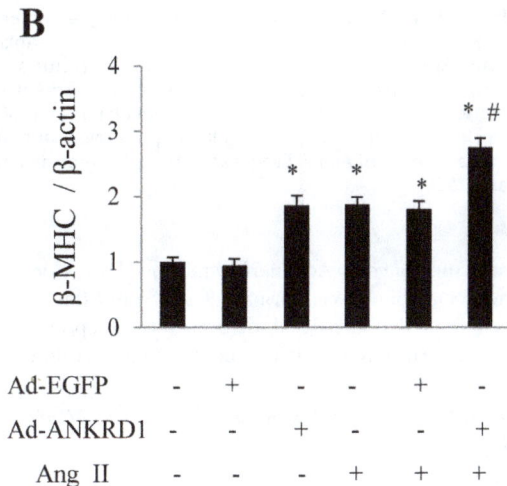

Ad-EGFP	-	+	-	-	+	-
Ad-ANKRD1	-	-	+	-	-	+
Ang II	-	-	-	+	+	+

D

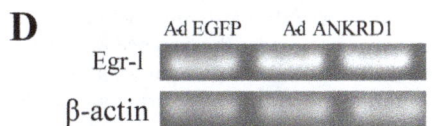

C

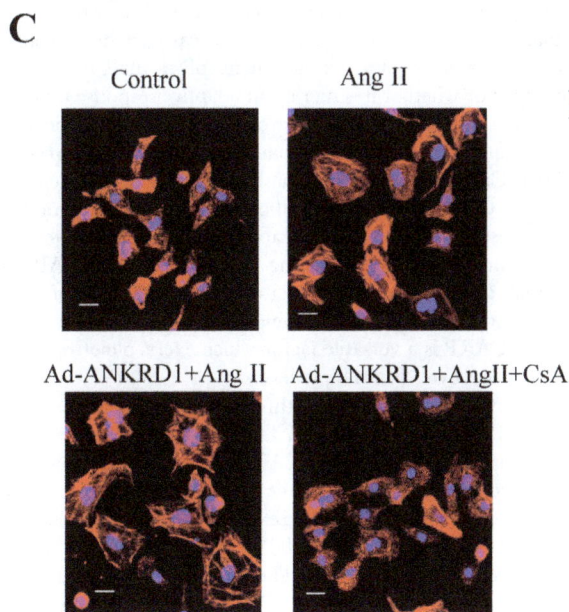

Control   Ang II

Ad-ANKRD1+Ang II   Ad-ANKRD1+AngII+CsA

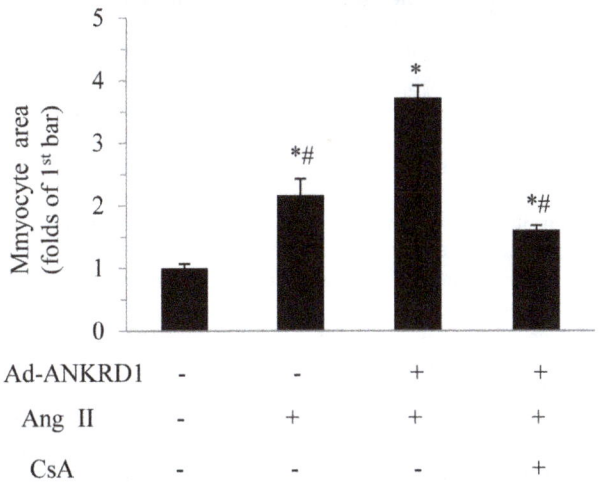

Ad-ANKRD1	-	-	+	+
Ang II	-	+	+	+
CsA	-	-	-	+

E

Calcineurin

β-actin

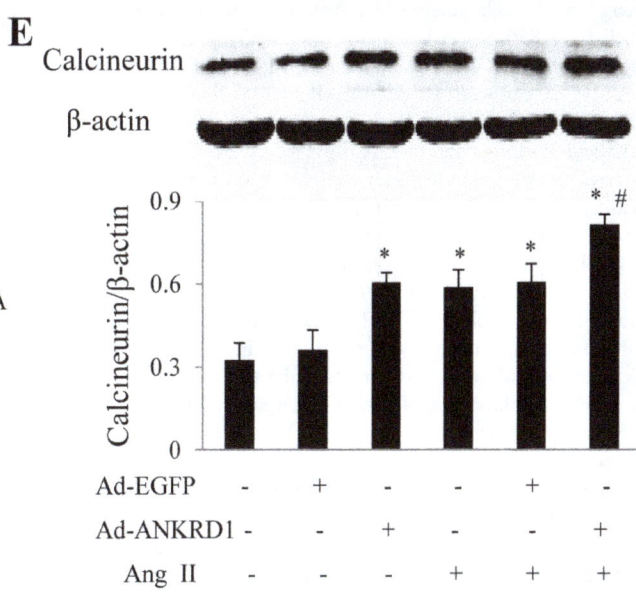

Ad-EGFP	-	+	-	-	+	-
Ad-ANKRD1	-	-	+	-	-	+
Ang II	-	-	-	+	+	+

F

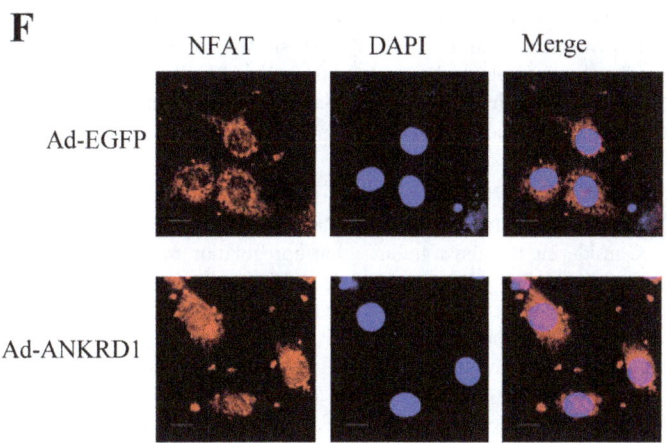

NFAT   DAPI   Merge

Ad-EGFP

Ad-ANKRD1

Figure 3. Effect of Ad-Ankrd1 transfection on myocyte hypertrophy in NRVCs. Hypertrophic markers of ANP *(A)* and β-MHC *(B)* gene expressions in response to Ang II stimulation in the presence of Ad-Ankrd1 or Ad-EGFP (10 MOI) were detected by Real-time PCR (*$P<$0.01 vs. control, #$P<$0.01 vs. Ad-EGFP + Ang II, n = 5). *(C)* Representative pictures of cultured cardiomyocytes used for calculation of cross section area and quantitative results (*$P<$0.01 vs. control (1st bar), #$P<$0.01 vs. Ad-Ankrd1+ Ang II, n = 100 in each group). *(D)* PCR results of early growth response 1 (egr-1) in response to Ad-Ankrd1 treatment. *(E)* Western blot analysis of calcineurin in cardiomyocytes in response to different treatment (*$P<$0.01 vs. control (1st bar), #$P<$0.01 vs. Ad-EGFP + Ang II group). *(F)* Nuclear translocation of nuclear factor of activated T cells (NFAT) induced by Ad-Ankrd1 transfection in the absence of Ang II. Every experiment was repeated at least 3 times. Dose of Ang II was 1 μM. Scale bar = 10 μm for panel *C* and *E*. Data are mean ± SEM.

cell surface area stimulated by Ad-Ankrd1 and Ang II was blocked by the calcineurin inhibitor cyclosporine A (CsA, Sigma) (Fig. 3C). These results indicate that forced Ankrd1 overexpression promotes cardiomyocyte hypertrophy via the calcineurin-NFAT pathway.

Effects of Ankrd1 overexpression or silence on cardiac hypertrophy

In the mice receiving sham operation, about 60% infection efficiency was obtained for the whole heart at 1 week after intramyocardial injection of Ad-Ankrd1 manifested by green fluorescence in cardiomyocytes under fluorescence microscopy as well as a significantly higher CARP expression level than in Ad-EGFP group (Fig. 2E and F). Cardiac overexpression of Ankrd1/CARP in TAC mice was achieved by intramyocardial injection of Ad-Ankrd1 at 2 weeks after TAC. Another 2 weeks later, total myocardial CARP expression was dramatically higher in Ad-Ankrd1-infected TAC mice than in Ad-EGFP-infected TAC mice (Fig. 4A and B), and overexpressed CARP largely localized in the cytoplasm (Fig. 4A). Furthermore, myocardial overexpression of Ankrd1 was found to promote TAC-induced cardiac hypertrophy (Fig. 4A). The heart weight/body weight (HW/BW) ratio was significantly higher in Ad-Ankrd1-TAC mice than in Ad-EGFP-TAC mice (8.69±0.38 mg/g in vs. 6.04±0.15 mg/g, $P<$0.01, Fig. 4C). Similarly, the TAC-induced increase of cardiomyocyte surface area and ANP expression was markedly enhanced by overexpression of Ankrd1 (Fig. 4A, D and E, all $P<$0.01). Myocardial calcineurin expression was higher in TAC mice than in shame group, while it was further enhanced in TAC mice treated with Ad-Ankrd1 (Fig. 4F and G). These findings indicated that myocardial overexpression of Ankrd1 exacerbates cardiac hypertrophy.

Silencing effect of sh-Ankrd1 was confirmed in cultured NRCs. AAV2/6 transfection for 96 h in cardiomyocytes led to about 60% transfection efficiency, while western blot showed that CARP was downregulated by 3 folds (Fig. 5A and B). AAV2/6 transfection for 5 weeks in murine heart resulted in more than 50% transduction efficiency (Fig. 5C). One week after TAC, we noted that myocardial transduction of AAV-sh-Ankrd1 could inhibit cardiac hypertrophy evidenced by that the HW/BW ratio was significantly smaller in AAV-sh-Ankrd1-TAC mice than in the scramble-TAC mice (Fig. 5D).

Olmesartan attenuates cardiac hypertrophy in TAC mice through down-regulation of Ankrd1/CARP

Considering the above findings that upregulation of myocardial Ankrd1/CARP in response to Ang II stimulation and pressure overload had a detrimental influence on myocyte hypertrophy, we investigated whether Ankrd1/CARP was a target of olmesartan, which is a selective angiotensin II type 1 receptor antagonist. Treatment with 1 μM RNH-6270 significantly prevented the Ang II-stimulated upregulation of CARP protein and ANP gene expression in cultured cardiomyocytes (Fig. 6A and B). Four weeks later, olmesartan significantly reduced the TAC-induced cardiac hypertrophy (Fig. 6C), and the HW/BW ratio in olmesartan-

treated TAC mice was significantly smaller than in vehicle-treated TAC group, while addition of Ad-Ankrd1 partially blocked the antihypertrophic effect of olmesartan ($P<$0.05 or 0.01, Fig. 6D). CARP expression was significantly lower in TAC mice treated with olmesartan than in untreated TAC mice (Fig. 6E).

Discussion

Although it has been demonstrated that Ankrd1/CARP expression is upregulated in response to myocardial damage and dysfunction regardless of the etiology [3,4,6], and elevation of Ankrd1/CARP expression is interpreted as an indicator of an unfavorable clinical outcome, it remains unclear whether myocardial overexpression of Ankrd1 in cardiac hypertrophy is causally related to the development of a malignant cardiac phenotype or whether it is merely an adaptive response that delays the progression of cardiac hypertrophy. This study provided both in vitro and in vivo evidence that myocardial overexpression of Ankrd1/CARP promotes cardiac hypertrophy. Cytosolic translocation of CARP induced by either pathological stress or forced overexpression, also contributed to the malignant cardiac phenotype. Another interesting finding was that Ankrd1/CARP is a potential pharmacological target for the treatment of cardiac remodeling. Our present findings support the concept that Ankrd1/CARP is a versatile factor which exerts pleiotropic effects on cardiomyocytes at multiple levels.

Arimura et al. detected three HCM-associated missense mutations (P52A, T123M, and I280V) in Ankrd1, all of which showing increased binding of CARP to titin and myopalladin in the I band region of the sarcomere [9], while a recent study by Crocini et al. showed that overexpression of either wildtype or mutant Ankrd1 (P52A and I280V) in cardiomyocytes led to a reduced cell contractility [14]. These lines of evidence imply that sarcomeric translocation of CARP and increased binding to titin and myopalladin are necessary for hypertrophy enhancement by CARP under pathological stress. The subcellular localization of CARP under physiological and pathophysiological conditions remains obscure or even controversial. Some studies indicated that CARP is a cardiac-restricted nuclear protein with a pivotal role in fetal development [23] or in failing and non-failing hearts of human [5,24], but CARP was also detected in the cytoplasm rather than the nucleus of cardiomyocytes from HF patients [6,25] or even in neonatal rat cardiomyocytes [9]. Generally, it is believed that CARP is both cytosolic and nuclear localization [8,10] which functions as stretching-sense component in the cytoplasm and a co-factor of cardiac gene expression in the nuclei, and their subcellular localization depends on physiological and pathological stresses. The present study showed that CARP was mainly located in the nucleus of neonatal cardiomyocytes under physiological conditions and underwent translocation to the cytoplasm in response to stimulation by Ang II. Moreover, we found that forced overexpression of CARP increased its cytosolic distribution and had several detrimental effects on cardiomyocytes. In adult mice receiving sham or TAC treatment, myocardial CARP is preferentially localized in cytoplasm. Therefore, it seems

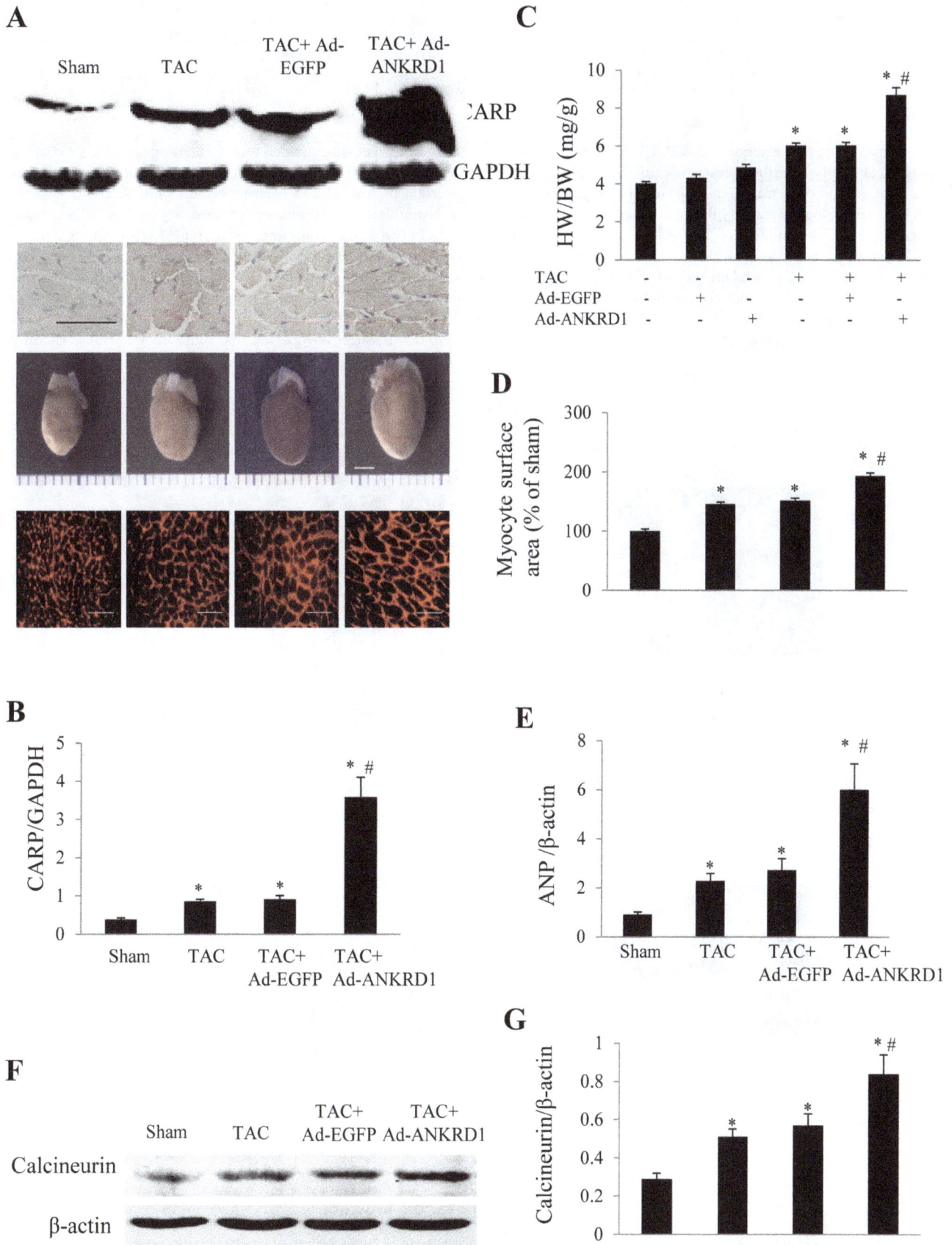

Figure 4. Myocardial injection of Ad-Ankrd1 in mice promotes cardiac hypertrophy. Cardiac overexpression of Ankrd1 was achieved by myocardial injection of Ad-Ankrd1 at 2 weeks after TAC, and the mice in each group were sacrificed at 4 weeks after the initial surgery. *(A)* Representative pictures of Western blot for CARP (upper panel), immunohistochemistry of myocardial CARP (2nd line, scale bar = 50 μm), whole hearts

(3rd line, scale bar = 3 mm) and myocyte cross-sectional area stained with rhodamine-conjugated wheat germ agglutinin (low panel, scale bar = 30 μm) from each group. *(B)* Expression levels of CARP in each group. *(C)* HW/BW ratio at 4 weeks after surgery in different groups. *(D)* Myocyte surface area was calculated from 100 cells in each group. *(E)* ANP gene expression detected by Real-time PCR using β-actin as an internal control. *(F)* Western blot analysis of calcineurin expression in heart from each group. *(G)* Semi-quantitative analysis of calcineurin expression. For panel *B-E, G,* *P<0.01 vs. sham, #P<0.01 vs. TAC + Ad-EGFP, n = 4–9 in each group. Data are mean ± SEM.

that cytoplasmic translocation of CARP in response to a pathological insult contributes to myocardial hypertrophy. Although there is no consensus about the subcellular distribution of CARP in pathological states [8,9,11,24], our results are in agreement with the findings of a previous clinical study that CARP immunoreactivity was localized to the cytoplasm in diseased myocardium and was barely detectable in the nucleus [6].

To date, the in vivo evidence concerning the role of CARP in myocardial hypertrophy are scant. HCM associated Ankrd1 mutations result in an increased binding of CARP to sacomeric

titin and myopalladin as well as a dual intracellular localization within sarcomere and nucleus [9]. On the other hand, overexpression of Ankrd1 has been reported to inhibit the phenylephrine-stimulated enlargement of neonatal rat cardiomyocytes [10,26], which is contradictory to our present findings and a consensus that "gain" of function (such as overexpression) for a sarcomeric gene usually results in hypertrophy [13]. One explanation for such discrepancy is the different intracellular localization of CARP dependent on the experimental conditions. Duboscq-Bidot et al reported that more nuclear translocation of

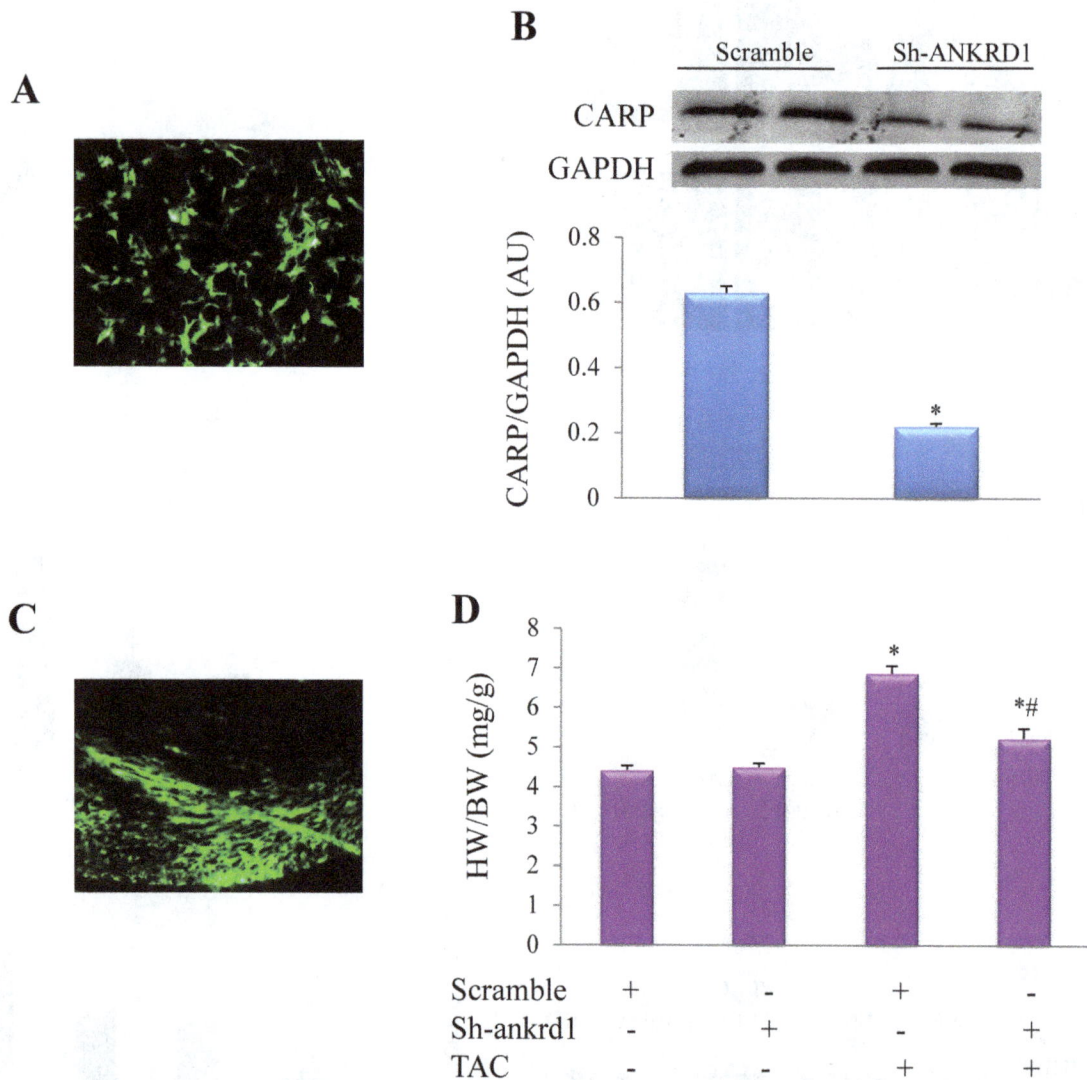

Figure 5. Myocardial injection of AAV-sh-Ankrd1 in mice inhibits cardiac hypertrophy. *(A)* Infective efficiency of AAV-sh-Ankrd1 in cultured NRVCs for 96 h detected by the green fluorescence of co-expressed EGFP (zsGreen). *(B)* Western blot analysis of CARP protein levels in response to AAV-sh-Ankrd1 or AAV-scramble infection (*P<0.01 vs. scramble group, n = 5). *(C)* Representative fluorescence microscopic pictures of left ventricular myocardium 5 weeks after intramyocardial AAV-sh-Ankrd1 delivery. *(D)* Heart weigh/body weight ratio (HW/BW) in TAC or Sham mice treated with AAV-scramble or AAV-sh-Ankrd1. *P<0.01 vs. the corresponding Sham (TAC -) group, #P<0.01 vs. TAC + scramble group, n = 5 in each group. TAC or Sham was persisted for 1 week.

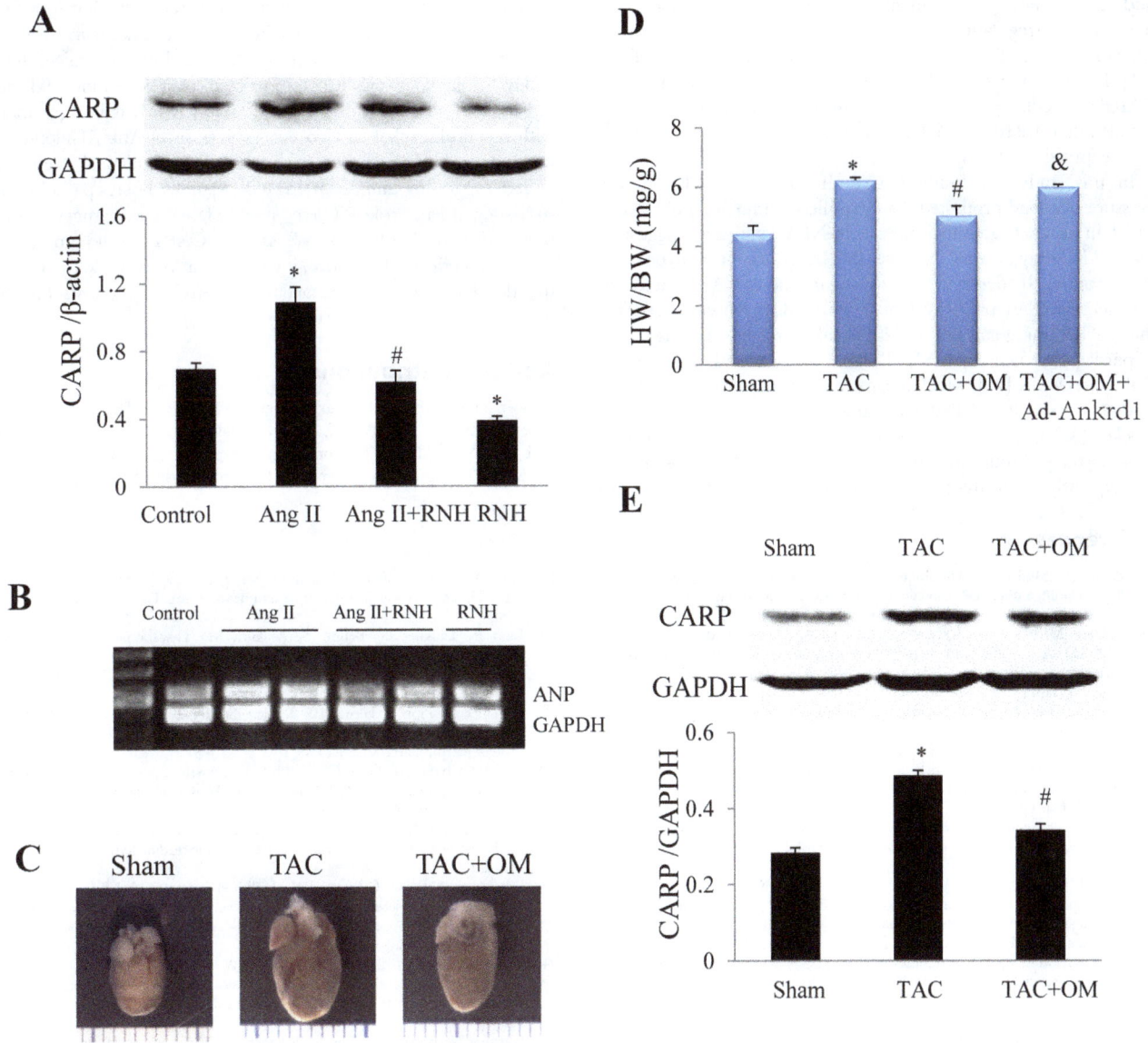

Figure 6. Olmesartan downregulates CARP and ameliorates cardiomyocyte hypertrophy. *(A)* Treatment with RNH6270 (RNH 1 μM, active form of olmesartan) reduced Ang II (1 μM) -induced increased of CARP protein in NRVCs (*P<0.05 vs. control, #P<0.05 vs. Ang II. n = 3). *(B)* ANP mRNA expression in NRVCs exposed to Ang II (1 μM) stimulation in the presence/absence of RNH (1 μM). *(C)* Representative picture of whole heart from different group (scale bar = 2 mm). *(D)* HW/BW ratio was significantly lower in TAC mice treated with olmesartan medoxomil (OM) in comparison with untreated TAC mice, while addition of Ad-Ankrd1 partially blocked the antihypertrophic effect of OM. (*P<0.01 vs. Sham, #P<0.01 vs. TAC, &P< 0.05 vs. TAC + OM, n = 4–6 in each group). *(E)* Olmesartan treatment for 4 weeks reduced the myocardial expression of CARP in TAC mice (*P<0.05 vs. Sham, #P<0.05 vs. TAC). Data are mean ± SEM.

CARP occurred upon phenylephrine stimulation [10], which is in contrast to our finding that cytosolic translocation occurred upon Ang-II stimulation. It seems that nuclear Y-box-binding protein (YB-1) can stimulate cell proliferation [27], whereas nuclear CARP can bind with YB-1 and inhibit its activity [11], implying that nuclear localization of CARP exerts anti-hypertrophic role. As the first in vivo evidence on the role of Ankrd1 in myocardial hypertrophy, Song et al recently reported that cardiac-specific overexpression of Ankrd1 attenuated pressure overload- or isoproterenol-induced cardiac hypertrophy in mice [26], which is in contrast to our present findings. The reasons for this discrepancy are unclear. Although in vivo evidence about the influence of CARP on the growth of cardiomyocytes is scant, there are several lines of evidence which suggest that Ankrd1/CARP

promotes non-cardiomyocyte cell growth rather than inhibiting it. For example, CARP was reported to promote neurite outgrowth in F11 cells [28], as well as the growth of cancer cells [29] and neovascularization in tissue wounds [30].

As reviewed by Mikhailov et al. [11], since the identification of Ankrd1/CARP in 1995, most investigations have focused on the induction of Ankrd1 expression in cultured primary cardiomyocytes or non-cardiomyocyte cell lines. Thus, there is little in vivo evidence about the effects of Ankrd1/CARP-mediated pathways in cardiomyocytes. Forced overexpression of wild type Ankrd1 in cultured NRVCs was reported to inhibit ANP gene promoter activity [23], while there are reports showed that no any significant influence on ANP levels was found when Ankrd1 or even HCM-associated Ankrd1 mutants were overexpressed [14]. These findings are not in agreement with the in vivo evidence that significant up-regulation of Ankrd1/CARP is associated with re-activation rather than inhibition of ANP in various types of HF [31]. In addition, we noted that forced overexpression of Ankrd1/CARP markedly upregulated calcineurin, which further challenges the idea that Ankrd1/CARP acts as a negative regulator of cardiac gene expression [24].

In this study, we found that both Ang II stimulation and pressure overload promoted the cytosolic accumulation of CARP, which in turn activated the calcineurin-NFAT pathway, suggesting that CARP may be a useful target for the treatment of myocardial hypertrophy. It deserves to investigate how CARP activates calcineurin-NFAT pathway. Coincidently, Boengler et al. reported that CARP upregulates egr-1 [20], while egr-1 has been reported to participate calcineurin-NFAT signal pathway-induced myocardial hypertrophy [21], which in agreement with our findings in this study. We also found that olmesartan, a selective AT1 receptor blocker (ARB), attenuated cardiac hypertrophy in TAC mice at least partially through down-regulation of CARP expression and consequently alleviating the accumulation of calcineurin. In

agreement with our findings, it has been reported that losartan, another ARB, markedly inhibits the increase of calcineurin activity in cardiomyocytes stimulated by Ang II [32]. In mice, total Ankrd1 knockout or cardiac-restricted overexpression did not produce an abnormal phenotype [26,33], which is in agreement with our finding that in vivo overexpression of Ankrd1 alone did not induce cardiac hypertrophy when no pathological stress was added, suggesting that Ankrd1 is redundant and plays pathological stress-dependent role. These lines of evidence suggest that pharmacological inhibition of Ankrd1/CARP would not cause severe side effects. Therefore, it would seem reasonable to attempt the development of pharmaceutical CARP antagonists for the treatment of cardiac hypertrophy.

Author Contributions

Conceived and designed the experiments: YL CC SC MK. Performed the experiments: CC LS XL WX. Analyzed the data: CC LS SC XL WX JZ XH JB DX GL MK YL. Contributed reagents/materials/analysis tools: YL MK. Contributed to the writing of the manuscript: YL CC JZ SC MK.

References

1. Bang ML, Mudry RE, McElhinny AS, Trombitas K, Geach AJ, et al. (2001) Myopalladin, a novel 145-kilodalton sarcomeric protein with multiple roles in Z-disc and I-band protein assemblies. J Cell Biol 153: 413–427.
2. Torrado M, Nespereira B, Lopez E, Centeno A, Castro-Beiras A, et al. (2005) ANKRD1 specifically binds CASQ2 in heart extracts and both proteins are co-enriched in piglet cardiac Purkinje cells. J Mol Cell Cardiol 38: 353–365.
3. Aihara Y, Kurabayashi M, Saito Y, Ohyama Y, Tanaka T, et al. (2000) Cardiac ankyrin repeat protein is a novel marker of cardiac hypertrophy: role of M-CAT element within the promoter. Hypertension 36: 48–53.
4. Gaussin V, Tomlinson JE, Depre C, Engelhardt S, Antos CL, et al. (2003) Common genomic response in different mouse models of beta-adrenergic-induced cardiomyopathy. Circulation 108: 2926–2933.
5. Wei YJ, Cui CJ, Huang YX, Zhang XL, Zhang H, et al. (2009) Upregulated expression of cardiac ankyrin repeat protein in human failing hearts due to arrhythmogenic right ventricular cardiomyopathy. Eur J Heart Fail 11: 559–566.
6. Nagueh SF, Shah G, Wu Y, Torre-Amione G, King NM, et al. (2004) Altered titin expression, myocardial stiffness, and left ventricular function in patients with dilated cardiomyopathy. Circulation 110: 155–162.
7. Kitakaze M, Asakura M, Kim J, Shintani Y, Asanuma H, et al. (2007) Human atrial natriuretic peptide and nicorandil as adjuncts to reperfusion treatment for acute myocardial infarction (J-WIND): two randomised trials. Lancet 370: 1483–1493.
8. Moulik M, Vatta M, Witt SH, Arola AM, Murphy RT, et al. (2009) ANKRD1, the gene encoding cardiac ankyrin repeat protein, is a novel dilated cardiomyopathy gene. J Am Coll Cardiol 54: 325–333.
9. Arimura T, Bos JM, Sato A, Kubo T, Okamoto H, et al. (2009) Cardiac ankyrin repeat protein gene (ANKRD1) mutations in hypertrophic cardiomyopathy. J Am Coll Cardiol 54: 334–342.
10. Duboscq-Bidot L, Charron P, Ruppert V, Fauchier L, Richter A, et al. (2009) Mutations in the ANKRD1 gene encoding CARP are responsible for human dilated cardiomyopathy. Eur Heart J 30: 2128–2136.
11. Mikhailov AT, Torrado M (2008) The enigmatic role of the ankyrin repeat domain 1 gene in heart development and disease. Int J Dev Biol 52: 811–821.
12. Laure L, Daniele N, Suel L, Marchand S, Aubert S, et al. (2010) A new pathway encompassing calpain 3 and its newly identified substrate cardiac ankyrin repeat protein is involved in the regulation of the nuclear factor-kappaB pathway in skeletal muscle. FEBS J 277: 4322–4337.
13. Mestroni L (2009) Phenotypic heterogeneity of sarcomeric gene mutations: a matter of gain and loss? J Am Coll Cardiol 54: 343–345.
14. Crocini C, Arimura T, Reischmann S, Eder A, Braren I, et al. (2013) Impact of ANKRD1 mutations associated with hypertrophic cardiomyopathy on contraction parameters of engineered heart tissue. Basic Res Cardiol 108: 349.
15. Letavernier E, Zafrani L, Perez J, Letavernier B, Haymann JP, et al. (2012) The role of calpains in myocardial remodelling and heart failure. Cardiovasc Res 96: 38–45.
16. Patterson C, Portbury AL, Schisler JC, Willis MS (2011) Tear me down: role of calpain in the development of cardiac ventricular hypertrophy. Circ Res 109: 453–462.
17. Yatabe J, Sanada H, Yatabe MS, Hashimoto S, Yoneda M, et al. (2009) Angiotensin II type 1 receptor blocker attenuates the activation of ERK and NADPH oxidase by mechanical strain in mesangial cells in the absence of angiotensin II. Am J Physiol Renal Physiol 296: F1052–1060.

18. Xuan W, Liao Y, Chen B, Huang Q, Xu D, et al. (2011) Detrimental effect of fractalkine on myocardial ischaemia and heart failure. Cardiovasc Res 92: 385–393.
19. Liao Y, Ishikura F, Beppu S, Asakura M, Takashima S, et al. (2002) Echocardiographic assessment of LV hypertrophy and function in aortic-banded mice: necropsy validation. Am J Physiol Heart Circ Physiol 282: H1703–1708.
20. Boengler K, Pipp F, Fernandez B, Ziegelhoeffer T, Schaper W, et al. (2003) Arteriogenesis is associated with an induction of the cardiac ankyrin repeat protein (carp). Cardiovasc Res 59: 573–581.
21. Hsu SC, Chang YT, Chen CC (2013) Early growth response 1 is an early signal inducing Cav3.2 T-type calcium channels during cardiac hypertrophy. Cardiovasc Res 100: 222–230.
22. Molkentin JD, Lu JR, Antos CL, Markham B, Richardson J, et al. (1998) A calcineurin-dependent transcriptional pathway for cardiac hypertrophy. Cell 93: 215–228.
23. Jeyaseelan R, Poizat C, Baker RK, Abdishoo S, Isterabadi LB, et al. (1997) A novel cardiac-restricted target for doxorubicin. CARP, a nuclear modulator of gene expression in cardiac progenitor cells and cardiomyocytes. J Biol Chem 272: 22800–22808.
24. Zolk O, Frohme M, Maurer A, Kluxen FW, Hentsch B, et al. (2002) Cardiac ankyrin repeat protein, a negative regulator of cardiac gene expression, is augmented in human heart failure. Biochem Biophys Res Commun 293: 1377–1382.
25. Ishiguro N, Baba T, Ishida T, Takeuchi K, Osaki M, et al. (2002) Carp, a cardiac ankyrin-repeated protein, and its new homologue, Arpp, are differentially expressed in heart, skeletal muscle, and rhabdomyosarcomas. Am J Pathol 160: 1767–1778.
26. Song Y, Xu J, Li Y, Jia C, Ma X, et al. (2012) Cardiac ankyrin repeat protein attenuates cardiac hypertrophy by inhibition of ERK1/2 and TGF-beta signaling pathways. PLoS One 7: e50436.
27. Kojic S, Radojkovic D, Faulkner G (2011) Muscle ankyrin repeat proteins: their role in striated muscle function in health and disease. Crit Rev Clin Lab Sci 48: 269–294.
28. Stam FJ, MacGillavry HD, Armstrong NJ, de Gunst MC, Zhang Y, et al. (2007) Identification of candidate transcriptional modulators involved in successful regeneration after nerve injury. Eur J Neurosci 25: 3629–3637.
29. Scurr LL, Guminski AD, Chiew YE, Balleine RL, Sharma R, et al. (2008) Ankyrin repeat domain 1, ANKRD1, a novel determinant of cisplatin sensitivity expressed in ovarian cancer. Clin Cancer Res 14: 6924–6932.
30. Shi Y, Reitmaier B, Regenbogen J, Slowey RM, Opalenik SR, et al. (2005) CARP, a cardiac ankyrin repeat protein, is up-regulated during wound healing and induces angiogenesis in experimental granulation tissue. Am J Pathol 166: 303–312.
31. Nanni L, Romualdi C, Maseri A, Lanfranchi G (2006) Differential gene expression profiling in genetic and multifactorial cardiovascular diseases. J Mol Cell Cardiol 41: 934–948.
32. Fu M, Xu S, Zhang J, Pang Y, Liu N, et al. (1999) Involvement of calcineurin in angiotensin II-induced cardiomyocyte hypertrophy and cardiac fibroblast hyperplasia of rats. Heart Vessels 14: 283–288.
33. Barash IA, Bang ML, Mathew L, Greaser ML, Chen J, et al. (2007) Structural and regulatory roles of muscle ankyrin repeat protein family in skeletal muscle. Am J Physiol Cell Physiol 293: C218–227.

Permissions

All chapters in this book were first published in PLOS ONE, by The Public Library of Science; hereby published with permission under the Creative Commons Attribution License or equivalent. Every chapter published in this book has been scrutinized by our experts. Their significance has been extensively debated. The topics covered herein carry significant findings which will fuel the growth of the discipline. They may even be implemented as practical applications or may be referred to as a beginning point for another development.

The contributors of this book come from diverse backgrounds, making this book a truly international effort. This book will bring forth new frontiers with its revolutionizing research information and detailed analysis of the nascent developments around the world.

We would like to thank all the contributing authors for lending their expertise to make the book truly unique. They have played a crucial role in the development of this book. Without their invaluable contributions this book wouldn't have been possible. They have made vital efforts to compile up to date information on the varied aspects of this subject to make this book a valuable addition to the collection of many professionals and students.

This book was conceptualized with the vision of imparting up-to-date information and advanced data in this field. To ensure the same, a matchless editorial board was set up. Every individual on the board went through rigorous rounds of assessment to prove their worth. After which they invested a large part of their time researching and compiling the most relevant data for our readers.

The editorial board has been involved in producing this book since its inception. They have spent rigorous hours researching and exploring the diverse topics which have resulted in the successful publishing of this book. They have passed on their knowledge of decades through this book. To expedite this challenging task, the publisher supported the team at every step. A small team of assistant editors was also appointed to further simplify the editing procedure and attain best results for the readers.

Apart from the editorial board, the designing team has also invested a significant amount of their time in understanding the subject and creating the most relevant covers. They scrutinized every image to scout for the most suitable representation of the subject and create an appropriate cover for the book.

The publishing team has been an ardent support to the editorial, designing and production team. Their endless efforts to recruit the best for this project, has resulted in the accomplishment of this book. They are a veteran in the field of academics and their pool of knowledge is as vast as their experience in printing. Their expertise and guidance has proved useful at every step. Their uncompromising quality standards have made this book an exceptional effort. Their encouragement from time to time has been an inspiration for everyone.

The publisher and the editorial board hope that this book will prove to be a valuable piece of knowledge for researchers, students, practitioners and scholars across the globe.

List of Contributors

Laszlo Deres, Eva Bartha, Anita Palfi, Krisztian Eros, Adam Riba, Kalman Toth and Robert Halmosi
First Department of Medicine, Division of Cardiology, University of Pécs, Pécs, Hungary

Laszlo Deres, Krisztian Eros, Adam Riba, Balazs Sumegi and Robert Halmosi
Szentagothai Janos Research Center, University of Pécs, Medical School, Pécs, Hungary

Janos Lantos
Department of Surgical Research and Techniques, University of Pécs, Pécs, Hungary

Tamas Kalai and Kalman Hideg
Department of Organic and Medicinal Chemistry, University of Pécs, Pécs, Hungary

Balazs Sumegi and Ferenc Gallyas
Department of Biochemistry and Medical Chemistry, Medical School, University of Pécs, Pécs, Hungary
MTA-PTE Nuclear-Mitochondrial Interactions Research Group, Pécs, Hungary

Jianchun Huang, Xingmei Liang, Qingwei Wen, Shijun Zhang, Feifei Xuan, Jie Jian, Xing Lin and Renbin Huang
Pharmaceutical College, Guangxi Medical University, Nanning, Guangxi, China

XiaoJun Tang
Department of Laboratory Medicine, Guangxi Medical College, Nanning, Guangxi, China

Li Li, Zhi-Guo Zhang, Hong Lei, Cheng Wang, Jin-Yu Wang and Li-Ling Wu
Department of Physiology and Pathophysiology, Peking University Health Science Center, and Key Laboratory of Molecular Cardiovascular Sciences, Ministry of Education, Beijing, China

Li-Peng Wu and Wei-Guo Zhu
Department of Biochemistry and Molecular Biology, Peking University Health Science Center, Beijing, China

Feng-Ying Fu
Key Laboratory of Cardiovascular Molecular Biology and Regulatory Peptides, Ministry of Health, Beijing, China

Jing Zong, Wei Deng, Heng Zhou, Zhou-yan Bian, Jia Dai, Yuan Yuan, Jie-yu Zhang, Rui Zhang, Yan Zhang, Qing-qing Wu, Hong-liang Li and Qi-zhu Tang
Department of Cardiology, Renmin Hospital of Wuhan University, Wuhan, China
Cardiovascular Research Institute of Wuhan University, Wuhan, China

Hai-peng Guo
The Key Laboratory of Cardiovascular Remodeling and Function Research, Chinese Ministry of Education and Chinese Ministry of Health, Qilu Hospital of Shandong University, Jinan, China

Xiaojian Wang, Jizheng Wang, Ming Su, Changxin Wang, Jingzhou Chen, Hu Wang and Rutai Hui
Sino-German Laboratory for Molecular Medicine, State Key Laboratory of Cardiovascular Disease, FuWai Hospital & Cardiovascular Institute, Chinese Academy of Medical Sciences, Peking Union Medical College, Beijing, People's Republic of China

Lei Song and Yubao Zou
Department of Cardiology, State Key Laboratory of Cardiovascular Disease, FuWai Hospital & Cardiovascular Institute, Chinese Academy of Medical Sciences, Peking Union Medical College, Beijing, People's Republic of China

Lianfeng Zhang
Key Laboratory of Human Disease Comparative Medicine, Ministry of Health, Institute of Laboratory Animal Science, Chinese Academy of Medical Sciences and Comparative Medical Center, Peking Union Medical College, Beijing, People's Republic of China

Youyi Zhang
Institute of Vascular Medicine, Peking University Third Hospital, Beijing, People's Republic of China

Polina Sysa-Shah, Yi Xu, Xin Guo, Frances Belmonte, Byunghak Kang, Djahida Bedja, Scott Pin, Noriko Tsuchiya and Kathleen Gabrielson
Johns Hopkins University, School of Medicine, Department of Molecular and Comparative Pathobiology, Baltimore, Maryland, United States of America

Noriko Tsuchiya
Drug Safety Evaluation, Drug Developmental Research Laboratories, Shionogi & Co., Ltd., Osaka, Japan

Hui Pang, Bing Han and Tao Yu
Department of Cardiovascular Medicine, Central Hospital of Xuzhou, Xuzhou Clinical School of Xuzhou Medical College, Affiliated Hospital of Southeast University, Xuzhou, Jiangsu, China

Zhen Peng
Department of Ultrasonography, Central Hospital of Xuzhou, Xuzhou Clinical School of Xuzhou Medical College, Affiliated Hospital of Southeast University, Xuzhou, Jiangsu, China

Juhee Shin, Min-Chul Kwon, Ha-Rim Seo, Yoon-Young Kim, Sun-Kyoung Im and Young-Yun Kong
Department of Biological Sciences, Seoul National University, Gwanak-gu, Seoul, Republic of Korea

Juhee Shin, Yoon- Young Kim, Sun-Kyoung Im and Kyong-Tai Kim
Department of Life Sciences, Pohang University of Science and Technology, Pohang, Kyungbuk, Republic of Korea

Seok Hong Lee and Jaetaek Kim
Division of Endocrinology and Metabolism, Department of Internal Medicine, College of Medicine, Chung-Ang University, Dongjak-gu, Seoul, Republic of Korea

Dong Kwon Yang and Woo Jin Park
Global Research Laboratory and Department of Life Science, Gwangju Institute of Science and Technology, Gwangju, Republic of Korea

Evan Dale Abel
Program in Molecular Medicine, University of Utah School of Medicine, Salt Lake City, Utah, United States of America

Oren Gordon, Zhiheng He and Eli Keshet
Departments of Developmental Biology and Cancer Research, The Hebrew University–Hadassah University Hospital, Jerusalem, Israel

Dan Gilon and Amit Oppenheim
Department of Cardiology, The Hebrew University–Hadassah University Hospital, Jerusalem, Israel

Sabine Gruener and Sherrie Pietranico-Cole
Department of Metabolic and Vascular Disease, Hoffmann-La Roche Pharmaceuticals, Basel, Switzerland

Jialin Xu, Yanfeng Li, Chunshi Jia, Lei Zhang, Yong Zhang and Dahai Zhu
Department of Biochemistry and Molecular Biology, Institute of Basic Medical Sciences, Chinese Academy of Medical Sciences and Peking Union Medical College, Beijing, China

Yao Song, Xiaowei Ma and Youyi Zhang
Institute of Vascular Medicine, Peking University Third Hospital, Key Laboratory of Cardiovascular Molecular Biology and Regulatory peptides, Ministry of Health and Key Laboratory of Molecular Cardiovascular Science, Ministry of Education, Beijing, China

Xiang Gao
National Resource Center for Mutant Mice Model Animal Research of Nanjing University, Pukou High-Tech District, Nanjing, China

Xiaojie Xie
Department of Cardiology, Second Affiliated Hospital, Zhejiang University College of Medicine, Hangzhou, China

Mohammad T. Elnakish, Mohamed D. H. Hassona, Mazin A. Alhaj and Hamdy H. Hassanain
Department of Anesthesiology, and Dorothy M. Davis Heart and Lung Research Institute, The Ohio State University, Columbus, Ohio, United States of America

Mohammad T. Elnakish and Paul M. L. Janssen
Department of Physiology and Cell Biology, and Dorothy M. Davis Heart and Lung Research Institute, The Ohio State University, Columbus, Ohio, United States of America

Leni Moldovan
Department of Pulmonary, Allergy, Critical Care and Sleep Medicine, and Dorothy M. Davis Heart and Lung Research Institute, The Ohio State University, Columbus, Ohio, United States of America

Mahmood Khan
Department of Internal Medicine, and Dorothy M. Davis Heart and Lung Research Institute, The Ohio State University, Columbus, Ohio, United States of America

Shijun Wang, Hui Gong, Aijun Sun, Junbo Ge and Yunzeng Zou
Shanghai Institute of Cardiovascular Diseases, Zhongshan Hospital, Fudan University, Shanghai, China,

Shijun Wang, Hui Gong, Guoliang Jiang, Yong Ye, Jian Wu, Jieyun You, Guoping Zhang, Aijun Sun, Junbo Ge and Yunzeng Zou
Institutes of Biomedical Science, Fudan University, Shanghai, China

Issei Komuro
Department of Cardiovascular Medicine, the University of Tokyo Graduate School of Medicine, Tokyo, Japan

Jia Dai, Di-Fei Shen, Zhou-Yan Bian, Heng Zhou, Hua-Wen Gan, Jing Zong, Wei Deng, Yuan Yuan, FangFang Li, Qing-Qing Wu, Rui Zhang, Zhen-Guo Ma, Hong-Liang Li and Qi-Zhu Tang
Department of Cardiology, Renmin Hospital of Wuhan University, Wuhan, China
Cardiovascular Research Institute of Wuhan University, Wuhan, China

Lu Gao
Department of Cardiology, Institute of Cardiovascular Disease, Union Hospital, Tongji Medical College, Huazhong University of Science and Technology, Wuhan, People's Republic of China

Andrea Iorga, Rod Partow-Navid and Mansoureh Eghbali
Department of Anesthesiology, Division of Molecular Medicine, David Geffen School of Medicine at University of California Los Angeles, Los Angeles, California, United States of America

Shannamar Dewey and Aldrin V. Gomes
Department of Neurobiology, Physiology and Behavior, University of California Davis, Davis, California, United States of America

Shenhong Gu, Ji Chen, Ruilian Ma, Xiang Xiao and Yanfang Chen
Department of Pharmacology and Toxicology, Boonshoft School of Medicine, Wright State University, Ohio, United States of America

Shenhong Gu
Department of Gerontology, the Affiliated Hospital of Hainan Medical College, Haikou, China

Wei Zhang, Ruilian Ma and Zhen Yao
Department of Cardiology, the People's Hospital of Sanya, Sanya, China

Ji Chen, Xiaotang Ma and Yanfang Chen
Department of Neurology, the Affiliated Hospital of Guangdong Medical College, Zhanjiang, Guangdong, China

Craig Bolte, Yufang Zhang, Tanya V. Kalin and Vladimir V. Kalinichenko
Division of Pulmonary Biology, Cincinnati Children's Hospital Research Foundation, Cincinnati, Ohio, United States of America

Allen York and Jeffery D. Molkentin
Molecular Cardiovascular Biology, Cincinnati Children's Hospital Research Foundation, Cincinnati, Ohio, United States of America

Jo El J. Schultz
Department of Pharmacology and Cell Biophysics, University of Cincinnati College of Medicine, Cincinnati, Ohio, United States of America

Raju Padiya and Sanjay K. Banerjee
Division of Medicinal Chemistry and Pharmacology, Indian Institute of Chemical Technology, Hyderabad, India

Debabrata Chowdhury and Manika Pal Bhadra
Division of Chemical Biology, Indian Institute of Chemical Technology, Hyderabad, India

Roshan Borkar and R. Srinivas
National Centre for Mass Spectrometry, Indian Institute of Chemical Technology, Hyderabad, India

Michal Mielcarek, Marie K. Bondulich, Linda Inuabasi, Sophie A. Franklin, Thomas Muller and Gillian P. Bates
Department of Medical and Molecular Genetics, King's College London, London, United Kingdom

Ahmadou M. Jingi and Samuel Kingue
Department of Internal Medicine and Specialties, Faculty of Medicine and Biomedical Sciences, University of YaoundéI, Yaoundé, Cameroon

Jean Jacques N. Noubiap
Internal Medicine Unit, Edéa Regional Hospital, Edéa, Cameroon

Philippe Kamdem
Centre Médical de la Trinité, Bafoussam, Cameroon

Samuel Kingue
Department of Internal Medicine, Yaoundé General Hospital, Yaoundé, Cameroon

Ci Chen, Liang Shen, Shiping Cao, Xixian Li, Wanling Xuan, Jingwen Zhang, Xiaobo Huang, Jianping Bin, Dingli Xu, Masafumi Kitakaze and Yulin Liao
State Key Laboratory of Organ Failure Research, Department of Cardiology, Nanfang Hospital, Southern Medical University, Guangzhou, China

Guofeng Li
Department of Pharmacy, Nanfang Hospital, Southern
Medical University, Guangzhou, China

Masafumi Kitakaze
Cardiovascular Division of the Department of Medicine,
National Cerebral and Cardiovascular Center, Osaka,
Japan

Index